Contents

Chapter 1: The Basics of Healthy Change
Rebecca Donatelle 1

Chapter 2: Managing Stress
Janet Hopson / Rebecca Donatelle / Tanya Littrell 29

Chapter 3: Psychosocial Health
Rebecca Donatelle 49

Chapter 4: Nutrition and You
Rebecca Donatelle 79

Chapter 5: Managing Your Weight
Janet Hopson / Rebecca Donatelle / Tanya Littrell 115

Chapter 6: Understanding Fitness Principles
Janet Hopson / Rebecca Donatelle / Tanya Littrell 137

Chapter 7: Cardiovascular Disease and Cancer
Rebecca Donatelle 155

Chapter 8: Infectious and Noninfectious Conditions
Rebecca Donatelle 191

Chapter 9: Addictions and Addictive Behavior: Threats to Wellness
Donatelle, Rebecca 227

Chapter 10: Savvy Health Care Consumerism
Rebecca Donatelle 251

Chapter 11: Environmental Health
Rebecca Donatelle 269

Index 290

PEARSON CUSTOM LIBRARY

HEALTH

Community College Health and Wellness

Pearson Learning Solutions

New York Boston San Francisco
London Toronto Sydney Tokyo Singapore Madrid
Mexico City Munich Paris Cape Town Hong Kong Montreal

Senior Vice President, Editorial and Marketing: Patrick F. Boles
Senior Sponsoring Editor: Natalie Danner
Development Editor: Mary Kate Paris
Editorial Assistant: Jill Johnson
Executive Marketing Manager: Nathan Wilbur
Operations Manager: Eric Kenney
Production Manager: Jennifer Berry
Art Director: Renée Sartell
Cover Designer: Tess Mattern

Cover Art: Bike—Courtesy of Bill Grove/iStockphoto; Orange Slices—Courtesy of Piet Mall/Getty Images; Salad—Courtesy of Photodisc/Getty Images; Tomatoes—Courtesy of Paul Taylor/Getty Images.

Printed in the United States of America

Please visit our website at *www.pearsoncustom.com*

Attention Bookstores: For permission to return any unsold stock, contact us at *pe-uscustomreturns@pearson.com.*

Pearson Learning Solutions, 501 Boylston Street, Suite 900, Boston, MA 02116
A Pearson Education Company
www.pearsoned.com

3 4 5 6 7 8 9 10 V0CR 14 13 12 11

PEARSON

ISBN 10: 0-558-62269-0
ISBN 13: 978-0-558-62269-5

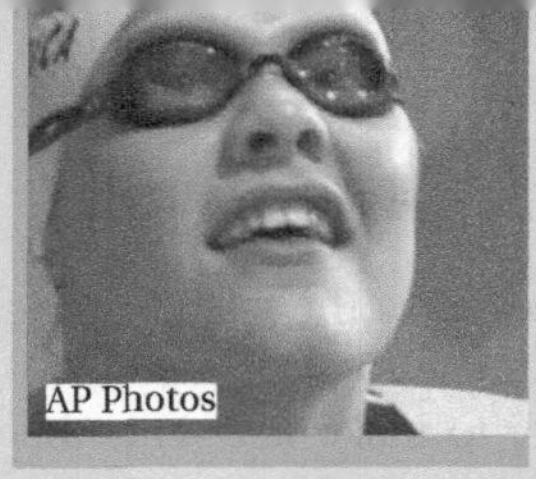

AP Photos

What is meant by "quality of life"?

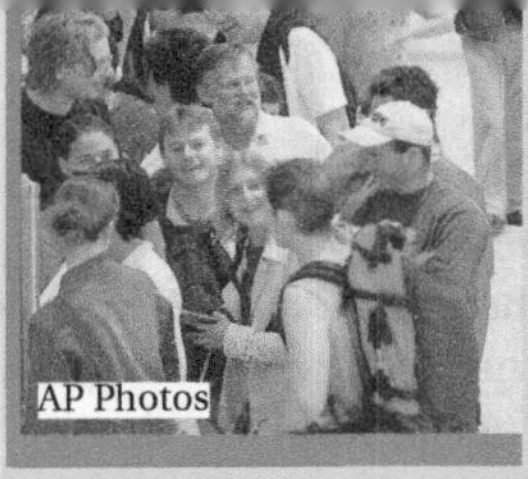

AP Photos

Why should I be concerned about health conditions in other places?

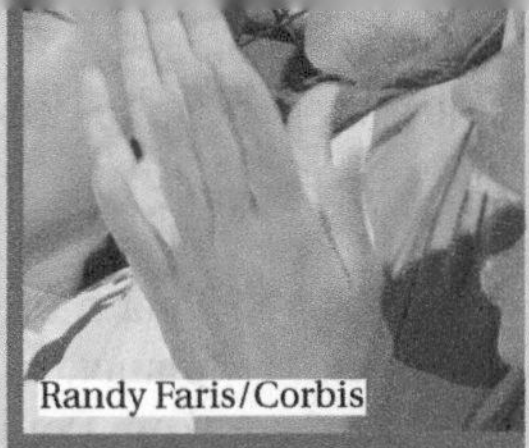

Randy Faris/Corbis

How do my friends and family influence my health?

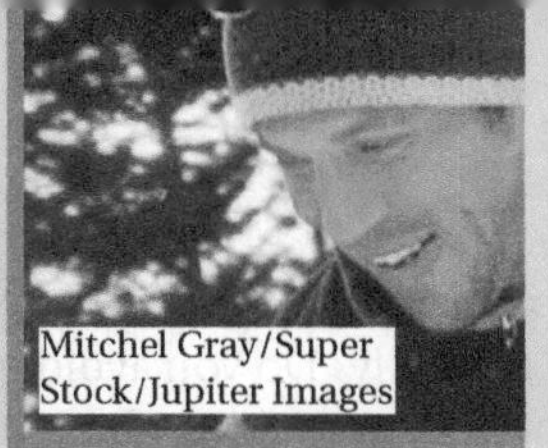

Mitchel Gray/Super Stock/Jupiter Images

What can I do to change an unhealthy habit?

The Basics of Healthy Change

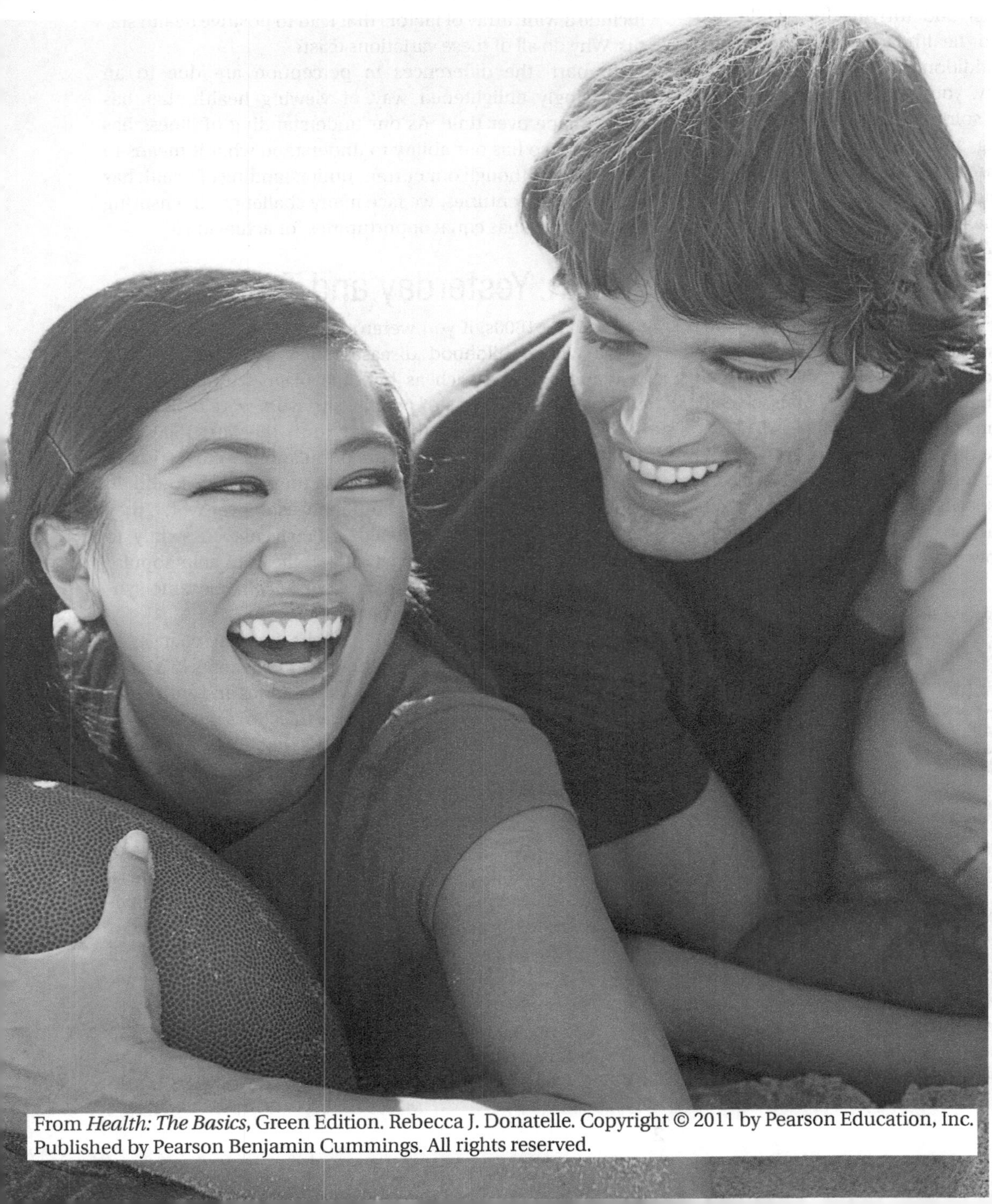

Laura Doss/Corbis

Objectives

* Discuss health in terms of its dimensions and historical, current, and future perspectives.
* Explain the importance of a healthy lifestyle in preventing premature disease and promoting wellness.
* Discuss the health status of Americans and the significance of *Healthy People 2010* and *2020* and other national initiatives to promote health.
* Understand the importance of a global perspective on health, and recognize how gender, racial, and cultural backgrounds influence disparities in health status, research, and risk.
* Examine your role in protecting global health through adoption of a green lifestyle.
* Evaluate sources of health information, particularly the Internet, to determine reliability.
* Focus on current risk behaviors, and realize how they can impact your current and future health.
* Learn how to apply behavior-change techniques to your own lifestyle.

Do you have health on your mind? Do you try to eat nutritious foods and exercise regularly? Do you avoid tobacco and alcohol use? Or do you prefer not to think about your health? Maybe you feel you have plenty of time to worry about it later in life, or maybe you just don't know where to begin. The health habits of college students, be they 19 or 39, vary widely. While many of you engage in less-than-healthy behaviors, many of you also take the opposite track and do your best to improve and maintain good health.

But what does it mean to be in good health? More importantly, do you think that you are healthy? If you feel fine and have no problems conducting your life from day to day, does that mean you enjoy optimal health?

You might be surprised to learn that *health* is much more complex than just the absence of disease. Optimal health habits can lead to a robust and thriving life, while marginal habits can lead to poor health later in life even though you may feel okay now. In addition to the physical health that helps ensure a sound body, your social, intellectual, emotional, environmental, and spiritual health all play a role in maintaining your well-being, and poor health in any of these areas can have negative impacts not just today, but next month, next year, and 20 years from now. Your health is affected by your environment, genetics, and, importantly, your lifestyle, and the choices you make every day help sustain, improve, or destroy it.

health The ever-changing process of achieving individual potential in the physical, social, emotional, mental, spiritual, and environmental dimensions.

wellness The achievement of the highest level of health possible in each of several dimensions.

The good news is that adopting healthy behaviors, while not necessarily easy, does not have to be painful, and achieving behavior change can be a fun and rewarding process. The purpose of this text is to explore the various areas of your life that affect your short- and long-term health. As you learn more about the health effects of specific behaviors, you are encouraged to consider how your actions today will affect you tomorrow, and you will learn how your behaviors also affect the health of the people around you, as well as the health of the planet. In the face of conflicting media messages and pressure from your peers, you have the power to make decisions that lead to better health for yourself, for others, and for the planet.

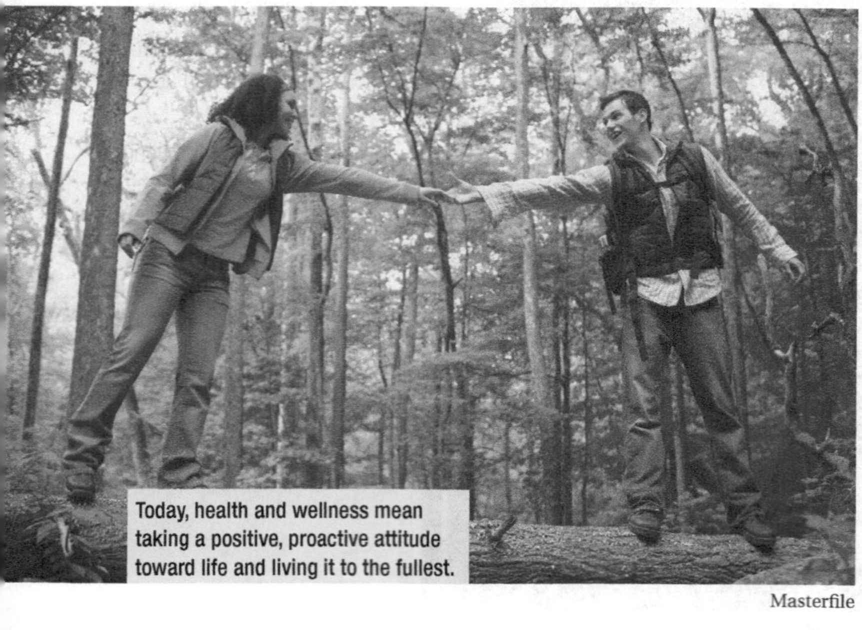

Today, health and wellness mean taking a positive, proactive attitude toward life and living it to the fullest.

Masterfile

Putting Your Health in Perspective

Although we use the term **health** almost unconsciously, few people understand the broad scope of the word. For some, health simply means the antithesis of sickness. To others, it means being in good physical shape and able to resist illness. Still others use terms such as **wellness,** or *well-being,* to include a wide array of factors that lead to positive health status. Why do all of these variations exist?

In part, the differences in perception are due to an increasingly enlightened way of viewing health that has taken shape over time. As our understanding of illness has improved, so has our ability to understand what it means to be healthy. Although our current understanding of health has evolved over centuries, we face many challenges in ensuring that everyone has equal opportunities for achieving it.

Health: Yesterday and Today

Prior to the 1800s, if you weren't sick, you were regarded as lucky. When childhood diseases such as diphtheria and deadly epidemics such as bubonic plague, influenza, and cholera killed millions of people, survivors were believed to be of hearty, healthy stock. Not until the late 1800s did researchers recognize that entire populations were victims of environmental factors (such as microorganisms found in contaminated water, air, and human waste) over which they had little control. Public health officials moved swiftly to clean water supplies and enact other policies to help populations at greatest risk. As a result, *health* became synonymous with *good hygiene.*

The twentieth century brought dramatic changes in life expectancy, with continued improvements in sanitation and the development of vaccinations and antibiotics that stopped the spread of many infectious diseases.

Today, scientists recognize that health is much more than the absence of disease. It includes the physical, social, and mental elements of life, as well as environmental, spiritual, emotional, and intellectual dimensions. To be truly healthy, a person must be capable of functioning at an optimal level in each of these areas, as well as interacting with others and the greater environment in a productive and healthy manner. Poor health and unhealthy habits involve and impact all areas of your life, from your relationships to your environment to your academic success (see Figure 1). Rather than simply looking at how long we live, or the number of disease-free years we enjoy, public health researchers know that the quality of those years is also vital. Today, *quality of life* is considered as important as years of life. It's not just how long we live, but also how *well* we live.

Improvements to health have not occurred just at the personal level. Over the past 100 years, numerous policies, individual actions, and public services have advanced our health status on a large scale (see Figure 2). Current **morbidity,** or illness rates, indicate that people are less likely to contract common infectious diseases that devastated previous generations. Today, most childhood diseases are preventable or curable because of improvements in education, socioeconomic conditions, medical technology, vaccinations, and other public health measures. For these reasons, people are now living longer than at any other time in our history. According to **mortality** statistics, the average life expectancy at birth in the United States has risen to 77.8 years (compare this to the average 47-year life expectancy of an individual born in the early 1900s).[1] Although the average life expectancy of Americans as a whole has increased over the past century, our average life expectancy at birth lags behind 49 other countries. Japan and other nations leading the pack have life expectancies of 82 years and higher.[2]

Will this trend continue? A recent study projects that today's newborns will be the first generation to have a lower life expectancy than that of their parents.[3] Largely attributable

The Ten Greatest Public Health Achievements of the 20th Century

- Vaccinations
- Motor vehicle safety
- Workplace safety
- Control of infectious diseases
- Reduction in cardiovascular disease (CVD) and stroke deaths
- Safe and healthy foods
- Maternal and infant care
- Family planning
- Fluoridated drinking water
- Recognition of tobacco as a health hazard

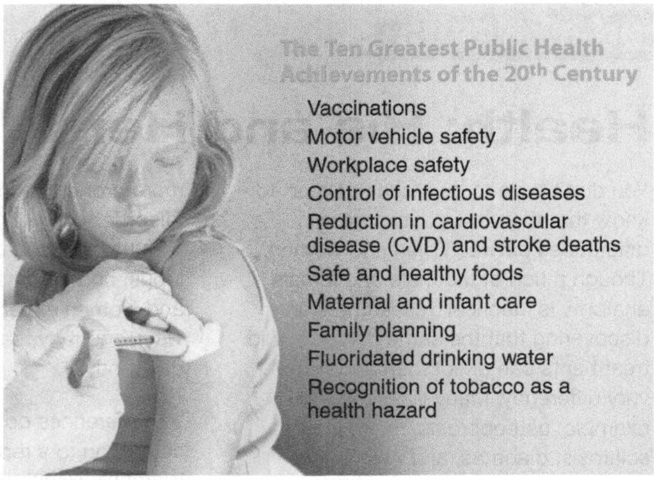

IT STOCK FREE/AGE Fotostock

FIGURE 2 **The Ten Greatest Public Health Achievements of the Twentieth Century**

Source: Adapted from Centers for Disease Control and Prevention, "Ten Great Public Health Achievements—United States, 1900–1999," *Morbidity and Mortality Weekly Report* 48, no. 12 (April 1999): 241–43.

to the consequences of obesity, researchers report that life expectancy could decline by as much as 5 years over the next few decades.[4] It is also important to note that life expectancy predictions are just an average of the total population and that there continue to be large disparities in life expectancy across different groups according to such factors as gender, race, and income. For example, a baby girl born in the United States in 2005 could expect to live 80.4 years, 5.2 years longer than her male counterpart, whose life expectancy is 75.2 years.[5] (See the Gender & Health box on the next page for more on the differences between men's and women's health status.) According to the same report, the life expectancy for a white girl born in 2005 was 80.8 years, but only 76.3 years for a black girl born the same year; for a white boy born in 2005, life expectancy was 75.7 years versus 69.5 for a black boy born the same year.

morbidity The relative incidence of disease.

mortality The proportion of deaths to population.

The Evolution toward Wellness

René Dubos, a twentieth-century biologist and philosopher, aptly summarized the thinking of his contemporaries by defining health as "a quality of life,

FIGURE 1 Top Ten Reported Impediments to Academic Performance—Past 12 Months
Your personal health and wellness can affect your academic success. In a recent National College Health Association survey, students indicated specific health problems that prevented them from performing at their best.

Source: Data are from American College Health Association. *American College Health Association—National College Health Assessment (ACHA-NCHA) Web Summary.* 2008. Available at www.acha-ncha.org.

Stress — 32.9%
Sleep difficulties — 25.4%
Cold/flu/sore throat — 24.8%
Concern for family/friend — 18.1%
Relationship difficulties — 15.5%
Depression/anxiety disorder — 15.5%
Internet use/games — 15.1%
Death of friend/family — 9.8%
Sinus infection — 9.4%
Alcohol use — 6.2%

Percent

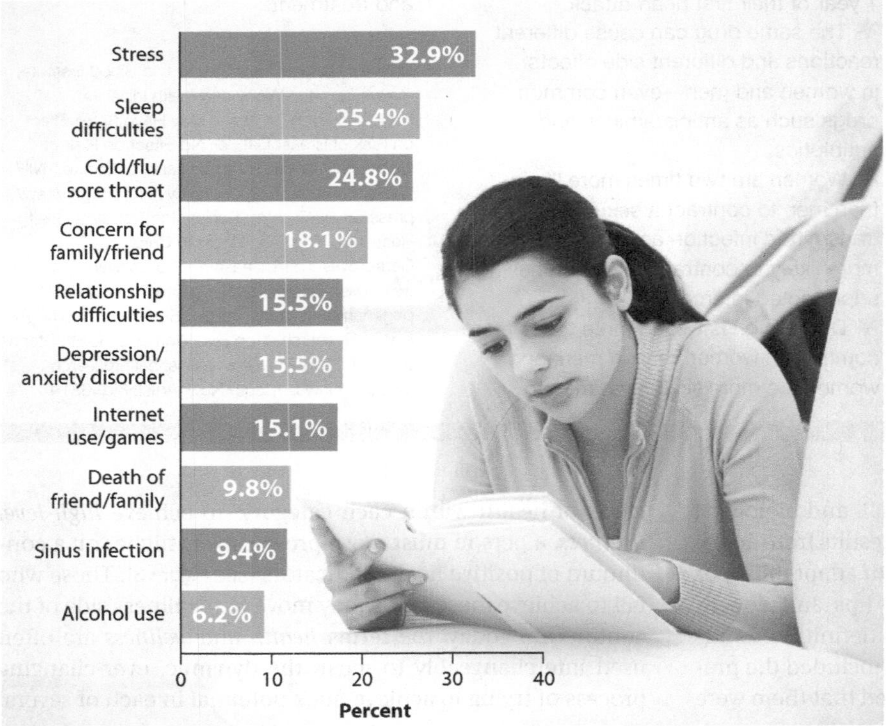

Ale Ventura/Jupiter Images

Gender&Health

Health: His and Hers

You don't have to be a health expert to know that there are physiological differences between men and women. Though much of the male and female anatomy is identical, researchers are discovering that the same diseases and treatments can affect men and women very differently. Many illnesses—for example, osteoporosis, multiple sclerosis, diabetes, and Alzheimer's disease—are much more common in women, even though rates for these diseases seem to be increasing in men. Why do these differences exist? Is it simply a matter of lifestyle? Clearly it is much more complicated than that. Consider the following:

- The size, structure, and function of the brain differ in women and men, particularly in areas that affect mood and behavior and in areas used to perform tasks. Reaction time is slower in women, but accuracy is higher.
- Bone mass in women peaks when they are in their twenties; in men, it increases gradually until age 30. At menopause, women lose bone at an accelerated rate, and 80 percent of osteoporosis cases are women.
- Women's cardiovascular systems are different in size, shape, and nervous system impulses; women have faster heart rates.
- Women's immune systems are stronger than men's, but women are more prone to autoimmune diseases (disorders in which the body attacks its own tissues, such as multiple sclerosis, lupus, and rheumatoid arthritis). Men and women experience pain in different ways and may react to pain medications differently.

Differences do not stop there, according to a report by the Society for Women's Health Research:

- When consuming the same amount of alcohol, women have a higher blood alcohol content than men, even allowing for size differences.
- Women who smoke are 20 to 70 percent more likely to develop lung cancer than men who smoke the same number of cigarettes.
- Women are more likely than men to suffer a second heart attack within 1 year of their first heart attack.
- The same drug can cause different reactions and different side effects in women and men—even common drugs such as antihistamines and antibiotics.
- Women are two times more likely than men to contract a sexually transmitted infection and are ten times more likely to contract HIV when having unprotected intercourse.
- Depression is two to three times more common in women than in men, and women are more likely than men to attempt suicide; however, men are more likely to succeed at suicide.

Surprisingly, although countless disparities in health have long been recognized, researchers largely ignored the unique aspects of women's health until the 1990s, when the National Institutes of Health (NIH) funded a highly publicized 15-year, $625 million study. Known as the Women's Health Initiative (WHI), this study was designed to focus research on the uniqueness of women when it came to drug trials, development of surgical instruments, and other health issues, rather than assuming that women were just like the men who had been studied. This research and the follow-up studies are providing invaluable information about women's health risks and potential strategies for prevention, intervention, and treatment.

Sources: National Heart, Lung and Blood Institute, "News from the Women's Health Initiative: Reducing Total Fat Intake May Have Small Effect on Risk of Breast Cancer, No Effect on Risk of Colorectal Cancer, Heart Disease, or Stroke," NIH News, February 7, 2006, www.nhlbi.nih.gov/new/press/06-02-07.htm; Society for Women's Health Research, "Sex Differences in Cardio/Cerebrovascular Diseases," 2007, www.womenshealthresearch.org/site/PageServer?pagename=hs_facts_cardio; Society for Women's Health Research, "Top Five Women's Health Stories of 2006," 2006, www.womenshealthresearch.org/site/News2?page=NewsArticle&id=6319.

involving social, emotional, mental, spiritual, and biological fitness on the part of the individual, which results from adaptations to the environment."[6] The concept of adaptability, or the ability to successfully cope with life's ups and downs, became a key element of the overall health definition. Eventually the term *wellness* became popular. It included the previously mentioned elements and also implied that there were levels of health within each category. To achieve *high-level wellness,* a person must move progressively higher on a continuum of positive health indicators (see Figure 3). Those who fail to achieve these levels may move to the illness side of the continuum. Today, the terms *health* and *wellness* are often used interchangeably to mean the dynamic, ever-changing process of trying to achieve one's potential in each of several

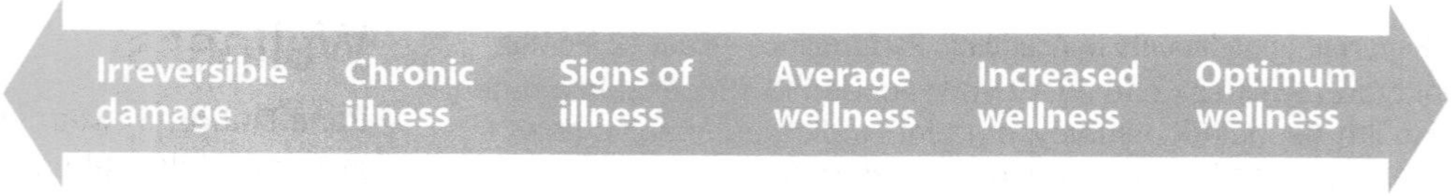

FIGURE 3 **The Wellness Continuum**

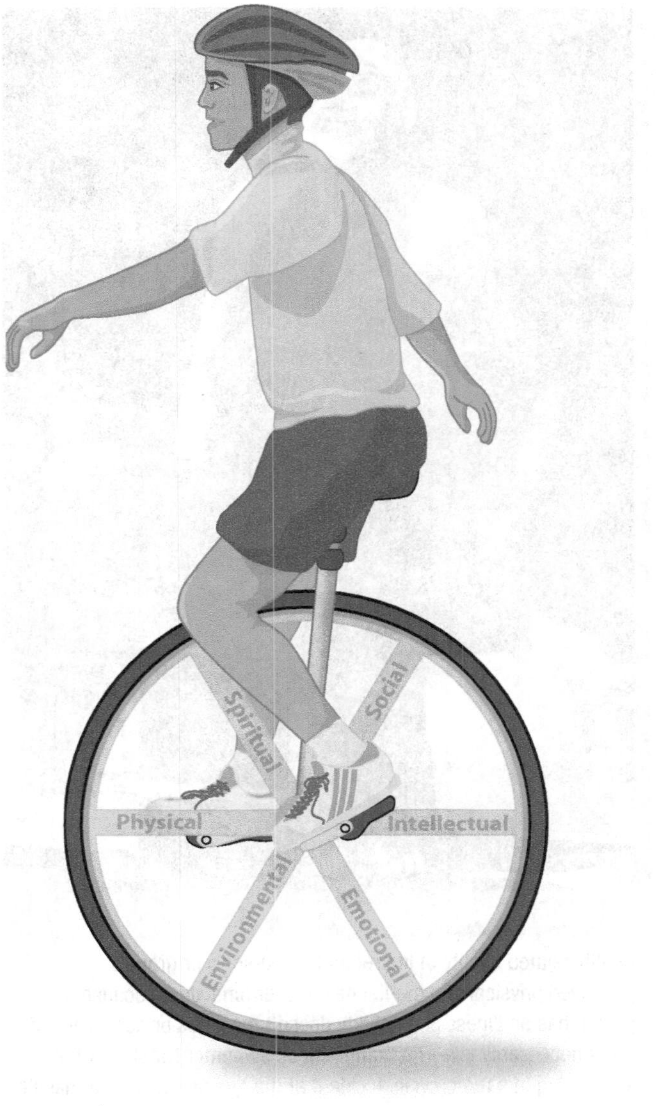

FIGURE 4 **The Dimensions of Health**
When all the dimensions are in balance and well developed, they can support your active and thriving lifestyle.

interrelated dimensions, which typically include the following (and are presented in Figure 4):

- *Physical health* includes characteristics such as body size and shape, sensory acuity and responsiveness, susceptibility to disease and disorders, body functioning, physical fitness, and recuperative abilities. Newer definitions of *physical health* also include our ability to perform normal *activities of daily living (ADLs)*, or those tasks that are necessary to normal existence in today's society.
- *Social health* refers to the ability to have satisfying interpersonal relationships, including interactions with others, adaptation to social situations, and appropriate daily behaviors in society.
- *Intellectual health* refers to the ability to think clearly, reason objectively, analyze critically, and use brain power effectively to meet life's challenges. It means learning from successes and mistakes and making responsible decisions that take into consideration all aspects of a situation.
- *Environmental health* refers to an appreciation of the external environment and the role individuals play to preserve, protect, and improve environmental conditions.
- *Emotional health* refers to the ability to express emotions when they are appropriate, controlling them when they are not, and avoiding expressing them inappropriately. Self-esteem, self-confidence, self-efficacy, trust, love, and many other emotional reactions and responses are all part of emotional health.
- *Spiritual health* involves subscribing to a way of life or a belief in a supreme being based on a particular religious doctrine or feeling of unity with a greater force and a guiding sense of meaning or value in all life. True spiritual health typically goes well beyond an organized religion and includes many more aspects of living a balanced, introspective, and meaningful life.

Although typically not considered a dimension in most wellness continuums, **mental health** is an important concept. Often confused with emotional, social, spiritual, or intellectual health, it is a broader concept that encompasses all of these dimensions. According to the U.S. surgeon general, this umbrella term refers to the "successful performance of mental function, resulting in productive activities, fulfilling relationships with others, and the ability to adapt to change and cope with adversity. From early childhood until late life, mental health is the springboard of thinking and communication skills, learning, emotional growth, resilience, and self-esteem."[7]

mental health The thinking part of psychosocial health; includes your values, attitudes, and beliefs.

Many people believe that the best way to achieve wellness is to adopt a *holistic* approach, which emphasizes the integration of and balance among mind, body, and spirit. Achieving wellness means attaining the optimal level of wellness for a person's unique limitations and strengths. A physically disabled person may function at his or her optimal level of performance; enjoy satisfying interpersonal relationships; maintain emotional, spiritual, and intellectual health; and have a strong interest in environmental concerns. In contrast, a person who spends hours lifting weights to perfect the size and shape of each muscle but pays little attention to nutrition may look healthy but not have a good balance in all areas of health. Although we often consider physical attractiveness and other external trappings in measuring overall health, these are only two indicators of wellness and indicate little about the other dimensions.

How healthy are you? Complete the **Assess Yourself** at the end of the chapter to gain perspective on your own level of wellness in each dimension.

what do you think?

Based on the wellness dimensions discussed, what are your key strengths in each dimension? ● What are your key deficiencies? ● What one or two things can you do to enhance your strong areas? ● To improve your weaknesses?

The *Healthy People* Initiatives

In 1990, the U.S. surgeon general proposed a national plan for promoting health among individuals and groups. Known as *Healthy People 2000,* the plan outlined a series of long-term objectives. Although many communities worked toward achieving these goals, as a nation we still had a long way to go by the new millennium, when a new plan, *Healthy People 2010,* came into effect.

Healthy People 2010 and Other Initiatives

The *Healthy People 2010* plan took the original initiative to the next level. *Healthy People 2010* is a nationwide program with two broad goals: (1) increase life span and quality of life and (2) eliminate health disparities. Each of these goals has the potential to make real changes in the population's health.

National Goal: Improving Quality of Life

For decades, we have looked at our steadily increasing life expectancy rates and proudly proclaimed that Americans' health has never been better. Recently, however, health organizations and international groups have attempted to quantify the number of years a person lives with a disability or illness, compared with the number of healthy years. The World Health Organization summarizes this concept as **healthy life expectancy.** Simply stated, *healthy life expectancy* refers to the number of years a newborn can expect to live in full health, based on current rates of illness and mortality and also on the quality of their lives. For example, if we could delay the onset of diabetes so that a person didn't develop the disease until he or she was 60 years old, rather than developing it at 30, there would be a dramatic increase in this individual's healthy life expectancy.

healthy life expectancy The number of years a newborn can expect to live in full health, based on current rates of illness and mortality

This new focus on *quality of life* has become increasingly important. By the year 2030, the number of older Americans is expected to reach 71 million, or roughly 20 percent of the U.S. population.[8] Will those Americans continue to be productive or suffer from largely avoidable, disabling chronic diseases? Will the numbers of persons in America disabled by mental illnesses, such as depression and anxiety disorders, or by substance abuse lead to nonproductive and destructive years of life for many? Will people be able to fully realize their dreams for happiness, education, healthy lifestyle, homes, families, and so on, or will large numbers of them report low quality of life? Concerns over health-related quality of life prompt health professionals to call for policies, programs, and services that emphasize health status, opportunity, and promotion of functional capacity at all ages and stages of life. A mentally and physically healthy population that can look forward to quality years of life is an important international health priority.

67 & 71 are the *healthy* life expectancies of men and women, respectively, in the U.S. Note that the average total life expectancies of men and women in the U.S. are 75 and 80, respectively, demonstrating that many people live their last years with significant health problems that affect their quality of life.

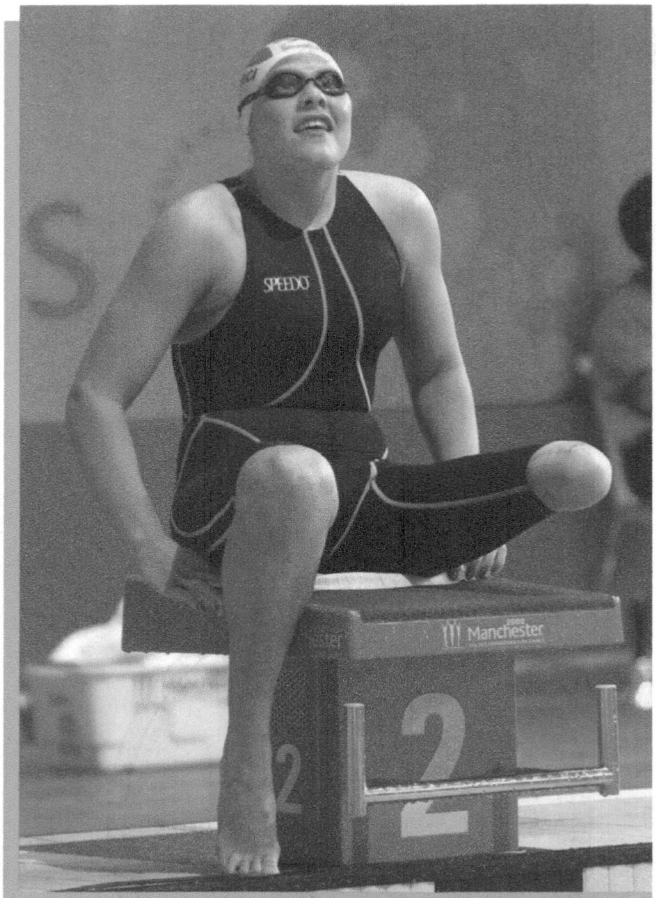

AP Photos

What is meant by "quality of life"?

Health-related quality of life refers to a person's or group's perceived physical and mental health over time. Just because a person has an illness or disability doesn't mean his or her quality of life is necessarily low. The South African swimmer Natalie du Toit lost her leg in a motorcycle accident at the age of 14, but that hasn't prevented her from achieving her goals and a high quality of life. In 2008 she swam in Beijing, the first amputee to qualify for and compete in the Olympic Games.

Healthy People 2010 also includes 28 focus areas, each representing a public health priority such as nutrition, tobacco use, substance abuse, access to quality health services, and common health conditions (for example, heart disease and diabetes). Under these focus areas is a list of leading health indicators (LHIs) that spell out specific health issues. For each focus area, the plan presents objectives for the nation to achieve during this decade. For instance, nutrition data show that only 42 percent of Americans aged 20 and older are at their healthy weight; the *Healthy People 2010* goal is to raise that number to 60 percent. In the focus area of physical activity and fitness, 40 percent of Americans aged 18 and older do not engage in any leisure-time physical activity. The objective is to reduce this number to 20 percent.[9] **Table 1** lists some of the objectives included in *Healthy People 2010*.

TABLE 1

A Sampling of *Healthy People 2010* Objectives

Objective	Baseline Statistic	Target 2010 Goal	Latest Statistic	Progress
Increase the proportion of persons with health insurance	83%	100%	83%*	No change
Increase the proportion of persons who use protective measures that may reduce the risk of skin cancer (e.g., sunscreen of SPF 15 or higher, sun-protective clothing, avoiding artificial sources of UV light)	59%	85%	71%‡	Moved toward target
Increase the proportion of adults with diabetes whose condition has been diagnosed	64%	78%	71%§	Moved toward target
Reduce the number of persons exposed to harmful air pollutants	137,019	0	115,149§	Moved toward target
Improve the nation's air quality by increasing the proportionate use of cleaner alternative fuels	0.8%	8%	2.4%†	Moved toward target
Reduce deaths caused by motor vehicle crashes	14.7 per 100,000 persons	8 per 100,000 persons	14.4 per 100,000 persons†	Moved toward target
Increase percentage of people using safety belts in motor vehicles	69%	92%	82%‡	Moved toward target
Reduce the annual rate of rape or attempted rape	0.9 per 1,000 persons	0.8 per 1,000 persons	0.6 per 1,000 persons*	Exceeded target
Increase the proportion of adults who are at a healthy weight	42%	60%	32%†	Moved away from target
Reduce the proportion of adults who are obese	23%	15%	33%†	Moved away from target
Increase the proportion of persons aged 2 years and older who consume at least three daily servings of vegetables	4%	50%	4%§	No change
Increase the proportion of adults who engage regularly, preferably daily, in moderate physical activity for at least 30 minutes per day	32%	50%	31%*	Moved away from target
Reduce deaths from HIV infection	5.3 deaths per 100,000 persons	0.7 deaths per 100,000 persons	4.0 deaths per 100,000 persons†	Moved toward target
Decrease the rate of binge drinking among college students	39%	20%	41%*	Moved away from target
Reduce proportion of adults who smoke cigarettes	24%	12%	20%*	Moved toward target
Increase the proportion of women smokers who stop smoking during their first trimester of pregnancy	14%	30%	11%‡	Moved away from target
Increase smoke-free and tobacco-free environments in schools, including all school facilities, property, vehicles, and school events	37%	100%	64%†	Moved toward target

*Latest data are from 2007.
†Latest data are from 2006.
‡Latest data are from 2005.
§Latest data are from 2004.

Sources: DATA2010 . . . *The Healthy People* 2010 Database, Centers for Disease Control and Prevention, http://wonder.cdc.gov/data2010/index.htm, updated September 2009; U.S. Department of Health and Human Services, *Healthy People 2010,* 2d ed., with *Understanding and Improving Health and Objectives for Improving Health,* 2 vols. (Washington, DC: U.S. Government Printing Office, November 2000), available at www.health.gov/healthypeople.

As 2010 arrives, health professionals have been taking input and planning for a whole new set of national objectives. Known as *Healthy People 2020,* these objectives are expected to have an even greater emphasis on diverse health needs and healthy disparities among selected populations and should be available soon. This increased focus on disparities is particularly important as we consider the increasingly diverse population in the United States. According to the 2000 U.S. Census, approximately 30 percent of the population currently belongs to a racial or ethnic minority group. It is projected that by the year 2060, non-Hispanic whites will make up less than 50 percent of the U.S. population.[10]

National Goal: Improving Health and Reducing Disparities

Are we making progress? From all indicators, national priorities are shifting, and health professionals and public and private organizations are beginning to work together to help people make better health decisions. For example, cities across the United States are passing legislation that bans *trans* fats from restaurant food items, and a majority of major cities have now gone "smoke-free." More and more states and cities are adopting green policies and programs in an effort to do their part in reducing global warming. Colleges and universities are ramping up their efforts to reduce waste, use less energy, and create more sustainable living environments on campus. These landmark actions and others are designed to improve life span, quality of life, and the state of our environment. On the flip side, there are still disparities in health care. Some populations are at a distinct disadvantage when it comes to getting and staying healthy. For example, if you are a college student without health insurance and are on a limited budget, you may put off visiting the doctor or not go at all. If you have a serious illness, this delay can lower your chance of successful treatment. Factors such as language barriers can also negatively impact an individual's health. Studies have shown that people whose primary language is not English or who cannot read prescription labels or follow written medical instructions have significant barriers to overall health.[11]

health disparities Differences in the incidence, prevalence, mortality, and burden of diseases and other health conditions among specific population groups.
health promotion Combined educational, organizational, policy, financial, and environmental supports to help people reduce negative health behaviors and promote positive change.
risk behaviors Actions that increase susceptibility to negative health outcomes.
sex The biological and physiological aspects that make an individual male or female.
gender The socially accepted roles and attributes of being male or female.

Recognizing the changing demographics of the U.S. population and the vast differences in health status based on racial or ethnic background, *Healthy People 2010* included strong language about the importance of reducing **health disparities.**[12] See the **Health in a Diverse World** box for examples of groups that often experience health disparities.

A New Focus on Health Promotion

The objectives of *Healthy People 2010* and *2020* and other programs are to promote health and to prevent premature disability through social, environmental, policy-related, and community-based programming. In addition, a new emphasis on assisting individuals in their pursuit of specific behavior changes is emerging. Although *change* seems to be a persistent buzzword at all levels of society today, making changes without knowledge, a plan, and appropriate resources is not easy. The term **health promotion** describes the educational, organizational, procedural, environmental, social, and financial supports that help individuals and groups reduce negative health behaviors and promote positive change. Health promotion programs identify healthy people who are engaging in **risk behaviors,** motivate them to change their actions, and provide support to increase chances of success. Effective stop-smoking programs, for instance, don't simply say, "Just do it." Instead, they provide information about possible consequences to smokers and the people they expose to secondhand smoke (educational support); encourage smokers to participate in smoking cessation classes and allow employees time off to attend or set up buddy systems to help them (organizational support); establish policies governing smokers' behaviors and supporting their decisions to change, such as banning smoking in the workplace and removing cigarettes from vending machines (environmental support); and provide monetary incentives to motivate people to participate (financial support).

46.3 million

Americans do not have health insurance.

Health promotion programs also encourage people with sound health habits to maintain them. By attempting to modify behaviors, increase skills, change attitudes, increase knowledge, influence values, and improve health decision making, health promotion goes well beyond the simple information campaign. By basing services in communities, organizations, schools, and other places where most people spend their time, health promotion programs increase the likelihood of long-term success on the road to health and wellness.

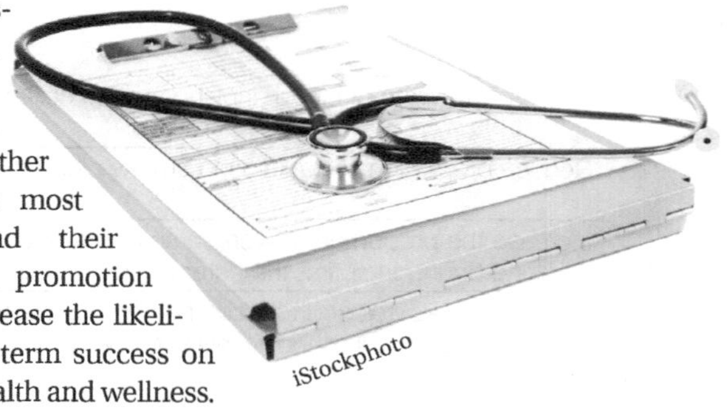

iStockphoto

Whether we use the term *health* or *wellness,* we are talking about a person's overall responses to the challenges of living. Occasional dips into the ice cream bucket and other deviations from optimal behavior should not be viewed as major failures. Actually, the ability to recognize that each of us is an imperfect being attempting to adapt in an imperfect world signals individual well-being.

Health In a DIVERSE World

The Challenge of Health Disparities

Among the factors that can affect an individual's ability to attain optimal health are the following:

✱ **Race and ethnicity.** Research indicates dramatic health disparities among people of certain racial and ethnic backgrounds. Socioeconomic differences, stigma based on "minority status," poor access to health care, cultural barriers and beliefs, discrimination, and limited education and employment opportunities can all impact health status. Some groups are also genetically predisposed to certain diseases; for example, sickle cell disease is most common among people of African ancestry, Tay-Sachs disease afflicts people of Eastern European heritage and French Canadians, and multiple sclerosis disproportionately afflicts Caucasians.

Although genes are clearly important to discussions of chronic disease susceptibility, there is considerable debate about the actual role of race and ethnicity in disparity research. One view approaches race as a biologically meaningful category and indicates that racial disparities in health reflect inherited susceptibility to disease. A second view treats race as a proxy for class and views socioeconomic status as the real culprit behind racial disparities. There are other views that combine various theories on why such disparities exist.

✱ **Inadequate health insurance.** A large and growing number of people are *uninsured* or *underinsured.* Those without adequate insurance coverage may face high copayments, high deductibles, or limited care in their area. In the past two decades, numerous health professionals, health-related groups, politicians, and government leaders have sought to address the looming crisis in health care in the United States. The complexity of the topic, the large numbers of special-interest groups that would be affected by any major changes, and concerns over economic and personal impacts of change have made significant progress difficult.

✱ **Sex and gender.** There are numerous instances of tremendous health disparities by **sex** and **gender,** not the least of which is the vast difference in life expectancy between men and women. At all ages and stages of life, men and women experience major differences in rates of disease and disability.

✱ **Lifestyle behaviors.** Persistent poverty may make it difficult to buy healthy food, get enough rest and exercise, cope with stress, and seek preventive medicine. Obesity, smoking, and lack of exercise are examples of health problems related directly to behavioral and cultural patterns we adopt from our families.

✱ **Geographic location/transportation access.** Whether you live in an urban or rural area and have access to public transportation or your own vehicle can have a huge impact on what you choose to eat and your ability to visit the doctor or dentist. Older people, people with disabilities, and people who lack the financial means to travel for preventive tests such as mammograms are clearly at a health disadvantage. In addition, persons who live in rural areas or small communities might not have ready access to high-tech diagnostic and treatment centers or may have difficulty getting referrals to specialists when facing chronic diseases.

✱ **Sexual orientation.** The 5 to 10 percent of Americans who identify themselves as gay, lesbian, bisexual, or transgender experience high levels of health disparities. These individuals may lack social support, are often denied health benefits due to unrecognized marital status, and face unusually high stress levels and stigmatization by other groups. They are also more likely to engage in risky behaviors such as smoking, unprotected sex, and drug and alcohol abuse and report higher levels of depression and suicide in adolescence.

✱ **Disability.** Today, over 50 million Americans, or 1 in 5 people, are living with at least one disability, and most Americans will experience a disability at some time in their lives. Although some are easy to recognize, such as a person using a wheelchair, others, such as autism or learning disabilities, are harder to detect. Regardless of the type of disability, problems with major life activities are often present. Disproportionate numbers of disabled individuals lack access to health care services, social support, and community resources that would enhance their quality of life.

Many people in the United States experience several impediments to receiving proper health care, such as geographic isolation, poverty, and lack of health insurance, One of the ways public health officials attempt to address this problem is to organize Remote Area Medical (RAM) clinics. At a clinic like this, rural families, most with little or no insurance, wait in line for hours to receive free health care from hundreds of professional doctors, nurses, dentists, and other health workers.

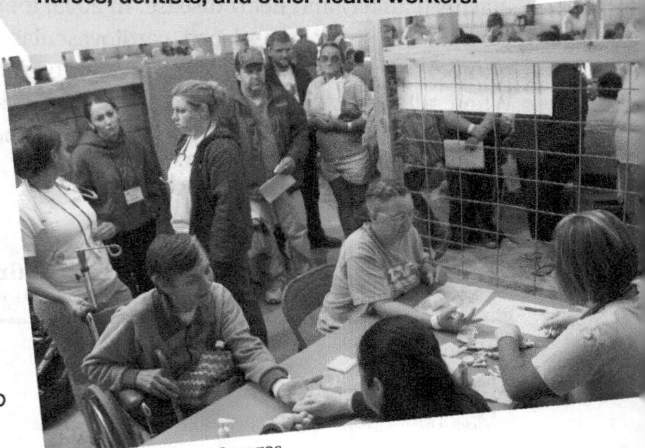

Suzy Allman / Getty Images

Sources: National Institutes of Health, *National Institutes of Health (NIH) Strategic Research Plan and Budget to Reduce and Ultimately Eliminate Health Disparities: Volume 1, Fiscal Years 2002–2006* (Bethesda, MD: National Institutes of Health, May 12, 2006); Centers for Disease Control and Prevention, "People with Disabilities Can Lead Long, Healthy Lives," www.cdc.gov/Features/Disabilities. Updated October 6, 2008; Centers for Disease Control and Prevention, "Uninsured Americans: Newly Released Health Insurance Statistics," www.cdc.gov/Features/Uninsured. Updated April 9, 2009; Centers for Disease Control and Prevention, "Lesbian, Gay, Bisexual and Transgender Health," www.cdc.gov/Features/LGBT. Updated August 7, 2008.

We must also remember to be tolerant of others. Rather than be warriors against pleasure in our zeal to change the health behaviors of others, we need to be supportive, non-judgmental, and helpful to people trying to achieve their own health goals. Ultimately, we all have to find our own best way to make change happen.

Health Status Report: How Are We Doing?

Table 2 summarizes the leading causes of death in the United States. Note that adolescents and young adults aged 15 to 24 are most likely to die from unintentional injuries, followed by homicide and suicide. Alcohol is a leading factor in many of these deaths. Unintentional injuries are also the major killer in the next age group, aged 25 to 44, followed by malignant neoplasms (cancer) and heart disease. In 2005, for the first time in U.S. history, cancer replaced cardiovascular disease as the number one cause of death for all persons under the age of 85.[13] When all age groups are included, cardiovascular disease remains the number one cause of death in the United States and worldwide.

In the United States, chronic diseases account for seven of the ten leading causes of death and are linked to preventable lifestyle behaviors such as tobacco use, poor nutrition, and lack of physical activity, all of which can lead to obesity, alcohol use, car crashes, risky sexual behavior, and drug use.[14] Currently, more than half of Americans suffer from one or more chronic diseases at a cost to our economy of over $1 trillion.[15] Many of these diseases are the result of preventable risk behaviors, and with earlier diagnosis and increased attention to reducing risks, billions of dollars could be saved each year. The modifiable behavioral risk factors in Figure 5 are the leading causes of preventable disease and death in the United States. By conservative estimates, these preventable risk behaviors affect quality of life for nearly 100 million Americans and account for 70 percent of total medical expenditures.[16] Primary and secondary

5.5 million

years of potential life are lost in the U.S. annually as a direct result of cigarette smoking.

TABLE 2 **Leading Causes of Death in the United States by Age (Years), 2006**

All Ages		**Aged 15–24**	
Diseases of the heart	629,191	Unintentional injuries	15,859
Malignant neoplasms (cancer)	560,102	Homicide	5,596
Cerebrovascular diseases	137,265	Suicide	4,097
Chronic lower respiratory diseases	124,614	Malignant neoplasms	1,643
Unintentional injuries	117,748	Diseases of the heart	1,021
Under 1 Year		**Aged 25–44**	
Congenital anomalies	5,827	Unintentional injuries	30,949
Short gestation or low birth weight	4,841	Malignant neoplasms	17,604
Sudden infant death syndrome	2,145	Diseases of the heart	14,873
Newborn affected by maternal complications	1,694	Suicide	11,240
Unintentional injuries	1,119	Homicide	7,525
Aged 1–4		**Aged 45–64**	
Unintentional injuries	1,591	Malignant neoplasms	151,654
Congenital anomalies	501	Diseases of the heart	101,588
Malignant neoplasms	372	Unintentional injuries	29,505
Homicide	350	Diabetes mellitus	17,012
Diseases of the heart	160	Cerebrovascular diseases	16,779
Aged 5–14		**Aged 65+**	
Unintentional injuries	2,228	Diseases of the heart	510,934
Malignant neoplasms	916	Malignant neoplasms	387,828
Homicide	387	Cerebrovascular diseases	117,284
Congenital anomalies	330	Chronic lower respiratory diseases	107,058
Diseases of the heart	242	Alzheimer's disease	72,135

Source: M. Heron, "Deaths: Preliminary Data for 2006," in *National Vital Statistics Reports* 56, no. 16 (Hyattsville, MD: National Center for Health Statistics, 2008).

FIGURE 5 **Leading Causes of Preventable Death in the United States**

Sources: Data are from A. Mokdad et al., "Actual Causes of Death in the United States, 2000," *Journal of the American Medical Association* 291, no. 10 (2004): 1238–45; A. Mokdad et al., "Actual Causes of Death in the United States, 2000—Correction," *Journal of the American Medical Association* 293, no. 3 (2005).

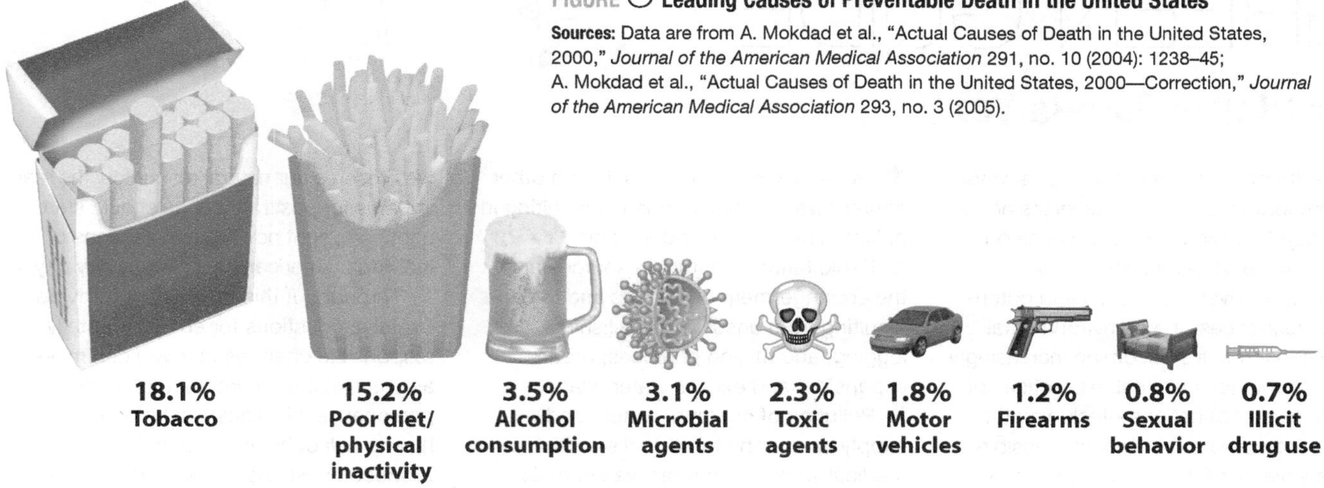

AP Photos

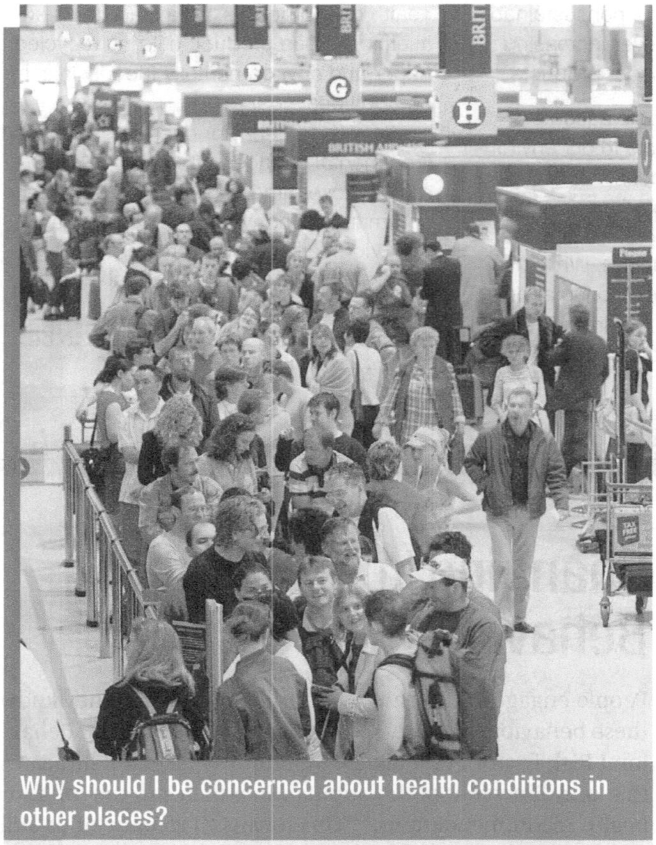

Why should I be concerned about health conditions in other places?

With the rise of global travel, commerce, and communication, we are living in an increasingly global society in which everyone's health and wellness is becoming interdependent. The health status of one nation—the environmental pollutants it produces, the diseases it harbors, even the eating habits it promotes—can impact the health of people in surrounding nations and around the world. For example, infectious disease can spread much more quickly now than in the past. The deadly flu pandemic of 1918 took over 1 year to travel around the globe, whereas people today could transmit illness globally in a matter of weeks.

preventions offer our best hope for reducing the **incidence** and **prevalence** of disease and disability.

Health educators in our schools and communities offer an effective delivery mechanism for prevention and intervention programs. **Certified Health Education Specialists (CHESs)** make up a trained cadre of public health educators with special credentials and competencies in developing prevention programs that offer scientifically and behaviorally sound methods to help individuals and communities increase the likelihood of success in achieving optimal health. These specialists have the skills and experience to greatly enhance the nation's health. A major shift in focus from treatment to prevention is necessary to achieve our national goals.

incidence The number of new cases.
prevalence The number of existing cases.
Certified Health Education Specialist (CHES) Academically trained health educator who has passed a national competency examination for prevention and intervention programming.

what do you think?

Think about your own health right now. On a scale from 1 to 10, with 1 being the lowest and 10 the highest, how would you rate your fitness level? ● Your ability to form and maintain healthy relationships? ● Your ability to cope with daily stressors?

Global Health Issues

Everyone's health is profoundly affected by economic, social, behavioral, scientific, and technological factors. The world economy has become increasingly interconnected and globalized; every day, millions of people move across national borders, leading to many new challenges for health around the world. Current concern over pandemic flu, resistant tuberculosis, and methicillin-resistant *Staphylococcus aureus* (MRSA) as well as the impact of global warming on health status provides a grim reminder for the need for a proactive international response to disease prevention. Health risks are not limited to

GREEN GUIDE

Our Planet Needs You!

The health of our environment has always been important, but today scientists agree that global environmental conditions pose dire threats to all living things. While debate rages over the causes and potential consequences of our environmental health concerns, it's becoming increasingly clear that the nonsustainable practices of an elite cluster of nations—including the United States—are primarily responsible for the severity of the problems we now face. Indeed, according to the Center for Environment and Population, the United States alone is responsible for 25 percent of the world's energy consumption—this in spite of the United States being home to only 5 percent of the global population.

Some of the greatest environmental challenges facing us are

- Climate change brought about by greenhouse gas emissions from the burning of fossil fuels in our homes; our factories; our businesses; and, perhaps most devastatingly, our cars, buses, trucks, and airplanes.
- Over-reliance on fossil fuels and other nonrenewable energy sources, resulting in pollution and resource depletion.
- Exploitation of natural resources and the endangerment of species and habitats resulting from unsustainable fishing, logging, and mining practices; urban expansion; and excess water usage.
- Pollution of our land, water, food supply, and air by fossil-fuel emissions, medical waste, electronic waste, toxic wastes, and nonbiodegradable trash.
- Deforestation and desertification driven by overpopulation, poverty, nonsustainable farming techniques, and ever-increasing demands for wood and paper products.

As more and more people become aware of these major threats to our environmental health, there has been an increasing recognition of the need to adopt environmentally responsible, or "green," practices in our homes and communities. While the next decade will undoubtedly bring about rapid changes in the cars we drive, the types of energy we develop, and the way we preserve our natural resources, the real impetus for positive change should start right here, right now, with the actions of individual Americans each and every day.

Throughout this text, we will provide useful suggestions for environmentally responsible changes that you can make as you explore different areas of your own personal health. These include ideas on how to select healthy foods that are produced sustainably, ways to reduce your environmental impact during your leisure time, and tips for locating green health care products. As a start, this text itself is a green product, utilizing recycled paper and environmentally friendly inks at no additional cost to you.

As with all behavior changes, small and incremental changes often reap huge rewards over time. If each of us makes the commitment today and initiates these behaviors for the rest of the term and beyond, it will help move us in the right direction. We hope to challenge you to be the change agent you want others to be.

disease—contaminants of food, air, and water supplies; climate change; and chemical toxins are modern health threats to the global community (see the **Green Guide** above).

Likewise, health disparities are not just a national concern. They exist in every nation around the globe. Those nations that lack adequate resources such as food, water, and shelter; have weak economies; or have ongoing political unrest are especially likely to experience extreme health disparities. In developed nations, the leading causes of death are ischemic heart disease, stroke, and chronic obstructive respiratory diseases. In developing nations, leading causes of death are HIV/AIDS, lower-respiratory infections, heart disease, and diarrheal diseases, which are largely a result of a lack of clean water.

what do you think?

What implications do developments in global health have for people living in the United States today? ● What international programs, policies, or services might help control the world's health problems in the next decade? ● Are there actions that individuals can take to help?

Changing Your Health Behaviors

People engage in unhealthy behaviors even when they know these behaviors are risky. In fact, a recent study of the Behavioral Risk Factor Surveillance System (BRFSS) data indicates that only 3 percent of the population adheres to the top four health recommendations.[17] This means that many of us still smoke, avoid exercise, and consume *trans* fats, even though we are bombarded with public health messages that tell us to do otherwise. While we may make resolutions every January 1 to lose weight, stop smoking, exercise more, eat better, and find more friends, usually by January 5 we've given up on these seemingly simple tasks. However, every individual has the potential to adopt healthier habits. The key is to do so one step at a time.

Major factors that influence behavior and behavior-change decisions can be divided into three general categories: predisposing, enabling, and reinforcing.

- **Predisposing factors.** Our life experiences, knowledge, cultural and ethnic heritage, and current beliefs and values are all *predisposing factors* that influence behavior. Factors that may predispose us to certain health conditions include age, sex, race, income, family background, educational background, and access to health care. For example, if your parents smoked, you are 90 percent more likely to start smoking than someone whose parents didn't. If your peers smoke, you are 80 percent more likely to smoke than someone whose friends don't.
- **Enabling factors.** Skills and abilities; physical, emotional, and mental capabilities; community and government priorities and commitment to health; and safe and convenient resources and facilities that make health decisions easy or difficult are *enabling factors*. Positive enablers encourage you to carry through on your intentions to change. Negative enablers work against your intentions to change. For example, if you would like to join a fitness center but discover that the closest one is 4 miles away, closes at 9:00 p.m., and the membership fee is $500, those negative enablers may convince you to stay home. By contrast, if your school's fitness center is two blocks away, stays open until midnight, and offers a special student membership, those positive enablers will probably convince you to join. Identifying positive and negative enabling factors and devising alternative plans when the negative factors outweigh the positive are part of planning for behavior change.

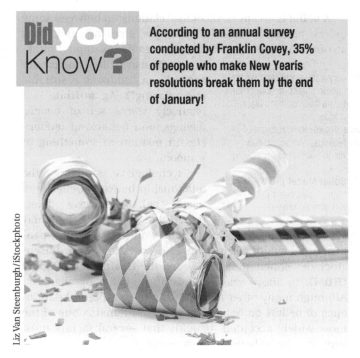

Skills for Behavior Change

How Many of These Healthy Behaviors Do You Practice?

- Get a good night's sleep (minimum of 7 hours)
- Maintain healthy eating habits and manage your weight
- Participate in physical recreational activities
- Practice safer sex
- Limit your intake of alcohol and avoid tobacco products
- Schedule regular self-exams and medical checkups

Several other actions may not add years to your life, but they can add significant life to your years:

- Control real and imaginary stressors
- Maintain meaningful relationships with family and friends
- Make time for yourself and be kind to others
- Participate in at least one fun activity each day
- Respect the environment and the people in it
- Consider alternatives when making decisions; view mistakes as learning experiences
- Value each day and make the best of opportunities
- Understand the health care system and use it wisely

Did you Know?

According to an annual survey conducted by Franklin Covey, 35% of people who make New Yearís resolutions break them by the end of January!

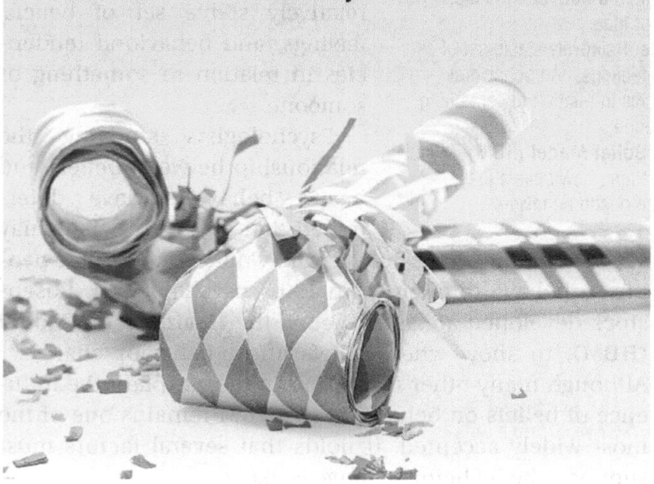

Liz Van Steenburgh/iStockphoto

- **Reinforcing factors.** *Reinforcing factors* include the presence or absence of support, encouragement, or discouragement that significant people in your life bring to a situation; employer actions and policies; health provider costs and access; community resources; and access to health education. For example, if you decide to stop smoking and your family and friends continue smoking in your presence, you may be tempted to start smoking again. In other words, your smoking behavior is reinforced. If, however, you are overweight, you lose a few pounds, and all your friends tell you how terrific you look, your positive behavior is reinforced, and you will likely continue your weight-loss plan.

The manner in which you reward or punish yourself in the process of change also plays a role. Accepting small failures and concentrating on your successes can foster further achievements. Berating yourself because you binged on potato chips or haven't found time to use that fitness club membership may create an internal environment in which failure becomes almost inevitable. Telling yourself that you're worth the extra effort and giving yourself a pat on the back for small accomplishments are often overlooked factors in positive behavior change.

Beliefs and Attitudes

We often assume that when rational people realize their behaviors put them at risk, they will change those behaviors and reduce that risk. But this is not necessarily true. Consider the number of health professionals who smoke, consume junk food, and act in other unhealthy ways. They surely know better, but their "knowing" is disconnected from their "doing." Why is this so? Two strong influences on behavior are beliefs and attitudes.

A **belief** is an appraisal of the relationship between some object, action, or idea (for example, smoking) and some attribute of that object, action, or idea (for example, "smoking is expensive, dirty, and causes cancer"—or, "smoking is sociable and relaxing"). An **attitude** is a relatively stable set of beliefs, feelings, and behavioral tendencies in relation to something or someone.

belief Appraisal of the relationship between some object, action, or idea and some attribute of that object, action, or idea.
attitude Relatively stable set of beliefs, feelings, and behavioral tendencies in relation to something or someone.
Health Belief Model (HBM) Model for explaining how beliefs may influence health behaviors.

Psychologists studying the relationship between beliefs and health behaviors have determined that although beliefs may subtly influence behavior, they may not actually cause people to behave differently. In 1966, psychologist I. Rosenstock developed a classic theory, the **Health Belief Model (HBM),** to show when beliefs affect behavior change.[18] Although many other models attempt to explain the influence of beliefs on behaviors, the HBM remains one of the most widely accepted. It holds that several factors must support a belief before change is likely:

- **Perceived seriousness of the health problem.** How severe would the medical and social consequences be if the health problem was to develop or be left untreated? The more serious the perceived effects, the more likely that action will be taken.
- **Perceived susceptibility to the health problem.** What is the likelihood of developing the health problem? People who perceive themselves at high risk are more likely to take preventive action.
- **Cues to action.** A person who is reminded or alerted about a potential health problem is more likely to take action. For example, having your doctor tell you that your blood sugar levels indicate a pre-diabetic state may be the cue that pushes you to lose weight and exercise.

People follow the Health Belief Model many times every day. Take, for example, smokers. Older smokers are likely to know other smokers who have developed serious heart or lung problems. They are thus more likely to perceive tobacco as a threat to their health than are teenagers who have just begun smoking. The greater the perceived threat of health problems caused by smoking, the greater the chance a person will quit.

However, many chronic smokers know the risks yet continue to smoke. Why do they miss these cues to action? According to Rosenstock, some people do not believe they will be affected by a severe problem—they act as though they are immune to it—and are unlikely to change their behavior. They also may feel that the immediate pleasure outweighs the long-range cost.

Our attitudes tend to reflect our emotional responses to situations and follow from our beliefs. The more consistent your attitude is toward an action and the more you are influenced by others to take that action, the more likely you are to be motivated to change the behavior and to ultimately succeed in doing so. The key is being able to recognize potential barriers that you may face as you try modifying your behaviors. Figure 6 lists some of the common barriers people encounter when trying to make behavior change and some suggested ways to overcome them.

If you think... then	try this strategy...
"I don't have enough time"	Chart your hourly activities for 1 day. What are your highest priorities? What can you eliminate? Plan to make some time for a healthy change next week.
"I'm too stressed"	Assess your major stressors right now. List those you can control and those you can change or avoid. Then identify two things you enjoy that can help you reduce stress now.
"I worry about what others may think"	Ask yourself how much others influence your decisions about drinking, sex, eating habits, etc. What is most important to you? What actions can you take to act in line with these values?
"I don't think I can do it"	Just because you haven't before doesn't mean you can't now. To develop some confidence, take baby steps and break tasks into small pieces.
"It's a habit I can't break"	Habits are difficult to break but not impossible. What triggers your behavior? List ways you can avoid these triggers. Ask for support from friends and family.

FIGURE 6 **Common Barriers to Behavior Change**
There are several types of obstacles that can make it difficult to succeed in making a behavior change. Each strategy shown can help overcome these obstacles.

Source: From D. L. Watson and R. G. Tharp, *Self-Directed Behavior: Self-Modification for Personal Adjustment.* 9th ed. © 2007 Reprinted with permission of Wadsworth Publishing, a division of Cengage Learning.

Self-Efficacy

Self-efficacy—an individual's belief that he or she is capable of achieving certain goals or of performing at a level that may influence events in life—is one of the most important factors that influence our health status. People who have it are more likely to take action to improve their health, stick to their plan of action, and experiment with other options for making improvements. In general, people who exhibit high self-efficacy are confident that they can succeed, and they approach challenges with a positive attitude. Prior success in academics, athletics, or social interactions will lead to expectations of success in the future. Self-efficacious people are more likely to feel a sense of personal control over situations. People who approach challenges, such as changing an unhealthy behavior, with confidence (that "I can do it" mentality) may be more motivated to change and achieve a greater level of success.

On the other hand, someone with low self-efficacy or with self-doubts about what they can and cannot do may give up easily or never even try to change a behavior. These people tend to shy away from difficult challenges. They may have failed before, and when the going gets tough, they are more likely to give up or revert to old patterns of behavior.

External versus Internal Locus of Control

The conviction that you have the power and ability to change is a powerful motivator. Individuals who feel that they have limited control over their lives often find it more difficult to initiate positive changes.[19] If they believe that someone or something else controls a situation or that they dare not act in a particular way because of peer repercussions, they may become easily frustrated and give up. People with these characteristics have an *external* **locus of control.** In contrast, people who have a stronger *internal* locus of control believe they have power over their own actions. They are more driven by their own thoughts and are more likely to state their opinions and be true to their own beliefs.

Having an internal or external locus of control can vary according to circumstance. For instance, someone who finds out that diabetes runs in their family may resign himself to one day facing the disease, instead of taking an active role in modifying his lifestyle to minimize his risk of developing diabetes. On this front, he would be demonstrating an external locus of control. However, the same individual might exhibit an internal locus of control when being pressured by friends to smoke. He knows that he does not want to smoke and does not want to risk the potential consequences of the habit, so he takes charge and resists the pressure. In general, developing and maintaining an internal locus of control can help you take charge of your health behaviors.

what do you think?

In general, do you have an internal or an external locus of control? ● Can you describe a situation where you demonstrated an internal locus of control? ● Can you think of some good friends who you'd describe as more internally controlled? Externally controlled? How have you seen these demonstrated?

Significant Others as Change Agents

Many of us are highly influenced by the approval or disapproval (real or imagined) of close friends, loved ones, and the social and cultural groups to which we belong. Such influences can support healthy behavior, or they can interfere with even the best intentions.

Your Family From the time of your birth, your parents and other family members have given you strong cues about which actions are and are not socially acceptable. Brushing your teeth, bathing, and chewing food with your mouth closed are behaviors that your family probably instilled in you long ago. Your family and local culture influenced your food choices, your religious beliefs, your political beliefs, and many of your other values and actions. If you deviated from your family's norms, a family member probably let you know fairly quickly. Strong and positive family units provide care, trust, and protection; are dedicated to the healthful development of all family members; and work to reduce problems.

self-efficacy Belief in one's ability to perform a task successfully.

locus of control The "location," *external* (outside oneself) or *internal* (within oneself), an individual perceives as the source and underlying cause of events in his or her life.

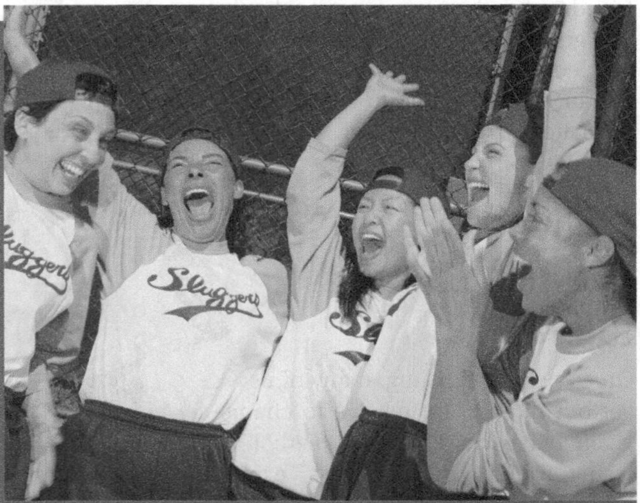

Randy Faris/Corbis

How do my friends and family influence my health?

The people in your life can play a huge role—both positive and negative—in the health choices you make. The behaviors of those around you can predispose you to certain health habits, at the same time enabling and reinforcing them. Seeking out the support and encouragement of friends who have similar goals and interests will strengthen your commitment to develop and maintain positive health behaviors.

When the loving family unit does not exist or when it does not provide for basic human needs, it becomes difficult for a child to learn positive health behaviors. Often, healthy behaviors get their start in healthy homes; unhealthy homes breed unhealthy habits. Healthy families provide the foundation for a clear and necessary understanding of what is right and wrong, what is positive and negative. Without this fundamental grounding, many young people have great difficulties.

Social Bonds and the Influence of Others Just as your family influences your actions during your childhood, your friends and significant others influence your behaviors as you grow older. Most of us desire to fit the "norm" and avoid hassles in our daily interactions with others. If you deviate from the actions expected in your hometown or among your friends, you may suffer ostracism, strange looks, and other negative social consequences. Understanding the subtle and not-so-subtle ways in which other people influence our actions is an important step toward changing our behaviors.

Transtheoretical Model of Health Behavior Change (Stages of Change model) Model of behavior change that identifies six distinct stages people go through in altering behavior patterns.

The influence of others serves as a powerful *social support* for positive change. If friends offer encouragement (subjective norms), for example, by becoming "workout buddies," you are more likely to remain motivated to change your behavior. However, if you believe your friends will think you are a "nerd" for going to the gym, you may quickly lose your motivation. The importance of cultivating and maintaining close *social bonds* with others is an important part of overall health. Finding friends who share your personal values can greatly affect your behaviors. The key people in our lives play a powerful role in our motivation to change for the better—or for the worse.

Motivation and Readiness to Change

On any given morning, many of us get out of bed and resolve to change a given behavior that day. Whether it be losing weight, drinking less, exercising more, being nicer to others, managing time better, or some other change, we start out with enthusiasm and high expectations. However, a vast majority of people return to their old behavior. Wanting to change is a prerequisite of the change process, but there is much more to the process than motivation. *Motivation* must be combined with common sense, commitment, and a realistic understanding of how best to move from point A to point B. *Readiness* is the state of being that precedes behavior change, and those who are ready are likely to make the actual effort. People who are ready to change possess the attitudes, knowledge, skills, and internal and external resources that make change possible.[20]

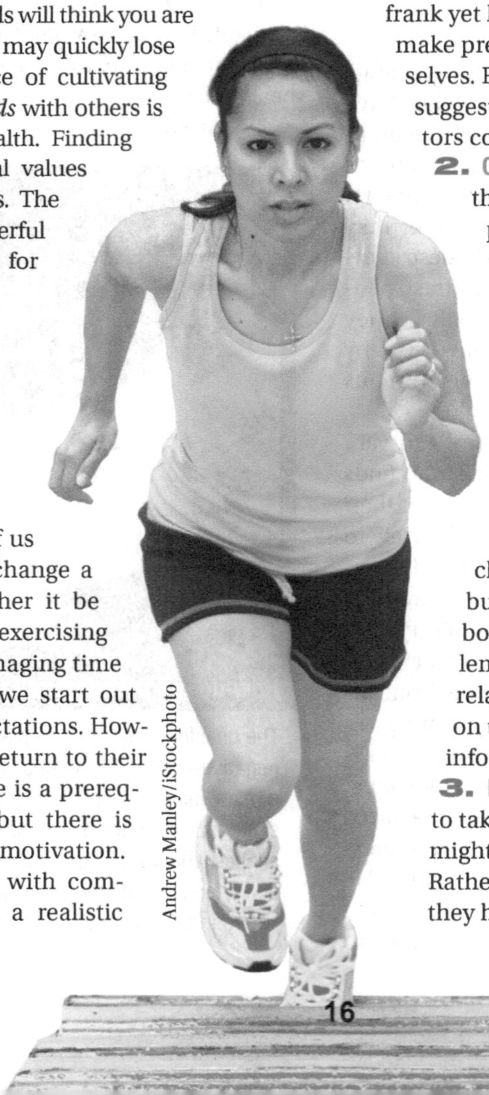

Andrew Manley/iStockphoto

Why do so many good intentions fail? According to Dr. James Prochaska of the University of Rhode Island and Dr. Carlos DiClemente of the University of Maryland, it's because we are going about things in the wrong way; fewer than 20 percent of us are really prepared to take action. After considerable research, they have concluded that behavior changes usually do not succeed if they start with the change itself. Instead, we must go through a series of stages to adequately prepare ourselves for that eventual change.[21] According to Prochaska and DiClemente's **Transtheoretical Model of Health Behavior Change** (also called the **Stages of Change model**), our chances of keeping those New Year's resolutions will be greatly enhanced if we have proper reinforcement and help during each of the following stages.

1. **Precontemplation.** People in the precontemplation stage have no current intention of changing. They may have tried to change a behavior before and given up, or they may be in denial and unaware of any problem. Sometimes a few frank yet kind words from friends may be enough to make precontemplators take a closer look at themselves. Recommending readings or making tactful suggestions can be useful in helping precontemplators consider making a change.
2. **Contemplation.** In this phase, people recognize that they have a problem and begin to contemplate the need to change. Acknowledgment usually results from increased awareness, often due to feedback from family and friends or access to information. Despite this acknowledgment, people can languish in this stage for years, realizing that they have a problem but lacking the time or energy to make the change.

   Often, contemplators need a little push to get them started. This may come in the form of someone helping them set up a change plan (for example, an exercise routine), buying a helpful gift (such as a low-fat cookbook), sharing articles about a particular problem, or inviting them to go hear a speaker on a related topic. See the **Consumer Health** box for tips on using the Internet to gather valuable health information.
3. **Preparation.** Most people at this point are close to taking action. They've thought about what they might do and may even have come up with a plan. Rather than thinking about why they can't begin, they have started to focus on what they can do.

There are some standard guidelines to follow when you are preparing for change. Set realistic goals (large and small), take small steps toward change, change only a couple of things at once, reward small milestones, and seek support from friends. Identify factors that have enabled or obstructed success in the past, and modify them where possible. Complete a Behavior Change Contract to help you commit to making these changes.

3 to 5 is the number of times most people will attempt to change an unhealthy behavior before succeeding.

4. Action. In this stage, people begin to follow their action plans. Those who have prepared for change, thought about alternatives, engaged social support, and made a plan of action are more ready for action than those who have given it little thought. Unfortunately, too many people start behavior change here rather than going through the first three stages. Without a plan, without enlisting the help of others, or without a realistic goal, failure is likely.

Publicly stating the desire to change helps ensure success. Encourage friends who are making a change to share their plans with you. Offer to help, and try to remove potential obstacles from the person's intended action plan. Social support and the buddy system can motivate even the most reluctant person.

5. Maintenance. Maintenance requires vigilance, attention to detail, and long-term commitment. Many people reach a goal, only to relax and slip back into the undesired behavior. In this stage, it is important to be aware of the potential for relapses and to develop strategies for dealing with such challenges. Common causes of relapse include overconfidence, daily temptations, stress or emotional distractions, and self-deprecation.

During maintenance, continue taking the same actions that led to success in the first place. Find fun and creative ways to maintain positive behaviors. This is where a willing and caring support group can be vital. Knowing where on your campus to turn for help when you don't have a close support network is also helpful.

6. Termination. By this point, the behavior is so ingrained that the current level of vigilance may be unnecessary. The new behavior has become an essential part of daily living. Do you know someone who has made a major behavior change that has now become an essential part of that person's life?

Choosing a Behavior-Change Technique

Once you have analyzed all the factors that influence your behaviors, consider what actions you can take to change the negative ones. Behavior-change techniques include shaping, visualization, modeling, controlling the situation, reinforcement, and changing self-talk. The options don't stop here, but these are the most common strategies.

Shaping

Regardless of how motivated you are, some behaviors are almost impossible to change immediately. To reach your goal, you may need to take a number of individual steps, each designed to change one small piece of the larger behavior. This process is known as **shaping.**

For example, suppose that you have not exercised for a while. You decide that you want to get into shape, and your goal is to jog 3 miles every other day. But you realize that you'd face a near-death experience if you tried to run even a few blocks in your current condition. So you decide to build up to your desired fitness level gradually. During week 1, you will walk for 1 hour every other day at a slow, relaxed pace. During week 2, you will walk for the same amount of time but speed up your pace and cover slightly more ground. During week 3, you will speed up even more and try to go even farther. You will continue taking such steps until you reach your goal.

Whatever the desired behavior change, all shaping involves the following actions:

- Start slowly, and try not to cause undue stress during the early stages of the program.
- Keep the steps small and achievable.
- Be flexible. If the original plan proves uncomfortable or you deviate from it, don't give up! Start again, and move forward.
- Don't skip steps or move to the next step until you have mastered the previous one.
- Reward yourself for meeting regular, previously-set goals.

Remember, behaviors don't develop overnight, so they won't change overnight.

Visualization

Mental practice can transform unhealthy behaviors into healthy ones. Athletes and others use a technique known as **imagined rehearsal** to reach their goals. By visualizing their planned action ahead of time, they are better prepared when they put themselves to the test.

For example, suppose you want to ask someone out on a date. Imagine the setting (walking together to class). Then practice in your mind and out loud exactly what you want to say. Mentally anticipate different responses ("Oh, I'd love to, but I'm busy that evening. . . .") and what you will say in reaction ("How about if I call you sometime this week?"). Careful mental and verbal rehearsal—you could even try out your scenario on a friend—will greatly improve the likelihood of success.

shaping Using a series of small steps to gradually achieve a particular goal.

imagined rehearsal Practicing, through mental imagery, to become better able to perform an event in actuality.

Modeling

Modeling, or learning behaviors by watching others perform them, is one of the most effective strategies for changing behavior. For example, suppose that you have trouble talking to people you don't know very well. One of the easiest ways to improve your communication skills is to select friends whose social skills you envy. Observe them. Do they talk more or listen more? How do people respond to them? Why are they such good communicators? If you observe behaviors you admire and isolate their components, you can model the steps of your behavior-change technique on a proven success.

Controlling the Situation

Sometimes, the right setting or the right group of people will positively influence your behaviors. Many situations and occasions trigger certain actions. For example, in libraries, houses of worship, and museums, most people talk softly. Few people laugh at funerals. The term **situational inducement** refers to an attempt to influence a behavior by using occasions and social settings to control it.

For example, you may be more apt to stop smoking if you work in a smoke-free office, a positive situational inducement. But working in a smoke-filled bar, a negative situational inducement, may tempt you to resume. By carefully considering which settings will help and which will hurt your effort to change, and by deciding to seek the first and avoid the second, you will improve your chances for change.

modeling Learning specific behaviors by watching others perform them.
situational inducement Attempt to influence a behavior through situations and occasions that are structured to exert control over that behavior.
positive reinforcement Presenting something positive following a behavior that is being reinforced.
self-talk The customary manner of thinking and talking to yourself, which can impact your self-image.

Reinforcement

Another way to promote positive behavior change is to reward yourself for it. This is called **positive reinforcement.** Each of us is motivated by different reinforcers.

Most positive reinforcers can be classified into five categories: consumable, activity, manipulative, possessional, and social.

- *Consumable reinforcers* are delicious edibles, such as candy, cookies, or gourmet meals.
- *Activity reinforcers* are opportunities to do something enjoyable, such as watching TV or going on vacation.
- *Manipulative reinforcers* are incentives, such as getting a lower rent in exchange for mowing the lawn or the promise of a better grade for doing an extra-credit project.
- *Possessional reinforcers* are tangible rewards, such as a new TV or a sports car.
- *Social reinforcers* are signs of appreciation, approval, or love, such as loving looks, affectionate hugs, and praise.

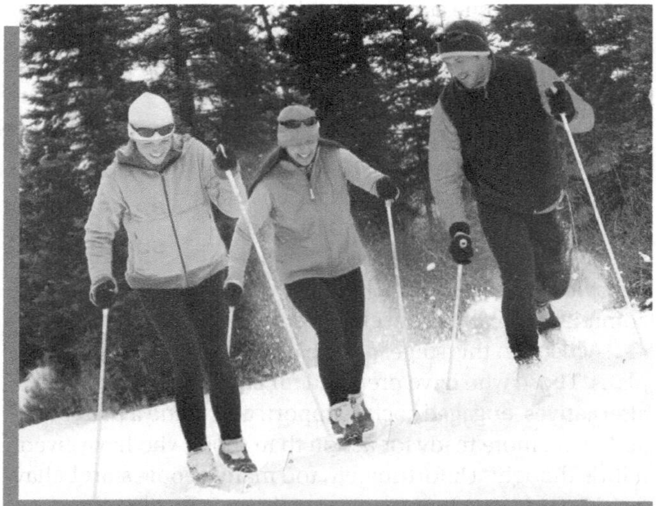
Mitchel Gray/Jupiter Images

What can I do to change an unhealthy habit?

Many people find it easiest to change an unhealthy habit by making small incremental changes, working toward a goal, and rewarding themselves along the way. The people in your life can help you change by modeling healthy behaviors, supporting your efforts to change, and offering reinforcement.

When choosing reinforcers, determine what would motivate you to act in a particular way. Research has shown that people can be motivated to change their behaviors, such as not smoking during pregnancy or abstaining from cocaine, if they set up a token economy system whereby they earn tokens or points that can be exchanged for meaningful rewards, such as money.[22] The difficulty often lies in determining which incentive will be most effective. Your reinforcers may initially come from others (extrinsic rewards), but as you see positive changes in yourself, you will begin to reward and reinforce yourself (intrinsic rewards). Although reinforcers should immediately follow a behavior, beware of overkill. If you reward yourself with a movie every time you go jogging, this reinforcer will soon lose its power. It would be better to give yourself this reward after, say, a full week of adhering to your jogging program.

what do you think?

What type of reinforcers would most likely get you to change a behavior? Money? Praise or recognition from someone in particular? ● Why would you find this reinforcer motivating? ● Can you think of some healthy options for reinforcing your own behavior changes?

Changing Self-Talk

Self-talk, the way you think and talk to yourself, can also play a role in modifying health-related behaviors. Self-talk can reflect your feelings of self-efficacy, discussed earlier in this chapter. When we don't feel self-efficacious, it's tempting to engage in negative self-talk, which can sabotage our

CONSUMER HEALTH

Surfing for the Latest in Health

The Internet can be a wonderful resource for rapid answers: 72 percent of college students obtain health information from the Web. However, the Web can also be a source of much *misinformation.* If you're not careful, you could end up feeling frazzled, confused, and—worst of all—misinformed. To ensure that the sites you visit are reliable and trustworthy, follow these tips:

* Look for websites sponsored by an official government agency, a university or college, or a hospital/medical center. These typically offer accurate, up-to-date information about a wide range of health topics. Government sites are easily identified by their *.gov* extensions (for example, the National Institute of Mental Health's website is www.nimh.nih.gov); college and university sites typically have *.edu* extensions (e.g., Johns Hopkins University's website is www.jhu.edu). Hospitals often have a *.org* extension (e.g., the Mayo Clinic's website is www.mayoclinic.org). Major philanthropic foundations, such as the Robert Wood Johnson Foundation, the Legacy Foundation, the Kellogg Foundation, and others, often provide information about selected health topics. In addition, national nonprofit organizations, such as the American Heart Association and the American Cancer Society, are often good, authoritative sources of information. Foundations and nonprofits usually have URLs ending with a .org extension.
* Search for well-established, professionally peer-reviewed journals such as the *New England Journal of Medicine* (http://content.nejm.org) or the *Journal of the American Medical Association (JAMA;* http://jama.ama-assn.org). Although some of these sites require a fee for access, you can often locate concise abstracts and information, such as a weekly table of contents, that can help you conduct a search. Other times, you can pay a basic fee for a certain number of hours of unlimited searching. Your college may have Internet access to these journals that they make available to students for no cost.
* Consult the Centers for Disease Control and Prevention (www.cdc.gov) for consumer news, updates, and alerts.
* For a global perspective on health issues, visit the World Health Organization (www.who.int/en).
* There are many government- and education-based sites that are independently sponsored and reliable. The following is just a sample. We'll provide more in each chapter as we cover specific topics:

1. Aetna Intelihealth: www.intelihealth.com
2. FamilyDoctor.org http://familydoctor.org
3. MedlinePlus: www.nlm.nih.gov/medlineplus
4. Go Ask Alice!: www.goaskalice.columbia.edu
5. WebMD health: http://my.webmd.com

* The nonprofit health care accrediting organization URAC (www.urac.org) has devised over 50 criteria that health sites must satisfy to display its seal. Look for the "URAC Accredited Health Web Site" seal on websites you visit. In addition to policing the accuracy of health claims, URAC evaluates health information and provides a forum for reporting misinformation, privacy violations, and other complaints.
* And, finally, don't believe everything you read. Cross-check information against reliable sources to see whether facts and figures are consistent. Be especially wary of websites that try to sell you something. Just because a source claims to be a physician or an expert does not mean that this is true. When in doubt, check with your own health care provider, health education professor, or state health division website.

best intentions. Here are some strategies for changing self-talk.

Rational-Emotive Therapy Rational-emotive therapy, a form of cognitive therapy or self-directed behavior change, is based on the premise that there is a close connection between what people say to themselves and how they feel. According to psychologist Albert Ellis, most emotional problems and related behaviors stem from irrational statements that people make to themselves when events in their lives are different from what they would like them to be.[23]

For example, suppose that after doing poorly on a test, you say to yourself, "I can't believe I flunked that easy exam. I'm so stupid." By changing this irrational, "catastrophic" self-talk into rational, positive statements about what is really going on, you increase the likelihood that you will make a positive behavior change. Positive self-talk might be phrased as follows: "I really didn't study enough for that exam, and I'm not surprised I didn't do well. I'm certainly not stupid. I just need to prepare better for the next test." Such self-talk will help you to recover quickly and take positive steps to correct the situation.

Blocking/Thought Stopping By purposefully blocking or stopping negative thoughts, a person can concentrate on taking positive steps toward behavior change. For example, suppose you are preoccupied with your ex-partner, who has recently deserted you for someone else. You consciously stop thinking about the situation and force yourself to think about something more pleasant (perhaps dinner tomorrow with your best friend). By refusing to dwell on negative images and forcing yourself to focus elsewhere, you can avoid wasting energy, time, and emotional resources and move on to positive change.

Planning Behavior Change

Before you begin the process of behavior change, take stock of the factors that have made you maintain the current behavior. Assessing the causes of your existing behaviors will help you determine where you need to make changes.

Self-Assessment: Antecedents and Consequences

Behaviors, thoughts, and feelings always occur in a context, that is, in a situation. Situations can be divided into two components: the events that come before and those that come after. *Antecedents* are the setting events for a behavior; they stimulate a person to act in certain ways. Antecedents can be physical events, thoughts, emotions, or the actions of other people. *Consequences*—the results of behavior—affect whether a person will repeat that action. Consequences also can consist of physical events, thoughts, emotions, or the actions of other people.

Suppose you are shy and must give a speech in front of a large class. The antecedents include walking into the class, feeling frightened, wondering whether you are capable of doing a good job, and being unable to remember a word of your speech. If the consequences are negative—if your classmates laugh or you get a low grade—your terror about speaking in public will be reinforced, and you will continue to dread this kind of event. In contrast, if you receive positive feedback from the class or instructor, you may actually learn to like speaking in public.

Learning to recognize the antecedents of a behavior and acting to modify them is one method of changing behavior. A diary noting your undesirable behaviors and identifying the settings in which they occur can be a useful tool.

Self-Assessment: Analyzing Personal Behavior

Successful behavior change requires determining what you want to change. All too often we berate ourselves by using generalities: "I'm lousy to my friends; I need to be a better person." Determining the specific behavior you would like to modify—in contrast to the general problem—will allow you to set clear goals. What are you doing that makes you a lousy friend? Are you gossiping or lying about your friends? Have you been a taker rather than a giver? Or are you really a good friend most of the time?

Let's say the problem is gossiping. You can analyze this behavior by examining the following components.

- **Frequency.** How often do you gossip—all the time or only once in a while?
- **Duration.** How long have you been doing this?
- **Seriousness.** Is your gossiping just idle chatter, or are you really trying to injure other people? What are the consequences for you? For your friends? For your relationships?
- **Basis for problem behavior.** Is your gossip based on facts, perceptions of facts, or deliberate embellishment of the truth?
- **Antecedents.** What kinds of situations trigger your gossiping? Do some settings or people bring it out in you more than others do? What triggers your feelings of dislike or irritation toward your friends? Why are you talking behind their backs?

Once you assess your actions and determine what motivates you, consider what you can do to change your behavior.

Setting Realistic Goals

Changing behavior is not easy, but sometimes we make it even harder by setting unrealistic and unattainable goals. To start making positive changes, ask yourself these questions:

1. **What do I want?** What is your ultimate goal—to lose weight? Exercise more? Reduce stress? Have a lasting relationship? Whatever it is, you need a clear picture of the target outcome.
2. **Which change is the greatest priority at this time?** Often people decide to change several things all at once. Suppose that you are gaining unwanted weight. Rather than saying, "I need to eat less, start jogging, and really get in shape," be specific about the current behavior you need to change. Are you eating too many sweets? Too many high-fat foods? Perhaps a realistic goal would be to try to eat less fat during dinner every day. Choose the behavior that constitutes your greatest problem, and tackle that first. You can always work on something else later. Take small steps, experiment with alternatives, and find the best way to meet your goals.
3. **Why is this important to me?** Think through why you want to change. Are you doing it because of your health? To look better? To win someone else's approval? Usually, doing something because it's right for you rather than to win others' approval is a sound strategy. If you are changing for someone else, what happens when that other person isn't around?
4. **What are the potential positive outcomes?** What do you hope to accomplish?
5. **What health-promoting programs and services can help me get started?** Nearly all campuses offer helpful resources. You might buy a self-help book at the campus bookstore, speak to a counselor, or enroll in an aerobics class at the local fitness center.

what do you think?

Do you think goal-setting is a useful strategy for behavior change? ● Can you think of a goal you've recently set that you did not accomplish? Why was this the case? ● What can you do in the future to help you achieve your goals?

6. Are there family or friends whose help I can enlist? Social support is one of your most powerful allies. Getting a friend to exercise with you, asking your partner to help you stop smoking by quitting at the same time you do, and making a commitment with a friend to never let each other drive if you've been drinking alcohol—these are all examples of how people can help each other make positive changes.

Decision Making: Choices for Change

Now it is time to make a decision that will lead to positive health outcomes. Try anticipating what might occur in a given setting and think through all possible safe alternatives.

For example, suppose you know you will likely be offered a drink at parties. What response would be okay in your social group? If someone is flirting with you and the situation takes on a distinct sexual overtone, how can you prevent the situation from turning unpleasant for you? Advance preparation will help you stick to your behavior plan.

Fill out the Behavior Change Contract at the beginning of this text to help you set a goal, anticipate obstacles, and create strategies to overcome those obstacles. Figure 7 shows an example of a completed contract. Remember that things typically don't "just happen." Making a commitment by completing a contract helps you stay alert to potential problems, to be aware of your alternatives, to maintain a good sense of your values, and to stick to your beliefs under pressure.

Behavior Change Contract

My behavior change will be:
To snack less on junk food and more on healthy foods.

My long-term goal for this behavior change is:
Eat junk food snacks no more than once a week.

These are three obstacles to change (things that I am currently doing or situations that contribute to this behavior or make it harder to change):

1. The grocery store is closed by the time I come home from school.
2. I get hungry between classes, and the vending machines only carry candy bars.
3. It's easier to order pizza or other snacks than to make a snack at home.

The strategies I will use to overcome these obstacles are:

1. I'll leave early for school once a week so I can stock up on healthy snacks in the morning.
2. I'll bring a piece of fruit or other healthy snack to eat between classes.
3. I'll learn some easy recipes for snacks to make at home.

Resources I will use to help me change this behavior include:
a friend/partner/relative: my roommates: I'll ask them to buy healthier snacks instead of chips when they do the shopping.
a school-based resource: The dining hall: I'll ask the manager to provide healthy foods we can take to eat between classes.
a community-based resource: The library: I'll check out some cookbooks to find easy snack ideas
a book or reputable website: The USDA nutrient database at www.ars.usda.gov: I'll use this site to make sure the foods I select are healthy choices.

In order to make my goal more attainable, I have devised these short-term goals:
short-term goal Eat a healthy snack 3 times per week target date September 15 reward new CD
short-term goal Learn to make a healthy snack target date October 15 reward concert tickets
short-term goal Eat a healthy snack 5 times per week target date November 15 reward new shoes

When I make the long-term behavior change described above, my reward will be:
ski lift tickets for winter break target date: December 15

I intend to make the behavior change described above. I will use the strategies and rewards to achieve the goals that will contribute to a healthy behavior change.

Signed: Elizabeth King Witness: Susan Bauer

FIGURE 7 **Example of a Completed Behavior Change Contract**

Assess yourself

How Healthy Are You?

PEARSON myhealthlab

Fill out this assessment online at www.pearsonhighered.com/myhealthlab or www.pearsonhighered.com/donatelle.

Jacob Wackerhausen/iStockphoto

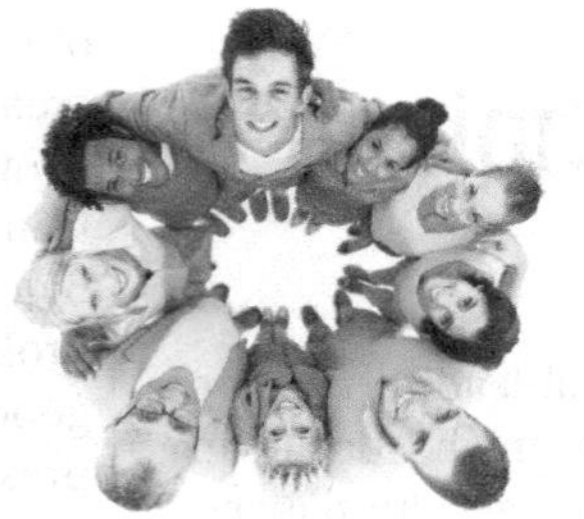

Although we all recognize the importance of being healthy, it can be a challenge to sort out which behaviors are most likely to cause problems or which ones pose the greatest risk. *Before* you decide where to start, it is important to look at your current health status.

By completing the following assessment, you will have a clearer picture of health areas in which you excel and those that could use some work. Taking this assessment will also help you to reflect on components of health that you may not have thought about.

Answer each question, then total your score for each section and fill it in on the Personal Checklist at the end of the assessment for a general sense of your health profile. Think about the behaviors that influenced your score in each category. Would you like to change any of them? Choose the area that you'd like to improve, then complete the Behavior Change Contract at the front of your text. Use the contract to think through and implement a behavior change over the course of this class.

Each of the categories in this questionnaire is an important aspect of the total dimensions of health, but this is not a substitute for the advice of a qualified health care provider. Consider scheduling a thorough physical examination by a licensed physician or setting up an appointment with a mental health counselor at your school if you need help making a behavior change.

For each of the following, indicate how often you think the statements describe you.

1 Physical Health

	Never	Rarely	Some of the Time	Usually or Always
1. I am happy with my body size and weight.	1	2	3	4
2. I engage in vigorous exercises such as brisk walking, jogging, swimming, or running for at least 30 minutes per day, three to four times per week.	1	2	3	4
3. I get at least 7 to 8 hours of sleep each night.	1	2	3	4
4. My immune system is strong, and my body heals itself quickly when I get sick or injured.	1	2	3	4
5. I listen to my body; when there is something wrong, I try to make adjustments to heal it or seek professional advice.	1	2	3	4

Total score for this section: ___________

2 Social Health

	Never	Rarely	Some of the Time	Usually or Always
1. I am open, honest, and get along well with others.	1	2	3	4
2. I participate in a wide variety of social activities and enjoy being with people who are different from me.	1	2	3	4
3. I try to be a "better person" and decrease behaviors that have caused problems in my interactions with others.	1	2	3	4
4. I am open and accessible to a loving and responsible relationship.	1	2	3	4
5. I try to see the good in my friends and do whatever I can to support them and help them feel good about themselves.	1	2	3	4

Total score for this section: ___________

3 Emotional Health

	Never	Rarely	Some of the Time	Usually or Always
1. I find it easy to laugh, cry, and show emotions like love, fear, and anger, and try to express these in positive, constructive ways.	1	2	3	4
2. I avoid using alcohol or other drugs as a means of helping me forget my problems.	1	2	3	4
3. I recognize when I am stressed and take steps to relax through exercise, quiet time, or other calming activities.	1	2	3	4
4. I try not to be too critical or judgmental of others and try to understand differences or quirks that I note in others.	1	2	3	4
5. I am flexible and adapt or adjust to change in a positive way.	1	2	3	4

Total score for this section: ___________

4 Environmental Health

	Never	Rarely	Some of the Time	Usually or Always
1. I buy recycled paper and purchase biodegradable detergents and cleaning agents, or make my own cleaning products, whenever possible.	1	2	3	4
2. I recycle paper, plastic, and metals; purchase refillable containers when possible; and try to minimize the amount of paper and plastics that I use.	1	2	3	4
3. I try to wear my clothes for longer periods between washing to reduce water consumption and the amount of detergents in our water sources.	1	2	3	4
4. I vote for proenvironment candidates in elections.	1	2	3	4
5. I minimize the amount of time that I run the faucet when I brush my teeth, shave, or shower.	1	2	3	4

Total score for this section: ___________

5 Spiritual Health

	Never	Rarely	Some of the Time	Usually or Always
1. I take time alone to think about what's important in life—who I am, what I value, where I fit in, and where I'm going.	1	2	3	4
2. I have faith in a greater power, be it a supreme being, nature, or the connectedness of all living things.	1	2	3	4
3. I engage in acts of caring and goodwill without expecting something in return.	1	2	3	4
4. I sympathize/empathize with those who are suffering and try to help them through difficult times.	1	2	3	4
5. I go for the gusto and experience life to the fullest.	1	2	3	4

Total score for this section: ___________

6 Intellectual Health

	Never	Rarely	Some of the Time	Usually or Always
1. I carefully consider my options and possible consequences as I make choices in life.	1	2	3	4
2. I learn from my mistakes and try to act differently the next time.	1	2	3	4
3. I have at least one hobby, learning activity, or personal growth activity that I make time for each week, something that improves me as a person.	1	2	3	4
4. I manage my time well rather than let time manage me.	1	2	3	4
5. My friends and family trust my judgment.	1	2	3	4

Total score for this section: ___________

Although each of these six aspects of health is important, there are some factors that don't readily fit in one category. As college students, you face some unique risks that others may not have. For this reason, we have added a section to this self-assessment that focuses on personal health promotion and disease prevention. Answer these questions and add your results to the Personal Checklist in the following section.

7 Personal Health Promotion/ Disease Prevention

	Never	Rarely	Some of the Time	Usually or Always
1. If I were to be sexually active, I would use protection such as latex condoms, dental dams, and other means of reducing my risk of sexually transmitted infections.	1	2	3	4
2. I can have a good time at parties or during happy hours without binge drinking.	1	2	3	4
3. I have eaten too much in the last month and have forced myself to vomit to avoid gaining weight.	4	3	2	1
4. If I were to get a tattoo or piercing, I would go to a reputable person who follows strict standards of sterilization and precautions against bloodborne disease transmission.	1	2	3	4
5. I engage in extreme sports and find that I enjoy the highs that come with risking bodily harm through physical performance.	4	3	2	1

Total score for this section: ___________

Personal Checklist

Now, total your scores for each section on the next page and compare them to what would be considered optimal scores. Are you surprised by your scores in any areas? Which areas do you need to work on?

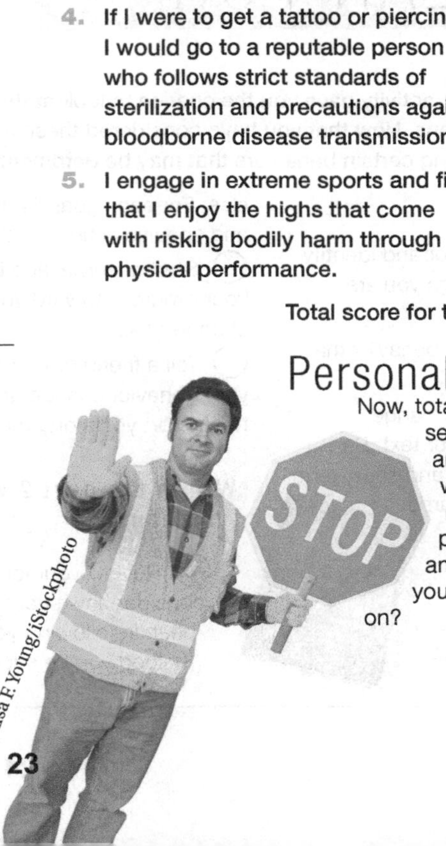

Lisa F. Young/iStockphoto

	Ideal Score	Your Score
Physical health	20	______
Social health	20	______
Emotional health	20	______
Environmental health	20	______
Spiritual health	20	______
Intellectual health	20	______
Personal health promotion/ disease prevention	20	______

What Your Scores in Each Category Mean

Scores of 15–20:

Outstanding! Your answers show that you are aware of the importance of these behaviors in your overall health. More important, you are putting your knowledge to work by practicing good health habits that should reduce your overall risks. Although you received a very high score on this part of the test, you may want to consider areas where your scores could be improved.

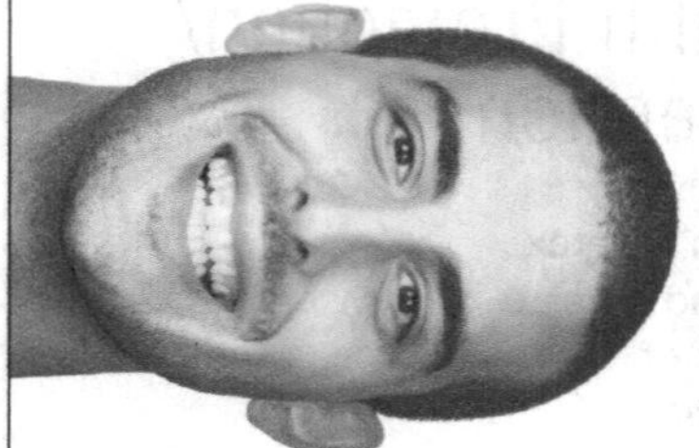

Boris Yankov/iStockphoto

Scores of 10–14:

Your health risks are showing! Find information about the risks you are facing and why it is important to change these behaviors. Perhaps you need help in deciding how to make the changes you desire. Assistance is available from this text, your professor, and student health services at your school.

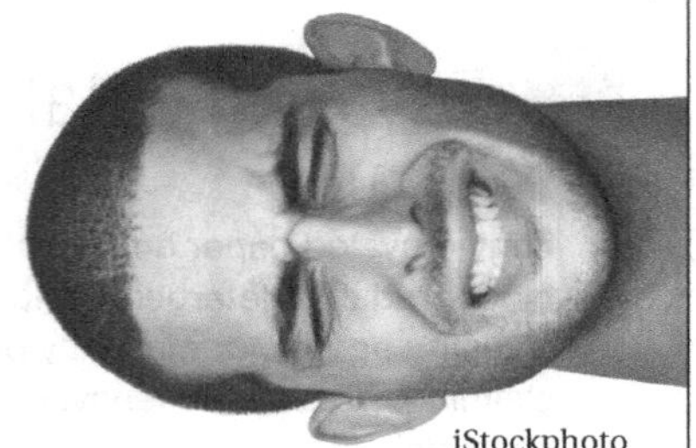

iStockphoto

Scores below 10:

You may be taking unnecessary risks with your health. Perhaps you are not aware of the risks and what to do about them. Identify each risk area and make a mental note as you read the associated chapter in the text. Whenever possible, seek additional resources, either on your campus or through your local community health resources, and make a serious commitment to behavior change. If any area is causing you to be less than functional in your class work or personal life, seek professional help. In this text you will find the information you need to help you improve your scores and your health. Remember that these scores are only indicators, not diagnostic tools.

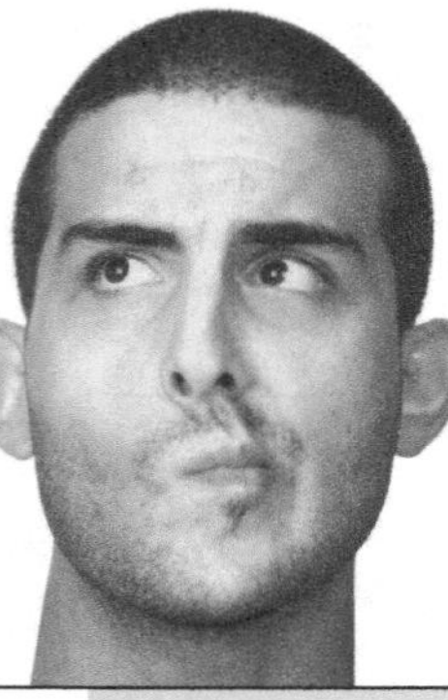

Boris Yankov/iStockphoto

YOUR PLAN FOR CHANGE

The Assess yourself activity gave you the chance to look at the status of your health in several dimensions. Now that you have considered these results, you can take steps toward changing certain behaviors that may be detrimental to your health.

Today, you can:

- ◯ Evaluate your behavior and identify patterns and specific things you are doing.
- ◯ Select one pattern of behavior that you want to change.
- ◯ Fill out the Behavior Change Contract at the front of your text. Be sure to include your long- and short-term goals for change, the rewards you'll give yourself for reaching these goals, the potential obstacles along the way, and the strategies for overcoming these obstacles. For each goal, list the small steps and specific actions that you will take.
- ◯ Start a journal and begin charting your progress toward your behavior change goal.
- ◯ Tell a friend or family member about your behavior change goal, and ask them to support you along the way.

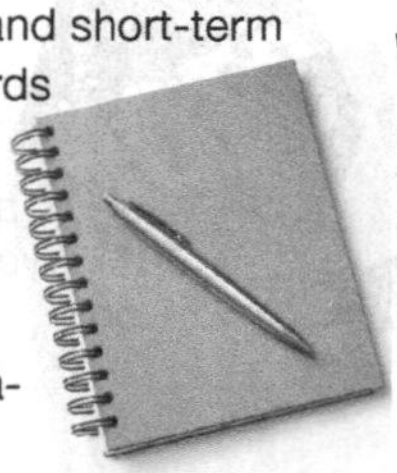

Within the next 2 weeks, you can:

- ◯ Review your journal entries and consider how successful you have been in following your plan. What helped you be successful? What made change more difficult? What will you do differently next week?
- ◯ Revise your plan as needed: Are the short-term goals attainable? Are the rewards satisfying?
- ◯ Practice safer sex.
- ◯ Maintain healthy eating habits and manage your weight.
- ◯ Control real and imaginary stressors.
- ◯ Maintain meaningful relationships with family and friends.

By the end of the semester, you can:

- ◯ Schedule a regular self-exam.
- ◯ Understand the health care system.
- ◯ Value each day and make the best of opportunities.

Summary

* Health encompasses the entire dynamic process of fulfilling one's potential in the physical, social, emotional, spiritual, intellectual, and environmental dimensions of life. Wellness means achieving the highest level of health possible in several dimensions.
* Although the average American life span has increased over the past century, we also need to increase the quality of life. Programs such as *Healthy People 2010* have established national objectives for achieving longer life and quality of life for all Americans through health promotion and disease prevention.
* Health disparities contribute to increased disease risks. Factors such as gender, race, and socioeconomic status continue to play a major role in health status and care. Women have longer lives but have more medical problems than do men. To close the gender gap in health care, researchers have begun to include more women in medical research and training.
* For the U.S. population as a whole, the leading causes of death are heart disease, cancer, and stroke. In the 15- to 24-year-old age group, the leading causes are unintentional injuries, homicide, and suicide. Many of the risks associated with cancer, heart disease, and stroke can be reduced through lifestyle changes. Many of the risks associated with accidents, homicide, and suicide can be reduced through preventive measures, particularly reductions in the use of alcohol and other drugs.
* Several factors contribute to a person's health status, and a number of them are within our control. Beliefs and attitudes, self-efficacy, locus of control, intentions to change, support from significant others, and readiness to change are factors over which individuals have some degree of control. Access to health care, genetic predisposition, health policies that support positive choices, and other factors are all potential reinforcing, predisposing, and enabling factors that may influence health decisions.
* Behavior-change techniques, such as shaping, visualization, modeling, controlling the situation, reinforcement, changing self-talk, and problem solving help people succeed in making behavior changes.
* Decision making has several key components. Each person must explore his or her own problems, the reasons for change, and the expected outcomes. The next step is to plan a course of action best suited to individual needs and fill out a Behavior Change Contract.

Pop Quiz

1. Our ability to perform everyday tasks, such as walking up the stairs or tying your shoes, is an example of
   a. improved quality of life.
   b. physical health.
   c. health promotion.
   d. activities of daily living.

2. Janice describes herself as confident and trusting, and she displays both high self-esteem and high self-efficacy. The dimension of health this relates to is the
   a. social dimension.
   b. emotional dimension.
   c. spiritual dimension.
   d. intellectual dimension.

3. What statistic is used to describe the number of new cases of AIDS in a given year?
   a. morbidity
   b. mortality
   c. incidence
   d. prevalence

4. Because Craig's parents smoked, he is 90 percent more likely to start smoking than someone whose parents didn't. This is an example of what factor influencing behavior change?
   a. circumstantial factor
   b. enabling factor
   c. reinforcing factor
   d. predisposing factor

5. Which of the following is likely to be a reinforcing factor in your efforts at healthy behavior change?
   a. Your friend tells you how great it is that you're sticking to your exercise plan and offers to take you to the movies if you keep it up.
   b. Your parents buy you a gym membership as it's too cold for you to exercise outdoors.
   c. Your parents tell you not to worry about a few extra pounds, because you're "big boned."
   d. Your friends agree not to allow you to "bum" cigarettes when you're at a party.

6. Suppose you want to lose 20 pounds. To reach your goal, you take small steps. You start by joining a support group and counting calories. After 2 weeks, you begin an exercise program and gradually build up to your desired fitness level. What behavior change strategy are you using?
   a. shaping
   b. visualization
   c. modeling
   d. reinforcement

7. After Kirk and Tammy pay their bills, they reward themselves by watching TV together. The type of positive reinforcement that motivates them to pay their bills is
   a. activity reinforcer.
   b. consumable reinforcer.
   c. manipulative reinforcer.
   d. possessional reinforcer.

8. The setting events for a behavior that cue or stimulate a person to act in certain ways are called
   a. antecedents.
   b. frequency of events.
   c. consequences.
   d. cues to action.

9. What strategy for change is advised for an individual in the preparation stage of change?
   a. seeking out recommended readings
   b. finding creative ways to maintain positive behaviors
   c. setting realistic goals
   d. publicly stating the desire for change

10. Spiritual health is
   a. exclusive to religiosity.
   b. optional for achieving wellness.
   c. related to one's purpose in life.
   d. finding fulfilling relationships.

Answers to Chapter Review Questions

1. d; 2. b; 3. c; 4. d; 5. a; 6. a; 7. a; 8. a; 9. a; 10. c

Think about It!

1. How are the terms *health* and *wellness* similar? What, if any, are important distinctions between these terms? What is health promotion? Disease prevention?
2. How healthy is the U.S. population today? Are we doing better or worse in terms of health status than we have done previously? What factors influence today's disparities in health?
3. What are some of the major differences in the way men and women are treated in the health care system? Why do you think these differences exist? How do race, sexual orientation, religion, marital status, and age affect how people are treated in the health care system?
4. What is the Health Belief Model? How may this model be working when a young woman decides to smoke her first cigarette? Her last cigarette?
5. Explain the predisposing, reinforcing, and enabling factors that might influence a young mother who is dependent on welfare as she decides whether to sell drugs to support her children.
6. Using the Stages of Change model, discuss what you might do (in stages) to help a friend stop smoking. Why is it important that a person be ready to change before trying to change?

Accessing Your Health on the Internet

The following websites explore further topics and issues related to personal health. For links to the websites below, visit the Companion Website for *Health: The Basics*, Green Edition at www.pearsonhighered.com/donatelle.

1. *CDC Wonder.* Clearinghouse for comprehensive information from the Centers for Disease Control and Prevention (CDC), including special reports, guidelines, and access to national health data. http://wonder.cdc.gov
2. *MayoClinic.com.* Reputable resource for specific information about health topics, diseases, and treatment options provided by the staff of the Mayo Clinic. Easy to navigate and consumer friendly. www.mayoclinic.com
3. *National Center for Health Statistics.* Outstanding place to start for information about health status in the United States. Links to key documents such as *Health, United States* (published yearly); national survey information; and information on mortality by age, race, gender, geographic location, and other important data. Includes comprehensive information provided by the CDC, as well as easy links to at least ten of the major health resources currently being used for policy and decision making about health in the United States. www.cdc.gov/nchs
4. *National Health Information Center.* Excellent resource for consumer information about health. www.health.gov/nhic
5. *World Health Organization.* Excellent resource for global health information. Provides information on the current state of health around the world, such as illness and disease statistics, trends, and illness outbreak alerts. www.who.int/en

References

1. National Center for Health Statistics, *Health, United States, 2008, with Chartbook on Trends in the Health of Americans* (Hyattsville, MD: National Center for Health Statistics, 2009).
2. Central Intelligence Agency, "Rank Order: Life Expectancy at Birth," in *The World Fact Book* (Washington, DC: CIA, 2009); National Center for Health Statistics, *Health, United States, 2007;* R. Dubos, *So Human an Animal* (New York: Scribners, 1968), 15.
3. S. J. Olshansky et al., "A Potential Decline in Life Expectancy in the United States in the 21st Century," *New England Journal of Medicine* 352, no. 11 (March 17, 2005): 1138–45.
4. Ibid.
5. U.S. Department of Health and Human Services, Health Resources and Services Administration, *Women's Health USA 2008* (Rockville, Maryland: U.S. Department of Health and Human Services, 2008).
6. R. Dubos, *So Human an Animal,* 15.
7. K. Braithwaite, "Mending Our Broken Mental Health Systems," *American Journal of Public Health* 96, no. 10 (2006): 1724.
8. Centers for Disease Control and Prevention and the Merck Company Foundation, *The State of Aging and Health in America 2007* (Whitehouse Station, NJ: The Merck Company Foundation, 2007).
9. National Center for Health Statistics, "About *Healthy People 2010,*" www.cdc.gov/nchs.
10. Centers for Disease Control and Prevention, Office of Minority Health and Health Disparities, "Racial and Ethnic Populations," 2009, www.cdc.gov/omhd/Populations/populations.htm.
11. G. F. Kominski et al., *Language Barriers Pose a Risk for California HMO Enrollees* (Los Angeles: UCLA Center for Health Policy Research, May 2006); G. Glores, "Language Barriers in Health Care in the

United States," *New England Journal of Medicine* 355, no. 3 (2006): 229–331.

12. National Institutes of Health, *National Institutes of Health (NIH) Strategic Research Plan and Budget to Reduce and Ultimately Eliminate Health Disparities: Volume 1, Fiscal Years 2002–2006* (Bethesda, MD: National Institutes of Health, May 12, 2006).
13. A. Jemal et al., "Cancer Statistics," *A Cancer Journal for Clinicians* 55 (January/February 2005): 10–30; E. Ward, News Conference: American Cancer Society, ACS (January 19, 2005).
14. Centers for Disease Control and Prevention, "Chronic Disease Prevention and Health Promotion," www.cdc.gov/nccdphp. Updated April 8, 2009.
15. R. DeVol et al., *An Unhealthy America: The Economic Burden of Chronic Disease—Charting a New Course to Save Lives and Increase Productivity and Economic Growth* (Santa Monica, CA: The Milken Institute, 2007).
16. Centers for Disease Control and Prevention, *The Burden of Chronic Diseases and Their Risk Factors: National and State Perspectives, 2004* (Atlanta: U.S. Department of Health and Human Services, 2004).
17. M. Reeves and A. Rafferty, "Healthy Lifestyle Characteristics Among Adults in the United States," *Archives of Internal Medicine* 165, no. 8 (2005): 854–57.
18. I. Rosenstock, "Historical Origins of the Health Belief Model," *Health Education Monographs* 2, no. 4 (1974): 328–35.
19. J. M. Twenge, Z. Liqing, and C. Im, "It's Beyond My Control: A Cross-Temporal Meta-Analysis of Increasing Externality in Locus of Control, 1960–2002," *Personality and Social Psychology Review* 8 (2004): 308–20.
20. M. Hesse, "The Readiness Ruler as a Measure of Readiness to Change Polydrug Use in Drug Abusers," *Journal of Harm Reduction* 3, no. 3 (2006): 1477–81; M. Cismaru, "Using Protection Motivation Theory to Increase the Persuasiveness of Public Service Communications," The Saskatchewan Institute of Public Policy, Public Policy Series paper no. 40 (February 2006); A. Fallon et al., "Health Care Provider Advice for African American Adults Not Meeting Health Behavior Recommendations," *Preventing Chronic Disease* 3, no. 2 (2006): A45; M. R. Chacko et al., "New Sexual Partners and Readiness to Seek Screening for Chlamydia and Gonorrhea: Predictors among Minority Young Women," *Sexually Transmitted Infections* 82 (2006): 75–79.
21. J. O. Prochaska and C. C. DiClemente, "Stages and Processes of Self-Change of Smoking: Toward an Integrative Model of Change," *Journal of Consulting and Clinical Psychology* 51 (1983): 390–95.
22. R. J. Donatelle et al., "Using Incentives and the 5A's in Clinical Practice to Motivate Pregnant Smokers to Quit: The Maternal Intervention to Stop Smoking (MISS) Trial" (forthcoming); S. Higgins et al., "The Effects of Monetary Value of Voucher-Based Incentives on Abstinence in Cocaine Users," *Addiction* 102, no. 2 (2007): 271–81.
23. A. Ellis and M. Benard, *Clinical Application of Rational Emotive Therapy* (New York: Plenum, 1985).

Yuka Kisugi/allead/amana images/Getty Images

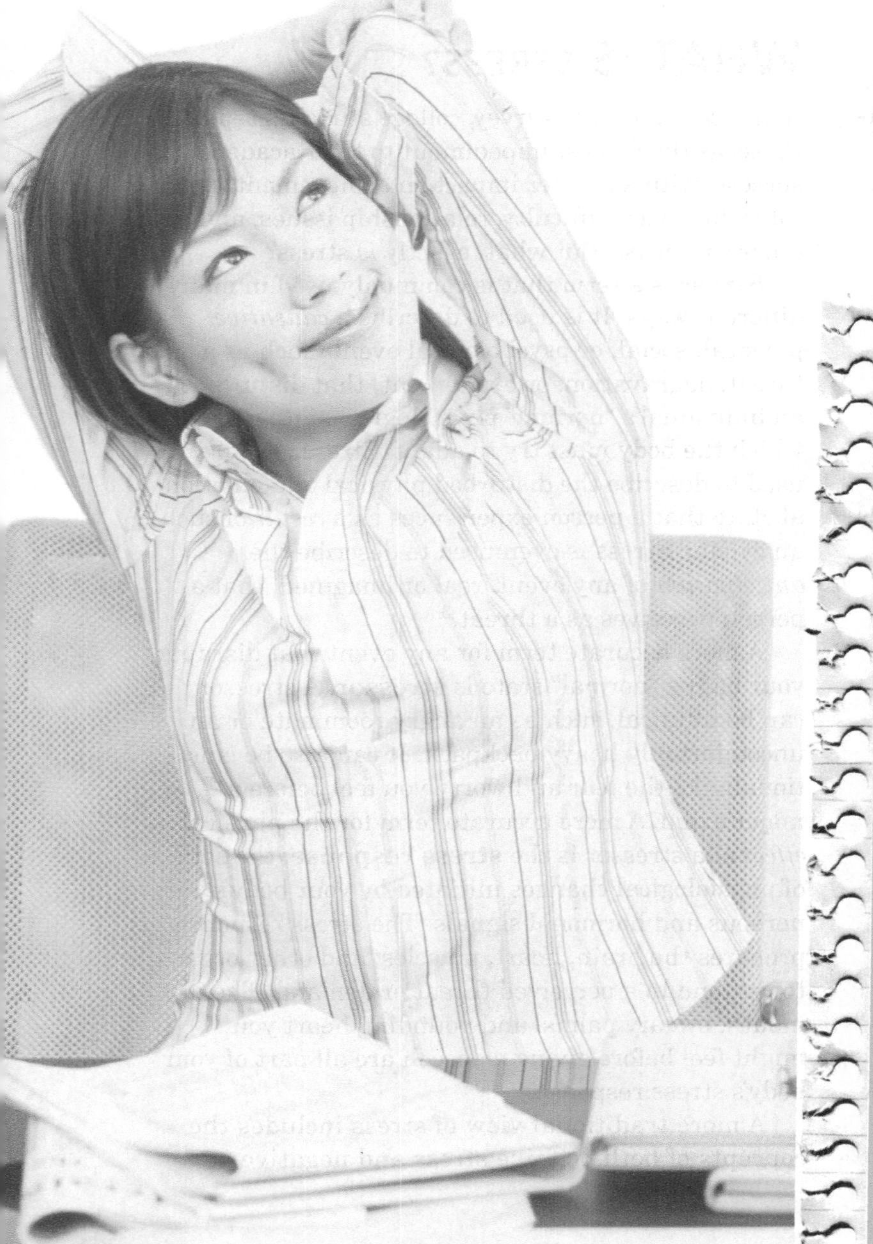

Managing Stress

OBJECTIVES

Understand how your body responds to stress.

Identify common sources of stress.

Describe effective tools for stress management.

Create your own stress management plan.

CASE STUDY

Cory

"Hi, I'm Cory. I'm a junior, majoring in biology. I'm from Denver, Colorado and just transferred schools in August to be closer to my dad, who lives alone and has diabetes. I take five classes, work part-time as a lab assistant, and I'm up late every night studying so that I can keep up my grades for applying to medical school. I've always felt like I was pretty good at working under pressure, but I have to admit, these past few months have been rough—I am constantly worn out, worried sick about my dad, and can hardly stay awake in class sometimes. I know that medical school will be even harder, so maybe I should just get used to living like this! But, man, I am so tired of being tired."

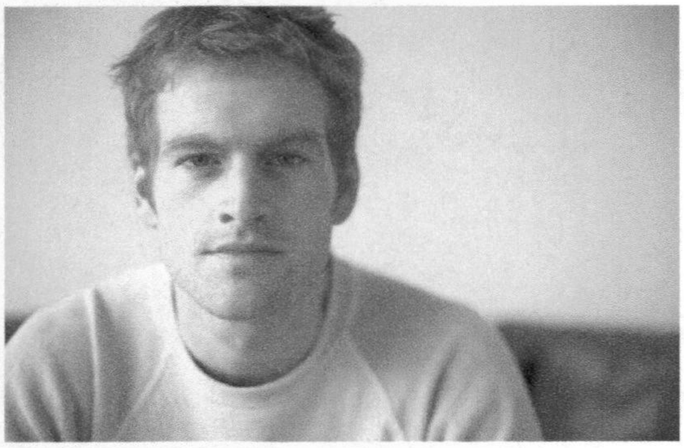

Larry Williams/Larry Williams and Associates/Corbis

Everyone feels stress at least some of the time, be it from traffic, crowding, competition for schools and jobs, fast-changing technology, and/or a hectic pace that seems to accelerate yearly. Often we do not even realize how great our stress levels have become. Over time, however, stress can diminish not just our enjoyment of life, but our health and well-being, too. Thus, learning effective stress-management techniques is an important part of any complete wellness program.

This chapter explains the stress response, details the ways accumulated stress can affect your health, and proposes several helpful strategies you can use to counteract stress. Using the stress-management tools you'll discover in this chapter, you can better face the pressures of college life and beyond.

stress A term used to describe a physical, social, or psychological event or circumstance that disturbs the body's "normal" state and to which the body must try to adapt. Also used to describe the disturbed physical or emotional state experienced as a result of such events/circumstances.

stressor A physical, social, or psychological event or circumstance to which the body tries to adapt; stressors are often threatening, unfamiliar, disturbing, or exciting

stress response A set of physical and emotional reactions initiated by your body in response to a stressor

WHAT IS STRESS?

In a recent national survey, college students reported stress as the biggest impediment to their academic success, with a greater impact on achievement than colds, flu, sleep difficulty, relationship issues, and all other concerns.[1] But what, exactly *is* stress?

Stress is a term that is commonly used in many different ways. It is used to describe a *causative* physical, social, or psychological event (such as a threat, aggravation, or excitement) that disturbs an individual's "normal" physiological state and to which the body must try to adapt. Stress is also used to describe the disturbed physical and emotional state that a person experiences as a *result* of such an event.[2] Stress is even used to describe the *anticipation* of any event, real or imagined, that a person perceives as a threat.[3]

A more accurate term for any event that disrupts your body's "normal" state is **stressor.** A stressor can be physical, such as an angry roommate or an uncomfortably heavy backpack. It can also be emotional, like the fear and worry you feel before a major exam. A more accurate term for the physical *effect* of a stressor is the **stress response:** the set of physiological changes initiated by your body's nervous and hormonal signals. The stress response prepares the brain, heart, muscles, and other organs to respond to a perceived threat or demand. The dry mouth, sweaty palms, and pounding heart you might feel before giving a speech are all part of your body's stress response.

A more traditional view of stress includes the concepts of both positive stress and negative stress. Positive stress, or **eustress,** presents an opportunity for personal growth, satisfaction, and enhanced well-being. Eustress can invigorate us and motivate us to work harder and achieve more. Entering college, starting a new job, and developing a new relationship are all challenges that can produce eustress. Negative stress, or **distress,** can result from a buildup of negative stressors such as academic pressures, relationship discord, or money problems. It can even result from an overload of positive stressors such as getting married, moving to a new state, and starting a new job all in the same week. Distress can reduce wellness by promoting cardiovascular disease, impairing immunity, or causing mental and emotional dysfunction.

HOW DOES YOUR BODY RESPOND TO STRESS?

You file into the lecture hall to take your hardest midterm, sit down in an aisle seat, and teaching assistants start passing out the exam papers. As you take one and pass the pile to your right, you realize your heart is pounding, your breathing has quickened, your hands are sweating, you have "butterflies" in your stomach, and you feel a sense of dread. You are experiencing a stress response: a reaction involving nervous and hormonal activities that prepare both body and mind to deal with the disturbance to your normal state.

THE STRESS RESPONSE

Here's a simplified version of what happens during the seconds that the body initiates a stress response and in the minutes and hours as the response continues (Figure 1):

1. Your senses perceive and your brain interprets something as a threat; for example, the arrival of a test that will determine half your grade.
2. The threat triggers a region of your brain called the *hypothalamus* to release a hormone that in turn triggers your pituitary gland to secrete **adrenocorticotropic hormone** (ACTH) into your blood.
3. ACTH travels through the bloodstream and reaches the outer zone of each adrenal gland (located on top of each kidney). ACTH causes the adrenal glands to secrete **cortisol,** your body's main stress hormone.

   At the same time, nerve signals from your brain and spinal cord reach and stimulate the central zone of each adrenal gland. Both adrenals respond by releasing **epinephrine** (also called *adrenalin*) and **norepinephrine,** two additional stress hormones that ready the body for quick action.
4. Traveling inside the bloodstream, cortisol reaches specific *target cells* within the body fat and within several organs, including the liver and intestines. Cortisol quickly triggers target cells to convert stored fat, protein, and carbohydrate molecules into glucose. Soon, more glucose is circulating in the blood, supplying the whole body—especially the brain and skeletal muscles—with the extra energy needed to respond to the stressor.
5. The epinephrine and norepinephrine released into the blood rapidly reach target cells in the heart, lungs, stomach, intestines, sense organs, and muscles. Along with signals from sympathetic nerves, these additional stress hormones ready the vital organs in ways that promote survival: fleeing from or confronting the threat. This physiological reaction is called the **fight-or-flight response.**

If you have ever jammed on the brakes to avoid an accident, you have probably felt a jolt of

eustress Stress based on positive circumstances or events; can present an opportunity for personal growth

distress Stress based on negative circumstances or events, or those perceived as negative; can diminish wellness

adrenocorticotropic hormone A hormone secreted by the pituitary gland that causes adrenal glands to secrete cortisol

cortisol Your body's main stress hormone, secreted by the cortex or outer layer of the adrenal glands located on top of the kidneys. Stimulates the sympathetic nervous system; can also damage or destroy neurons

epinephrine Also called *adrenaline;* one of two stress hormones released by adrenal glands that readies your body for quick action by stimulating sympathetic nerves

norepinephrine One of two stress hormones secreted by adrenal glands that readies your body for quick action by increasing arousal

fight-or-flight response A physiological reaction induced by nervous and hormonal signals that readies the heart, lungs, brain, muscles, and other vital organs and systems in ways that promote survival: fleeing from or confronting a threat

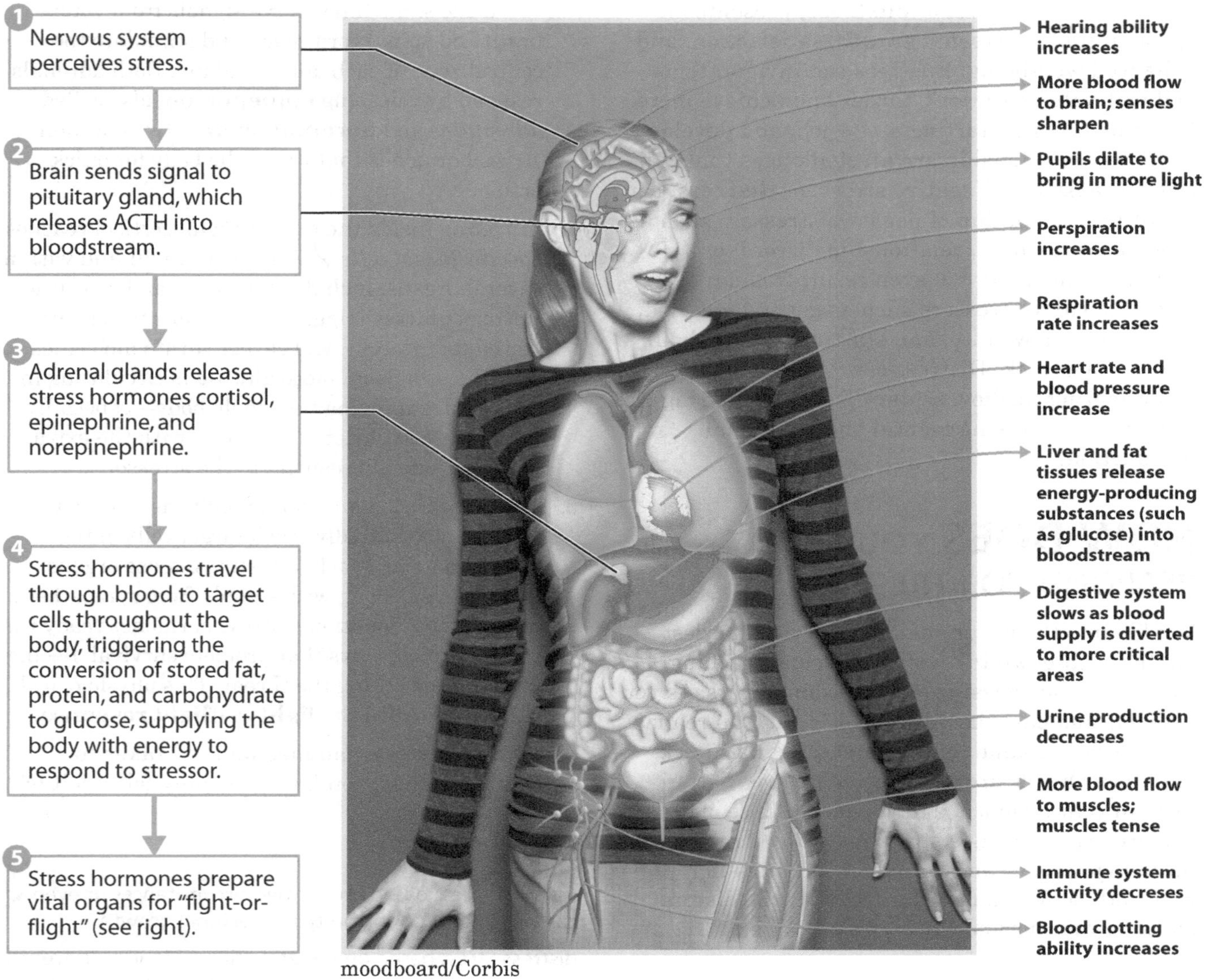
1 Nervous system perceives stress.
2 Brain sends signal to pituitary gland, which releases ACTH into bloodstream.
3 Adrenal glands release stress hormones cortisol, epinephrine, and norepinephrine.
4 Stress hormones travel through blood to target cells throughout the body, triggering the conversion of stored fat, protein, and carbohydrate to glucose, supplying the body with energy to respond to stressor.
5 Stress hormones prepare vital organs for "fight-or-flight" (see right).
Hearing ability increases
More blood flow to brain; senses sharpen
Pupils dilate to bring in more light
Perspiration increases
Respiration rate increases
Heart rate and blood pressure increase
Liver and fat tissues release energy-producing substances (such as glucose) into bloodstream
Digestive system slows as blood supply is diverted to more critical areas
Urine production decreases
More blood flow to muscles; muscles tense
Immune system activity decreses
Blood clotting ability increases
moodboard/Corbis

FIGURE 1
The stress response.

epinephrine. As part of the fight-or-flight response, your pupils dilate, enabling you to see more clearly. The air passages in your lungs also dilate, allowing more oxygen to enter. Your heart beats faster and pumps more blood to your muscles and brain. Your sweat glands release more sweat, and blood is directed away from your hands and feet toward your large muscles and body core; this can make your hands feel cold and clammy. Your digestive action slows or stops, and your bladder function slows, since neither process is crucial to short-term survival. Primed in all these ways, your body is ready to handle the stressor. Confronted by a car speeding toward you, your fight-or-flight response could save your life. Faced with financial hardship or excessive work pressures for years on end, your stress response can become chronic and start to harm your health.

After a perceived stressor subsides, your nervous system returns the body to its "normal" state with slower heartbeats, normal breathing rate, normal digestion, and so on. The stress-reduction techniques you will learn later deliberately encourage the body's return to this more relaxed state.

WHY DOES STRESS CAUSE HARM?

Why is chronic stress harmful? Two insightful models help explain how sustained stress can cause damage over time.

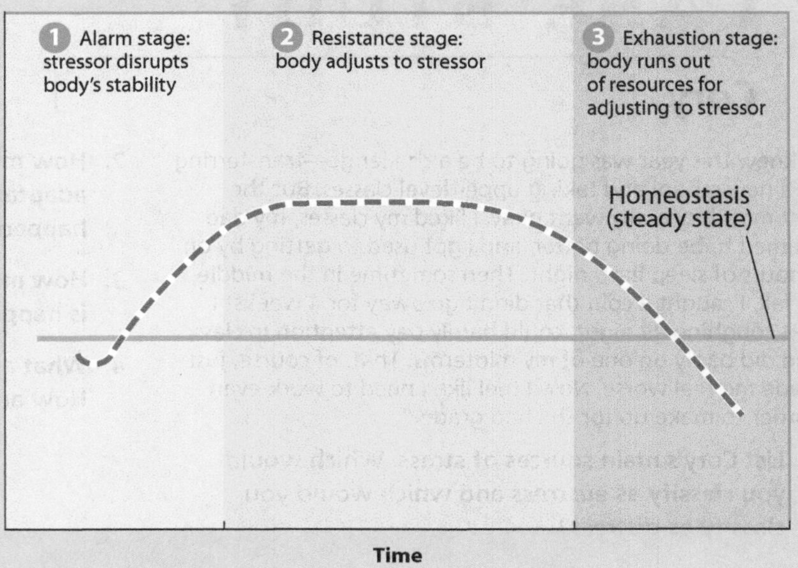

FIGURE 2
Hans Seyle's general adaptation syndrome.

THE GENERAL ADAPTATION SYNDROME

In the 1930s, biologist Hans Selye studied the response of laboratory rats to painful physical or emotional stressors. He discovered that a wide variety of stressors—such as extreme heat, extreme cold, forced exercise, or surgery—all seemed to provoke the same general set of changes in the rats' bodies. Selye proposed a model he called the **general adaptation syndrome (GAS),** based on the reactions of the rats he observed.

Central to Seyle's GAS model is the idea that stress disrupts the body's stable internal environment, or *steady state.* Physiological mechanisms work to keep internal conditions (such as body temperature, blood-oxygen content, blood pH, and blood sugar levels) within certain "normal" ranges. Life scientists use the term **homeostasis** to describe the body's steady state. Seyle's general adaptation syndrome characterizes the stages of the body's response to stress as follows:

1. In the *alarm stage,* a stressor disrupts the steady state and triggers a *fight-or-flight response.* The body starts adapting to the stressor, but the effort can lower one's resistance to injury or disease (see Figure 2).[4]
2. In the *resistance stage,* a person's physiology and behavior adjusts, and resistance builds to the stressor. The body establishes a new level of homeostasis, despite the continued presence of the stressor.
3. In the hypothetical *exhaustion stage,* the body runs out of resources to successfully adapt to the stressor, resulting in physiological harm in the form of reduced immunity and increased susceptibility to physical or mental illness.

The general adaptation syndrome recognized that sustained stress can take a toll on wellness. However, scientists have since modified Seyle's concept of an "exhaustion stage" and the idea that illness results from running out of resources to adapt to a stressor. Rather, they now believe that over time, the stress response *itself* can damage the body and increase one's risk of developing illness, as we will examine in the next section.

ALLOSTATIC LOAD

Today's stress researchers use the term **allostasis** to describe the many simultaneous changes that

general adaptation syndrome (GAS) A historical model proposed by Hans Selye attempting to explain the body's stress response, consisting of alarm, resistance, and exhaustion stages

homeostasis A state of physiological equilibrium wherein various physiological mechanisms maintain internal conditions (such as pH, salt concentration, and temperature) within certain viable ranges

allostasis The many simultaneous changes that occur in the body to maintain homeostasis

CASE STUDY

Cory

"I knew this year was going to be a challenge—transferring to a new school and taking upper-level classes. But the first month actually went okay. I liked my classes, my dad seemed to be doing better, and I got used to getting by on 5 hours of sleep each night. Then sometime in the middle of fall, I caught a cold that didn't go away for 4 weeks! I was coughing all night, could barely pay attention in class, and did badly on one of my midterms. That, of course, just made me feel worse. Now I feel like I need to work even harder to make up for the bad grade."

1. **List Cory's main sources of stress. Which would you classify as *eustress* and which would you classify as *distress*?**
2. **How might Hans Seyle have used general adaptation syndrome to explain what is happening with Cory?**
3. **How might the allostatic load model explain what is happening with Cory?**
4. **What are your own major sources of stress? How are you dealing with them?**

occur in the body to maintain homeostasis, and they use the term **allostatic load** to refer to the long-term wear and tear on the body that is caused by prolonged allostasis.[5]

Allostatic load can result if your body's ability to shut off the stress response (after a stressor has disappeared) is impaired, allowing high levels of stress hormones to remain in the bloodstream. It can also develop when your body releases too *few* stress hormones and cannot mount an adequate stress response.[6] And it can build up if you experience a sustained string of stressful events over a long period of time. A classic example of a consequence of allostatic load is the development of stress-induced high blood pressure (hypertension.) As you will see shortly, chronically high blood pressure can damage arteries and increase one's risk of developing cardiovascular disease.[7]

A person's behavior and choices can also result in allostatic load. For example, some people respond to stress by exercising more, meditating, getting extra sleep, and avoiding drugs and alcohol. Others respond by exercising less, staying up late, drinking more, or starting smoking or taking drugs. Such counterproductive measures can result in allostatic load and increase one's susceptibility to developing illness.

allostatic load The long-term wear and tear on the body that is caused by prolonged allostasis

WHAT KINDS OF HARM CAN STRESS CAUSE?

Studies indicate that 40 percent of deaths and 70 percent of disease in the United States are related, in whole or in part, to stress.[8] The list of ailments related to chronic stress includes heart disease, diabetes, cancer, headaches, ulcers, low back pain, depression, and the common cold.

STRESS AND CARDIOVASCULAR DISEASE RISKS

Perhaps the most studied and documented health consequence of unresolved stress is cardiovascular disease (CVD). Research on this topic has demonstrated the impact of chronic stress on heart rate, blood pressure, heart attack, and stroke.[9] Historically, the increased risk of CVD from chronic stress has been linked to increased plaque buildup due to elevated cholesterol, hardening of the arteries, alterations in heart rhythm, and increased and fluctuating blood pressure. Recent research also points to metabolic abnormalities, insulin resistance, and inflammation in blood vessels as major contributors to heart disease.[10] In the past 15 to 20 years, researchers have identified direct links between the incidence and progression of CVD and stressors such as job strain, caregiving, bereavement, and natural disasters.[11] Whatever the mechanism, the evidence is clear that stress is a significant contributor to CVD morbidity and mortality.

SPOTLIGHT

STRESS AND DEPRESSION

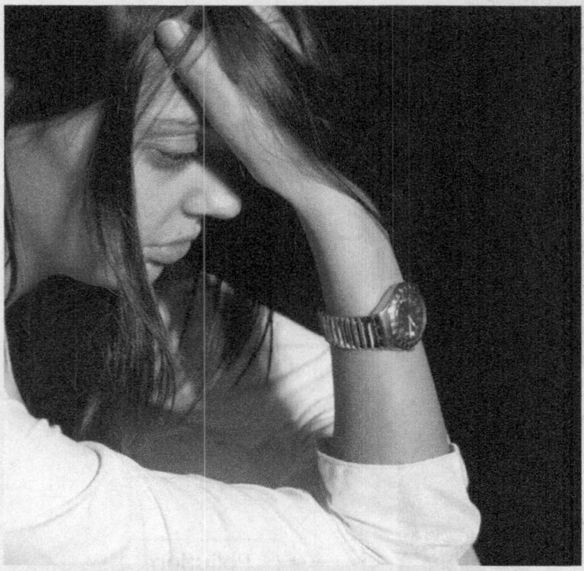

David De Lossy/Getty Images

Stress and depression have complicated interconnections based on emotional, physiological, and biochemical processes. Prolonged stress can trigger depression in susceptible people, and prior periods of depression can leave individuals more susceptible to stress.[1]

The *physical* links between stress and depression are strong. During the stress response, the body is flooded with cortisol and with chemicals called *cytokines.* These factors promote inflammation as part of the body's immune response. Researchers think that exposure to both kinds of chemicals can damage or kill neurons in a part of the brain called the *hippocampus* and can alter nerve transmission within the brain. One result of hippocampal damage is impaired learning and memory.[2] Another is the onset of depression symptoms in genetically susceptible individuals.[3] Research confirms that loss of hippocampal neurons is present in many who suffer depression.[4]

Realizing the important interconnections between stress and depression can help you take appropriate steps to handling one or both. Because stress and depression symptoms overlap, applying the stress-management techniques outlined in this chapter may help alleviate depression. If depression symptoms become severe enough to interfere with studying or other aspects of daily life, you should seek help. Potential sources are the student health service, the campus counseling center, a doctor or mental health professional in your community, and your local depression or suicide hotline.

Sources:

1. M. A. Ilgen and K. E. Hutchison, "A History of Major Depressive Disorder and the Response to Stress," *Journal of Affective Disorders* 86, no. 2–3 (June 2005): 143–50.
2. F. A. Scorza and others, "Neurogenesis and Depression: Etiology or New Illusion?" *Review of Brazilian Psychiatry* 27, no. 3 (September 2005): 249–53.
3. See reference 1.
4. Prentiss Price, "Stress and Depression," *All About Depression* (September 9, 2004). www.allaboutdepression.com; David G. Myers, *Psychology.* 5th ed. (New York: Worth Publishers, 1998).

STRESS AND THE IMMUNE SYSTEM

A growing area of scientific investigation known as **psychoneuroimmunology (PNI)** explores the intricate relationship between the mind's response to stress and the immune system's ability to function effectively. Research suggests that too much stress over a long period can negatively regulate various aspects of the cellular immune response.[12] Whereas a short-term stress response is usually protective, prolonged fight-or-flight depresses the immune system. During prolonged stress, elevated levels of adrenal hormones (like cortisol) destroy or reduce the ability of certain white blood cells, known as killer T cells, to aid the immune response. When killer T cells aren't working correctly, the body becomes more susceptible to illness.

STRESS AND THE MIND

Stress may be one of the single greatest contributors to mental disability and emotional dysfunction in industrialized nations. Studies have shown that the rates of mental disorders, particularly depression and anxiety, are associated with various environmental stressors, including divorce, marital conflict, and economic hardship (see **Spotlight: Stress and Depression**).[13]

In severe cases, an individual's response to stress may develop into **post-traumatic stress disorder (PTSD).** PTSD generally develops within the first hours or days after a traumatic event, but in some cases symptoms do not begin until months or years later. Traumas that can trigger PTSD include wartime experiences, rape, near-death experiences in accidents, witnessing a

psychoneuroimmunology (PNI) Science of the interaction between the mind and the immune system

post-traumatic stress disorder (PTSD) An acute stress disorder caused by experiencing an extremely traumatic event

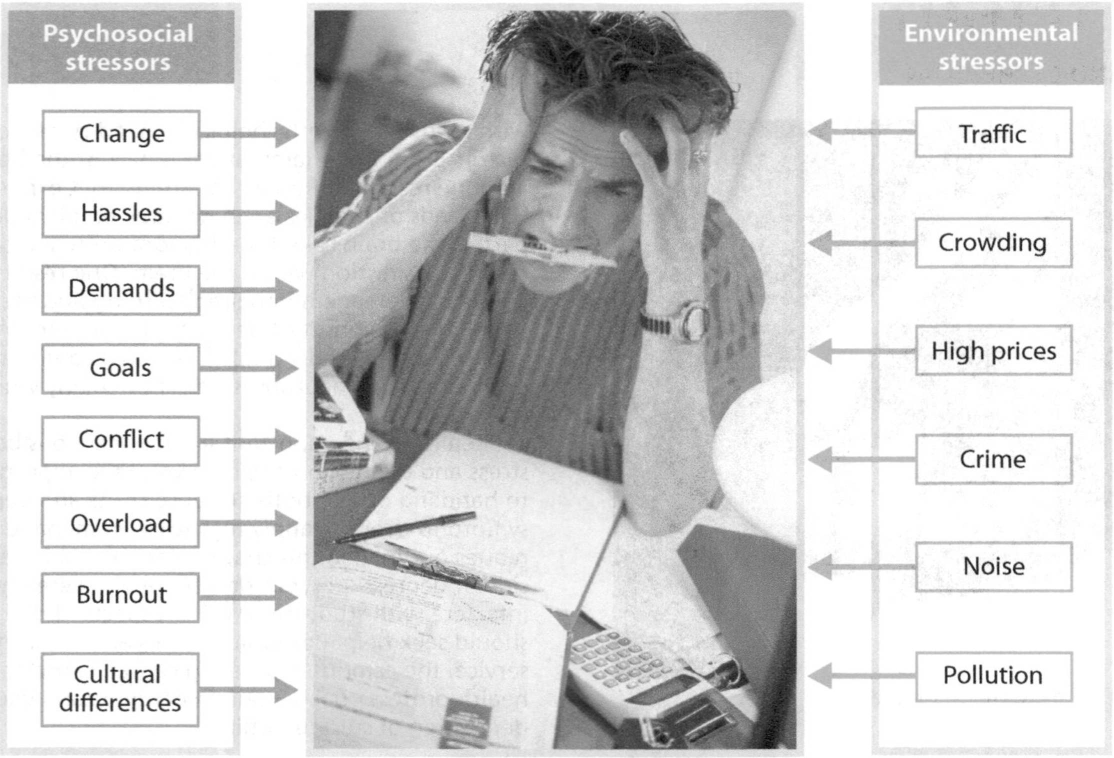

Sw Productions/Photolibrary

FIGURE 3
Stressors are often psychosocial or environmental in nature.

murder or death, being caught in a natural disaster, or a terrorist attack.

WHAT ARE THE MAJOR SOURCES OF STRESS?

College students tend to experience different stressors depending on age, sex, and year in school. First-year students, for example, primarily feel academic pressure.[14] Female freshmen also tend to report dieting and weight gain as stressful, while male students worry more about being underweight, relationship issues, and substance use (drugs, alcohol).[15] In addition, nontraditional students may experience other sources of stress, as described in the box **Understanding Diversity: Stress in Traditional and Nontraditional Students.**

What are your main sources of stress? Examining the many psychological, social, and environmental causes of stress may help you identify them (Figure 3).

PSYCHOSOCIAL SOURCES OF STRESS

Interactions with others, expectations we and others have of ourselves, and the social conditions we live in force us to readjust constantly. Some key psychosocial factors are:

Change Alterations from your normal routine can cause stress. The greater the change and your necessary adjustments to it, the more stress and the greater the potential impact on your immune system.[16] Certain kinds of life events predict increased risk for stress-related illness.

Hassles Petty annoyances and frustrations may seem unimportant if taken one by one: getting stuck in a long line at the bookstore, for example, or finding out that a school administrator has lost all your paperwork. However, minor hassles can build to major stress, if you perceive them negatively and let the feelings mount.[17] Regular release through stress management can counter this buildup.

UNDERSTANDING DIVERSITY

STRESS IN TRADITIONAL AND NONTRADITIONAL STUDENTS

As currently defined, *traditional students* are 18 to 24 years old, go right to college after high school, and are fully or partially supported by parents. *Nontraditional students* are 25 or older; have interrupted their educational sequence with working, traveling, or military service; are often married with children; and are self-supporting. Researchers have found notable differences in the way students in the two categories experience stressors at college.

Traditional students tend to experience stress mainly from course work, academic performance, and relationships.[1] Nontraditional students tend to be more stressed by juggling family responsibilities and schoolwork, commuting from off-campus, working at jobs, and feeling less involved with fellow students and detached from the institution they attend.[2] Research shows that wives or husbands who are supportive about the time demands on their college student spouses can help buffer some of the stress. According to those same studies, college and university counselors can and should play an increasingly important role in helping both traditional and nontraditional students overcome their unique stressors and thus complete their degrees.[3]

Sources:

1. H. Li and W. Kam, "Types and Characteristics of Stress on College Campus," *Psychological Science* 25, no. 4 (2002): 398–401.
2. Dawna-Cricket-Martita Meehan and Charles Negy, "Undergraduate Students' Adaptation to College: Does Being Married Make a Difference?" *Journal of College Development* (September–October 2003): 567–78.
3. Ibid.

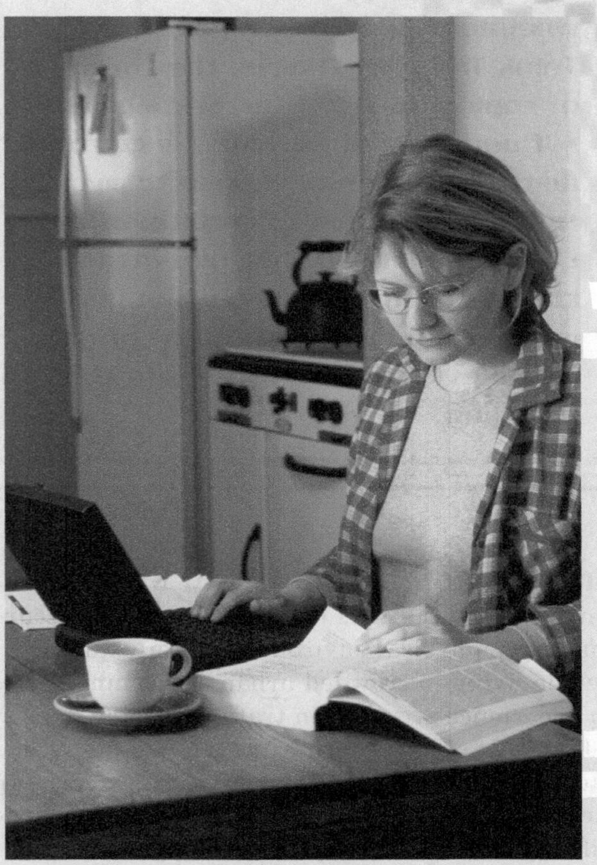

Scott T. Baxter/Getty Images

Performance Demands We experience stress when we must speed up, intensify, or alter our behavior to meet higher standards or unfamiliar demands. We can lessen the impact of such demands by setting priorities and realistic deadlines.

Inconsistent Goals and Behaviors The negative effects of stress can be magnified when we don't match our goals with our actions. For instance, you may want good grades, and your family may expect them. But if you party and procrastinate throughout the term, your goals and behaviors are inconsistent. Behaviors that are consistent with your goals—for example, studying harder and partying less to achieve good grades—can help alleviate stress.

Conflict Conflict occurs when we have to choose between competing motives, behaviors, or impulses, or when we must face incompatible demands, opportunities, needs, or goals. For example, what if your best friend wanted you to help her cheat on an exam, but you didn't feel right about it? College students often experience stress because their own developing set of beliefs conflicts with the values they learned from their parents.

Overload and Burnout Time pressure, responsibilities, course work, tuition, and high expectations for yourself and those around you—coupled with a lack of support—can lead to *overload:* a state of feeling overburdened, unable to keep up, and longing for escape. Overload pushes some students toward depression or substance abuse; others respond by using stress-management tools to alleviate tension before it piles up. Unrelieved overload can lead to *burnout,* a state of stress-induced physical and mental exhaustion. Teachers, nurses, and law enforcement officers, for example, experience high levels of burnout, and highly pressured professionals often apply stress-management techniques to avoid reaching this point.

Try it NOW! **Feeling overwhelmed? Experiencing overload? Think Triple A—that is, the three As of coping: avoid, alter, and abolish.** • **If your school workload is causing distress, you may choose to *avoid* taking more than 15 credits, *alter* your schedule so that you attend classes in the morning when you are most alert, or *abolish* a few of your social events to devote more time to studying.**

Environmental Sources of Stress

Environmental stress results from events occurring in the physical environment. For example, people living in crowded urban environments tend to experience stress from traffic, housing density, a high cost of living, crime, noise, and pollution. Meanwhile, people living in rural areas may experience different stresses, including transportation difficulties, limited employment opportunities, reduced availability of services, and greater impact from weather and climatic events such as floods, fires, and tornadoes.

RACIAL, ETHNIC OR CULTURAL ISOLATION

Imagine what it would be like to come to campus and find yourself isolated, lacking friends, and ridiculed on the basis of who you are or how you look. Often, those who act, speak, or dress differently face additional pressures that do not affect more "typical" students. Students perceived as different—whether due to race, ethnicity, religious affiliation, age, physical handicap, or sexual orientation—may become victims of subtle and not-so-subtle forms of bigotry, insensitivity, harassment, or hostility.

appraisal The interpretation and evaluation of information provided to the brain by the senses

INTERNAL SOURCES OF STRESS

When you perceive that your coping resources are sufficient to meet life's demands, you experience little or no stress. By contrast, when you perceive that life's demands exceed your coping resources, you are likely to feel strain and distress.

Low Self-Esteem and Self-Efficacy

Several coping resources influence your **appraisal** of stress. Two of the most important are *self-esteem* and *self-efficacy.* Self-esteem is a sense of positive self-regard, or how you feel about yourself. Self-efficacy is a belief or confidence in personal skills and performance abilities. Researchers consider self-efficacy one of the most important personality traits that influence psychological and physiological stress responses.[18] Low self-esteem or low self-efficacy can lead you to feel helpless to cope with the stress in your life.

Type A Personality So-called "Type A" personalities are characterized as hard-driving, competitive, time-driven perfectionists. "Type B" personalities, in contrast, are more relaxed, noncompetitive, and more tolerant of others. Historically, researchers believed that people with Type A characteristics were more prone to heart attacks than their Type B counterparts.[19] Researchers today believe that personality types are more complex than previously thought—most people are not one personality type all the time, and other variables must be explored.

According to psychologist Susanne Kobasa, *psychological hardiness* may negate self-imposed stress associated with Type A behavior. Psychologically hardy people are characterized by control, commitment, and an embrace of challenge.[20] People with a sense of control are able to accept responsibility for their behaviors and change those that they discover to be debilitating. People with a sense of commitment have good self-esteem and understand their purpose in life. People who embrace challenge see change as a stimulating opportunity for personal growth. The concept of hardiness has been studied extensively, and many researchers believe it is the foundation of an individual's ability to cope with stress and remain healthy.[21]

What stresses do you face, and how heavily are they affecting you?

WHAT ARE EFFECTIVE TOOLS FOR STRESS MANAGEMENT?

Most college students do best with a low-key, multipronged approach to stress management.

EXERCISE AND PHYSICAL ACTIVITY

Improving your overall level of fitness may be the most helpful thing you can do to combat stress. Interestingly, research shows that exercise actually *stimulates* the stress response,[22] but that a well-exercised body adapts to the *eustress* of exercise, and as a result is able to tolerate greater levels of *distress* of all kinds. Compared to an unfit person, a fit individual develops a milder stress response to any given stressor.[23] Research also shows that exercise reduces both psychosocial stress and metabolic disturbances leading to belly fat, high blood pressure, high blood cholesterol, and vascular disease.[24]

Many physical activities relieve the feeling of stress and tension, while others—especially those that involve competition, high skill levels, or physical risk—may add to your stress load. Some activities are high in one value and low in the other, but many can build fitness and promote relaxation at the same time. The trick is to balance exercise, fun, and recreational activities in your free time so that you can stay fit and reduce chronic stress.

BASIC WELLNESS MEASURES

Many of the habits you cultivate to improve your wellness can also fight the negative effects of stress.

Eating Well Eating nutrient-dense foods rather than fast foods and junk foods gives you more mental and physical energy, improves your immune responses, and helps you stay at a healthy weight. Undereating, overeating, or eating nutrient-poor foods can contribute to your stress levels by diminishing your overall wellness. Most claims about vitamins and supplements that reduce stress are unsupported. Vitamin and mineral supplementation beyond your daily requirements may only add to your stress—financial stress, that is!

Getting Enough Sleep Sleep is a central wellness component. As explained in the box **Spotlight: Sleep, Performance, and Stress,** sleep loss hinders learning, memory, academic work, and

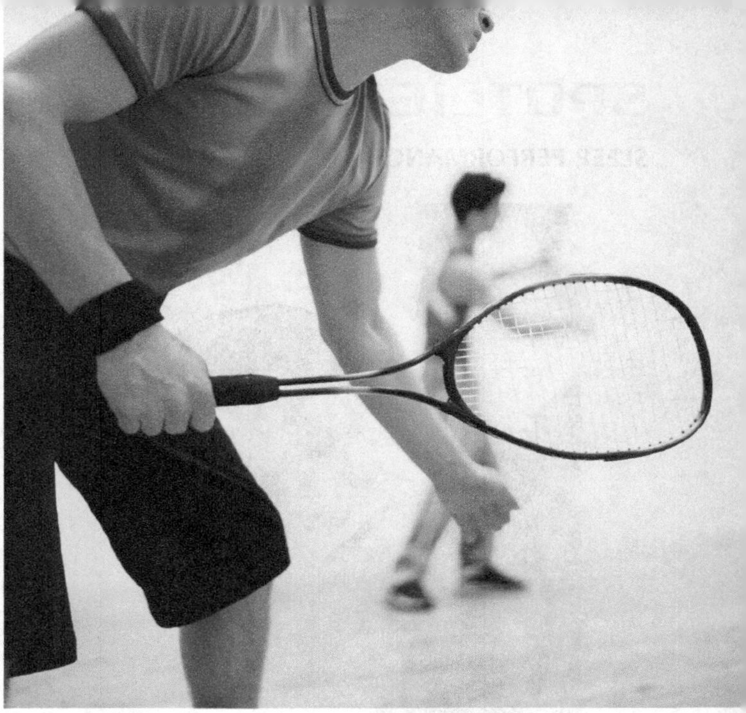

Stockyte/Getty Images

physical performance. It can also depress mood and prompt feelings of stress, anger, and sadness. *Sound* sleep is important, too. Some people find that inexpensive earplugs or eye masks from a drugstore block sleep-disturbing sound and light. Others require a quieter, darker room or more considerate roommates to solve their sleep problems.

Avoiding Tobacco and Alcohol Both drinking and smoking can disrupt sleep patterns during the night. The nicotine in tobacco is highly addictive and acts as a mild stimulant. Tobacco use also impairs normal breathing and diminishes your ability to fight off colds and other infections.

CHANGING YOUR BEHAVIORAL RESPONSES

Realizing that stress is harming your fitness, wellness, relationships, or productivity is often the first step toward making positive changes. Start by assessing all aspects of a stressor, examining your typical response, determining ways to change it, and learning to cope. Often, you cannot change the stressors you face: the death of a loved one, the stringent requirements of your major, stacked-up course assignments, and so on. You can, however, change your reactions to them, and in so doing, help manage your stress.

Assess the Stressor List and evaluate the stressors in your life. Can you change the stressor itself? If not, you can still change your behavior

SPOTLIGHT

SLEEP, PERFORMANCE, AND STRESS

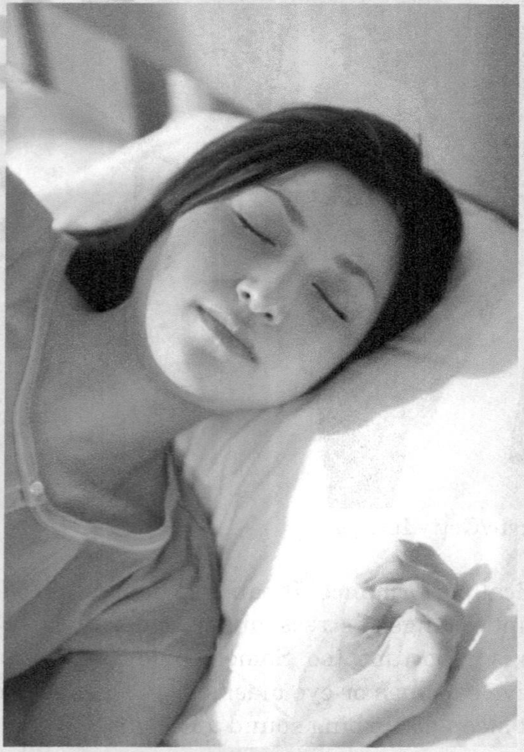

Dex Image/Jupiter Images

Sleep experts suggest that 18- to 20-year-olds need about 8.5 to 9.25 hours of sleep per night, while adults over 21 need about 7 to 9 hours of sleep (depending on individual physiology.)[1] In the 1980s, college students got an average of 7 to 7.5 hours of sleep per night. Today, however, that has slid to between 6 to 6.9 hours. In addition, the typical student sleeps less at the end of a semester than at the beginning due to the accumulation of assignments and exams.[2]

Losing an hour or two of sleep actually does matter, even to young, active, healthy college students. Research shows that sleep loss degrades learning and memory, physical performance, and mood in both young and older adults. One piece of evidence for this is a German study that presented students with a math puzzle to work out. Most of those who "slept on it" realized a shortcut to solving the problem by morning and could solve the task much more quickly. Three-quarters of those who didn't "sleep on it" failed to intuit the way to a faster, simpler solution.[3] This was the first scientific proof that sleep can promote insight and problem solving.

Sleep deprivation can also increase feelings of stress, anger, and sadness. These emotional states can, in turn, make sleeping even harder. Feeling extremely stressed out and having a negative emotional response to that stress is, in fact, the best predictor that a student will have sleep problems.[4] Loneliness and limited social contacts are also correlated with higher stress levels and poorer sleep.[5]

Poor sleep is defined as getting fewer-than-recommended hours of sleep, having irregular bedtimes and rising times, and experiencing interrupted sleep. To improve your sleep and adopt better sleep habits,

- go to bed and wake up at as regular a time as possible;
- sleep in a room that is as quiet and dark as possible;
- get regular exercise but not too close to bedtime;
- avoid caffeine in the afternoon or evening;
- avoid taking naps;
- sleep where it is cool (not cold) and ventilated (but not drafty);
- avoid excess alcohol.

Sources:
1. National Sleep Foundation, "How Much Sleep Is Enough?" 2005. www.sleepfoundation.org.
2. J. Hawkins and P. Shaw, "Self-Reported Sleep Quality in College Students: A Repeated Measures Approach," *Sleep* 15, no. 6 (December 1992): 545–9.
3. Bruce Bower, "Sleeper Effects," *Science News* 165 (January 24, 2004): 53–54.
4. L. A. Verlander, J. O. Benedict, and D. P. Hanson, "Stress and Sleep Patterns of College Students," *Perceptual Motor Skills* 88, no. 3, pt. 1 (June 1999): 893–8.
5. S. D. Pressman and others, "Loneliness, Social Network Size, and Immune Response to Influenza Vaccination in College Freshman," *Health Psychology* 24, no. 3 (May 2005): 297–306.

and reactions to reduce the levels of stress you experience. For example, if you have a heavy academic workload, such as five term papers due for five different courses during the same quarter or semester, make a plan to start the papers early and space your work evenly so you can avoid panic over deadlines and all-night sessions to finish papers on time.

Change Your Response If something causes you distress—a habitually messy roommate, for example—you can (1) express your anger by yelling; (2) pick up the mess yourself but then leave a nasty note; or (3) use humor to get your point across. Your first inclination may be counterproductive, so stop and ask yourself, "What will I gain from this approach?" Then think through the most effective choice. This technique requires practice and emotional control but reaps a large benefit.

Cognitive Coping Strategies Thinking things through before acting may help you avoid destructive or ineffective responses to potentially stressful events. Forethought and planning can also help you tolerate increasingly higher stress levels while limiting physical and mental wear and tear.

Prepare *Before* Stressful Events Preparing yourself for an event that you know will be stressful can diminish its impact. For example, suppose you are nervous about giving a speech. Practicing in front of friends or taping yourself with a video camera may help you find and correct rough spots, and in turn, lower your levels of stress during the actual speech. The important thing is making the effort to plan and prepare.

Downshift You may experience stress because you want to "have it all": a college diploma, a successful career, a family, a wide circle of friends, possessions, status in the community, and so on. But many people are starting to **downshift:** to step back to a simpler life by, for example, moving from a large urban area to a smaller town, from a hectic high-pressure career to a quieter one, or by scaling back to fewer, less-expensive possessions.

Consider some immediate and longer-term steps for simplifying your life:

- List and prioritize your goals. What must you do to reach your selected goals?
- Learn to say no. Decide who you want and need to spend time with, and which requests you can and cannot accommodate.
- Write out a financial plan for paying off credit cards and existing debt, and avoid unnecessary spending.
- Choose a career that you enjoy for itself, not primarily for the salary it commands. Some lower-paying jobs are less stressful and allow more free time for relaxation.
- Establish a savings plan, no matter how small; having a reserve for emergencies and future plans can ease tension.
- Clean drawers, closets, and desktops of clutter. Having fewer unnecessary, unused items means keeping track and taking care of that much less.

SEEKING SOCIAL SUPPORT

Making, keeping, and spending time with friends is a central stress-management tool that helps protect you against harmful stressors. Social interactions are such important buffers against the effects of stress that a person who is well-integrated socially is only half as likely to die from any cause at any age than is a person with few or no sources of social support.[25] This makes social connections a factor as large as being a nonsmoker versus a smoker! Married people are healthier and live longer than single or divorced people, and researchers attribute most of this effect to stress reduction.[26] Compared to students with a network of friends, lonely students experience more stress, poorer moods, and lower quality sleep.[27]

While friends can be important stress reducers, people sometimes need the help of a counselor or support group. Most colleges and universities offer counseling services at no cost for short-term crises. Clergy, instructors, and dorm supervisors also may be helpful resources. If university services are unavailable or if you are concerned about confidentiality, most communities offer low-cost counseling through mental health clinics. You may also be able to find and join a stress-reduction program or stress support group through one of these professional resources. Many individual counselors and stress-reduction classes teach tools like relaxation breathing, progressive muscle relaxation, mindfulness meditation, and cognitive stress reduction techniques to help you learn to change your thinking, behavior, or emotions. These help control your experience of stress and actually reduce stress hormone levels, and by so doing, slow the heart rate, relax the muscles, boost immunity, and help balance brain chemistry.

RELAXATION TECHNIQUES

Relaxation techniques tend to focus the mind and breathing while the body remains fairly stationary. Here are some of the most popular examples.

Relaxation Breathing When we're tense, we often breathe shallowly in the upper chest or even hold our breath, but this kind of breathing can increase anxiety.[28] **Relaxation breathing**—inhaling deeply, rhythmically, and involving the abdominal muscles—can help relieve tension and increase oxygen levels in the blood. This, in turn, can boost energy and sharpen thinking. Relaxation breathing, also called

downshifting Forging new values that include stepping back to a simpler life

relaxation breathing Inhaling deeply and rhythmically, and expanding then relaxing the abdomen; this breathing technique can help relieve tension and increase oxygen intake

TOOLS FOR CHANGE

MINDFULNESS MEDITATION

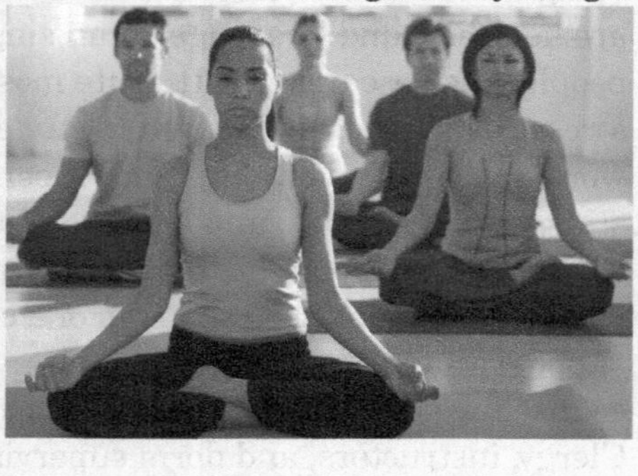
Tetra Images/Getty Images

Meditation is a centuries-old practice that can promote relaxation, lessen damage from chronic stress, and help prevent stress-related illnesses. One of the easiest forms of meditation is called *mindfulness meditation,* which cultivates awareness, calms the body, and stops the mind from racing—at least for a while. You can start learning mindfulness meditation with 5-minute sessions, then build to frequent or daily sessions of 30 minutes or more. Many people find that meditating with a partner or in a small group helps reinforce their practice.

The following specific steps work for many beginning and experienced meditators.[1]

1. In a quiet place, sit cross-legged on the floor or upright in a chair, back straight but not stiff.
2. With eyes closed, breathe in slowly and fully and notice the sensation of air moving in and out of your nose, breathing passages, and lungs. Focus carefully on the abdomen rising. Then breathe out and note the abdomen falling. It helps some people to say silently, "Rising, rising . . . falling, falling . . ."
3. As you sit, you will inevitably experience sounds, smells, tastes, and other sensations. As they come up, notice them and label them (for example, "hearing, hearing . . ."). Then, gently return your concentration to your breathing and the rising and falling of your abdomen.
4. As you sit, your mind will inevitably become active with thoughts, images, plans, or worries. Notice them and label them (for example, "thinking, thinking . . .") and then return your focus to your breathing.
5. After meditating, open your eyes. Rise slowly and carefully, being aware of all the small changes in posture, movement, and effort.

Source: Sayadaw U Pandita Bhivamsa, "The Way to Practice Vipassana Meditation," www.Realization.org, May 20, 2000.

diaphragmatic breathing, is easy and can be done sitting in a chair or lying down, alone or in a small group, and for a few minutes or for a half hour or more. The object is to expand the chest fully by drawing downward with the diaphragm and outward with the abdomen, then releasing fully. Yoga, tai chi, meditation, and most other relaxation techniques rely on this or some similar form of deep, rhythmic breathing.

Progressive Muscle Relaxation **Progressive muscle relaxation (PMR)** identifies tension stored in the muscles and releases it, muscle group by muscle group. To do PMR, lie down in a quiet, comfortable place and devote 10 or 20 minutes to gradually letting go of accumulated stiffness and tension in the affected muscles.

progressive muscle relaxation (PMR) A stress-management technique that identifies tension stored in the muscles and releases it, one muscle group at a time

biofeedback A stress-management technique that teaches you to alter automatic physiological responses such as body temperature, heart rate, or sweating; uses a machine to monitor such responses and measure the success of conscious control attempts

Meditation There are dozens of forms of meditation, but most involve sitting quietly for 15 to 30 minutes and focusing on deep breathing. Some involve assuming a particular posture like sitting cross-legged with back straight and hands resting gently on the thighs. Researchers have confirmed that meditation reduces the stress response and boosts the immune response.[29] Meditation also shifts brain activity from the right prefrontal lobe, associated with unhappiness, anger, and distress, and toward the left prefrontal lobe, associated with happiness and enthusiasm. The box **Tools for Change: Mindfulness Meditation** presents one of the easiest-to-learn meditation techniques.

Biofeedback **Biofeedback** involves monitoring physical stress responses such as brain activity, blood pressure, muscle tension, or heart rate with a special machine and then learning to consciously alter these responses. Biofeedback is effective for several stress-related conditions, including high blood pressure, headaches, irritable bowel syndrome, and asthma.[30]

Hypnosis **Hypnosis** trains people to focus on one thought, object, or voice and to become unusually responsive to suggestion. A qualified hypnotherapist can implant a suggestion that directs a patient to resist habits such as smoking or overeating or to lessen phobias such as fear of snakes or air travel. The patient then learns to induce a state of self-hypnosis as a way to relax deeply and reinforce the behavioral changes.

People who get regular physical exercise and also practice one or more of these relaxation methods—relaxation breathing, progressive muscle relaxation, meditation, biofeedback, and hypnosis—can achieve very effective relief from stress symptoms.[31] Many will also see improvement in medical conditions that are worsened by stress.

MANAGING YOUR TIME, THOUGHTS, AND EMOTIONS

The world presents us with plenty of stressors. But we create some of our own as well through our ineffective time-management habits and our ways of thinking and reacting to events. Habits are learned behaviors, and you can *unlearn* or replace them with new habits that serve you better in managing stress. Here is what to aim for.

Manage Your Time Time—or our perceived lack of it—is one of our biggest stressors. If you learn to handle demands in a more streamlined, efficient way, you can leave more time for other things, such as studying and having fun. The following tips can help:

- **Assess how you spend your time.** How do you spend the 168 hours in your week? Try keeping a time journal for 1 week. Tabulate the time you spend in productive pursuits, the time spent relaxing, and the time you may be wasting. Look for ways to tip the balance toward productivity.
- **Prioritize your tasks.** Make a daily "to do" list of things you must do today, must do soon, or could do later, if at all. Rank and assign deadlines to the more important tasks.
- **Single-task or multitask when appropriate.** It is usually unproductive to try to make phone calls, clean the bathroom, and write your term paper all at once. Term papers are singular tasks. Save multitasking for things that take less concentration such as doing the laundry and paying bills.
- **Break up big tasks.** Divide big tasks like finishing a term paper into smaller segments, then allocate a certain amount of time to each piece. If you find yourself floundering in a task, move on and come back to it when you are refreshed.
- **Clean your desk.** Periodically weed out unneeded papers and file the useful ones in separate folders. Try to handle papers just once: When bills come in, for example, take care of them immediately. Promptly read, respond to, file, or toss the other mail into the recycle bin.
- **Accommodate your natural rhythms.** Schedule activities to coincide with the time you are at your best. If you are a morning person, study and write papers in the morning, and take breaks when you start to slow down.
- **Avoid overcommitment.** Set your school and personal priorities and don't be afraid to say no to things you cannot or should not agree to do.
- **Avoid interruptions.** When you have a project that requires total concentration, schedule uninterrupted time. Go to a quiet room in the library or student union where no one will find you. Shut off your cell phone and let it take messages.
- **Reward yourself.** When you finish a task early, take a break and do something enjoyable that helps you recharge and refresh your energy levels.

Manage Your Thinking Our "negative scripts" about ourselves contribute to our stress. When we see ourselves as unable to cope (that is, when we have low self-efficacy), we tend to handle life's problems and stresses more poorly. You can change negative scripts to more positive ones, however, and in the process reduce your stress responses. Successful stress management involves developing and practicing self-esteem skills, such as applying positive thinking and examining self-talk to reduce negative and irrational responses. Focus on your current capabilities rather than on past problems.

Here are specific actions you can take to develop better mental skills for stress management:

- **Worry constructively.** Don't waste time and energy worrying about things you can't change or events that may never happen.

hypnosis A medical and psychiatric tool that trains people to focus on one thought, object, or voice and to become unusually responsive to suggestion

- **Perceive life as changeable.** If you accept that change is a natural part of living and growing, the jolt of changes will become less stressful.
- **Consider alternatives.** Remember, there is seldom only one appropriate action. Anticipating options will help you plan for change and adjust more rapidly.
- **Moderate your expectations.** Aim high but be realistic about your circumstances and motivation.
- **Don't rush into action.** Think before you act. Tolerate mistakes by yourself and others. Rather than getting angry and stressed by mishaps, evaluate what happened, learn from them, and plan to avoid future occurrences.
- **Live simply.** Eliminate unnecessary possessions and obligations.
- **Take things less seriously.** Think about the times that you have spent getting all worked up about some perceived interpersonal slight, or concerns over what others may think or say. Lighten up—try to keep the real importance of these things in perspective. Ask yourself: How much will this matter in two weeks? Six months?

Manage Negative Emotions and Anger

Stress management involves learning to identify emotional reactions that are based on irrational beliefs and negative self-talk. Identifying those can allow you to deal with the belief or emotion in a healthy and appropriate way.

Learning how to manage anger is particularly important. Anger can be constructive if it mobilizes us to stand up for ourselves or to accomplish something others think we are incapable of. However, a habit of responding angrily when our wants or desires are thwarted can be destructive. Because anger triggers the fight-or-flight response, people who manage anger poorly operate with the stress response turned on longer than necessary.

Hotheaded, short-fused people are at risk for health problems. Numerous studies show that anger can significantly increase the risk of heart disease. Stress hormones released during anger may constrict blood vessels in the heart or actually promote clot formation, which can trigger a heart attack.[32] Strategies for controlling and redirecting anger include learning to forgive and forget; practicing problem-solving techniques in place of complaining; seeking objective opinions and constructive advice from friends; anticipating situations that trigger your anger and brainstorming solutions in advance; learning to express your feelings constructively; learning to de-escalate from anger by taking deep breaths or counting to 10; and keeping a journal to observe your own reactions and progress in controlling anger.

SPIRITUAL PRACTICE

Several medical studies have discovered correlations between spirituality and wellness. For example, prayer elicits the same relaxation response attained through other stress-management techniques: lowered blood pressure, heart rate, breathing and metabolism, and a more vigorous immune response.[33] Spirituality is also correlated with a reduced *perception* of stress in one's life.

Developing one's spirituality can be more than just an internal process. It can also be a social process that enhances your relationships with others. The ability to give and take, speak and listen, and forgive and move on is integral to any process of spiritual development.

The above techniques are summarized in Figure 4.

CASE STUDY

Cory

"Life was getting ridiculous. I was exhausted but would have trouble falling asleep, so that was a vicious cycle. I gained weight because I stopped working out—which I used to do twice a week but just didn't have the time for anymore. And I caught another cold at the end of October. My dad started joking that he was healthier than I was! Something had to give, so I dropped my one elective—Spanish, which I love. And I started going back to the gym, which actually seemed to give me some energy back. I honestly think just those two things alone helped me to get through the rest of the semester. Now, if I can just ace my MCATs . . ."

1. **What kinds of stress-related problems was Cory exhibiting?**
2. **Review the section on stress-management tools. Which strategies did Cory employ?**
3. **Which stress-management strategies do you use? What techniques seem to be the most effective for you?**

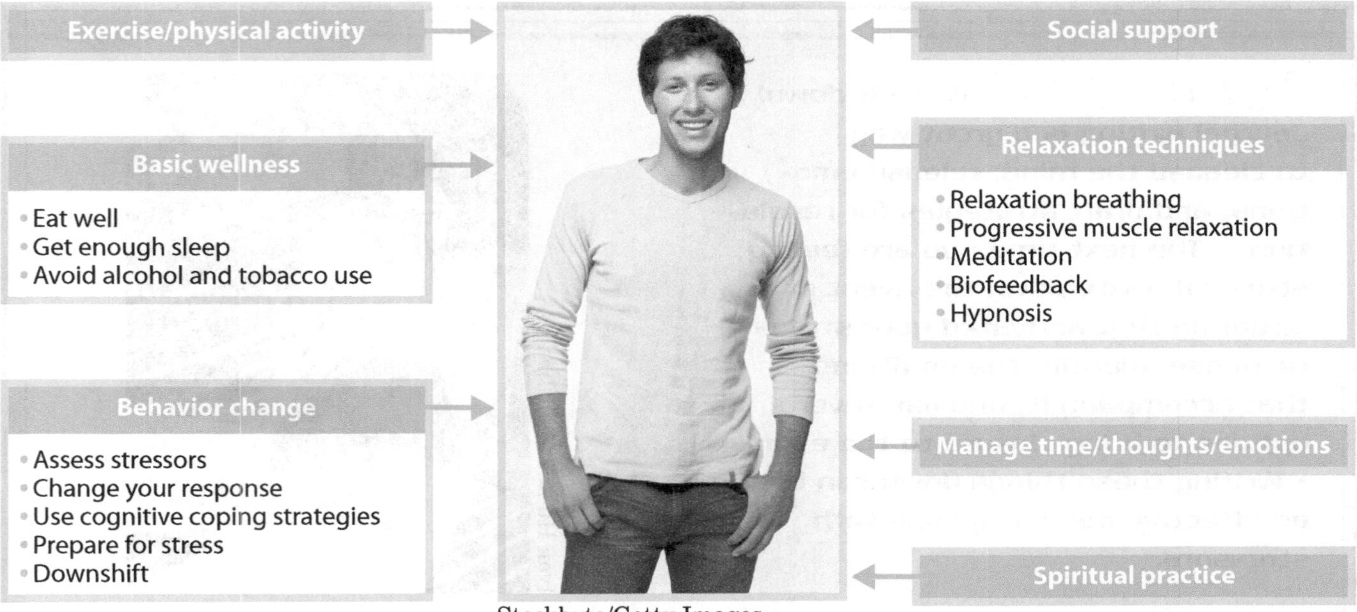

Stockbyte/Getty Images

FIGURE 4

There are many effective techniques for helping you manage stress.

HOW CAN YOU CREATE YOUR OWN STRESS-MANAGEMENT PLAN?

You can use many of the fitness and wellness tools you read about in earlier chapters to help reduce your stress levels. These tools include self-assessment, drawing up a behavior change contract, and journaling.

STEP ONE: ASSESS YOURSELF

Target for change one or more behaviors that contribute to your increased stress.

Then, evaluate the behavior(s) you have chosen. Identify your stress-producing behavior patterns. What can you change now? What can you change in the near future?

STEP TWO: PLAN FOR CHANGE

Select one stress-producing behavior pattern that you want to change. As you learned earlier, your behavior change contract should include your long-term goal for change, your short-term goals, the rewards you will give yourself for reaching these goals, potential obstacles along the way, and strategies for overcoming these obstacles. Look for ways to apply wellness tools such as meditation, relaxation breathing, and progressive muscle relaxation.

STEP THREE: CHART YOUR PROGRESS

Chart your progress in your journal. At the end of a week, evaluate how successful you were in following your plan. What helped you be successful? What obstacles to change did you encounter? What will you do differently next week?

After you assess yourself, make a plan and revise it as needed. Are your short-term goals attainable? Are the rewards satisfying? Do you need to go beyond your own self-efforts and enlist the help of your peers or professionals? If you think you need professional support, start by consulting the student health service for advice and direction on finding suitable counselors, therapists, or stress-management support groups.

Try it NOW! **Write it down!** Journal writing is a great way to cleanse the mind, release emotions, and draft strategies for resolution. • The next time you are feeling stressed, write down the event or situation that activated your stress response, identify the emotions that accompany it, and list several options to bring closure to the event. • Writing these things down can be an effective means to cope with stressors.

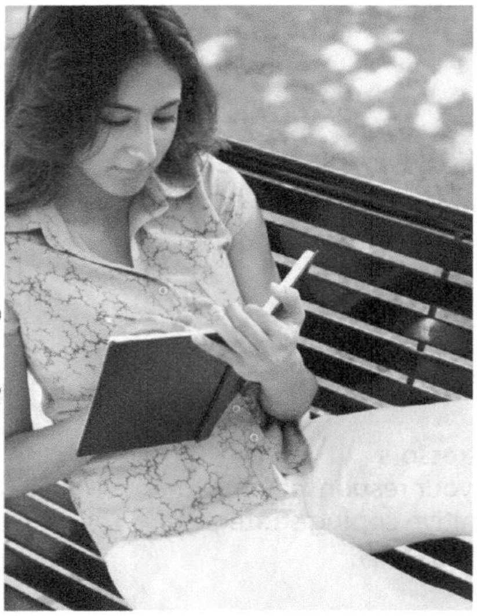

Ivan Hunter/Getty Images

CHAPTER IN REVIEW

REVIEW QUESTIONS

1. Graduating from college and moving to a new city can create stress as well as provide an opportunity for growth. This type of stress is called
   a. strain.
   b. distress.
   c. eustress.
   d. adaptive response.
2. The physiological instinct to flee from or confront a threat is called
   a. homeostasis.
   b. the fight-or-flight response.
   c. allostasis.
   d. allostatic load.
3. *Homeostasis* describes
   a. the body's "normal" or "steady state."
   b. long-term wear-and-tear on the body.
   c. sustained stress.
   d. the exhaustion stage of the general adaptation syndrome.
4. Hans Selye's general adaptation syndrome includes all of the following stages except
   a. the alarm stage.
   b. the resistance stage.
   c. the allostasis stage.
   d. the exhaustion stage.
5. Stress has been linked to all of the following except
   a. cardiovascular disease.
   b. immune system impairment.
   c. mental disorders.
   d. greater health.
6. Change, hassles, performance demands, and burnout are all examples of
   a. psychosocial sources of stress.
   b. environmental sources of stress.
   c. internal sources of stress.
   d. homeostasis.
7. *Allostatic load* refers to
   a. changes that occur in the body to maintain homeostasis.
   b. long-term wear-and-tear on the body caused by stress.
   c. the first stage of the general adaptation syndrome.
   d. eustress.
8. Effective tools for stress management include all of the following except
   a. getting by on little sleep.
   b. exercise and physical activity.
   c. eating well.
   d. avoiding alcohol and tobacco.

9. *Relaxation breathing* refers to
   a. inhaling deeply and rhythmically to relieve tension and increase oxygen levels in the blood.
   b. progressive muscle relaxation.
   c. monitoring physical stress responses and then consciously working to alter those responses.
   d. biofeedback.

10. What stress-fighting technique allows people to become unusually responsive to suggestion?
   a. Meditation
   b. Massage
   c. Biofeedback
   d. Hypnosis

CRITICAL THINKING QUESTIONS

1. Compare and contrast distress and eustress. In what ways are both types of stress potentially harmful?
2. Describe the body's physiological response to stress.
3. What are some of the health risks that result from chronic stress? Summarize the main points of the general adaptation syndrome and the allostatic load model.
4. What major factors seem to influence the nature and extent of a person's susceptibility to stress? Explain how social support, self-esteem, and personality may make a person more or less susceptible.

ONLINE RESOURCES

Please visit this book's website at **www.aw-bc.com/hopson** to access links related to topics in this chapter.

REFERENCES

1. American College Health Association, "National College Health Assessment. Reference Group Executive Summary Fall 2006," Baltimore: American College Health Association, 2007.
2. Mark A. Staal, "Stress, Cognition, and Human Performance: A Literature Review and Conceptual Framework," *National Aeronautics and Space Administration* (May 2004): NASA/TM-2004–212024.
3. Robert Sapolsky, *Why Zebras Don't Get Ulcers: An Updated Guide to Stress, Stress-Related Diseases, and Coping* (New York: Owl Books, 2004).
4. David G. Myers, *Psychology.* 5th ed. (New York: Worth Publishers, 1998): 518.
5. Bruce McEwen and Teresa Seeman, "Allostatic Load and Allostasis," John D. and Catherine T. MacArthur Research Network on Socioeconomic Status and Health (University of California at San Francisco 1999).
6. Ibid.
7. Robert Sapolsky, *Why Zebras Don't Get Ulcers: An Updated Guide to Stress, Stress-Related Diseases, and Coping* (New York: Owl Books, 2004).
8. A. Mokdal and others, "Actual Causes of Death in the United States 2000," *Journal of the American Medical Association* 291 (2004): 1238–45.
9. S. Das and J. H. O'Keefe, "Behavioral Cardiology: Recognizing and Addressing the Profound Impact of Psychosocial Stress on Cardiovascular Health," *Current Atherosclerosis Reports* 8, no. 2 (2006): 111–18; A. K. Ferketich and P. F. Binkley, "Psychological Distress and Cardiovascular Disease: Results from the 2002 National Health Interview Study," *European Heart Journal* 26, no. 18 (2005): 1923–29; S. Yusef and others, "Effect of Potentially Modifiable Risk Factors Associated with Myocardial Infarction in 52 Countries (The INTERHEART Study): Case-Control Study," *The Lancet* 364, no. 9438 (2004): 937–52.
10. J. R. Hapuarachchi and others, "Changes in Clinically Relevant Metabolites with Psychological Stress Parameters," *Behavioral Medicine* 29 (2003): 52–60; C. N. Merz and others, "Psychosocial Stress and Cardiovascular Disease: Pathophysiological Links," *Behavioral Medicine* 27 (2002): 141–48.
11. S. A. Everson-Rose and T. T. Lewis, "Psychosocial Risk Factors and Cardiovascular Disease," *Annual Review of Public Health* 26 (2005): 469–500.
12. S. C. Segerstrom and G. E. Miller, "Psychological Stress and the Human Immune System," *Psychological Bulletin* 130, no. 4 (2004): 601–30.
13. D. A. Katerndahl and M. Parchman, "The Ability of the Stress Process Model to Explain Mental Health Outcomes," *Comprehensive Psychiatry* 43 (2002): 351–60; R. C. Kessler and others, "The Epidemiology of Major Depressive Disorder," *Journal of the American Medical Association* 289 (2003): 3095–3105.
14. P. Jackson and M. Finney, "Negative Life Events and Psychological Distress Among Young Adults," *Social Psychology Quarterly* 65, no. 2 (June 2002): 186–201.
15. Ibid.
16. T. Holmes and R. Rahe, "The Social Readjustment Rating Scale," *Journal of Psychosomatic Research* 11 (1967): 213–18.
17. R. Lazarus, "The Trivialization of Distress," in *Preventing Health*

Risk Behaviors and Promoting Coping with Illness, eds. J. Rosen and L. Solomon (Hanover, NH: University Press of New England, 1985): 279–98.

18. A. D. Von and others, "Predictors of Health Behaviors in College Students," *Journal of Advanced Nursing* 48, no. 5 (2004): 463–74.
19. M. Friedman and R. H. Rosenman, *Type A Behavior and Your Heart* (New York: Knopf, 1974).
20. S. Kobasa, "Stressful Life Events, Personality, and Health: An Inquiry Into Hardiness," *Journal of Personality and Social Psychology* 37 (1979): 1–11.
21. B. J. Crowley and others, "Psychological Hardiness and Adjustment to Life Events in Adulthood," *Journal of Adult Development* 10 (2003): 237–48; S. R. Maddi, "The Story of Hardiness: Twenty Years of Theorizing, Research, and Practice," *Consulting Psychology Journal: Practice and Research* 54 (2002): 173–86.
22. A. Leal-Cerro and others, "Mechanisms Underlying the Neuroendocrine Response to Physical Exercise," *Journal of Endocrinological Investigation* 26, no. 9 (September 2003): 879–85.
23. U. Rimmele and others, "Trained Men Show Lower Cortisol, Heart Rate, and Psychological Responses to Psychosocial Stress Compared with Untrained Men," *Psychoneuroendocrinology* 32, no. 6 (July 2007): 627–35.
24. A. Tsatsoulis and S. Fountoulakis, "The Protective Role of Exercise on Stress System Dysregulation and Comorbidities," *Annals of the New York Academy of Sciences* 1083 (November 2006): 196–213.
25. S. Levine, D. M. Lyons, and A. F. Schatzberg, "Psychobiological Consequences of Social Relationships," *Annals of the New York Academy of Sciences* 89, no. 7 (1999): 210–18.
26. J. Holmes, "Healthy Relationships: Their Influence on Physical Health," BC Council for Families, 2004. www.bccf.bc.ca/learn/health_relations.htm.
27. S. D. Pressman and others, "Loneliness, Social Network Size, and Immune Response to Influenza Vaccination in College Freshmen," *Health Psychology* 24, no. 4 (July 2005): 348.
28. A. Conrad and others, "Psychophysiological Effects of Breathing Instructions for Stress Management," *Applied Psychophysiology and Biofeedback* 32, no. 2 (June 2007): 89–98.
29. S. Jain and others, "A Randomized Controlled Trial of Mindfulness Meditation Versus Relaxation Training: Effects on Distress, Positive States of Mind, Rumination, and Distraction," *Annals of Behavioral Medicine* 33, no. 1 (February 2007): 11021, R. J. Davidson and others, "Alterations in Brain and Immune Function Produced by Mindfulness Meditation," *Psychosomatic Medicine* 65, no. 4 (July–August 2003): 564–70.
30. Mayo Clinic, "Biofeedback: Using Your Mind to Improve Your Health," January 26, 2006. www.mayoclinic.com/health/biofeedback/SA00083.
31. Mayo Clinic, "Relaxation Techniques: Learn Ways to Calm Your Stress," March 7, 2007. www.mayoclinic.com/health/relaxation-technique/SR00007. Also, "Exercise: Rev Up Your Routine to Reduce Stress," MayoClinic.com, July 20, 2006. www.mayoclinic.com/print/exercise-and-stress/SR00036/METHOP=print.
32. L. D. Kubzansky and others, "Shared and Unique Contributions of Anger, Anxiety, and Depression to Coronary Heart Disease: A Prospective Study in the Normative Aging Study," *Annals of Behavioral Medicine* 31, no. 1 (February 2006): 21–9; I. Kawachi and others, "A Prospective Study of Anger and Coronary Heart Disease. The Normative Aging Study," *Circulation* 94, no. 9 (November 1, 1996): 2090–5.
33. D. K. Reibel and others, "Mindfulness-Based Stress Reduction and Health-Related Quality of Life in a Heterogeneous Patient Population," *General Hospital Psychiatry* 23, no. 4 (July–August 2001): 183–92, R. Sethness and others, "Cardiac Health: Relationships Among Hostility, Spirituality, and Health Risk," *Journal of Nursing Care Quality* 20, no. 1 (January–March 2005): 81–9. And L. E. Carlson and others, "Mindfulness-Based Stress Reduction in Relation to Quality of Life, Mood, Symptoms of Stress and Levels of Cortisol, Dehyroepiandrosterone Sulfate (DHEAS) and Melatonin in Breast and Prostate Cancer Outpatient," *Psychoneuroendocrinology* 29, no. 4 (May 2004): 448–74.

ANSWERS TO END-OF-CHAPTER QUESTIONS

1.c; 2.b; 3.a; 4.c; 5.d; 6.a; 7.b; 8.a; 9.a; 10.d

Psychosocial Health

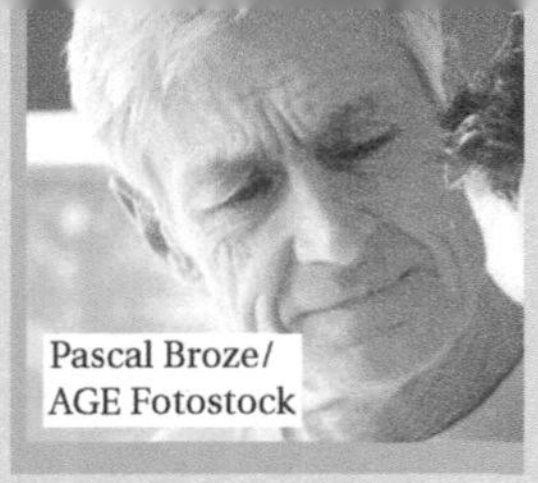
Pascal Broze/ AGE Fotostock

How do others influence my psychosocial health?

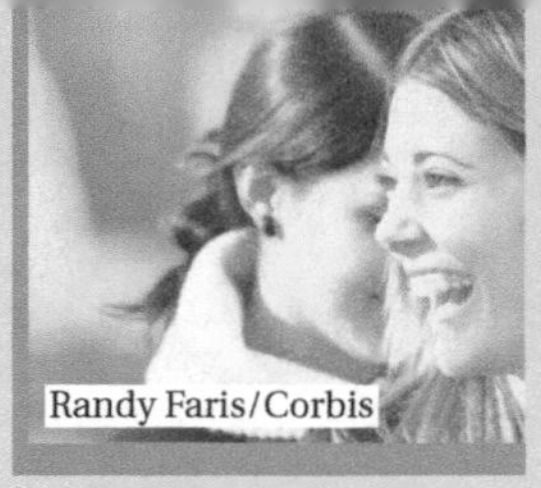
Randy Faris/Corbis

Is laughter really the best medicine?

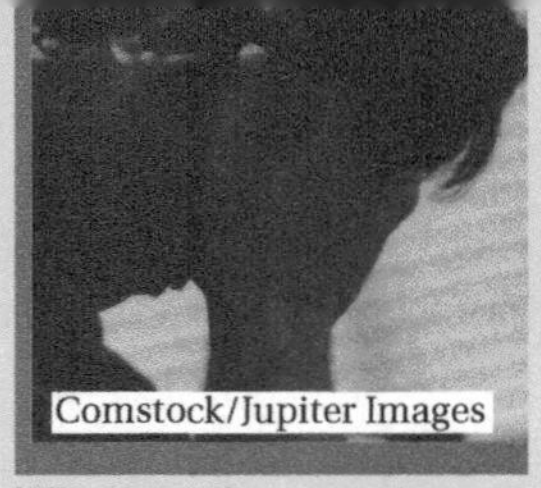
Comstock/Jupiter Images

What are the symptoms of depression?

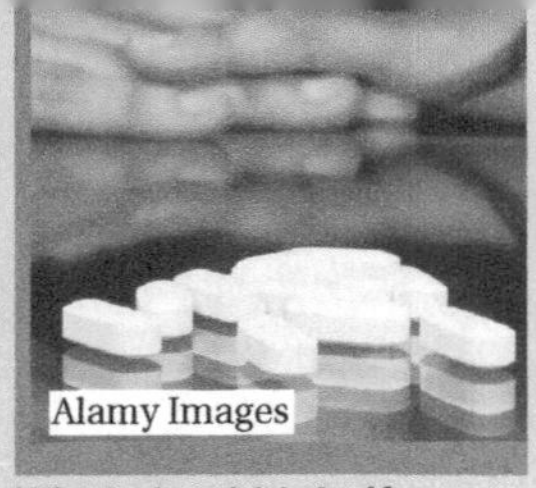
Alamy Images

What should I do if someone I know is suicidal?

Psychosocial Health

Objectives

* Define each of the four components of psychosocial health, and identify the basic traits shared by psychosocially healthy people.
* Learn what factors affect your psychosocial health; discuss the positive steps you can take to enhance your psychosocial health.
* Identify common psychosocial problems, such as anxiety disorders and depression, and explain their causes and treatments.
* Explain the methods of different types of mental health professionals, and examine how they can play a role in preventing specific types of psychosocial health problems.

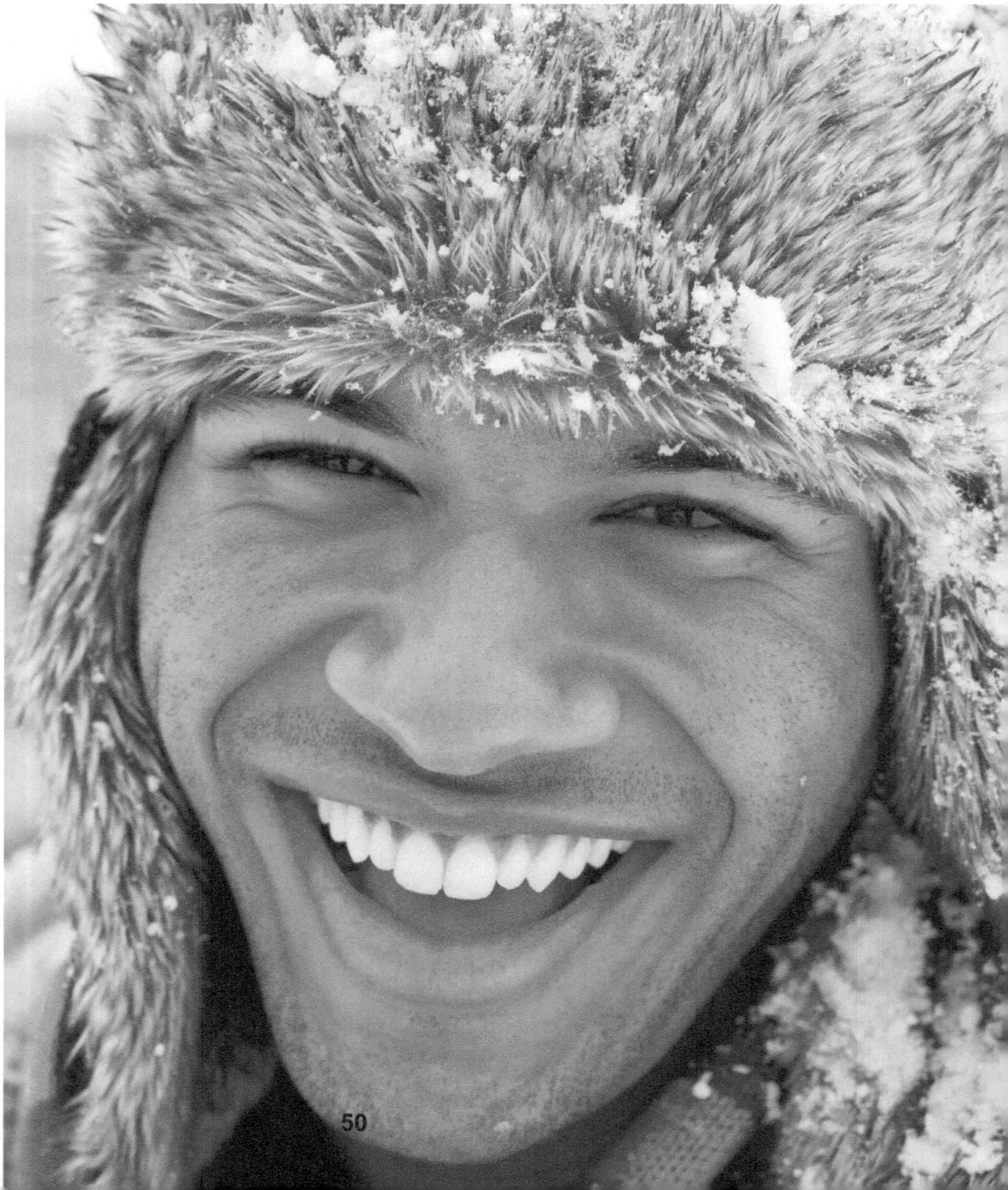
RubberBall/SuperStock

Although the vast majority of college students describe their college years as among the best of their lives, many find the pressure of grades, financial concerns, relationship problems, and the struggle to understand who they are to be extraordinarily difficult. Steven Hyman, provost of Harvard University and former director of the National Institutes of Mental Health, sounded this alarm about student mental health: "The mental state of many students is so precarious that it is interfering with the core mission of the university."[1] Psychological distress caused by relationship issues, family issues, academic competition, and college life adjustment is rampant on college campuses today. Experts believe that the anxiety-prone campus environment is a major contributor to poor health decisions such as high alcohol consumption and, in turn, to health problems that ultimately affect academic success and success in life.

Fortunately, even though we often face seemingly insurmountable pressures, human beings possess a resiliency that enables us to cope, adapt, and thrive, regardless of life's challenges. How we feel and think about ourselves, those around us, and our environment can tell us a lot about our psychosocial health and whether we are healthy emotionally, spiritually, and mentally. Increasingly, health professionals recognize that having a solid social network, being emotionally and mentally healthy, and developing spiritual capacity don't just add years to life—they put life into years.

What Is Psychosocial Health?

Psychosocial health encompasses the mental, emotional, social, and spiritual dimensions of what it means to be healthy (Figure 1). It is the result of a complex interaction between a person's history and his or her thoughts about and interpretations of the past and what it means to the present. Psychosocially healthy people are emotionally, mentally, socially, intellectually, and spiritually resilient. They respond to challenges and frustrations in appropriate ways most of the time, despite occasional slips (Figure 2). When they do slip, they recognize it and take action to rectify the situation. Once they are informed about the resources that are available to help them get through tough situations, they use them. Most authorities identify several basic characteristics shared by psychosocially healthy people.[2]

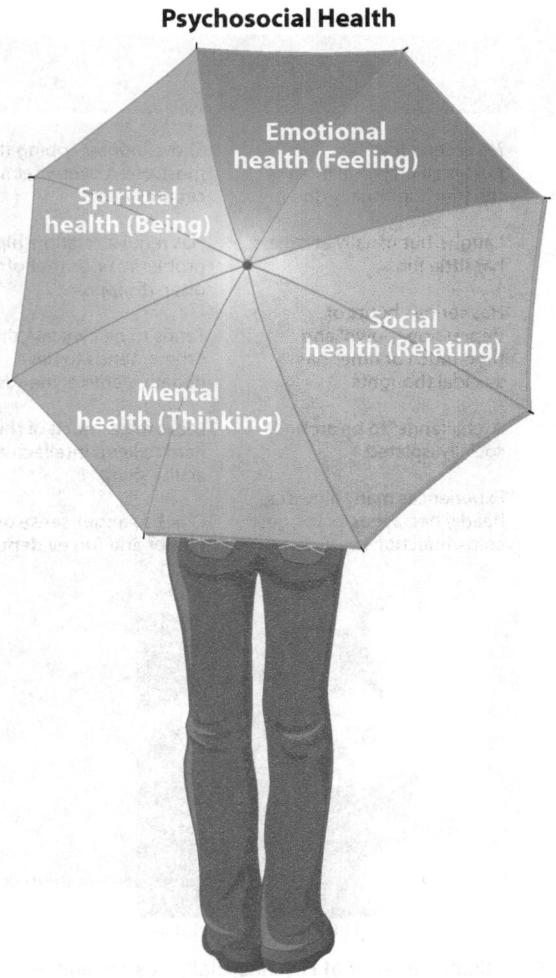

FIGURE 1 **Psychosocial Health**
Psychosocial health is a complex interaction of mental, emotional, social, and spiritual health. Possessing strength and resiliency in these dimensions can maintain your overall well-being and help you weather the storms of life.

- **They feel good about themselves.** They typically are not overwhelmed by fear, love, anger, jealousy, guilt, or worry. They know who they are, have a realistic sense of their capabilities, and respect themselves even though they realize they aren't perfect.
- **They feel comfortable with other people.** They enjoy satisfying and lasting personal relationships and do not take advantage of others or allow others to take advantage of them. They recognize that there are others whose needs are greater than their own. They can give love, consider others' interests, take time to help others, respect personal differences, and feel responsible for their fellow human beings.
- **They control tension and anxiety.** They recognize the underlying causes and symptoms of stress in their lives and consciously avoid irrational thoughts, hostility, excessive excuse making, and blaming others for their problems. They use resources and learn skills to control reactions to stressful situations.
- **They meet the demands of life.** They try to solve problems as they arise, accept responsibility, and plan ahead. They set realistic goals, think for themselves, and make independent decisions. Acknowledging that change is inevitable, they welcome new experiences.
- **They curb hate and guilt.** They acknowledge and combat tendencies to respond with anger, thoughtlessness, selfishness, vengeful acts, or feelings of inadequacy. They do not try

psychosocial health The mental, emotional, social, and spiritual dimensions of health.

Psychosocially unhealthy			Psychosocially healthy
No zest for life; pessimistic/cynical most of the time; spiritually down	Shows poorer coping than most, often overwhelmed by circumstances	Works to improve in all areas, recognizes strengths and weaknesses	Possesses zest for life; spiritually healthy and intellectually thriving
Laughs, but usually at others, has little fun	Has regular relationship problems, finds that others often disappoint	Healthy relationships with family and friends, capable of giving and receiving love and affection	High energy, resilient, enjoys challenges, focused
Has serious bouts of depression, "down" and tired much of time; has suicidal thoughts	Tends to be cynical/critical of others; tends to have negative/critical friends	Has strong social support, may need to work on improving social skills but usually no major problems	Realistic sense of self and others, sound coping skills, open minded
A "challenge" to be around, socially isolated	Lacks focus much of the time, hard to keep intellectual acuity sharp	Has occasional emotional "dips" but overall good mental/emotional adaptors	Adapts to change easily, sensitive to others and environment
Experiences many illnesses, headaches, aches/pains, gets colds/infections easily	Quick to anger, sense of humor and fun evident less often		Has strong social support and healthy relationships with family and friends

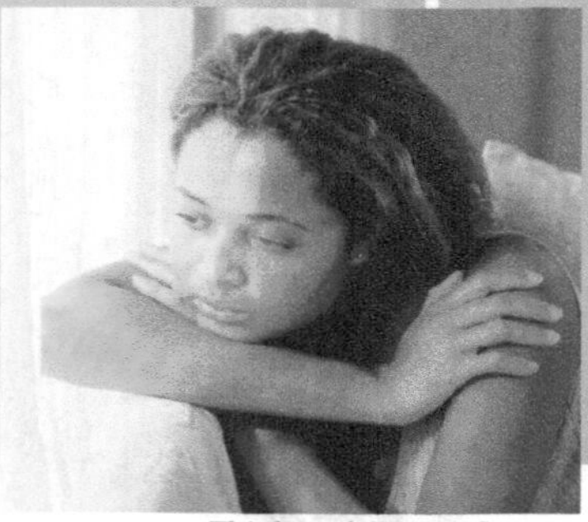

Thinkstock/Jupiter Images

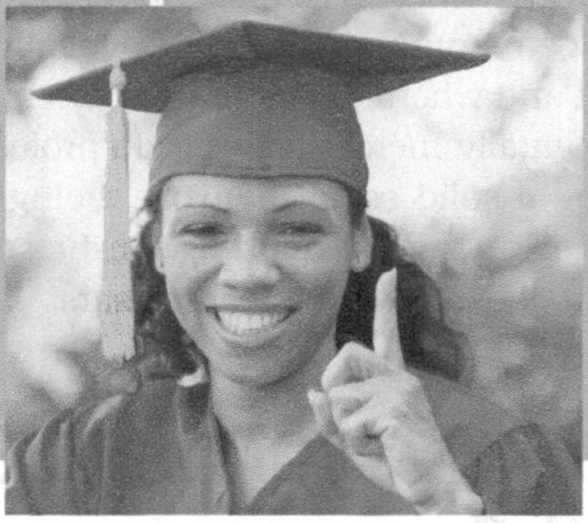

Terry Vine/Blend Images/Getty Images

FIGURE 2 **Characteristics of Psychosocially Healthy and Unhealthy People**
Where do you fall on this continuum?

to knock others aside to get ahead but rather reach out to help others—even people they don't particularly like.

- **They maintain a positive outlook.** They approach each day with a presumption that things will go well. They look to the future with enthusiasm rather than dread. Reminders of good experiences brighten their day. Fun and making time for themselves are integral parts of their lives.
- **They value diversity.** They do not feel threatened by people of a different race, gender, religion, sexual orientation, ethnicity, or political party. They are nonjudgmental and do not force their beliefs and values on others.
- **They appreciate and respect nature.** They take the time to enjoy their surroundings, are conscious of their place in the universe, and act responsibly to preserve their environment.
- **They enrich the lives of others.** They "tune in," and rather than being narcissistic and self-serving, they often think of others' needs and try to help whenever possible.

Psychologists have long argued that before we can achieve any of the above characteristics of psychologically and socially healthy people, we must have certain basic needs met in our lives. In the 1960s, human theorist Abraham Maslow developed a *hierarchy of needs* to describe this idea (Figure 3): At the bottom of his hierarchy are basic *survival needs,* such as food, sleep, and water; at the next level are *security needs,* such as shelter and safety; at the third level—*social needs*—is a sense of belonging and affection; at the fourth level are *esteem needs,* self-respect and respect for others; and at the top are needs for *self-actualization* and self-transcendence.

According to Maslow's theory, a person's needs must be met at each of these levels before that person can ever truly be healthy. Failure to meet one of the lower levels of needs will interfere with a person's ability to address the upper-level ones. For example, someone who is homeless or worried about threats from violence will be unable to focus on fulfilling social, esteem, or actualization needs. Maslow believed that people are more likely to behave badly if they are frustrated by a lack of need fulfillment.[3]

what do you think?

Which psychosocial qualities do you value most in your friends? ● What area do you think is your greatest psychosocial strength? Your greatest weakness? ● Do you agree with Maslow's assessment that people behave badly socially when their needs are not being met? Can you think of an example?

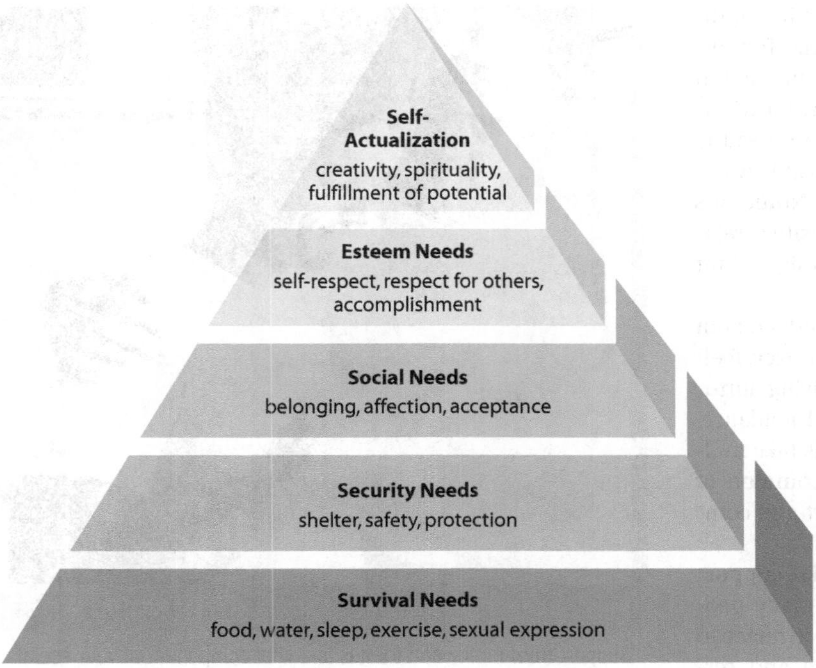

FIGURE 3 **Maslow's Hierarchy of Needs**

Attaining psychosocial health and wellness involves many complex processes. This chapter will help you understand not only what it means to be psychosocially well, but also why we may run into problems in our psychosocial health. Learning how to assess your own health and take action to help yourself are important aspects of psychosocial health.

Mental Health: The Thinking You

The term **mental health** is often used to describe the "thinking" or "rational" part of psychosocial health. It is defined as the successful performance of mental function and results in productive activities, fulfilling relationships, and the ability to cope with life's challenges. Mental health plays a role in the way we think, communicate, express emotion, and feel about ourselves. A mentally healthy person has the intellectual ability to sort through information, messages, and life events, to attach meaning, and to respond appropriately.

A mentally healthy person is likely to respond to life's challenges constructively. For example, suppose you spend your spring break with friends on the beaches of Mexico, knowing that you have a major term paper due on the first day back from vacation. The night before the paper is due, you quickly throw it together. Rather than falling off the deep end and blaming the instructor if you get a D on the paper, as a mentally healthy student you would accept responsibility for the choices you made, learn from mistakes, and plan differently next time.

When mentally healthy individuals realize that they are getting into trouble with classes, relationships, and life in general, they know when they are still okay and when they are starting to slide. Knowing when to seek help, talk to a trusted friend, or take time out for rest and regrouping are all part of healthy adapting and coping.

Emotional Health: The Feeling You

The term **emotional health** is often used interchangeably with *mental health.* Although the two are closely intertwined, emotional health more accurately refers to the feeling, or subjective, side of psychosocial health that includes emotional reactions to life. **Emotions** are intensified feelings or complex patterns of feelings that we experience on a regular basis. Love, hate, frustration, anxiety, and joy are only a few of the many emotions we feel.

Emotionally healthy people usually respond appropriately to upsetting events. Rather than respond in an extreme fashion or behave inconsistently or offensively, they are able to express their feelings, communicate with others, and show emotions in appropriate ways. Have you ever seen someone react with extreme anger by shouting or punching a wall? Ex-lovers who become jealous of new relationships and who then damage cars or property are classic examples of people exhibiting unhealthy and dangerous emotional reactions. Such violent responses and emotional volatility have become a problem of epidemic proportions in the United States.

Emotional health also affects *social health.* People who feel hostile, withdrawn, or moody may become socially isolated.[4] Because they are not much fun to be around, their friends may avoid them at the very time they are most in need of emotional support. For students, a more immediate concern is the impact of emotional trauma on academic performance. Have you ever tried to study for an exam after a fight with a close friend or family member? Emotional turmoil may seriously affect your ability to think, reason, and act rationally. Many otherwise rational, mentally healthy people do ridiculous things when they are going through a major emotional upset. Mental functioning and emotional responses are intricately connected.

mental health The thinking part of psychosocial health; includes your values, attitudes, and beliefs.
emotional health The feeling part of psychosocial health; includes your emotional reactions to life.
emotions Intensified feelings or complex patterns of feelings we constantly experience.
social health Aspect of psychosocial health that includes interactions with others, ability to use social supports, and ability to adapt to various situations.

Social Health: Interactions with Others

Social health, an important part of the broader concept of psychosocial health, includes your interactions with others on an individual and group basis, your ability to use social resources and support in times of need, and your ability to adapt to a variety of social situations. Socially healthy individuals have a wide range of interactions with family, friends, and acquaintances and are able to have a healthy interaction with an intimate partner. Typically, socially healthy individuals are able to listen, express themselves, form healthy attachments, act in socially acceptable and responsible ways, and find the best fit for themselves in society. Numerous studies have documented the importance of positive relationships with family members, friends, and one's significant other in overall well-being and healthy longevity.[5]

Social bonds reflect the level of closeness and attachment that we develop with individuals. They provide intimacy, feelings of belonging, opportunities for giving and receiving nurturance, reassurance of one's worth, assistance and guidance, and advice. Social bonds take multiple forms, the most common of which are social support and community engagements.

social bonds Degree and nature of interpersonal contacts.
social support Network of people and services with whom you share ties and from whom you get support.
spiritual health The aspect of psychosocial health that relates to having a sense of meaning and purpose to one's life, as well as a feeling of connection with others and with nature.

The concept of **social support** is more complex than many people realize. In general, it refers to the networks of people and services with whom and which we interact and share social connections. These ties can provide *tangible support,* such as babysitting services or money to help pay the bills, or *intangible support,* such as encouraging you to share intimate thoughts. Sometimes, support can be felt as perceiving that someone would be there for us in a crisis. Generally, the closer and the higher the quality of the social bond, the more likely a person is to ask for and receive social support. For example, if your car broke down on a dark country road in the middle of the night, whom could you call for help and know that they would do everything possible to get there? Common descriptions of strong social support include the following:[6]

- Being cared for and loved, with shared intimacy
- Being esteemed and valued; having a sense of self-worth
- Sharing companionship, communication, and mutual obligations with others; having a sense of belonging
- Having "informational" support—access to information, advice, community services, and guidance from others

Social health also reflects the way we react to others. In its most extreme forms, a lack of social health may be represented by aggressive acts of prejudice toward other individuals or groups.

Spiritual Health: An Inner Quest for Well-Being

Although mental health and emotional health are key factors in overall psychosocial functioning, it is possible to be mentally and emotionally healthy and still not achieve optimal well-being. What is missing? For many people, the difficult-to-describe element that gives meaning to life is the spiritual dimension.

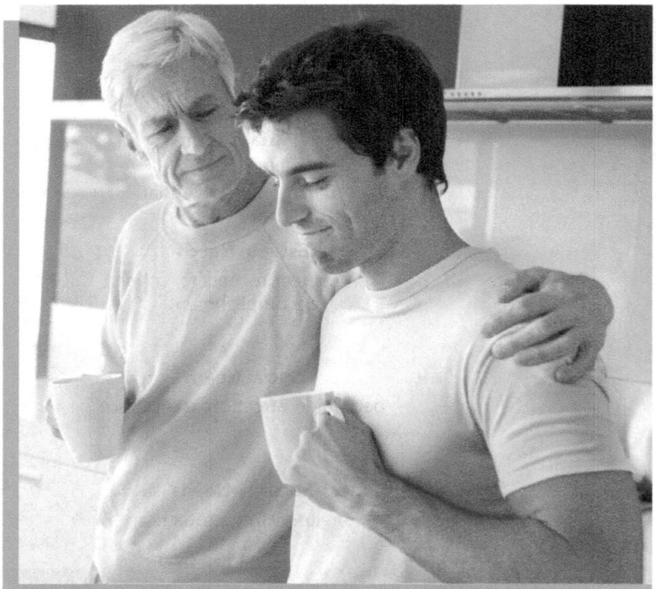

Pascal Broze/AGE Fotostock

How do others influence my psychosocial health?

Support from family and friends is a vital component of your social health. Your general sense of well-being can be strongly affected by the positive or negative nature of your social bonds.

According to the National Center for Complementary and Alternative Medicine, *Spirituality* is broader than religion and is defined as an individual's sense of purpose and meaning in life; it goes beyond material values.[7] Spirituality may be practiced in many ways, including religion; however, religion does not have to be part of a spiritual person's life. **Spiritual health** refers to the sense of belonging to something greater than the purely physical or personal dimensions of existence. For some, this unifying force is nature; for others, it is a feeling of connection to other people; for still others, the unifying force is a god or other higher power.

On a day-to-day basis, many of us focus on acquiring material possessions and satisfying basic needs. But there comes a point when we discover that material possessions do not automatically bring happiness or a sense of self-worth. As we develop into spiritually healthy beings, we recognize our identity as unique individuals and gain a better appreciation of our strengths and shortcomings and our place in the universe.

Factors Influencing Psychosocial Health

Most of our mental, emotional, and social reactions to life are a direct outcome of our experiences and social and cultural expectations. Our psychosocial health is based, in part, on how we perceive life experiences.

Skills for Behavior Change

Build Your Self-Esteem

* Pay attention to your own needs and wants. Listen to what your body, mind, and heart are telling you.
* Take good care of yourself. Eat healthy foods, get plenty of sleep, exercise, and plan fun activities for yourself.
* Take time to do things you enjoy. Make a list of things that make you happy and do something from that list every day.
* Do something that you have been putting off, such as cleaning out your closet or paying a bill that you've been ignoring, to give yourself sense of accomplishment.
* Give yourself rewards. Acknowledge that you are a great person by rewarding yourself occasionally.
* Spend time with people who make you feel good about yourself. Avoid people who treat you badly or make you feel bad about yourself.
* Display or keep close by items that you like and that remind you of your achievements, your friends, or special times.
* Take advantage of any opportunity to learn something new—you'll feel better about yourself and be more productive.
* Do something nice for another person. There is no greater way to feel better about yourself than to help someone in need.

The Family

Families have a significant influence on psychosocial development. Children raised in healthy, nurturing, happy families are more likely to become well-adjusted, productive adults. Children raised in **dysfunctional families,** in which there is violence; negative behavior; distrust; anger; dietary deprivation; drug abuse; parental discord; or sexual, physical, or emotional abuse, may have a harder time adapting to life and run an increased risk of psychosocial problems. In dysfunctional families, love, security, and unconditional trust are so lacking that children often become confused and psychologically bruised. Yet, not all people raised in dysfunctional families become psychosocially unhealthy, and not all children from healthy environments become well adjusted. Obviously, more factors are involved in our "process of becoming" than just our family.

The Macro Environment

Although isolated negative events may do little damage to psychosocial health, persistent stressors, uncertainties, and threats can cause significant problems. Drugs, neighborhood crime and threats to safety, injury, school failure, unemployment, financial problems, natural disasters, and a host of other bad things can happen to good people. But it is believed that certain protective factors, such as having a positive role model in the midst of chaos, or certain positive personality traits can help children from even the worst environments remain healthy and well adjusted. They are often more resilient in the face of adversity and are more likely to have the resources to cope more effectively.

Another important influence is access to health services and programs designed to enhance psychosocial health. Attending a support group or seeing a trained therapist is often a crucial first step in prevention and intervention efforts. Memberships in church groups, athletics, or other socially bonding situations can also help a person feel connected and supported. Individuals from poor socioeconomic environments who cannot afford professional help and who don't have community and social networks of support, often find it difficult to secure help in improving their psychosocial health.

Self-Efficacy and Self-Esteem

During our formative years, successes and failures in school, athletics, friendships, intimate relationships, our jobs, and every other aspect of life subtly shape our beliefs about our own personal worth and abilities. These beliefs are internal influences on our psychosocial health.

Self-efficacy describes a person's belief about whether he or she can successfully engage in and execute a specific behavior. **Self-esteem** refers to one's sense of self-respect or self-worth. It can be defined as one's evaluation of oneself and one's personal worth as an individual. People with a high sense of self-efficacy and self-esteem tend to express a positive outlook on life. People with low self-esteem may demean themselves and doubt their ability to succeed.

Our self-esteem is a result of the relationships we have with our parents and family during our formative years; with our friends as we grow older; with our significant others as we form intimate relationships; and with our teachers, coworkers, and others throughout our lives. How can you build up your self-esteem? The **Skills for Behavior Change** box on this page suggests small things you can do every day that can significantly impact the way you feel about yourself.

dysfunctional families Families in which there is violence; physical, emotional, or sexual abuse; parental discord; or other negative family interactions.
self-efficacy Belief in one's own ability to perform a task successfully.
self-esteem Sense of self-respect or self-worth.
learned helplessness Pattern of responding to situations by giving up because of repeated failure in the past.

Learned Helplessness versus Learned Optimism

Psychologist Martin Seligman has proposed that people who continually experience failure may develop a pattern of responding known as **learned helplessness,** in which they give up and fail to take any action to help themselves. Seligman

what do you think?

What impact has your family had on your psychosocial health? ● Are you primarily an optimist or a pessimist? Why do you think you have this outlook? ● Do you ever struggle with low self-esteem or feelings of helplessness?

ascribes this response in part to society's tendency toward victimology, blaming one's problems on other people and circumstances.[8] Although viewing ourselves as victims may make us feel better temporarily, it does not address the underlying causes of a problem. Ultimately, it can erode self-efficacy and foster learned helplessness by making us feel that we cannot do anything to improve the situation.

Today, many people have developed self-help programs that utilize elements of Seligman's principle of **learned optimism.** Foundational to these self-help programs is the thought that just as we learn to be helpless, so can we teach ourselves to be optimistic. By changing our self-talk, examining our reactions and the way we assess what happens to us in life, and blocking negative thoughts, we can "unlearn" negative thought processes that have become habitual. Some programs practice "positive affirmations" with clients, teaching them the sometimes difficult task of learning to write and/or verbalize positive things about themselves. Often we are our own worst critics, and taking praise from others and learning to be kinder to ourselves are difficult.

learned optimism Teaching oneself to think positively.

Personality

Your personality is the unique mix of characteristics that distinguish you from others. Heredity, environment, culture, and experience influence how each person develops. Personality determines how we react to the challenges of life, interpret our feelings, and resolve conflicts.

Most of the recent schools of psychosocial theory promote the idea that we have the power not only to understand our behavior, but also to change it and thus mold our own personalities. Although much has been written about the importance of a healthy personality, there is little consensus on what that concept really means. In general, people who possess the following traits often appear to be psychosocially healthy:[9]

- **Extroversion,** the ability to adapt to a social situation and demonstrate assertiveness as well as power or interpersonal involvement
- **Agreeableness,** the ability to conform, be likable, and demonstrate friendly compliance as well as love
- **Openness to experience,** the willingness to demonstrate curiosity and independence (also referred to as inquiring intellect)
- **Emotional stability,** the ability to maintain social control
- **Conscientiousness,** the qualities of being dependable and demonstrating self-control, discipline, and a need to achieve
- **Resiliency,** the ability to adapt to change and stressful events in healthy and flexible ways

Life Span and Maturity

Our temperaments change as we move through life, as illustrated by the extreme emotions that many young teens experience. Most of us learn to control our emotions as we advance toward adulthood.

75% **of the general U.S. population is estimated to be extroverted, as measured by the Myers–Briggs Type Indicator personality test.**

The college years mark a critical transition period for young adults as they move away from families and establish themselves as independent adults. The transition to independence will be easier for those who have successfully accomplished earlier developmental tasks, such as learning how to solve problems, make and evaluate decisions, define and adhere to personal values, and establish both casual and intimate relationships. People who have not fulfilled these earlier tasks may find their lives interrupted by recurrent "crises" left over from earlier stages. For example, if they did not learn to trust others in childhood, they may have difficulty establishing intimate relationships as adults.

Strategies to Enhance Psychosocial Health

As we have seen, psychosocial health involves four dimensions. Attaining self-fulfillment is a lifelong, conscious process that involves enhancing each of these components. Strategies include building self-efficacy and self-esteem, understanding and controlling emotions, maintaining support networks, and learning to solve problems and make decisions.

Ed Bock/Corbis

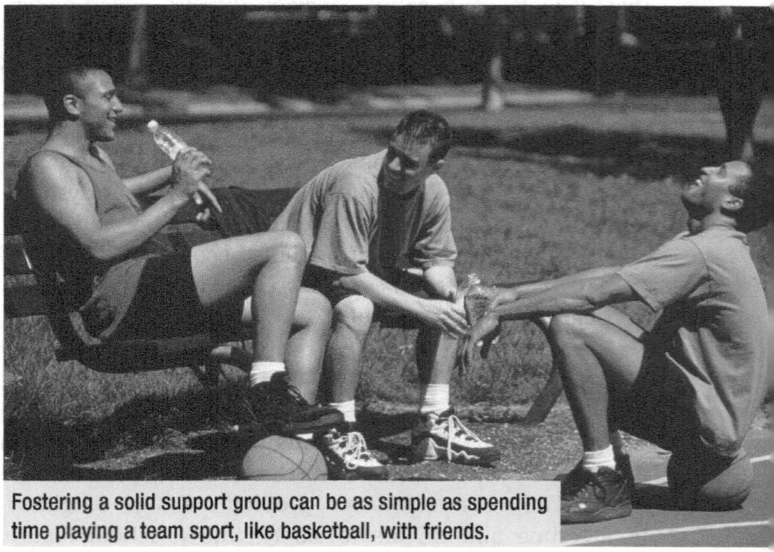

Fostering a solid support group can be as simple as spending time playing a team sport, like basketball, with friends.

- **Find a support group.** A support group of peers who share your values can make you feel good about yourself and encourage you to take an honest look at your actions and choices. Keeping in contact with old friends and important family members can provide a foundation of unconditional love that will help you through life's transitions.
- **Complete required tasks.** A good way to boost your sense of self-efficacy is to learn new skills and develop a history of success. Most college campuses provide study groups and learning centers that can help you manage time, develop study skills, and prepare for tests.
- **Form realistic expectations.** If you expect perfect grades, a steady stream of Saturday-night dates, and the perfect job, you may be setting yourself up for failure. Assess your current resources and the direction in which you are heading. Set small, incremental goals that you can actually meet.
- **Make time for you.** Taking time to enjoy yourself is another way to boost your self-esteem and psychosocial health. View a new activity as something to look forward to and an opportunity to have fun. Anticipate and focus on the fun things you have to look forward to each day.
- **Maintain physical health through exercise.** Regular exercise fosters a sense of well-being. A growing body of research supports the role of exercise in improved mental health.
- **Examine problems and seek help when necessary.** Knowing when to seek help from friends, support groups, family, or professionals is another important factor in boosting self-esteem. Sometimes you can handle life's problems alone; at other times, you need assistance.
- **Get adequate sleep.** Getting enough sleep on a daily basis is a key factor in physical and psychosocial health. Not only do our bodies need to rest to conserve energy for our daily activities, but we also need to restore supplies of many of the neurotransmitters that we use up during our waking hours.

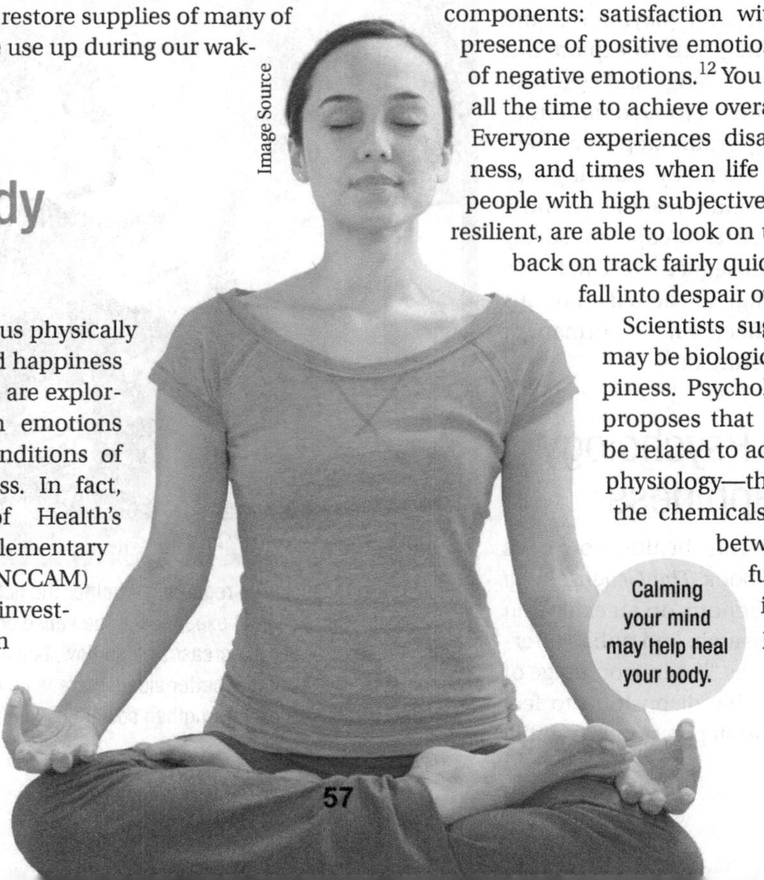

Image Source

Calming your mind may help heal your body.

The Mind–Body Connection

Can negative emotions make us physically ill? Can positive emotions and happiness help us stay well? Researchers are exploring the interaction between emotions and health, especially in conditions of uncontrolled, persistent stress. In fact, the National Institutes of Health's National Center for Complementary and Alternative Medicine (NCCAM) and other organizations are investing more and more dollars in large research projects designed to explore the link between mind and body.

At the core of the mind–body connection is the study of **psychoneuroimmunology (PNI),** or how the brain and behavior affect the body's immune system. The science of PNI focuses on the relationship between emotions, psychosocial factors, the central nervous system, the immune system, and disease and illness.

Happiness and Health

One area of study that appears to be particularly promising in enhancing physical health is happiness—defined as a kind of placeholder for several positive states in which individuals actively embrace the world around them.[10] In examining the characteristics of happy people, scientists have found that this emotion can have a profound impact on the body. Happiness, or related mental states like hopefulness, optimism, and contentment, appears to reduce the risk or limit the severity of cardiovascular disease, pulmonary disease, diabetes, hypertension, colds, and other infections. Laughter can promote increases in heart and respiration rates and can reduce levels of stress hormones in much the same way as light exercise. For this reason, it has been promoted as a possible risk reducer for people with hypertension and other forms of cardiovascular disease.[11]

psychoneuroimmunology (PNI) The science that examines the relationship between the brain and behavior and how this affects the body's immune system.

subjective well-being An uplifting feeling of inner peace.

Subjective well-being refers to that uplifting feeling of inner peace or an overall "feel-good" state, which includes happiness. Subjective well-being is defined by three central components: satisfaction with present life, relative presence of positive emotions, and relative absence of negative emotions.[12] You do not have to be happy all the time to achieve overall subjective well-being. Everyone experiences disappointments, unhappiness, and times when life seems unfair. However, people with high subjective well-being are typically resilient, are able to look on the positive side and get back on track fairly quickly, and are less likely to fall into despair over setbacks.

Scientists suggest that some people may be biologically predisposed to happiness. Psychologist Richard Davidson proposes that happiness may, in part, be related to actual differences in brain physiology—that *neurotransmitters,* the chemicals that transfer messages between neurons, may function more efficiently in happy people.[13] Other psychologists suggest that we can develop happiness by practicing positive psychological actions.[14]

Whereas positive emotions appear to benefit physical health, evidence is accumulating that negative emotions can impair it. Studies of widowed and divorced people reveal below-normal immune-system functioning and higher rates of illness and death than among married people. Other studies have shown unusually high rates of cancer among depressed people.[15] Some researchers suggest that people who are divorced, widowed, or depressed are more likely to drink and smoke, use drugs, eat and sleep poorly, and be sedentary—all of which may affect the immune system. In fact, the immune system changes measured in studies of the mind–body connection are relatively small. The health consequences of such minute changes are difficult to gauge, and researchers continue to seek the answer to this question.[16]

Does Laughter Enhance Health? Do you remember the last time you laughed so hard that you cried? Remember how relaxed you felt afterward? Scientists are just beginning to understand the role of humor in our lives and health. For example, researchers have found that stressed-out people with a strong sense of humor become less depressed and anxious than those whose sense of humor is less well developed. Couples who reminisce and laugh about positive shared experiences have more stable, lasting relationships, while students who use humor as a coping mechanism report that it predisposes them to a positive mood.[17]

Learning to laugh puts more joy into everyday experiences and increases the likelihood that fun-loving people will keep company with us. Psychologist Barbara Fredrickson argues that positive emotions such as joy, interest, and contentment serve valuable life functions.[18] Joy is associated with playfulness and creativity. Interest encourages us to explore our world, which enhances knowledge and cognitive ability. Contentment allows us to savor and integrate experiences, an important step in achieving mindfulness and insight. By building our physical, social, and mental resources, these positive feelings empower us to cope effectively with life's challenges. Subsequent research has demonstrated that although the actual emotions may be transient, their effects can be permanent and provide lifelong enrichment.[19]

Using Positive Psychology to Enhance Happiness

If happiness is good for your health, how does one "get happy"? In his book *The Geography of Bliss,* author Eric Weiner reports on an explosion in happiness writings, research, and public interest. He defines happiness as "the mirror image of depression. . . . It is a stable disposition to feel good in the same way that depression is a stable disposition to feel sad or melancholy."[20] The emerging discipline of *positive psychology* focuses on helping us achieve the happiness we desire, find meaning in life, build our character strengths, and in general approach life from a more "positivistic" perspective.[21] Though this body of research is still in its early stages, several key aspects have emerged. You can implement the following strategies to enhance happiness and employ a more positive outlook on life:[22]

- **Develop gratitude.** Gratitude is a sense of thankfulness and appreciation for the good things in your life as well as for life's lessons. In one study, Seligman required individuals to write down three positive occurrences that happened each day for 1 week, then write an answer to the question, "Why did this good thing happen?" Try this yourself for 1 week.
- **Use capitalization.** Capitalization refers to the process by which we focus on the good things that happen to us and share those things with others. Research in this area indicates that telling others about a positive experience increases the positive emotion associated with the event and prolongs the good feelings.
- **Know when to say when.** Researchers have found that people who are always trying to do their absolute best and are not meeting their own high expectations may be more prone to depression, frustration, anxiety, and other problems. Find a level of achievement that you will be satisfied with, make sure it is realistic, and stick to it.
- **Grow a signature strength.** Traits such as wisdom, courage, humanity, hope, vitality, curiosity, and love are all considered virtues one should work hard to develop. These

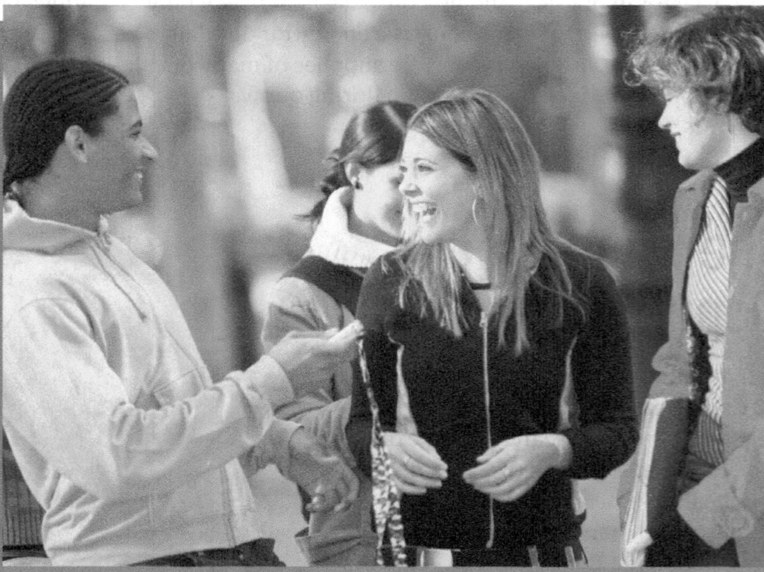

Randy Faris/Corbis

Is laughter really the best medicine?

Research is inconclusive regarding whether the act of laughing actually improves your health, but we've all experienced the sense of well-being that a good laugh can bring. Whether or not it increases blood flow, boosts immune response, lowers blood sugar levels, or facilitates better sleep, there is no doubting that sharing laughter and fun with others can strengthen social ties and bring joy to your everyday life.

strengths are believed to be among the most important to one's overall health.

When Psychosocial Health Deteriorates

57.7 million

U.S. adults suffer from a diagnosable mental disorder in any given year.

Sometimes circumstances overwhelm us to such a degree that we need outside assistance to help us get back on track toward healthful living. Abusive relationships, stress, anxiety, loneliness, financial upheavals, and other traumatic events can sap our spirits, causing us to turn inward or to act in ways that are outside what might be considered normal. Chemical imbalances, drug interactions, trauma, neurological disruptions, and other physical problems also may contribute to these behaviors. **Mental illnesses** are disorders that disrupt thinking, feeling, moods, and behaviors and cause a varying degree of impaired functioning in daily life. They are believed to be caused by life events in some cases and by biochemical or brain dysfunction in others.[23] As with physical disease, mental illnesses can range from mild to severe and exact a heavy toll on the quality of life, both for people with the illnesses and for those who come in contact with them.

Mental disorders are common in the United States and worldwide. An estimated 26.2 percent of Americans aged 18 and older—about 1 in 4 adults—suffer from a diagnosable mental disorder in a given year. This translates to 57.7 million people. Out of these, about 6 percent, or 1 in 17, suffer from a serious mental illness requiring close monitoring, residential care in many instances, and medication. Mental disorders are the leading cause of disability in the United States and Canada for people aged 15 to 44. Nearly half (45 percent) of those with any mental disorder meet criteria for two or more disorders at the same time.[24] In the United States, mental disorders are diagnosed based on the American Psychiatric Association's *Diagnostic and Statistical Manual of Mental Disorders,* Fourth Edition, Text Revision *(DSM-IV-TR).*

Mental Health Threats to College Students

Today's students face increasing threats from difficulties in relationships, anxiety, depression, sexual assaults, pressures to take drugs, and a swirling morass of social and environmental problems. The pressures to succeed in an increasingly fast-paced and depersonalized environment often result in significant mental health problems for students. According to a recent American College Health Association survey of students from across the United States, 18.2 percent had been diagnosed with depression at some time in their lives.[25] Figure 4 shows more results from this survey. The **Health Headlines** box on the next page highlights one growing mental health concern among young adults, attention deficit/hyperactivity disorder.

mental illnesses Disorders that disrupt thinking, feeling, moods, and behaviors and that impair daily functioning.

Although there are many types of mental illness, we will focus here on those most likely to be experienced by large numbers of college students. For information about other disorders, consult the websites at the end of this chapter, or ask your instructor for local resources.

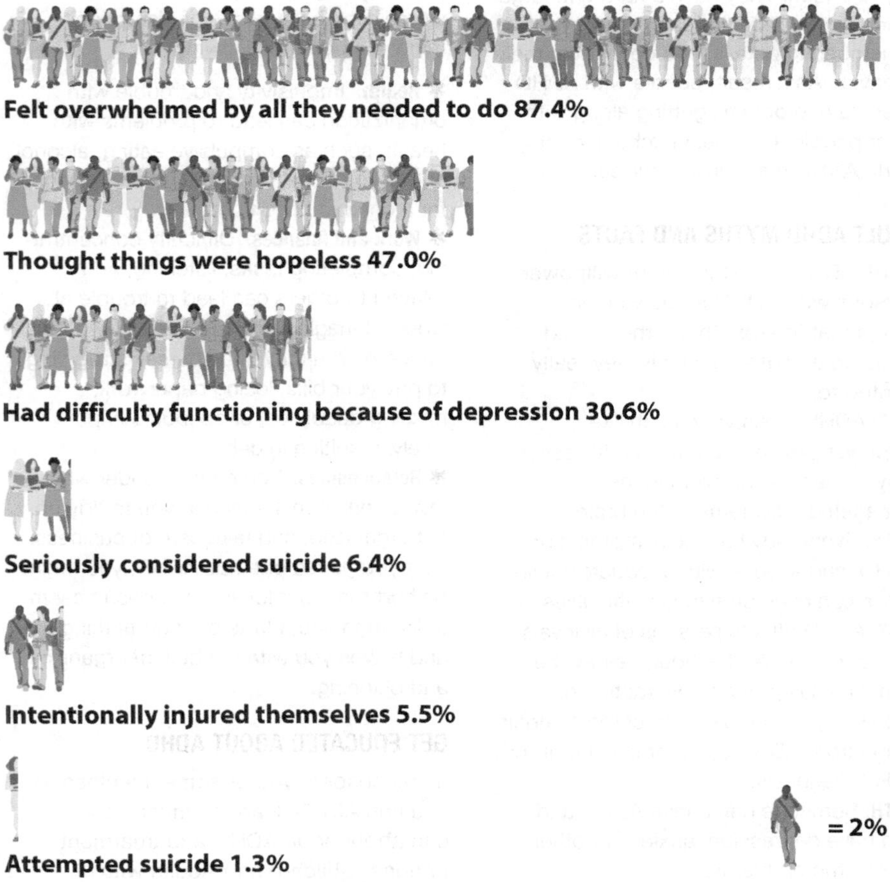

FIGURE 4 **Mental Health Concerns of American College Students, Past 12 Months**

Source: Data are from American College Health Association (ACHA), *ACHA-National College Health Assessment II, Reference Group Data Report, Fall 2008.* (Baltimore: ACHA, 2009).

Health Headlines

WHEN ADULTS HAVE ADHD

Attention deficit/hyperactivity disorder (ADHD) is a common neurobehavioral disorder that affects 5 to 8 percent of school-aged children. In as many as 60 percent of cases, symptoms persist into adulthood. In any given year, 4.1 percent of adults are identified as having ADHD.

People with ADHD are hyperactive or distracted most of the time. Even when they try to concentrate, they find it hard to pay attention. They have a hard time organizing things, listening to instructions, remembering details, and controlling their behavior. As a result, people with ADHD often have problems getting along with other people at home, at school, or at work. ADHD may run in families.

ADULT ADHD MYTHS AND FACTS

MYTH: ADHD is just a lack of willpower. Persons with ADHD focus well on things that interest them; they could focus on any other tasks if they really wanted to.
FACT: ADHD looks very much like a willpower problem, but it isn't. It's essentially a chemical problem in the management systems of the brain.
MYTH: Everybody has the symptoms of ADHD, and anyone with adequate intelligence can overcome these difficulties.
FACT: ADHD affects persons of all levels of intelligence. And although everyone sometimes is prone to distraction or impulsivity, only those with chronic impairments from ADHD symptoms warrant an ADHD diagnosis.
MYTH: Someone can't have ADHD and also have depression, anxiety, or other psychiatric problems.
FACT: A person with ADHD is six times more likely to have another psychiatric or learning disorder than most other people. ADHD usually overlaps with other disorders.
MYTH: Unless you have been diagnosed with ADHD as a child, you can't have it as an adult.
FACT: Many adults struggle all their lives with unrecognized ADHD impairments. They haven't received help because they assumed that their chronic difficulties, like depression or anxiety, were caused by other impairments that did not respond to usual treatment.

EFFECTS OF ADULT ADHD

Left untreated, ADHD can disrupt everything from your career to your relationships and financial stability. Although most of us sometimes have challenges in these areas, the persistent chaos and disorganization of ADHD can make managing the problems worse and worse. Some key areas of disruption might include the following:

* **Health.** Impulsivity and trouble with organization can lead to problems with health, such as compulsive eating, alcohol and drug abuse, or forgetting medication for a chronic condition.
* **Work and finances.** Difficulty concentrating, completing tasks, listening, and relating to others can lead to trouble at work. Managing finances also may be a concern. You may find yourself struggling to pay your bills, losing paperwork, missing deadlines, or spending impulsively, resulting in debt.
* **Relationships.** You might wonder why loved ones constantly nag you to tidy up, get organized, and take care of business. Or if your loved one has ADHD, you might be hurt that your loved one doesn't seem to listen to you, blurts out hurtful things, and leaves you with the bulk of organizing and planning.

GET EDUCATED ABOUT ADHD

If you suspect you or someone close to you has ADHD, learn as much as you can about adult ADHD and treatment options. Children and Adults with Attention-Deficit Hyperactivity Disorder (CHADD) is a good source of information and support (www.chadd.org). Adult ADHD can be a challenge to diagnose, as there is no simple test for it. Many symptoms of ADHD overlap with other conditions, and ADHD often occurs concurrently with other conditions, such as depression or anxiety disorders. To ensure that you have the best treatment plan, secure a diagnosis and treatment plan from a qualified professional with experience in ADHD.

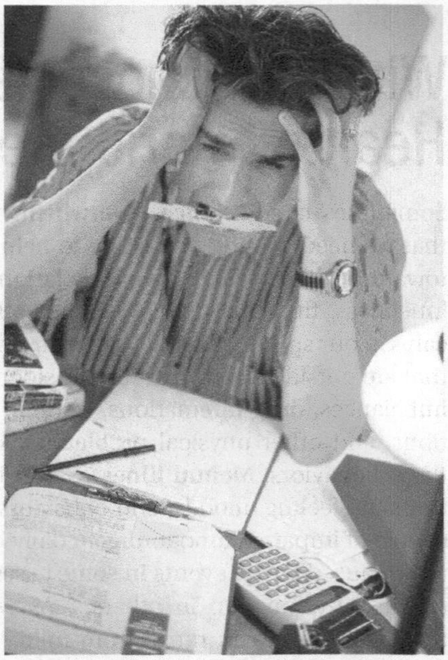
Photolibrary.com

Disorder and chaos can be headaches for us all, but ADHD sufferers may find them insurmountable obstacles.

Sources: Centers for Disease Control and Prevention, "Attention-Deficit Hyperactivity Disorder," www.cdc.gov/ncbddd/adhd, accessed March 8, 2009; National Institute of Mental Health, "The Numbers Count," www.nimh.nih.gov/health/publications/the-numbers-count-mental-disorders-in-america/index.shtml, 2008; H. R. Searight, J. M. Burke, and F. Rottnek, "Adult ADHD: Evaluation and Treatment in Family Medicine," *American Family Physician* 62, no. 9 (2000): 2091–92; J. Saisan, J. Jaffe, T. de Benedictis, M. Smith, and R. O. Segal, "Adult ADD/ADHD: Signs, Symptoms, Effects, and Getting Help," Helpguide.org, updated March 2009, www.helpguide.org/mental/adhd_add_adult_symptoms.htm; T. Brown, *Attention Deficit Disorder: The Unfocused Mind in Children and Adults* (New Haven, CT: Yale University Press, 2005).

Mood Disorders

30 years old is the median age of onset for mood disorders.

Chronic mood disorders are disorders that affect how you feel, such as persistent sadness or feelings of euphoria. They include depression, dysthymia, bipolar disorder, and seasonal affective disorder. In any given year, approximately 10 percent of Americans aged 18 or older—or 20.9 million people—suffer from a mood disorder.[26]

Depressive disorders are the most common mood disorders. The president of the American Psychological Association once remarked, "Depression has been called the common cold of psychological disturbances, which underscores its prevalence, but trivializes its impact."[27] Each year, depression affects approximately 14.8 million American adults, or about 7 percent of the U.S. population, and it is the leading cause of disability in the United States for people aged 15 to 44.[28] These numbers may reflect just the tip of the iceberg when it comes to determining how many people suffer from depression. Many more are misdiagnosed or underdiagnosed, are not receiving treatment, or are not treated with the right combinations of therapy.[29] Some people experience one bout of depression and never have problems again, but others suffer recurrences throughout their lives. Stressful life events are often catalysts for these recurrences.

Depressive Disorders

Sometimes life throws us down the proverbial stairs. We experience loss, pain, disappointment, and frustration, and we can be left feeling beaten and bruised. How do we know whether those emotions are really signs of a **major depressive disorder**? It's important to note that true depressive disorders are not the same as having a bad day or feeling down after a negative experience. It also isn't something that can be willed or wished away, or just a matter of learning to "grow a thicker skin." True depressive disorders are characterized by a combination of symptoms that interfere with work, study, sleep, eating, relationships, and enjoyment of life. Symptoms can last for weeks, months, or years and vary in intensity.[30]

Sadness and despair are the main symptoms of depression. Other common signs include the following:

- Loss of motivation or interest in pleasurable activities
- Preoccupation with failures and inadequacies; concern over what others are thinking
- Difficulty concentrating; indecisiveness; memory lapses
- Loss of sex drive or interest in close interactions with others
- Fatigue and loss of energy; slow reactions
- Sleeping too much or too little; insomnia
- Feeling agitated, worthless, or hopeless
- Withdrawal from friends and family
- Diminished or increased appetite
- Significant weight loss or weight gain
- Recurring thoughts that life isn't worth living; thoughts of death or suicide

Although most people only think of major depression when they think of depression, many people suffer from **dysthymic disorder,** a less severe syndrome of chronic, mild depression. Dysthymia can be harder to recognize than major depression. Dysthymic individuals may appear to function okay, but they may lack energy or may fatigue easily; be short-tempered, overly pessimistic, and ornery; or just not quite feel up to par without having any really overt symptoms. People with dysthymia may cycle into major depression over time. For a diagnosis, symptoms must persist for at least 2 years in adults (1 year in children). This disorder affects approximately 1.5 percent of the U.S. population aged 18 and older in a given year, or about 3.3 million American adults.[31]

Another type of depressive mood disorder is **bipolar disorder,** also called *manic depression.* People with bipolar disorder often have severe mood swings, ranging from extreme highs (mania) to extreme lows (depression). Sometimes these swings are dramatic and rapid; other times they are slow and gradual. When in the manic phase, people may be overactive, talkative, and have tons of energy; in the depressed phase, they may experience some or all of the typical major depressive symptoms.

Although the exact cause of bipolar disorder is unknown, biological, genetic, and environmental factors, such as drug abuse and stressful or psychologically traumatic events, seem to be involved in triggering episodes of the illness. Once diagnosed, persons with bipolar disorder have several counseling and pharmaceutical options, and most will be able to live a healthy, functional life while being treated.

An estimated 6 percent of Americans suffer from another form of depression called **seasonal affective disorder (SAD),** and an additional 14 percent experience a milder form of the illness known as the *winter blues.* SAD strikes during the winter months and is associated with reduced exposure to sunlight. People with SAD suffer from irritability, apathy, carbohydrate craving and weight gain, increased sleep time, and general sadness. Several factors are implicated in SAD development, including disruption in the body's natural circadian rhythms and changes in levels of the hormone melatonin and the brain chemical serotonin.[32]

The most beneficial treatment for SAD is light therapy, in which patients are exposed to lamps that simulate sunlight. Eighty percent of patients experience relief from their symptoms within 4 days. Other treatments for SAD include diet change (eating more complex carbohydrates), increased

chronic mood disorder Experience of persistent emotional states, such as sadness, despair, and hopelessness.

major depressive disorder Severe depression that entails chronic mood disorder, physical effects such as sleep disturbance and exhaustion, and mental effects such as the inability to concentrate.

dysthymic disorder A less severe type of depression than major depressive disorder that is milder, chronic, harder to recognize, and often characterized by fatigue, pessimism, or a short temper.

bipolar disorder Form of mood disorder characterized by alternating mania and depression.

seasonal affective disorder (SAD) A type of depression that occurs in the winter months, when sunlight levels are low.

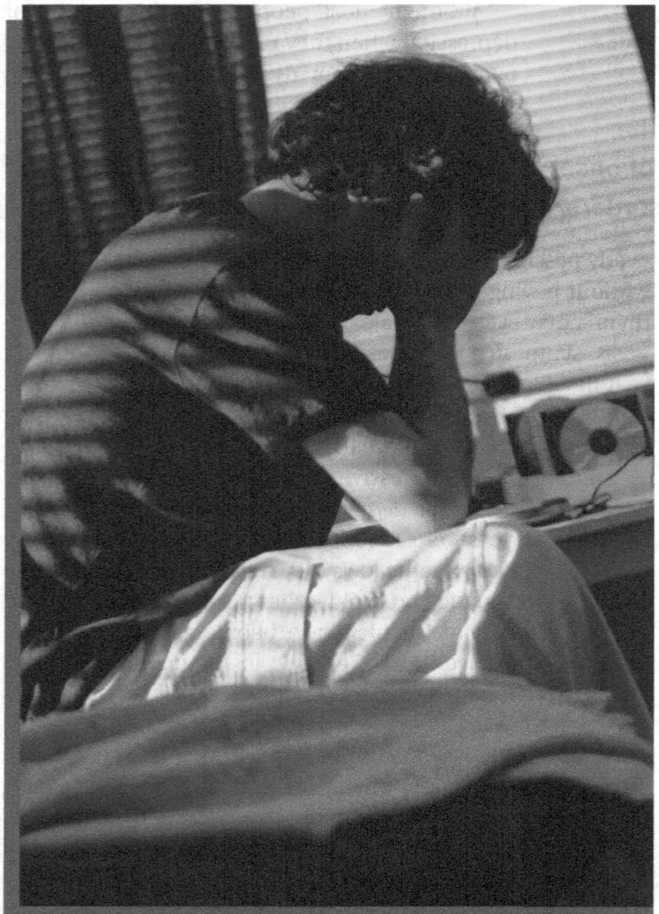

Comstock/Jupiter Images

What are the symptoms of depression?

There is more to depression than simply feeling blue. When a person is clinically depressed, he finds it difficult to function, sometimes struggling just to get out of bed in the morning or to follow a conversation.

exercise, stress-management techniques, sleep restriction (limiting the number of hours slept in a 24-hour period), psychotherapy, and prescription medications.

Causes of Depressive Disorders Depressive disorders are caused by the interaction between biology, learned behavioral responses, cognitive factors, environment, and situational triggers and stressors. The biology of mood disorders is related to individual levels of brain chemicals called *neurotransmitters.* Some types of depression, such as bipolar disorder, appear to have a genetic component and to run in families. People who have low self-esteem, who consistently view themselves and the world with pessimism, or who are readily overwhelmed by stress are prone to depression. Depression can also be triggered by a serious loss, difficult relationships, financial problems, and pressure to get good grades or succeed in athletics. In recent years, researchers have shown that changes in the body's physical health can be accompanied by mental changes, particularly depression. Stroke, heart attack, cancer, Parkinson's disease, problems with chronic pain, type 2 diabetes, certain medications, alcohol, hormonal disorders, and a wide range of afflictions can cause you to become depressed, frustrated, and angry. When this happens, recovery is often more difficult. A person who feels exhausted and defeated may lack the will to fight illness and do what is necessary to optimize recovery.

Depression in College Students Mental health problems, particularly depression, have gained increased recognition as major obstacles to success and healthy adjustment on campuses throughout the country. Students who have weak communication skills; who find that college isn't what they expected; or who find that people they've known seem different, causing them to lose their "lifeboats" in a sea of strangers, often have difficulties. Stressors such as anxiety over relationships, pressure to get good grades and win social acceptance, abuse of alcohol and other drugs, poor diet, and lack of sleep can create a toxic cocktail that can overwhelm even the most resilient students.

The National College Health Assessment found that over a 6-year period, from 2002 to 2008, the number of students who reported "having been diagnosed with depression" increased from 11 percent to 15 percent. Predictably, stress and depression are among students' top five impediments to academic success.[33] See the **Health Today** box on the next page for information on another, often related, psychological disorder of growing concern among young people—self-mutilation.

International students are particularly vulnerable to depression and other mental health concerns. Being far from home without the security of family and friends can exacerbate problems and make coping difficult. Most campuses have counseling centers, cultural centers, and other services available; however, many students do not use them because of persistent stigma about going to a counselor.

Depression in Women Women are almost twice as likely as men to experience depression. Hormonal changes related to the menstrual cycle, pregnancy, miscarriage, postpartum period, premenopause, and menopause may be factors in this increased rate.[34] Additionally, women face various stressors in their lives related to multiple responsibilities—work, child-rearing, single parenthood, household work, and caring for older parents—at rates that are higher than those of men. New research indicates that women have more difficulties obtaining restorative sleep, which may contribute to these problems.[35]

Researchers have observed gender differences in coping strategies (responses to certain events or stimuli) and have proposed that some women's strategies make them more vulnerable to depression. Presented with a list of things people do when depressed, college students were asked to indicate how likely they were to engage in each behavior. Men were

HEALTH Today: Cutting through the Pain

When some people are unable to deal with the pain, pressure, and stress they experience in everyday life, they may resort to self-injury in order to cope. *Self-injury,* also termed *self-mutilation, self-harm,* or *nonsuicidal self-injury* (NSSI), is the act of deliberately harming one's body in an attempt to cope with overwhelming negative emotions. Self-injury is a coping mechanism; it is not an attempt at suicide.

The most common method of self-harm is cutting (with razors, glass, knives, or other sharp objects). Other methods include burning, bruising, excessive nail biting, breaking bones, pulling out hair, and embedding sharp objects under the skin. Seventy-five percent of those who harm themselves do so in more than one way.

Researchers estimate that between 2 and 8 million Americans have engaged in self-harm at some point in their lives and the prevalence of NSSI in college students is reported between 17 and 38 percent. Many people who inflict self-harm suffer from larger mental health conditions and have experienced sexual, physical, or emotional abuse as children or adults. Self-harm is also commonly associated with mental illnesses such as borderline personality disorder, depression, anxiety disorders, substance abuse disorders, post-traumatic stress disorder, and eating disorders.

Signs of self-injury include multiple scars, current cuts and abrasions, and implausible explanations for wounds and ongoing injuries. A self-injurer may attempt to conceal scars and injuries by wearing long sleeves and pants. Other symptoms can include difficulty handling anger, social withdrawal, sensitivity to rejection, or body alienation. If you or someone you know is engaging in self-injury, seek professional help. Treatment is challenging; not only must the self-injurious behavior be stopped, but the sufferer must learn to recognize and manage the feelings that triggered the behavior.

Recovering cutters use some of the following steps in their treatment:

1. Start by being aware of feelings and situations that trigger your urge to cut.
2. Identify a plan of what you can do instead of cutting when you feel the urge.
3. Create a list of alternatives, including:
   * Things that might distract you
   * Things that might soothe and calm you
   * Things that might help you express the pain and deep emotion
   * Things that might help release physical tension and distress
   * Things that might help you feel supported and connected
   * Things that might substitute for the cutting sensation

For more information, try these resources: American Self-Harm Information Clearinghouse, www.selfinjury.org; S. A. F. E. Alternatives, www.selfinjury.com; and Self-Injury Support, www.sisupport.org.

Previously, self-injury was thought to be more common in females, but recent research indicates that rates are generally the same for men and women.

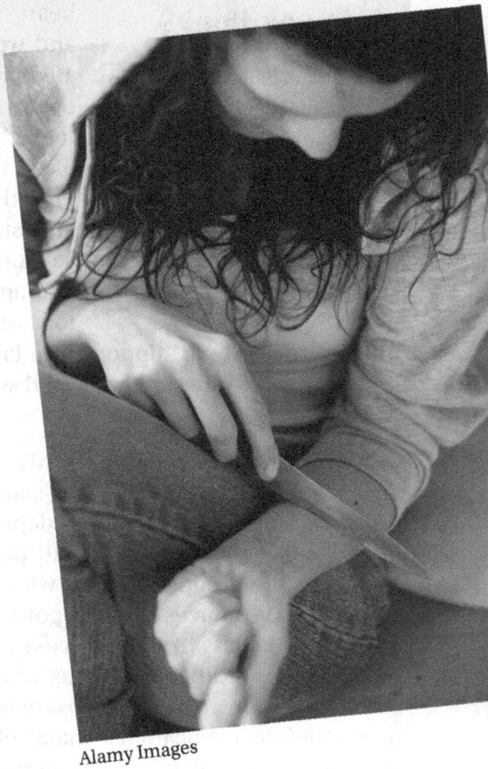

Alamy Images

Sources: J. Bennett, "Why She Cuts," *Newsweek* Web Exclusive, December 29, 2008, www.newsweek.com/id/177135; M. J. Prinstein, "Introduction to the Special Section on Suicide and Nonsuicidal Self-Injury: A Review of Unique Challenges and Important Directions for Self-Injury Science," *Journal of Consulting and Clinical Psychology* 76, no. 1 (2008): 1–8; Mayo Clinic Staff, "Self-Injury/Cutting," August 2, 2008, www.mayoclinic.com.

more likely to assert, "I avoid thinking of reasons why I am depressed," "I do something physical," or "I play sports." Women were more likely to answer, "I try to determine why I am depressed," "I talk to other people about my feelings," and "I cry to relieve the tension." In other words, the men tried to distract themselves from a depressed mood, whereas the women focused on it. If focusing obsessively on negative feelings intensifies these feelings, women who do this may predispose themselves to depression. This hypothesis has not been directly tested recently, but some early supporting evidence suggested its validity.[36]

Depression in Men Six million men in the United States are currently in treatment for depression, and countless others suffering from the disorder are untreated. Depression in men is often masked by alcohol or drug abuse or by the socially acceptable habit of working excessively long hours. Typically, depressed men present not as hopeless and helpless, but as irritable, angry, and discouraged, often personifying a "tough guy" image. Men are less likely to admit they are depressed, and doctors are less likely to suspect it, based on what men report during doctor's visits.[37]

Depression can also affect men's physical health differently from women's. Although depression is associated with an increased risk of coronary heart disease in both men and women, it is also associated with a higher risk of death by heart disease in men.[38] Men are also more likely to act on suicidal feelings than women, and they are usually more successful at suicide as well; suicide rates among depressed men are four times those of women.[39] Encouragement and support from families and friends may help men recognize symptoms and seek treatment.

> **what do you think?**
>
> Why do you think that women experience more depression than men? ● Do you think men and women cope with depression differently? In what ways? ● Who is most likely to seek counseling for depression on campus? Why?

Depression in Older Adults Many adults in their middle and older years are emotionally stable and lead active and satisfying lives. However, when depression does occur, it is often undiagnosed or untreated, particularly in people in lower income groups or those who do not have access to community resources and supports or medications. Older adults may be less likely to discuss feelings of sadness, loss, helplessness, or other symptoms, or they may attribute their own depression to aging. Those who have insurance may take multiple medications, many of which may result in depression symptoms and may increase their risks for related problems.

Depression in Children Today, depression in children is an increasingly reported phenomenon, with shocking cases of suicide and other outcomes in children as young as 4 and 5 years old. Depressed children may pretend to be sick, refuse to go to school, sleep incessantly, engage in self-mutilation, get into trouble with drugs or alcohol, and attempt suicide. Parents of children who are depressed may find it difficult to find therapists trained in working with depressed children or physicians skilled in determining which adult antidepressants may be best for children.

Treating Mood Disorders

The best treatment for mood disorders involves determining the person's type and degree of depression and its possible causes. Both psychotherapeutic and pharmacological modes of treatment are recommended for clinical (severe and prolonged) depression. Drugs often relieve the symptoms of depression, such as loss of sleep or appetite, and psychotherapy can be equally helpful by improving the ability to function.

Psychotherapeutic Treatment In some cases, psychotherapy alone may be the most successful treatment. The two most common psychotherapeutic treatments for depression are cognitive therapy and interpersonal therapy.

Cognitive therapy helps a patient look at life rationally and correct habitually pessimistic thought patterns. It focuses on the present rather than analyzing a patient's past. To pull a person out of depression, cognitive therapists usually need 6 to 18 months of weekly sessions that include reasoning and behavioral exercises.

Interpersonal therapy, sometimes combined with cognitive therapy, also addresses the present but focuses on correcting chronic relationship problems. Interpersonal therapists focus on patients' relationships with their families and other people.

Pharmacological Treatment Antidepressent drugs offer several options for treating depressive disorders. The most common antidepressants are the selective serotonin reuptake inhibitors (SSRIs), but in the past few years new drugs with different methods of action have also become available. **Table 1** lists some of the common psychiatric medications prescribed to treat depression as well as those commonly prescribed to treat the other mental disorders discussed later in this chapter.

The potency, dosage, and side effects of each drug vary greatly. Antidepressants should be prescribed only after a thorough psychological and physiological examination. In 2004, the U.S. Food and Drug Administration asked the makers of antidepressant drugs to add a warning to the labels advising that patients taking these drugs be monitored for "worsening depression or the emergence of suicidality." Recent reports of suicidal tendencies among some youth taking antidepressants have stirred controversy over the use of these drugs in certain populations.[40]

If your doctor suggests an antidepressant, ask these questions first:

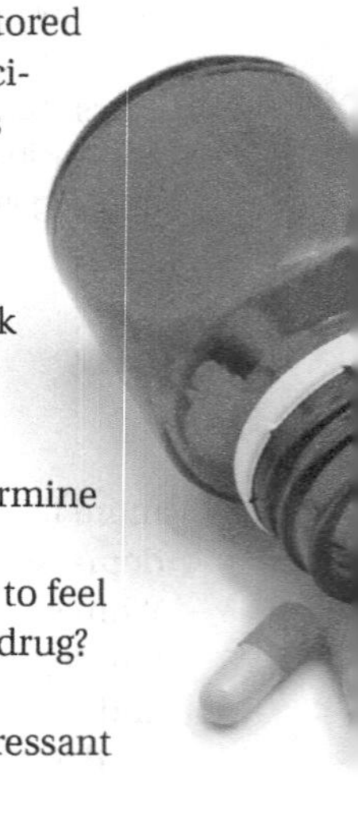

- What biological indicators are you using to determine whether I really need this drug?
- What is the action of this drug? When will I start to feel the benefits? What are the side effects of using this drug? What happens if I stop taking it?
- What is your rationale for selecting this antidepressant over others?

TABLE 1

Types of Medications Used to Treat Various Mental Illnesses

Antidepressants	**Used to treat depression, panic disorders, anxiety disorders**	
Selective serotonin reuptake inhibitors (SSRIs)	*Examples:* fluoxetine (Prozac), paroxetine (Paxil, Seroxat), escitalopram (Lexapro, Esipram), citalopram (Celexa), and sertraline (Zoloft)	The current standard drug treatment for depression; also frequently prescribed for anxiety disorders
Noradrenergic and specific serotonergic antidepressants (NaSSAs)	*Examples:* mirtazapine (Avanza, Zispin, Remeron)	Reportedly have fewer sexual dysfunction side effects than SSRIs
Serotonin-norepinephrine reuptake inhibitors (SNRIs)	*Examples:* venlafaxine (Effexor), duloxetine (Cymbalta)	Also sometimes prescribed for ADHD
Norepinephrine-dopamine reuptake inhibitors (NDRIs)	*Examples:* bupropion (Wellbutrin, Zyban)	Also used in smoking cessation; fewer weight gain or sexual dysfunction side effects than SSRIs
Tricyclic antidepressants (TCAs)	*Examples:* imipramine, amitriptyline, nortriptyline, and desipramine	Negative side effects; usually used as a 2nd or 3rd line of treatment when other medications prove ineffective
Monoamine oxidase inhibitors (MAOIs)	*Examples:* phenelzine (Nardil), tranylcypromine (Parnate), and isocarboxazid (Marplan)	Dangerous interactions with many other drugs and substances in food; generally no longer prescribed
Anxiolytics (antianxiety drugs)	**Used to treat anxiety disorders including OCD, GAD, panic disorders, phobias, PTSD**	
Benzodiazepines	*Examples:* lorazepam (Ativan), clonazepam (Klonopin), alprazolam (Xanax), diazepam (Valium)	Short-term relief, sometimes taken on an as-needed basis; dangerous interactions with alcohol; possible to develop tolerance or dependence
Serotonin 1A agonists	*Examples:* buspirone (BuSpar)	Longer-term relief; must be taken for at least 2 weeks to achieve antianxiety effects
Mood stabilizers	**Used to treat bipolar disorder, schizophrenia**	
Lithium	*Examples:* lithium carbonate	Drug most commonly used to treat bipolar disorder; blood levels must be closely monitored to determine proper dosage and avoid toxic effects
Anticonvulsants	*Examples:* valproic acid (Depakene), divalproex sodium (Depakote), sodium valproate (Depacon)	Used more frequently for acute mania than for long-term maintenance of bipolar disorder
Antipsychotics (neuroleptics)	**Used to treat schizophrenia, mania, bipolar disorder**	
Atypical antipsychotics	*Examples:* clozapine (Clozaril), risperidone (Risperdal)	First line of treatment for schizophrenia; fewer adverse effects than earlier antipsychotics
First-generation antipsychotics	*Examples:* haloperidol (Haldol), chlorpromazine (Thorazine)	Earliest forms of antipsychotics; unpleasant side effects such as tremor and muscle stiffness
Stimulants	**Used to treat ADHD, narcolepsy**	
Methylphenidate	*Brand names:* Ritalin, Metadate, Concerta	Can lead to tolerance and dependence; frequently abused for both performance enhancement and recreational use
Amphetamines	*Examples:* amphetamine (Adderall), dextroamphetamine (Dexedrine, Dextrostat), pemoline (Cylert)	Can lead to tolerance and dependence; frequently abused for both performance enhancement and recreational use

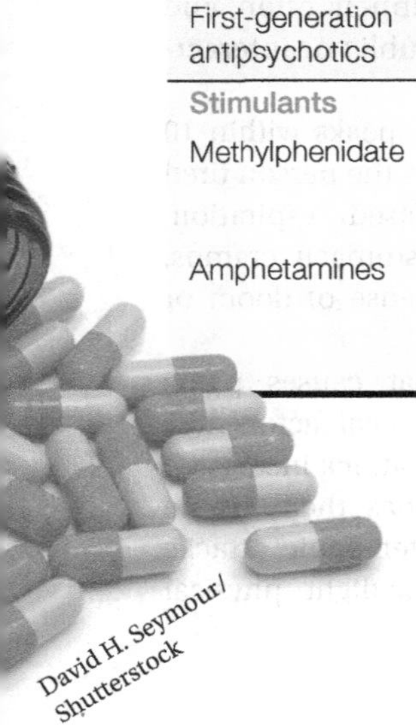

David H. Seymour/ Shutterstock

- How long can I be on this medication without significant risk to my health?
- How will you follow up or monitor the levels of this drug in my body? How often will I need to be checked?

You may not feel the therapeutic effects of antidepressants for several weeks, so patience is important. Also, you should not stop taking medication all at once, but rather gradually, and always under your doctor's supervision. In addition, be careful when taking antidepressant medications to avoid alcohol or illicit drug consumption, as the interactions between these drugs can be life threatening.

Anxiety Disorders

Anxiety disorders include generalized anxiety disorder, panic disorders, obsessive-compulsive disorder, and phobic disorders. They are characterized by persistent feelings of threat and worry. Consider John Madden, former head coach of the Oakland Raiders and a true "man's man," who outfitted his own bus and, for many years, drove every weekend across the country to serve as commentator on NFL football games. What was the reason behind this exhausting driving schedule? Madden is terrified of getting on a plane.

anxiety disorders Disorders characterized by persistent feelings of threat and worry in coping with everyday problems.
generalized anxiety disorder (GAD) A constant sense of worry that may cause restlessness, difficulty in concentrating, tension, and other symptoms.
panic attack Severe anxiety reaction in which a particular situation, often for unknown reasons, causes terror.

Anxiety disorders are the number-one mental health problem in the United States, affecting over 40 million people aged 18 to 54 each year, or about 18 percent of all adults.[41] Anxiety is also a leading mental health problem among adolescents, affecting 13 million youngsters aged 9 to 17. Costs associated with an overly anxious populace are growing rapidly; conservative estimates cite nearly $50 billion a year spent in doctors' bills and workplace losses in America. These numbers don't begin to address the human costs incurred when a person is too fearful to leave the house or talk to anyone outside the immediate family.

Generalized Anxiety Disorder

One common form of anxiety disorder, **generalized anxiety disorder (GAD),** is severe enough to significantly interfere with daily life. Generally, the person with GAD is a consummate worrier who develops a debilitating level of anxiety. Often multiple sources of worry exist, and it is hard to pinpoint the root cause of the anxiety. To be diagnosed with GAD, one must exhibit at least three of the following symptoms for more days than not during a 6-month period: restlessness or feeling keyed up or on edge; being easily fatigued; difficulty concentrating or mind going blank; irritability; muscle tension; and sleep disturbances.[42] Often GAD runs in families and is readily treatable with benzodiazepines such as Librium, Valium, and Xanax, which calm the person for short periods. Individual therapy can be a more effective long-term treatment.

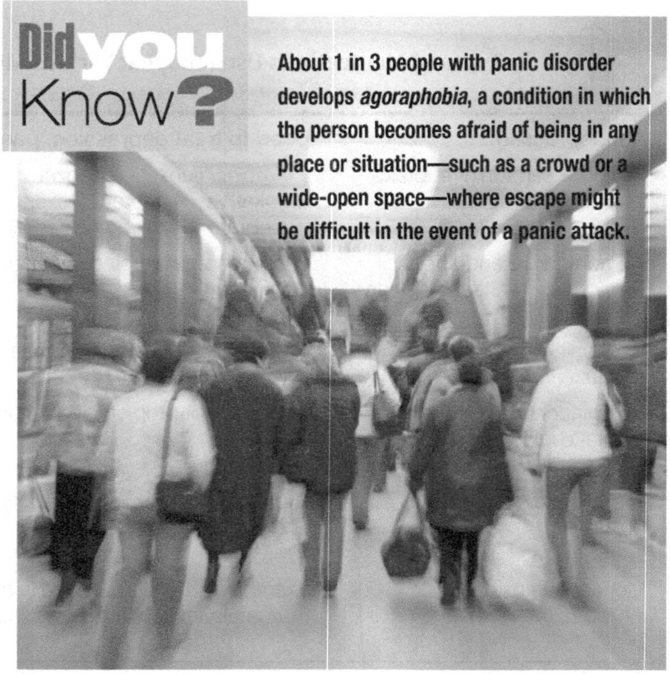

Did you Know?
About 1 in 3 people with panic disorder develops *agoraphobia*, a condition in which the person becomes afraid of being in any place or situation—such as a crowd or a wide-open space—where escape might be difficult in the event of a panic attack.

Losevsky Pavel/Shutterstock

Panic Disorders

Panic disorders are characterized by the occurrence of **panic attacks,** a form of acute anxiety reaction that brings on an intense physical reaction. You may dismiss the feelings as the jitters from too much stress, or the reaction may be so severe that you fear you will have a heart attack and die. Approximately 6 million Americans aged 18 and older experience panic attacks each year, usually in early adulthood. Panic attacks and disorders are increasing in incidence, particularly among young women. Although highly treatable, panic attacks may become debilitating and destructive, particularly if they happen often and cause the person to avoid going out in public or interacting with others.

A panic attack typically starts abruptly, peaks within 10 minutes, lasts about 30 minutes, and leaves the person tired and drained.[43] Symptoms include increased respiration, chills, hot flashes, shortness of breath, stomach cramps, chest pain, difficulty swallowing, and a sense of doom or impending death.

Although researchers aren't sure what causes panic attacks, heredity, stress, and certain biochemical factors may play a role. Your chances of having a panic attack increase if you have a close family member who has them. Some researchers believe that people who suffer panic attacks are experiencing an overreactive fight-or-flight physical response.

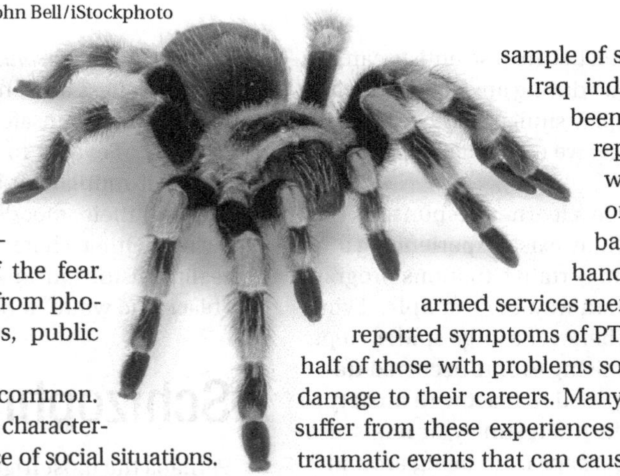
John Bell/iStockphoto

Phobic Disorders

Phobias, or phobic disorders, involve a persistent and irrational fear of a specific object, activity, or situation, often out of proportion to the circumstances. Phobias result in a compelling desire to avoid the source of the fear. About 13 percent of Americans suffer from phobias, such as fear of spiders, snakes, public speaking, and so on.

Social phobias are perhaps the most common. A **social phobia** is an anxiety disorder characterized by the persistent fear and avoidance of social situations. Essentially, the person dreads these situations for fear of being humiliated, embarrassed, or simply looked at. These disorders vary in scope. Some cause difficulty only in specific situations, such as getting up in front of the class to give a report. In more extreme cases, a person avoids all contact with others.

Obsessive-Compulsive Disorder

People who feel compelled to perform rituals over and over again; are fearful of dirt or contamination; have an unnatural concern about order, symmetry, and exactness; or have persistent intrusive thoughts that they can't shake may be suffering from **obsessive-compulsive disorder (OCD).** Approximately 2 million Americans aged 18 or over have OCD.[44] Not to be confused with being a perfectionist, a person with OCD often knows the behaviors are irrational and senseless yet is powerless to stop them. According to the *DSM-IV-TR,* to be diagnosed as OCD, the obsessions must consume more than 1 hour per day and interfere with normal social and/or life activities. Although the exact cause is unknown, genetics, biological abnormalities, learned behaviors, and environmental factors have all been considered. OCD usually begins in adolescence or early adulthood, and the median age of onset is 19.

As with other anxiety-based disorders, medication and cognitive behavioral therapy are often the keys to treatment. Some individuals are given antidepressants, antianxiety drugs, or other drug combinations, which often prevent future attacks. Cognitive therapy can help sufferers recognize and avoid triggers or deal with triggers through meditation, deep breathing, and other relaxation techniques.

Post-Traumatic Stress Disorder

According to the American Psychiatric Association, one-third to one-half of individuals exposed to a traumatic life event will develop some form of psychopathology. In severe cases, an individual may develop **post-traumatic stress disorder (PTSD).** PTSD generally develops within the first hours or days after a traumatic event, but occasionally symptoms do not begin until months or years later.

Often PTSD affects soldiers returning home from war, particularly those who saw friends killed or mangled or who experienced terrible wounds. Responses from a survey given to a sample of service personnel deployed to Iraq indicated that 90 percent had been shot at and a high percentage reported knowing someone who was injured or had been killed, or had killed an enemy combatant. Almost 50 percent had handled dead bodies. This study of armed services members found that one in eight reported symptoms of PTSD.[45] Unfortunately, less than half of those with problems sought help, fearing stigma and damage to their careers. Many of these soldiers continue to suffer from these experiences for decades afterward. Other traumatic events that can cause PTSD include rape or other physical attacks, severe accidents, witnessing a murder or death, being caught in a natural disaster, or terrorist attacks.

Symptoms of PTSD include the following:

- Dissociation, or perceived detachment of the mind from the emotional state or even the body. The person may have a sense of the world as a dreamlike or unreal place and have little memory of the events—a form of dissociative amnesia.
- Acute anxiety or nervousness, in which the person is hyperaroused; may cry easily or experience mood swings; and experience flashbacks, nightmares, and recurrent thoughts or visual images. Some people may sense vague uneasiness or feel like the traumatic event is happening again and again. Others may experience intense physiological reactions, such as shaking or nausea, when something reminds them of the event. In some cases, they may have difficulty returning to areas that remind them of the trauma.

phobia A deep and persistent fear of a specific object, activity, or situation that results in a compelling desire to avoid the source of the fear.

social phobia A phobia characterized by fear and avoidance of social situations.

obsessive-compulsive disorder (OCD) A form of anxiety disorder characterized by recurrent, unwanted thoughts and repetitive behaviors.

post-traumatic stress disorder (PTSD) A collection of symptoms that may occur as a delayed response to a serious trauma.

As our knowledge about this disorder grows, therapies designed to help trauma victims recover are becoming increasingly effective. Schools, communities, and workplaces now routinely bring in crisis experts immediately after a traumatic event to help survivors talk through their feelings and gain support from others. New generations of antianxiety drugs can help individuals who have difficulties. Sleep aids and other options are available to ease short-term symptoms.

Sources of Anxiety Disorders

Because anxiety disorders vary in complexity and degree, scientists have yet to find clear reasons why one person develops them and another doesn't. The following factors are often cited as possible causes.[46]

- **Biology.** Some scientists trace the origin of anxiety to the brain and brain functioning. Using sophisticated positron emission tomography scans (PET scans), scientists can analyze areas of the brain that react during anxiety-producing events. Families appear to display similar brain and physiological reactivity, indicating that we may inherit our tendencies toward anxiety disorders.

- **Environment.** Anxiety can be a learned response. Although genetic tendencies may exist, experiencing a repeated pattern of reacting to certain situations programs the brain to respond in a certain way. For example, if your mother or father screamed whenever a large spider crept into view or if other anxiety-raising events occurred frequently, you might be predisposed to react with anxiety to similar events later in your life. Interestingly, animals also experience such anxieties—perhaps from being around their edgy owners.
- **Social and cultural roles.** Cultural and social roles also may be a factor in risks for anxiety. Because men and women are taught to assume different roles in society (for example, man as protector, woman as victim), women may find it more acceptable to scream, shake, pass out, and otherwise express extreme anxiety. Men, by contrast, may have learned to suppress such anxieties rather than act on them.

Personality Disorders

According to the *DSM-IV-TR,* **personality disorders** are "enduring patterns of inner experience and behavior that deviate markedly from the expectation of the individual's culture and are pervasive and inflexible."[47] Researchers at the National Institutes of Mental Health have found that about 9 percent of adults in the United States have some form of personality disorder as defined by the *DSM-IV-TR.*[48] People who live, work, or are in relationships with individuals suffering from personality disorders often find them to be very challenging and destructive interactions.

Common types of personality disorders include *paranoid personality disorders,* which involve pervasive, unfounded suspicion and mistrust of other people, irrational jealousy, and secretiveness. Persons with this illness have delusions of being persecuted by everyone, from their family members and loved ones to the government. *Narcissistic personality disorders* involve an exaggerated sense of self-importance and self-absorption. Persons with narcissistic personalities are fascinated with themselves and are preoccupied with fantasies of how wonderful they are.[49] Typically they are overly needy and demanding and believe that they are "entitled" to nothing but the best. Most are so self-absorbed that they don't have time to be supportive of anyone else.

personality disorders A class of mental disorders that is characterized by inflexible patterns of thought and beliefs that lead to socially distressing behavior.

schizophrenia A mental illness with biological origins that is characterized by irrational behavior, severe alterations of the senses (hallucinations), and often an inability to function in society.

Borderline personality disorder (BPD) is characterized by impulsiveness and engaging in risky behaviors such as gambling sprees, unsafe sex, use of illicit drugs, and risky driving.[50] Seventy to 80 percent of persons diagnosed with BPD self-mutilate or self-harm.[51] Sufferers have trouble stabilizing their moods and can experience erratic mood swings. Other characteristics of this mental illness include reality distortion and the tendency to see things in only "black and white" terms.

Schizophrenia

Perhaps the most frightening of all psychological disorders is **schizophrenia,** which affects about 1 percent of the U.S. population. Schizophrenia is characterized by alterations of the senses (including auditory and visual hallucinations); the inability to sort out incoming stimuli and make appropriate responses; an altered sense of self; and radical changes in emotions, movements, and behaviors. Typical symptoms of schizophrenia include fluctuating courses of such things as delusional behavior, hallucinations, incoherent and rambling speech, inability to think logically, erratic movement and odd gesturing, and difficulty with normal activities of daily living.[52] The net effect is that such individuals are often regarded by an unknowing society as being "odd;" as such, they have difficulties in social interactions and may withdraw. Contrary to popular belief, schizophrenia is not the same as split personality or multiple personality disorder.

For decades, scientists believed that schizophrenia was an environmentally provoked form of madness. They blamed abnormal family interactions or early childhood traumas. Since the mid-1980s, however, when magnetic resonance imaging (MRI) and positron-emission tomography (PET)

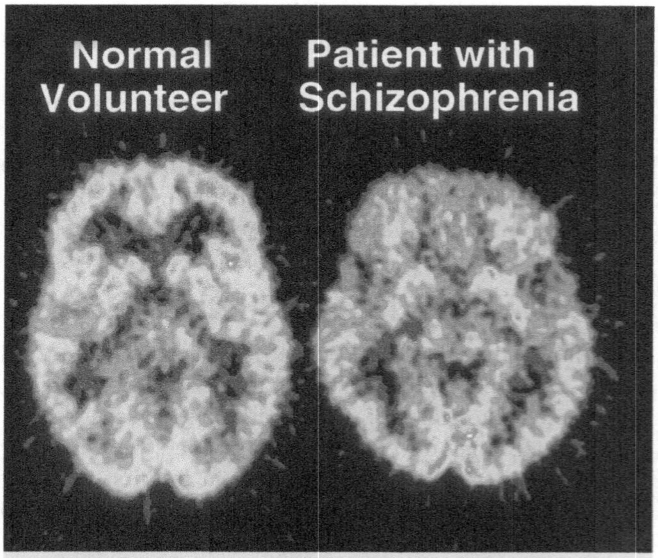

Monte S. Buchsbaum, MD, Mt. Sinai School of Medicine, New York, NY

These brain images reveal significant differences between normal brain activity and that of a person with schizophrenia. Yellow and red identify areas of greatest activity, and blue signifies reduced activity.

allowed us to study brain function more closely, scientists have recognized that schizophrenia is a biological disease of the brain. The brain damage occurs early in life, possibly as early as the second trimester of fetal development. Fetal exposure to toxic substances, infections, or medications have all been studied as possible risks. In addition, possible hereditary links are being explored. Symptoms usually appear in men in their late teens and twenties and in women in their late twenties and early thirties.[53]

90% **of people who kill themselves have a diagnosable mental disorder, most commonly a depressive disorder or a substance abuse disorder.**

Even though environmental theories of the causes of schizophrenia have been discarded in favor of biological ones, a stigma remains attached to the disease. Families of people with schizophrenia frequently experience anger and guilt. They often need information, family counseling, and advice on how to meet the schizophrenic person's needs for shelter, medical care, vocational training, and social interaction.

At present, schizophrenia is treatable but not curable. Treatments usually include some combination of hospitalization, medication, and supportive psychotherapy. Supportive psychotherapy, as opposed to psychoanalysis, can help the patient acquire skills for living in society. With proper medication, public understanding, support of loved ones, and access to therapy, many schizophrenics lead normal lives. In the absence of these forms of assistance and treatment, they may have great difficulty.

Suicide: Giving Up on Life

Each year there are over 32,000 reported suicides in the United States.[54] Experts estimate that there may actually be closer to 100,000 cases; the discrepancy is due to the difficulty in determining the causes of many suspicious deaths. More lives are lost to suicide than to any other single cause except cancer and cardiovascular disease. It is the third leading cause of death for 15- to 24-year-olds and the fourth leading cause of death for 10- to 14-year-olds.[55]

College students are more likely than the general population to attempt suicide; it is the second leading cause of death on college campuses (accidents are the first). The pressures, joys, disappointments, challenges, and changes of the college environment are believed to be partially responsible for the emotional turmoil that can lead a young person to contemplate suicide. However, young adults who choose not to go to college but who are searching for direction in careers, relationships, and other life goals are also at risk. Specific risk factors include a family history of suicide, previous suicide attempts, excessive drug and alcohol use, prolonged depression, financial difficulties, serious illness in oneself or a loved one, and loss of a loved one through death or rejection. Societal pressures often serve as a catalyst.

Recent studies indicate that suicide is the eighth leading cause of death for men and the sixteenth leading cause of death for women. Whether they are more likely to attempt suicide or are more often successful in their attempts, nearly four times as many men die by suicide than women. Overall, firearms, suffocation, and poison are by far the most common methods of suicide. However, men are almost twice as likely as women to commit suicide with firearms, while women are almost three times as likely as men to commit suicide by poisoning.[56]

Warning Signs of Suicide

In most cases, suicide does not occur unpredictably. In fact, 75 to 80 percent of people who commit suicide give a warning of their intentions, though they are not always recognized as such by the people around them. Anyone who expresses a desire to kill himself or herself or who has made an attempt is at risk. Common signs that a person may be contemplating suicide include the following:[57]

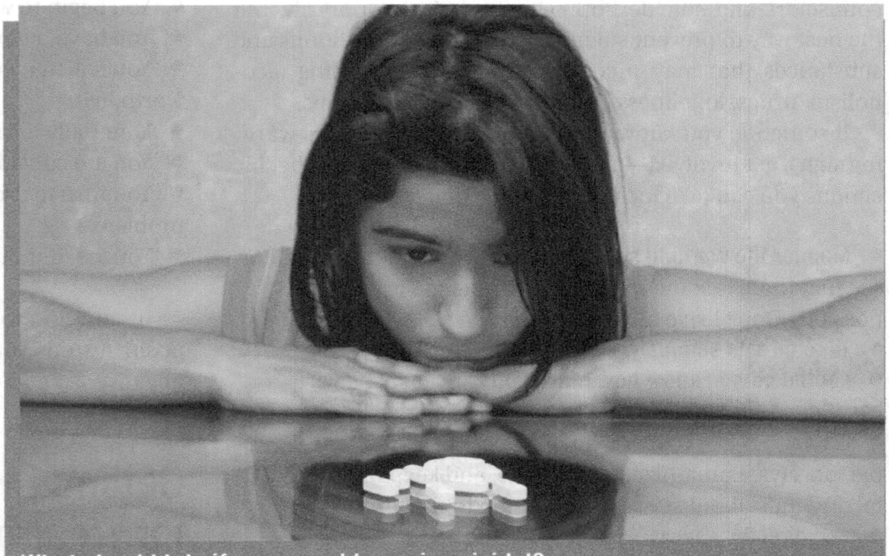

Alamy Images

What should I do if someone I know is suicidal?

If you notice warning signs of suicide in someone you know, it is imperative that you take action. Suicidal people urgently need professional assistance; your willingness to talk to the person about depression and suicide in a nonjudgmental way can be the encouragement he or she needs to seek help. Remember: always take thoughts of or plans for suicide seriously; a life may depend on it.

- Recent loss and a seeming inability to let go of grief
- A history of depression
- Change in personality, such as sadness, withdrawal, irritability, anxiety, tiredness, indecisiveness, apathy
- Change in behavior, such as inability to concentrate, loss of interest in classes or work, unexplained demonstration of happiness following a period of depression
- Sexual dysfunction (such as impotence) or diminished sexual interest
- Expressions of self-hatred, excessive risk taking, or an "I don't care what happens to me" attitude
- Change in sleep patterns or eating habits
- A direct statement about committing suicide, such as, "I might as well end it all"
- An indirect statement, such as, "You won't have to worry about me anymore"
- Final preparations, such as writing a will, repairing poor relationships with family or friends, giving away prized possessions, or writing revealing letters
- A preoccupation with themes of death
- Marked changes in personal appearance

what do you think?

If your roommate showed warning signs of suicide, what action would you take? ● Whom would you contact first? ● Where on campus might your friend get help? ● What if someone in class whom you hardly know gave warning signs of suicide? What would you do then?

Preventing Suicide

Most people who attempt suicide really want to live but see suicide as the only way out of an intolerable situation. Crisis counselors and suicide hotlines may help temporarily, but the best way to prevent suicide is to get rid of conditions and substances that may precipitate attempts, including alcoholism, drugs, loneliness, isolation, and access to guns.

If someone you know threatens suicide or displays warning signs, get involved—ask questions and seek help. Specific actions you can take include the following:[58]

- **Monitor the warning signals.** Keep an eye on the person or see that there is someone around the person as much as possible. Don't leave him or her alone.
- **Take threats seriously.** Don't brush them off.
- **Let the person know how much you care about him or her.** State that you are there to help.
- **Listen.** Try not to discredit or be shocked by what the person says. Empathize, sympathize, and keep the person talking. Talk about stressors and listen to the responses.
- **Ask directly,** "Are you thinking of hurting or killing yourself?"
- **Do not belittle the person's feelings.** Don't say that he or she doesn't really mean it or couldn't succeed at suicide. To some people, these comments offer the challenge of proving you wrong.
- **Help the person think about alternatives to suicide.** Offer to go for help together. Call your local suicide hotline, and use all available community and campus resources. Recommend a counselor or other person to talk to.
- **Tell your friend's spouse, partner, parents, siblings, or counselor.** Do not keep your suspicions to yourself. Don't let a suicidal friend talk you into keeping your discussions confidential. If your friend succeeds in a suicide attempt, you may find that others will question your decision, and you may blame yourself.

Seeking Professional Help for Psychosocial Problems

A physical ailment will readily send most of us to the nearest health professional, but many people view seeking professional help for psychosocial problems as an admission of personal failure. However, increasing numbers of Americans are turning to mental health professionals, and nearly one in five seeks such help. Researchers cite breakdown in support systems, high societal expectations of the individual, and dysfunctional families as three major reasons why more people are asking for assistance than ever before.

Consider seeking help if

- You feel like you need help.
- You experience wild mood swings or inappropriate emotional responses.
- Your fears or feelings of guilt frequently distract your attention.
- You begin to withdraw from others.
- You have hallucinations.
- You feel inadequate or worthless or feel that life is not worth living.
- Your daily life seems to be nothing but repeated crises.
- You are considering suicide.
- You turn to drugs or alcohol to escape from your problems.
- You feel out of control.

In addition to seeking professional help, there are other positive steps you can take now to help pull yourself out of negative thoughts and feelings (see the **Skills for Behavior Change** box).

Getting Evaluated for Treatment

If you are considering treatment for a psychosocial problem, schedule a complete evaluation first. Consult a credentialed health professional for a thorough examination, which should include three parts.

1. **A physical checkup,** which will rule out thyroid disorders, viral infections, and anemia—all of which can result in

depressive-like symptoms—and a neurological check of coordination, reflexes, and balance to rule out brain disorders

2. **A psychiatric history,** which will attempt to trace the course of the apparent disorder, genetic or family factors, and any past treatments

3. **A mental status examination,** which will assess thoughts, speaking processes, and memory, and will include an in-depth interview with tests for other psychiatric symptoms.

Once physical factors have been ruled out, you may decide to consult a professional who specializes in psychosocial health.

Mental Health Professionals

Several types of mental health professionals are available to help you; Table 2 compares several of the most common. When choosing a therapist to work with, the most important criterion is not how many degrees this person has, but whether you feel you can work together. A qualified mental health professional should be willing to answer all your questions during an initial consultation. Questions to ask the therapist and yourself include the following:

- **Can you interview the therapist before starting treatment?** An initial meeting will help you determine whether this person will be a good fit for you.
- **Do you like the therapist as a person?** Can you talk to him or her comfortably?
- **Is the therapist watching the clock or easily distracted?** You should be the main focus of the session.
- **Does the therapist demonstrate professionalism?** Be concerned if your therapist is frequently late or breaks appointments, suggests social interactions outside your therapy sessions, talks inappropriately about himself or herself, has questionable billing practices, or resists releasing you from therapy.
- **Will the therapist help you set your own goals?** A good professional should evaluate your general situation and help you set small goals to work on between sessions. The therapist should not tell you how to help yourself, but rather help you discover the steps.

Remember, in most states, the use of the titles *therapist* and *counselor* are unregulated. Make your choice carefully.

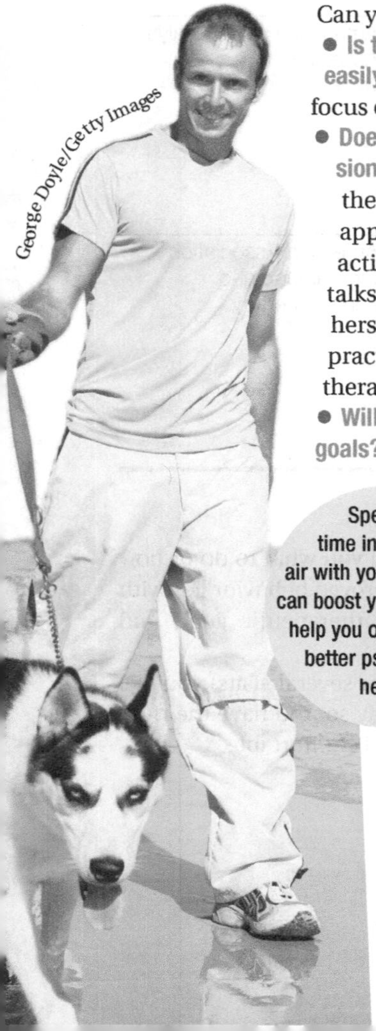

George Doyle/Getty Images

Spending time in the fresh air with your best friend can boost your spirits and help you on the road to better psychosocial health.

Skills for Behavior Change

Dealing with and Defeating Depression

The first step in defeating depression is recognizing it. If you feel you have depression symptoms, setting up an appointment with a counselor is key. Depression is often a biological condition that you can't just get over on your own. Talk therapy, sometimes combined with antidepressant medication, may be necessary to help you reach a place where you are able to play a greater role in getting well. Once you've started along a path of therapy and healing, the following strategies may help you feel better faster.

* Set realistic goals in light of the depression and assume a reasonable amount of responsibility.
* Break large tasks into small ones, set some priorities, and do what you can as you can.
* Try to be with other people and to confide in someone; it is usually better than being alone and secretive.
* Participate in activities that may make you feel better.
* Mild exercise, going to a movie or a ballgame, or participating in religious or social activities may help.
* Take a course in meditation, yoga, tai chi, or some other mind–body practice. These disciplines can help you connect with your inner feelings, release tension, and empty your mind to make room for positive thoughts.
* Expect your mood to improve gradually, not immediately. Feeling better takes time.
* Consider postponing important decisions until the depression has lifted. Before deciding to make a significant transition, change jobs, or get married or divorced, discuss it with others who know you well and have a more objective view of your situation.
* Let your family and friends help you.
* Continue working with your counselor. If you find he or she isn't helpful, look for another one.

What to Expect in Therapy

Many different types of counseling exist, ranging from individual therapy, which involves one-on-one work between therapist and client, to group therapy, in which two or more clients meet with a therapist to discuss problems. The first trip to a therapist can be difficult. Most of us have misconceptions about what therapy is and what it can do. That first visit is a verbal and mental sizing up between you and the therapist. You may not accomplish much in that first hour. If you decide that this professional is not for you, you will at least have learned how to present your problem and what qualities you need in a therapist.

TABLE 2 **Mental Health Professionals**

What are they called?	What kind of training do they have?	What kind of therapy do they do?	Professional association
Psychiatrist	Medical doctor (MD) degree, followed by 4 years of specialized mental health training	As a licensed MD, a psychiatrist can prescribe medications and may have admitting privileges at a local hospital. Some psychiatrists are affiliated with hospitals, while others are in private practice.	American Psychiatric Association www.psych.org
Psychologist	PhD degree in counseling or clinical psychology followed by several years of supervised practice to earn license	Psychologists are trained in various types of therapy, including behavior and insight therapy. Most can conduct both individual and group sessions. They may be trained in certain specialties, such as family counseling or sexual counseling.	American Psychological Association www.apa.org
Clinical/psychiatric social worker	Master's degree in social work (MSW) followed by 2 years of experience in a clinical setting to earn license	Social workers may be trained in certain specialties, such as substance abuse counseling or child counseling. Some social workers are employed in clinics, schools, or agencies; others have private practices.	National Association of Social Workers www.socialworkers.org
Counselor	Master's degree in counseling, psychology, educational psychology, or related human service. Generally must complete at least 2 years of supervised practice before obtaining a license	Many counselors are trained to do individual and group therapy. They often specialize in one type of counseling, such as family, marital, relationship, children, drug, divorce, behavioral, or personal counseling.	American Counseling Association www.counseling.org
Psychoanalyst	Postgraduate degree in psychology or psychiatry (PhD or MD), followed by 8 to 10 years of training in psychoanalysis, which includes undergoing analysis themselves	Psychoanalysis is a form of therapy based on the theories of Freud and his successors. It focuses on patterns of thinking and behavior and the recall of early traumas that have blocked personal growth. Treatment is intensive, lasting 5 to 10 years, with 3 or 4 sessions per week.	American Psychoanalytic Association www.apsa.org
Licensed marriage and family therapist (LMFT)	Master's or doctoral degree in psychology, social work, or counseling, specializing in family and interpersonal dynamics; generally must complete at least 2 years of supervised practice before obtaining a license	LMFTs treat individuals or families in the context of family relationships. Treatment is typically brief (20 sessions or less) and focused on finding solutions to specific relational problems. Some LMFTs work in clinics, schools, or agencies; others have private practices.	American Association for Marriage and Family Therapy www.aamft.org

Before meeting, briefly explain your needs. Ask what the fee is. Arrive on time, wear comfortable clothing, and expect to spend about an hour during your first visit. The therapist will want to take down your history and details about the problems that have brought you to therapy. Answer as honestly as possible. He or she may ask how you feel about aspects of your life. Do not be embarrassed to acknowledge your feelings. It is critical to the success of your treatment that you trust this person enough to be open and honest.

Do not expect the therapist to tell you what to do or how to behave. The responsibility for improved behavior lies with you. Ask if you can set your own therapeutic goals and timetables.

If after your first visit (or even after several visits) you feel you cannot work with this person, say so. You have the right to find a therapist with whom you feel comfortable.

Assess yourself

What Is Your Psychosocial Health Status?

PEARSON myhealthlab

Fill out this assessment online at www.pearsonhighered.com/myhealthlab or www.pearsonhighered.com/donatelle.

Being psychosocially healthy requires both introspection and the willingness to work on areas that need improvement. Begin by completing the following assessment scale. Use it to determine how much each statement describes you. When you're finished, ask someone who is very close to you to take the same test and respond with their perceptions of you. Carefully assess areas where your responses differ from those of your friend or family member. Which areas need some work? Which are in good shape?

	Never	Rarely	Fairly Frequently	Most of the Time	All of the Time
1. My actions and interactions indicate that I am confident in my abilities.	1	2	3	4	5
2. I am quick to blame others for things that go wrong in my life.	1	2	3	4	5
3. I am spontaneous and like to have fun with others.	1	2	3	4	5
4. I am able to give love and affection to others and show my feelings.	1	2	3	4	5
5. I am able to receive love and signs of affection from others without feeling uneasy.	1	2	3	4	5
6. I am generally positive and upbeat about things in my life.	1	2	3	4	5
7. I am cynical and tend to be critical of others.	1	2	3	4	5
8. I have a large group of people whom I consider to be good friends.	1	2	3	4	5
9. I make time for others in my life.	1	2	3	4	5
10. I take time each day for myself for quiet introspection, having fun, or just doing nothing.	1	2	3	4	5
11. I am compulsive and competitive in my actions.	1	2	3	4	5
12. I handle stress well and am seldom upset or stressed out by others.	1	2	3	4	5

	Never	Rarely	Fairly Frequently	Most of the Time	All of the Time
13. I try to look for the good in everyone and every situation before finding fault.	1	2	3	4	5
14. I am comfortable meeting new people and interact well in social settings.	1	2	3	4	5
15. I would rather stay in and watch TV or read than go out with friends or interact with others.	1	2	3	4	5
16. I am flexible and can adapt to most situations, even if I don't like them.	1	2	3	4	5
17. Nature, the environment, and other living things are important aspects of my life.	1	2	3	4	5
18. I think before responding to my emotions.	1	2	3	4	5
19. I am selfish and tend to think of my own needs before those of others.	1	2	3	4	5
20. I am consciously trying to be a "better person."	1	2	3	4	5
21. I like to plan ahead and set realistic goals for myself and others.	1	2	3	4	5
22. I accept others for who they are.	1	2	3	4	5
23. I value diversity and respect others' rights, regardless of culture, race, sexual orientation, religion, or other differences.	1	2	3	4	5

Jon Helgason/iStockphoto

	Never	Rarely	Fairly Frequently	Most of the Time	All of the Time
24. I try to live each day as if it might be my last.	1	2	3	4	5
25. I have a great deal of energy and appreciate the little things in life.	1	2	3	4	5
26. I cope with stress in appropriate ways.	1	2	3	4	5
27. I get enough sleep each day and seldom feel tired.	1	2	3	4	5
28. I have healthy relationships with my family.	1	2	3	4	5
29. I am confident that I can do most things if I put my mind to them.	1	2	3	4	5
30. I respect others' opinions and believe that others should be free to express their opinions, even when they differ from my own.	1	2	3	4	5

Interpreting Your Scores

Look at items 2, 7, 11, 15, and 19. Add up your score for these 5 items and divide by 5. Is your average for these items above or below 3? Did you score a 5 on any of these items? These may indicate areas where your attitudes and patterns of behavior and thought could use improvement. Now look at your scores for the remaining items (there should be 25 items). Total these scores and divide by 25. Is your average above or below 3? On which items did you score a 5? Obviously you're doing well in these areas. Now remove these items from this grouping of 25 (scores of 5), and add up your scores for the remaining items. Then divide your total by the number of items included. Now what is your average?

Do the same for the scores completed by your friend or family member. How do your scores compare? Which ones, if any, are different, and how do they differ? Which areas do you need to work on? What actions can you take now to improve your ratings in these areas?

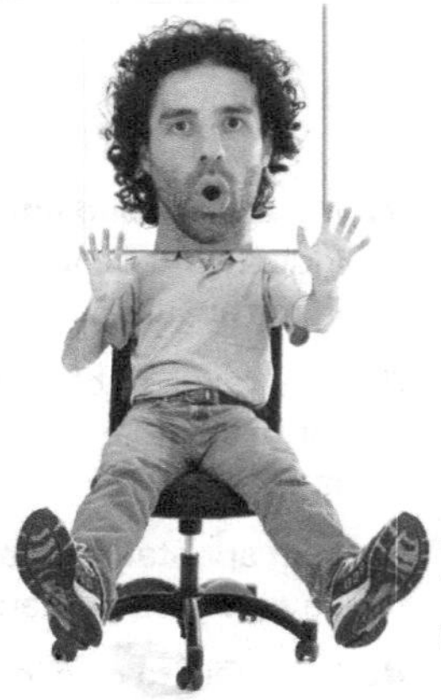

iStockphoto

YOUR PLAN FOR CHANGE

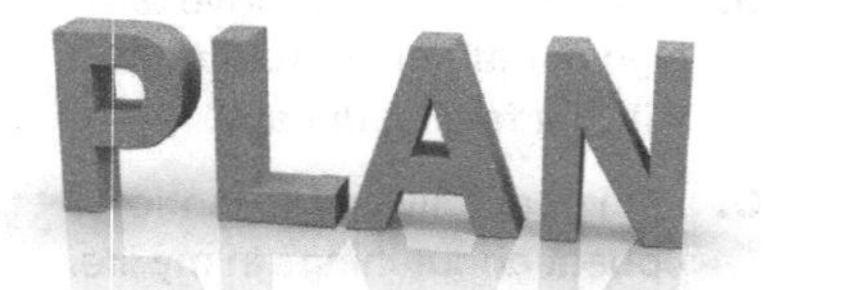

The Assessyourself activity gave you the chance to look at various aspects of your psychosocial health and compare your self-assessment with a friend's perceptions. Now that you have considered these results, you can take steps to change behaviors that may be detrimental to your psychosocial health.

Today, you can:

◯ Develop a plan. Evaluate your behavior and identify patterns and specific things you are doing that negatively affect your psychosocial health. What can you change now? What can you change in the near future?

◯ Start a journal in which you note changes in your mood. Look for trends and think about ways you can change your behavior to address them.

◯ Make a list of the things that bring you joy—friends, family, activities, entertainment, nature. Commit yourself to making more room for these joy-givers in your life.

Within the next 2 weeks, you can:

◯ Visit your campus health center and find out about the counseling services they offer. If you are feeling overwhelmed, depressed, or anxious, make an appointment with a counselor.

◯ Pay attention to the negative thoughts that pop up throughout the day. Note times when you find yourself devaluing or undermining your abilities, and notice when you project negative attitudes on others. Bringing your awareness to these thoughts gives you an opportunity to stop and reevaluate them.

By the end of the semester, you can:

◯ Make a commitment to an ongoing therapeutic practice aimed at improving your psychosocial health. Depending on your current situation, this could mean anything from seeing a counselor or joining a support group to practicing meditation or attending religious services.

◯ Volunteer regularly with a local organization you care about. Focus your energy and gain satisfaction by helping to improve others' lives or the environment.

Summary

* Psychosocial health is a complex phenomenon involving mental, emotional, social, and spiritual health.
* Many factors influence psychosocial health, including life experiences, family, the environment, other people, self-esteem, self-efficacy, and personality. Some of these are modifiable; others are not.
* Developing self-esteem and self-efficacy, making healthy connections, having a positive outlook on life, enhancing your spiritual nature, and getting enough sleep are key to maintaining psychosocial health.
* Happiness is a key factor in determining overall reaction to life's challenges. The mind–body connection is an important link in overall health and well-being.
* Indicators of deteriorating psychosocial health include depression, difficulty sleeping, and emotional volatility. College life is a high-risk time for developing depression because of high stress and pressures for grades, financial problems, and other problems. Identifying symptoms of depression is the first step in treating this disorder.
* Other psychosocial problems are mood disorders, including major depressive disorder, dysthymic disorder, bipolar disorder, and seasonal affective disorder; anxiety disorders, including generalized anxiety disorder, panic attacks, social phobias, obsessive-compulsive disorder, and post-traumatic stress disorder; and personality disorders.
* Schizophrenia is a disorder once believed to be the result of environmental causes. Now brain function studies have shown that it is instead a biological disease of the brain.
* Suicide is a result of negative psychosocial reactions to life. People considering suicide often give warning signs of their intentions. Such people often can be helped.
* Mental health professionals include psychiatrists, psychologists, clinical/psychiatric social workers, counselors, psychoanalysts, and licensed marriage and family therapists. Many therapy methods exist, including group and individual therapy. It is wise to interview a therapist carefully before beginning treatment.

Pop Quiz

1. A person with high self-esteem
   a. possesses feelings of self-respect and self-worth.
   b. believes he or she can successfully engage in a specific behavior.
   c. believes external influences shape one's psychosocial health.
   d. has a high altruistic capacity.
2. All of the following traits have been identified as characterizing psychosocially healthy people *except*
   a. conscientiousness.
   b. introversion.
   c. openness to experience.
   d. agreeableness.
3. Subjective well-being has all of the following components *except*
   a. psychological hardiness.
   b. satisfaction with present life.
   c. relative presence of positive emotions.
   d. relative absence of negative emotions.
4. People who have experienced repeated failures at the same task may eventually give up and quit trying altogether. This pattern of behavior is termed
   a. post-traumatic stress disorder.
   b. learned helplessness.
   c. self-efficacy.
   d. introversion.
5. The term that most accurately refers to the feelings or subjective side of psychosocial health is
   a. social health.
   b. mental health.
   c. emotional health.
   d. spiritual health.
6. Which statement below is false?
   a. One in four adults in the United States suffers from a diagnosable mental disorder in a given year.
   b. Mental disorders are the leading cause of disability in the United States.
   c. Dysthymia is an example of an anxiety disorder.
   d. Bipolar disorder can also be referred to as manic depression.
7. This disorder is characterized by a need to perform rituals over and over again; fear of dirt or contamination; or an unnatural concern with order, symmetry, and exactness.
   a. personality disorder
   b. obsessive-compulsive disorder
   c. phobic disorder
   d. post-traumatic stress disorder
8. What is the number-one mental health problem in the United States?
   a. depression
   b. anxiety disorders
   c. alcohol dependence
   d. schizophrenia
9. Every winter, Stan suffers from irritability, apathy, carbohydrate craving, weight gain, increased sleep time, and sadness. He most likely has
   a. panic disorder.
   b. generalized anxiety disorder.
   c. seasonal affective disorder.
   d. chronic mood disorder.
10. A person with a PhD in counseling psychology and training in various types of therapy is a
    a. psychiatrist.
    b. psychologist.
    c. social worker.
    d. psychoanalyst.

Answers to Chapter Review Questions

1. a; 2. b; 3. a; 4. b; 5. c;
6. c; 7. b; 8. b; 9. c; 10. b

Think about It!

1. What is psychosocial health? What indicates that you are or aren't psychosocially healthy? Why might the college environment provide a challenge to your psychosocial health?
2. Discuss the factors that influence your overall level of psychosocial health. Which factors can you change? Which ones may be more difficult to change?
3. What steps could you take today to improve your psychosocial health? Which steps require long-term effort?
4. Why is laughter therapeutic? How can humor help you better achieve wellness?
5. What factors appear to contribute to psychosocial difficulties and illnesses? Which of the common psychosocial illnesses is likely to affect people in your age group?
6. What are the warning signs of suicide? Of depression? Why is depression so pervasive among young Americans today? Why are some groups more vulnerable to suicide and depression than are others? What would you do if you heard a friend in the cafeteria say to no one in particular that he was going to "do the world a favor and end it all"?
7. Discuss the different types of health professionals and therapies. If you felt depressed about breaking off a long-term relationship, which professional therapy do you think would be most beneficial? Explain your answer. What services does your student health center provide? What fees are charged to students?
8. What psychosocial areas do you need to work on? Which are most important to you, and why? What actions can you take today?

Accessing Your Health on the Internet

The following websites explore further topics and issues related to personal health. For links to the websites below, visit the Companion Website for *Health: The Basics,* Green Edition at www.pearsonhighered.com/donatelle.

1. *American Foundation for Suicide Prevention.* Resources for suicide prevention and support for family and friends of those who have committed suicide. www.afsp.org
2. *American Psychological Association Help Center.* Includes information on psychology at work, the mind–body connection, psychological responses to war, and other topics. http://apahelpcenter.org
3. *Anxiety Disorders Association of America.* Offers links to treatment resources, self-help tools, information on clinical trials, and other information. www.adaa.org
4. *National Alliance on Mental Illness.* A support and advocacy organization of families and friends of people with severe mental illnesses. Over 1,200 state and local affiliates; local branches can often help with finding treatment. www.nami.org
5. *National Institute of Mental Health (NIMH).* Overview of mental health information and new research relating to mental health. www.nimh.nih.gov
6. *Mental Health America.* Works to promote mental health through advocacy, education, research, and services. www.nmha.org
7. *Helpguide.* Resources for improving mental and emotional health as well as specific information on topics such as self-injury, sleep, depressive disorders, and anxiety disorders. www.helpguide.org

References

1. H. Marano, "A Nation of Wimps," *Psychology Today* 37, no. 6 (2004): 58–68.
2. National Institute of Mental Health, National Survey of Counseling Center Directors, 2005.
3. A. H. Maslow, *Motivation and Personality.* 2nd ed. (New York: Harper and Row, 1970).
4. T. M. Chaplin, "Anger, Happiness, and Sadness: Association with Depressive Symptoms in Late Adolescence," *Journal of Youth and Adolescence* 35, no. 6 (2006): 977–86.
5. A. F. Jorm, "Social Networks and Health: It's Time for an Intervention Trial," *Journal of Epidemiology and Community Health* 59 (2005): 537–39; C. Huang, "Elderly Social Support System and Health Status in the Urban and Rural Areas," paper presented at the American Public Health Association Annual Meeting (New Orleans, 2005); C. Alarie, *Impact of Social Support on Women's Health: A Literature Review,* Women's Center of Excellence, www.pwhce.ca/limpactDuSupport.htm; A. Sherman, J. Lansford, and B. Volling, "Sibling Relationships and Best Friendships in Young Adulthood: Warmth, Conflict and Well-Being," *Personal Relationships* 13, no. 2 (2006): 151–65; N. Stevens, "Marriage, Social Integration, and Loneliness in the Second Half of Life," *Research on Aging* 28, no. 2 (2006): 713–29.
6. K. Karren et al., *Mind/Body Health.* 4th ed. (San Francisco: Benjamin Cummings, 2010).
7. NCCAM, "Prayer and Spirituality in Health: Ancient Practices, Modern Science," *CAM at the NIH: Focus on Complementary and Alternative Medicine* 12, no. 1 (2005), available at http://nccam.nih.gov/news/newsletter/pdf/2005winter.pdf. Updated October 2007.
8. M. Seligman and C. Peterson, "Learned Helplessness," in *International Encyclopedia for the Social and Behavioral Sciences,* vol. 13, ed. N. Smelser (New York: Elsevier, 2002), 8583–866.
9. M. Seligman, *Learned Optimism: How to Change Your Mind and Your Life* (New York: Free Press, 1998); J. H. Martin, "Motivation Processes and Performance: The Role of Global and Facet Personality," PhD dissertation, University of North Carolina at Chapel Hill, 2002.
10. M. Lemonick, "The Biology of Joy," *Time* (January 17, 2005): A12–A14; P. Herschberger, "Prescribing Happiness: Positive Psychology and Family Medicine," *Family Medicine* 37, no. 9 (2005): 630–34.
11. J. Kluger, "The Funny Thing about Laughter," *Time* (January 17, 2005): A25–A29.

12. Ibid.
13. R. Davidson et al., "The Privileged Status of Emotion in the Brain," *Proceedings of the National Academy of Sciences of the United States of America* 101, no. 33 (2004): 11915–16.
14. E. Diener and M. E. P. Seligman, "Beyond Money: Toward an Economy of Well-Being," *Psychological Science in the Public Interest* 5 (2004): 1–31; C. Peterson and M. Seligman, *Character Strengths and Virtues* (London: Oxford University Press, 2004).
15. D. Grady, "Think Right, Stay Well," *American Health* 11 (1992): 50–54.
16. Ibid.
17. D. Bazzini et al., "The Effect of Reminiscing about Laughter on Relationship Satisfaction," *Motivation and Emotion* 31, no. 1 (March 2007): 25–34; K. Taber et al., "Functional Anatomy of Humor: Positive Affect and Chronic Mental Illness," *Journal of Neuropsychiatry and Clinical Neuroscience* 19 (2007): 358–62.
18. B. Fredrickson, "Cultivating Positive Emotions to Optimize Health and Well-Being," *Prevention and Treatment* 3 (March 7, 2000), article 0001a.
19. N. Ross, "Health, Happiness, and Higher Levels of Social Organization," *Journal of Epidemiology and Community Health* 59 (2005): 614; A. J. Bishop, P. Martin, and L. Poon, "Happiness and Congruence in Older Adulthood: A Structural Model of Life Satisfaction," *Aging and Mental Health* 10, no. 5 (2006): 445–53.
20. E. Weiner, *The Geography of Bliss: One Grump's Search for the Happiest Places in the World* (New York: Hachette Book Group USA, 2008).
21. P. Herschberger, "Prescribing Happiness: Positive Psychology and Family Medicine," *Family Medicine* 37, no. 9 (2005): 630–34; M. E. Seligman et al., "Positive Psychology Progress: Empirical Validation of Interventions," *American Psychologist* 60, no. 5 (2005): 410–21.
22. M. Seligman, "Positive Interventions: More Evidence of Effectiveness," *Authentic Happiness Newsletter* (September 2004), www.authentichappiness.sas.upenn.edu/newsletter.aspx?id=45; S. I. Gable et al., "What Do You Do When Things Go Right? The Intrapersonal and Interpersonal Benefits of Sharing Positive Events," *Journal of Personal and Social Psychology* 87, no. 2 (2004): 228–45; B. Swartz, *The Paradox of Choice: Why More Is Less* (New York: HarperCollins, 2004); P. C. Seligman, *Character Strengths and Virtues: A Handbook and Classification* (New York: Oxford University Press, 2004).
23. MayoClinic.com, "Mental Health Definitions," 2008, www.mayoclinic.com.
24. National Institute of Mental Health, "The Numbers Count: Mental Disorders in America," www.nimh.nih.gov/health/publications/the-numbers-count-mental-disorders-in-america/index.shtml. Updated March 2008.
25. American College Health Association, *American College Health Association—National College Health Assessment (ACHA-NCHA): Reference Group Data Report Fall 2008* (Baltimore: American College Health Association, 2009).
26. National Institute of Mental Health, "The Numbers Count," 2008.
27. L. A. Lefton, *Psychology.* 8th ed. (Boston: Allyn & Bacon, 2002).
28. National Institute of Mental Health, "The Numbers Count," 2008.
29. R. C. Kessler et al., "Lifetime Prevalence and Age-of-Onset Distributions of *DSM-IV* Disorders in the National Comorbidity Survey Replication (NCS-R)," *Archives of General Psychiatry* 62, no. 6 (2005): 593–602.
30. National Institute of Mental Health, "Depression," www.nimh.nih.gov/publicat/depression.cfm, 2009.
31. National Institute of Mental Health, "The Numbers Count," 2008.
32. American Psychiatric Association, "Let's Talk about Seasonal Affective Disorder," www.healthyminds.org/Main-Topic/Seasonal-Affective-Disorder.aspx. Accessed October 2009.
33. American College Health Association, *ACHA-NCHA: Reference Group Data Report Fall 2008.*
34. National Institute of Mental Health, "Depression," 2009; N. Gavin et al., "Perinatal Depression: A Systematic Review of Prevalence and Incidence," *Obstetrics and Gynecology* 106 (2005): 1071–83.
35. National Sleep Foundation, "NSF's 2007 Sleep in America Poll: Stressed-Out American Women Have No Time for Sleep," March 6, 2007, www.sleepfoundation.org.
36. A. K. Ferketick et al., "Depression as an Antecedent to Heart Disease among Women and Men in the NHANES I Study," National Health and Nutrition Examination Survey," *Archives of Internal Medicine* 160, no. 9 (2002): 1261–68.
37. National Institute of Mental Health, "The Numbers Count," 2008.
38. A. K. Ferketick et al., "NHANES I Study," 2002.
39. National Institute of Mental Health, "Depression," 2009.
40. U.S. Food and Drug Administration (FDA), "Anti-depressant Drug Use in Pediatric Populations," September 23, 2004, www.fda.gov/NewsEvents/Testimony/ucm113265.htm; U.S. FDA, Center for Drug Evaluation and Research, "Antidepressant Use in Children, Adolescents, and Adults," www.fda.gov/cder/drug/antidepressants/default.htm. Updated May 2007; National Institute of Mental Health, "The Numbers Count," 2008.
41. National Institute of Mental Health, "The Numbers Count," 2008.
42. National Institute of Mental Health, "Generalized Anxiety Disorder, GAD," www.nimh.nih.gov/health/publications/anxiety-disorders/generalized-anxiety-disorder-gad.shtml. Reviewed July 7, 2009.
43. MayoClinic.com, "Panic Attacks," www.mayoclinic.com/health/panic-attacks/DS00338. Updated July 1, 2008.
44. National Institute of Mental Health, "The Numbers Count," 2008.
45. C. W. Hoge, et al., "Combat Duty in Iraq and Afghanistan, Mental Health Problems, and Barriers to Care," *New England Journal of Medicine* 351 (2004): 13–22.
46. National Institute of Mental Health, "Generalized Anxiety Disorder, GAD," 2009.
47. W. T. O'Donohue, K. A. Fowler, and S. O. Lilienfeld, *Personality Disorders: Toward the DSM-V* (Thousand Oaks, CA: Sage, 2007).
48. National Institute of Mental Health, "National Survey Tracks Prevalence of Personality Disorders in U.S. Population" (October 18, 2007), www.nimh.nih.gov/science-news/2007/national-survey-tracks-prevalence-of-personality-disorders-in-us-population.shtml.
49. C. Wade and C. Tavries, *Invitation to Psychology.* 4th ed. (Upper Saddle River, NJ: Prentice Hall, 2008), 384–85.
50. Mayo Clinic Staff, "Borderline Personality Disorder" (May 14, 2008), www.mayoclinic.com/health/borderline-personality-disorder/DS00442.
51. J. Cole, "Facts," BPDWORLD (2009), www.bpdworld.org/demo-category/106-facts.
52. National Institute of Mental Health, "Schizophrenia," www.nimh.nih.gov/health/topics/schizophrenia/index.shtml. Updated March 2008.
53. Ibid.
54. National Institute of Mental Health, "Suicide in the U.S.: Statistics and Prevention," www.nimh.nih.gov/publicat/harmsway.cfm. Last reviewed May 18, 2009.
55. B. Hamilton et al., "Annual Summary of Vital Statistics: 2005," *Pediatrics* 119, no. 2 (2007): 336–37.
56. National Institute of Mental Health, "Suicide in the U.S.: Statistics and Prevention."
57. Ibid.
58. National Institute of Mental Health, "The Numbers Count," 2008.

Nutrition and You

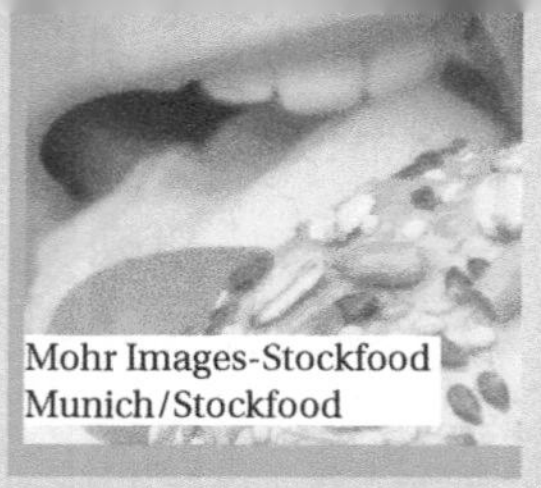

Mohr Images-Stockfood Munich/Stockfood

Why are whole grains better than refined ones?

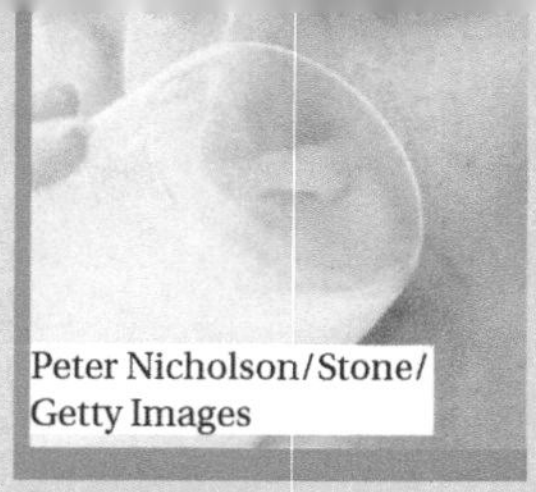

Peter Nicholson/Stone/Getty Images

Do teenagers really need to drink milk?

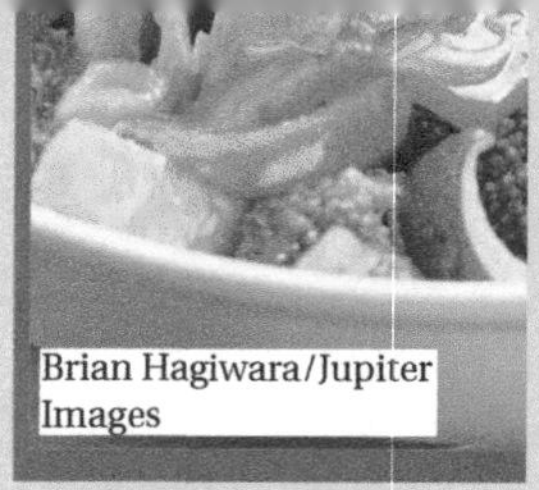

Brian Hagiwara/Jupiter Images

Is vegetarianism healthy?

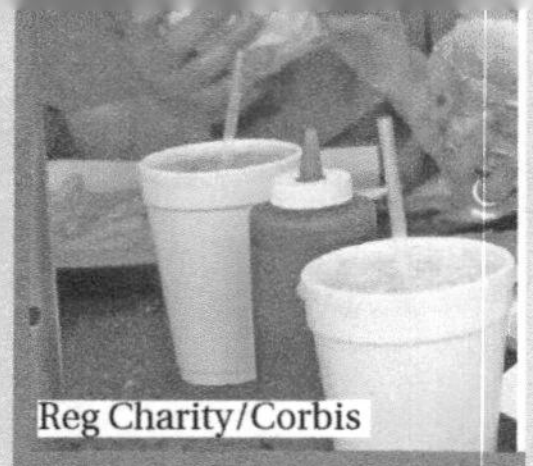

Reg Charity/Corbis

How can I eat well when I'm in a hurry?

Nutrition and You

Objectives

* List the six classes of nutrients, and explain the primary functions of each and their roles in maintaining long-term health.
* Understand the factors that influence dietary choices.
* Discuss how to change old eating habits, improve dietary behaviors, and use the USDA MyPyramid Plan to make the best nutritional choices.
* Distinguish fact from fiction about trends in nutrition, potential risks versus benefits of food supplements, and the role of nutrition in fighting various diseases.
* Discuss issues surrounding gender, culture, and other factors that influence decision making about healthy nutrition.
* Discuss the unique challenges that college students face when trying to eat healthy foods and the actions they can take to eat healthfully.
* Explain food safety concerns facing Americans and people in other regions of the world.

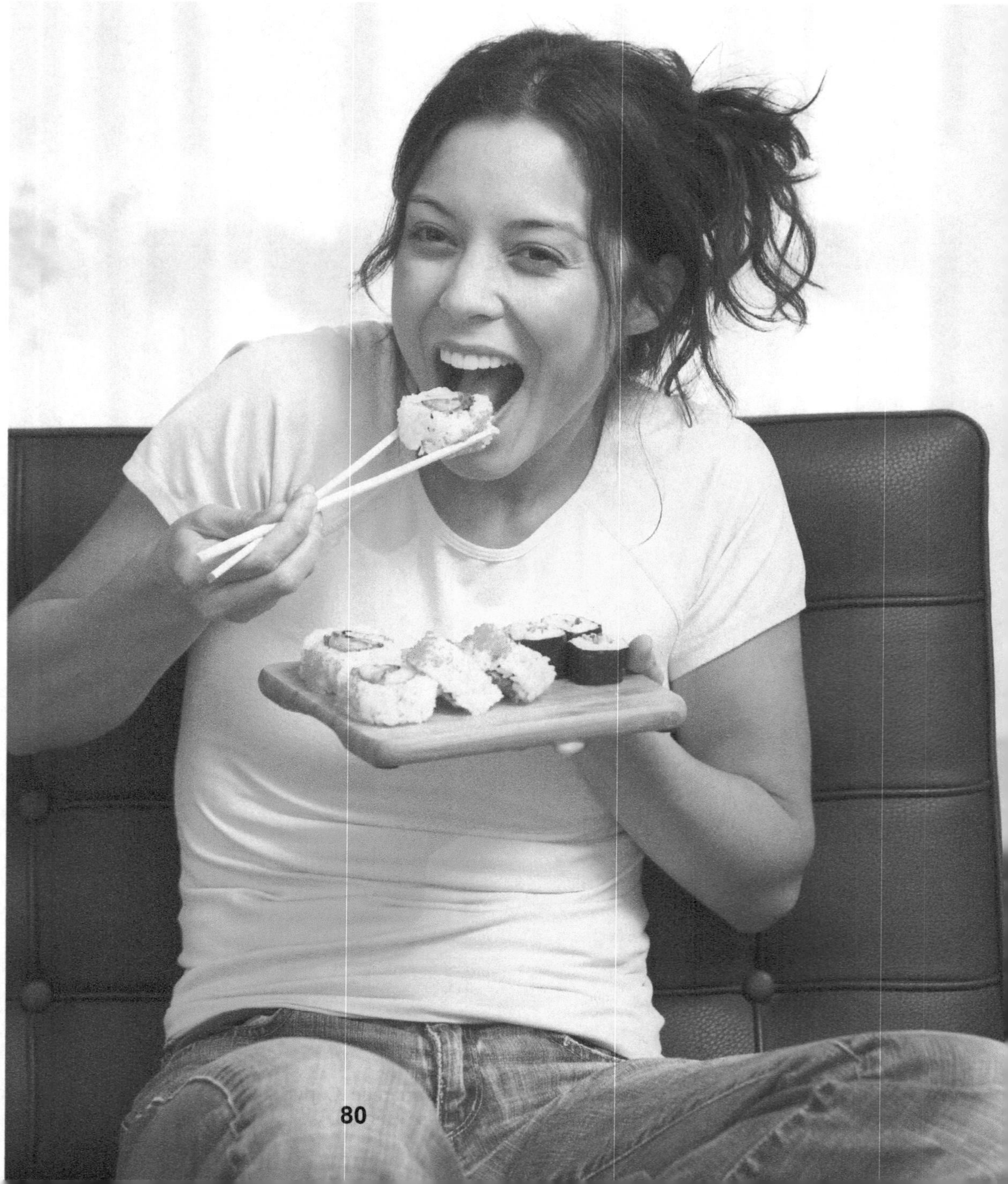

Radius Images/Getty Images

When was the last time you ate something without regard for its fat or calorie content? Can you remember when you last went out to dinner with friends and didn't think twice before ordering the fried foods or high-calorie desserts? Do you eat differently around your health-conscious friends than when by yourself? If so, you are not alone. Clearly, Americans are trying to heed expert advice and the multiple pressures to eat low-fat, high-fiber foods, and to consume fewer calories overall. However, knowing what to eat, how much to eat, and how to choose from a media-driven array of foods and nutrition advice can be mind-boggling.

The good news is that in survey after survey, 60 to 80 percent of food shoppers say they read food labels before selecting products; they consume more vegetables, fruits, and lower-fat foods; and they are cutting down on portion sizes and total calories.[1] Diet-book sales are at an all-time high as millions of people make the leap toward what they think is healthy eating. But we still have a long way to go. In fact, although reports indicate that increasing numbers of us read labels and are trying to eat more healthfully, nearly 78 percent of all adults indicate that they are not eating the recommended servings of fruits and vegetables and that they are still eating too many refined carbohydrates and high-fat foods.

Just how important is sound nutrition? Thousands of individual studies have shown associations between what we eat and a wide range of chronic diseases, such as diabetes, heart disease, hypertension, stroke, and many types of cancer.[2] A landmark review of over 4,500 research studies concluded that widespread consumption of five to six servings of fruits and vegetables daily would lower cancer rates by more than 20 percent in the global population.[3] Newer reviews have focused on specific chronic diseases, and all have shown an important link between diet and risks for certain diseases.[4]

Many documented studies indicate that undernutrition and overnutrition play major roles in global population health (See the **Health in a Diverse World** box on the next page). Indeed, undernutrition, overnutrition, and diet-related chronic diseases account for more than half of the world's diseases and hundreds of millions of dollars in public expenditures.[5] The evidence is compelling and clear. Your health depends largely on what you eat, how much you eat, and the amount of exercise that you get throughout your life.

Family mealtimes and the traditions they involve can reinforce the cultural and social meanings we often attach to food.

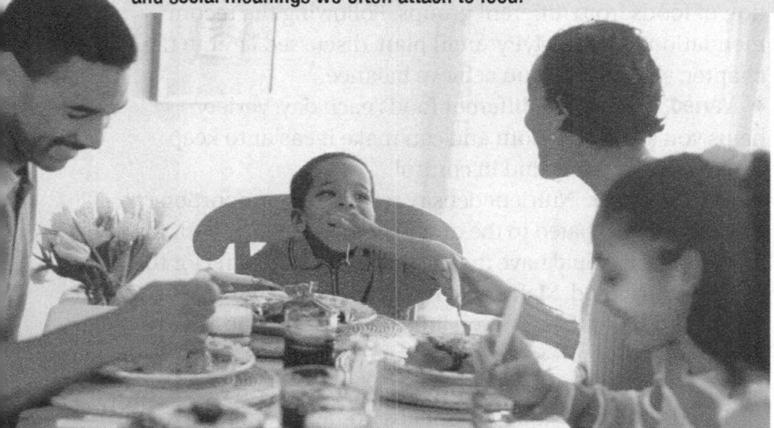

Ariel Skelley/Corbis

Assessing Eating Behaviors: Are You What You Eat?

True **hunger** occurs when there is a lack or shortage of basic foods needed to provide the energy and nutrients that support health.[6] When we are hungry, chemical messages in the brain, especially in the hypothalamus, initiate a physiological response that prompts us to seek food. Few Americans have experienced the type of hunger that continues for days and threatens survival. Most of us eat because of our **appetite,** a learned psychological desire to eat that may or may not have anything to do with feeling hungry. Appetite can be triggered by smells, tastes, and other triggers such as certain times of day, special occasions, or proximity to a favorite food.

hunger The physiological impulse to seek food, prompted by the lack or shortage of basic foods needed to provide the energy and nutrients that support health.

appetite The desire to eat; normally accompanies hunger but is more psychological than physiological.

nutrition The science that investigates the relationship between physiological function and the essential elements of foods eaten.

Hunger and appetite are not the only forces involved in our physiological drive to eat. Other factors that influence when, how, and what we eat include the following:

- **Cultural and social meanings attached to food.** Cultural traditions and food choices give us many of our *food preferences.* We learn to like the tastes of certain foods, especially the foods we grew up eating. A yearning for sweet, salty, or high-fat foods can evolve from our earliest days.
- **Convenience and advertising.** That juicy burger on TV looked really good. You've got to have it.
- **Habit or custom.** Often we select foods because they are familiar and fit religious, political, or spiritual views.
- **Emotional comfort.** Eating makes you feel better—a form of reward and security. We derive pleasure or sensory delight from eating specific foods and reward ourselves with foods.
- **Nutritional value.** You think the food is good or bad for you, or it may help you maintain your weight.
- **Social interaction.** Eating out or having company over for a meal is an enjoyable social event.
- **Regional/seasonal trends.** Some foods may be favored in your area by season or overall climate.

With all the factors that influence our dietary choices and the wide array of foods available, the challenge of eating for health increases daily. Fortunately, we have a wealth of solid information that serves as a foundation for our decisions.

Eating for Health

Nutrition is the science that investigates the relationship between physiological function and the essential elements

Health In a DIVERSE World

Global Nutrition: Threats to World Populations

Although it's widely accepted that in general good nutrition means stronger immune systems, better productivity, fewer illnesses, and better health, millions of people in the developed and developing world suffer from food scarcity, food insecurity, and malnutrition. Just how much of an impact does poor nutrition have on the health of global populations? Consider this:

* Poor nutrition contributes to one out of two deaths (53 percent) associated with infectious diseases among children under age 5 in developing countries.
* One out of four preschool children suffers from undernutrition in the global population.
* One in three people in developing countries are affected by vitamin and mineral deficiencies and therefore are more at risk for infection, birth defects, and impaired physical and intellectual development.
* In the United States, nearly 12 percent of the population suffers from *food insecurity,* meaning that they are unable to provide sufficient food for themselves or their families.

Ironically, at the same time that food insecurity and insufficient food levels plague the world, the global population is also seeing a dramatic increase in other forms of malnutrition. These are characterized by obesity and the long-term implications of unbalanced dietary and lifestyle practices that result in chronic diseases such as cardiovascular disease, cancer, and diabetes. Although we often think that obesity is a problem of excess and affluence, this isn't always the case. In fact, obesity flourishes in populations where acute hunger also persists.

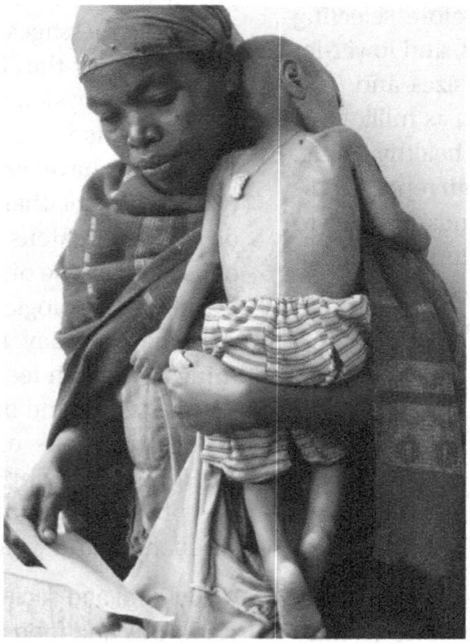

HO/Reuters/Corbis

Drought, high food prices, and political unrest all contribute to the severe malnutrition experienced by millions of people worldwide.

* Two out of three overweight and obese people now live in developing countries, the vast majority in emerging markets and transition economies.
* Under- and overnutrition problems and diet-related chronic diseases (including obesity-related diseases) account for more than half of the world's diseases and hundreds of millions of dollars in public expenditure to combat them.

Sources: World Health Organization, "Nutrition for Health and Development: Challenges," 2009, www.who.int/nutrition/challenges/en/index.html; M. Nord, M. Andrews, and S. Carlson, *Household Food Security in the United States, 2007,* Economic Research Report no. 66, U.S. Department of Agriculture, Economic Research Service, November 2008, www.ers.usda.gov/Publications/ERR66.

of the foods we eat. Generally, a healthful diet provides the proper combination of energy and **nutrients,** the compounds in food that your body requires to sustain proper functioning. A healthful diet should be

- **Adequate.** It provides enough of the energy, nutrients, and fiber to maintain health and essential body functions. A **calorie** is the unit of measurement used to quantify the amount of energy we obtain from a particular food. Everyone's energy needs differ (Table 1). For example, a small woman who has a sedentary lifestyle may need only 1,700 calories of energy to support her body's functions, whereas a professional biker may need several thousand calories of energy to be up for his competition.
- **Moderate.** The quantity of food you consume can cause you to gain weight. Moderate caloric consumption, portion control, and awareness of the total amount of nutrients in the foods you eat are key aspects of dietary health.
- **Balanced.** Your diet should contain the proper combination of foods from different groups. Following the recommendations for the MyPyramid plan, discussed later in the chapter, should help you achieve balance.
- **Varied.** Eat a lot of different foods each day. Variety helps you avoid boredom and can make it easier to keep your diet interesting and in control.
- **Nutrient dense.** Nutrient density refers to the proportion of nutrients compared to the number of calories. In short, the foods you eat should have the biggest nutritional bang for the calories consumed. Making each bite count and not wasting calories on foods that give you little nutritional value are key to healthful eating.

nutrients The constituents of food that sustain humans physiologically: proteins, carbohydrates, fats, vitamins, minerals, and water.
calorie A unit of measure that indicates the amount of energy obtained from a particular food.

Trends indicate that Americans today overall eat more food than ever before (see Figure 1). In a 30-year study of changes in consumption, women's overall caloric intake

TABLE 1 **Estimated Daily Calorie Needs**

	Calorie Range		
	Sedentary[a]	→	Active[b]
Children			
2–3 years old	1,000	→	1,400
Females			
4–8 years old	1,200	→	1,800
9–13	1,600	→	2,200
14–18	1,800	→	2,400
19–30	2,000	→	2,400
31–50	1,800	→	2,200
51+	1,600	→	2,200
Males			
4–8 years old	1,400	→	2,000
9–13	1,800	→	2,600
14–18	2,200	→	3,200
19–30	2,400	→	3,000
31–50	2,200	→	3,000
51+	2,000	→	2,800

[a] A lifestyle that includes only the light physical activity associated with typical day-to-day life.

[b] A lifestyle that includes physical activity equivalent to walking more than 3 miles per day at 3 to 4 miles per hour, in addition to the light physical activity associated with typical day-to-day life.

Source: Center for Nutrition Policy & Promotion, April 2005, www.MyPyramid.gov.

increased by 22 percent and men's by 7 percent.[7] Are we eating more food, or is it what we are eating? Trends indicate that it isn't actual amounts of food, but the number of calories in the foods we choose to eat.[8] When these trends are combined with our increasingly sedentary lifestyle, it is not surprising that we have seen a dramatic rise in obesity.

1/3 **of the calories Americans consume come from junk foods with no nutritional value such as sweets, soft drinks, and alcoholic beverages.**

Americans typically get approximately 38 percent of their calories from fat, 15 percent from proteins, 22 percent from complex carbohydrates, and 24 percent from simple sugars.[9] Nearly one-third of the calories we consume come from junk foods with no real nutritional value. Sweets and desserts, soft drinks, sugary fruit juice beverages, and alcoholic beverages make up 25 percent of those calories, and another 5 percent come from salty snacks and fruit-flavored drinks. In sharp contrast, healthy foods such as vegetables and fruit make up only 10 percent of our total calories.[10]

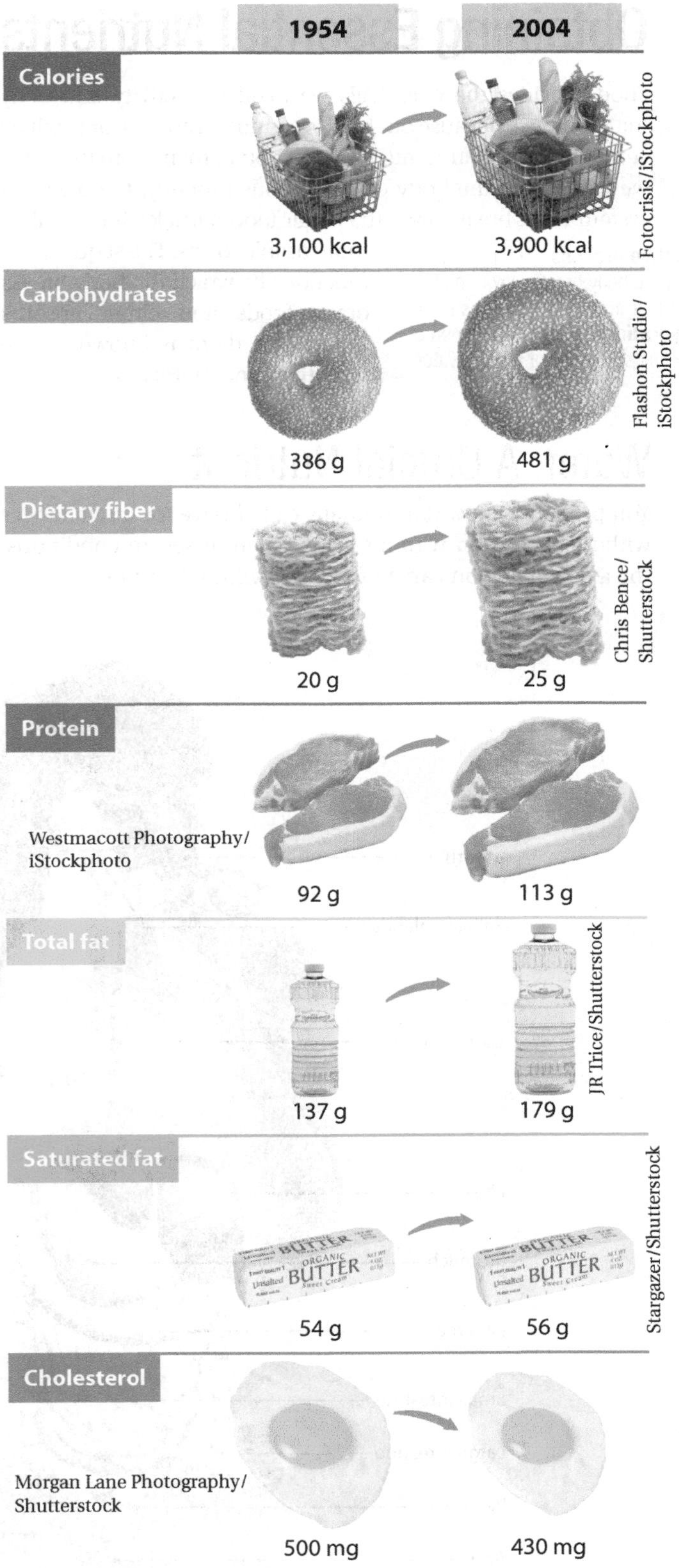

FIGURE 1 **Trends in Per Capita Nutrient Consumption**
Since 1954, Americans' daily caloric intake has increased by about 25%, as has daily consumption of carbohydrates, fiber, and protein. Daily total fat has increased by 30%.
Source: Data are from USDA Economic Research Service, Food Availability (Per Capita) Data System, 2008, www.ers.usda.gov/data/foodconsumption.

Obtaining Essential Nutrients

Food provides the chemicals we need for activity and body maintenance. Because our bodies cannot synthesize or produce certain essential nutrients, we must obtain them from the foods we eat. Before the body can use foods properly, the digestive system must break down the larger food particles into smaller, more usable forms. The sequence of functions by which the body breaks down foods and either absorbs or excretes them is known as the **digestive process** (Figure 2).

digestive process The process by which the body breaks down foods and either absorbs or excretes them.
dehydration Abnormal depletion of body fluids; a result of lack of water.

Water: A Crucial Nutrient

You probably know that humans can survive for much longer without food than without water. Even in severe conditions, the average person can go for weeks without certain vitamins and minerals before experiencing serious deficiency symptoms. However, **dehydration** (abnormal depletion of body fluids), can cause serious problems within a matter of hours, and death after a few days. Too much water can also pose a serious risk to your health, a condition known as *hyponatremia.*

The human body consists of 50 to 60 percent water by weight. The water in our system bathes cells, aids in fluid and electrolyte balance, maintains pH balance, and transports molecules and cells throughout the body. Water is the major component of our blood, which carries oxygen and nutrients to the tissues, removes metabolic wastes, and is responsible for maintaining cells in working order.

Individual needs for water vary drastically according to dietary factors, age, size, overall health, environmental temperature and humidity levels, and exercise. For the most part, scientists now refute the conventional wisdom that we need 8 cups of water per day. There is little scientific evidence to support carrying that water bottle with you (see the **Green Guide** at right for some environmental reasons *not* to). Extra

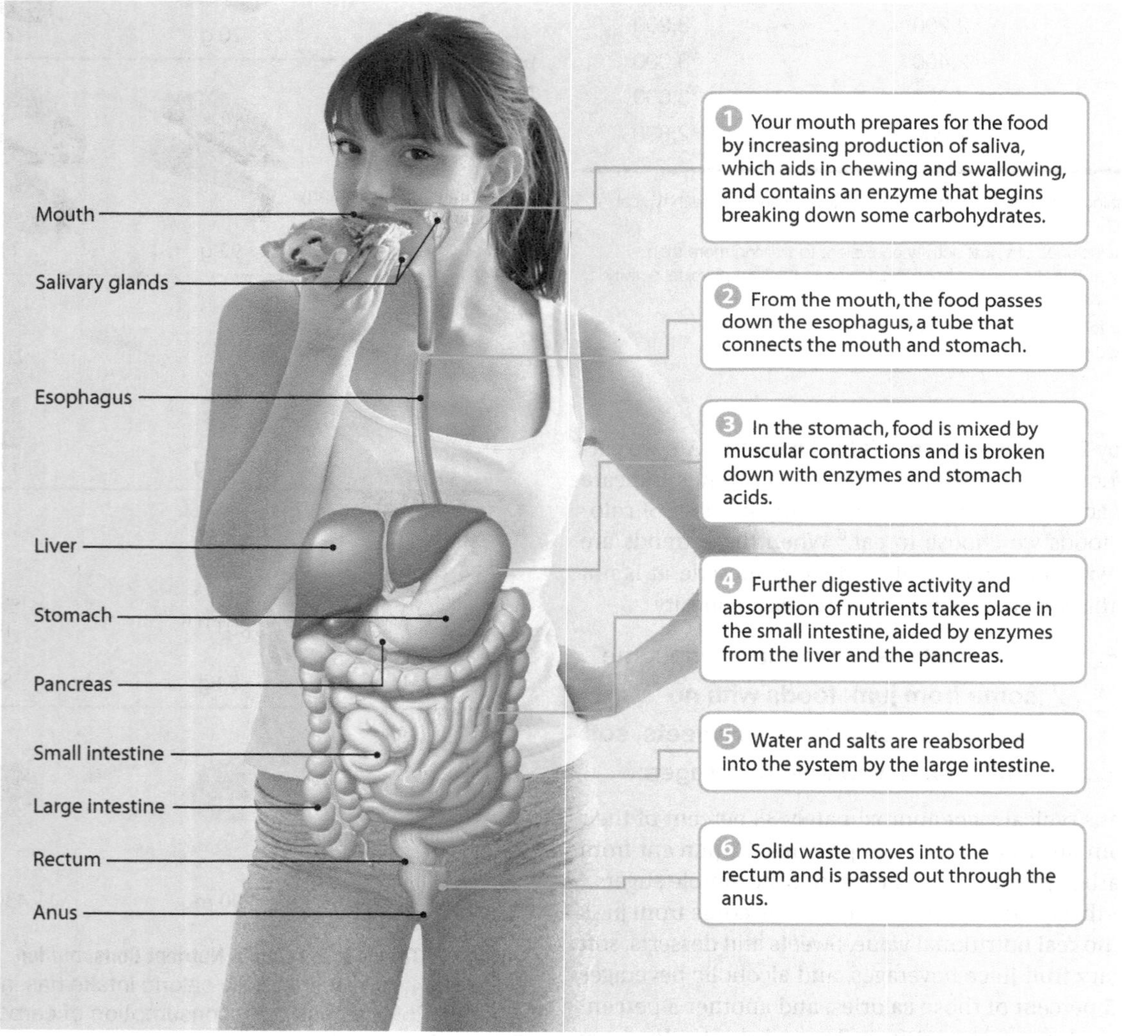

Mouth
Salivary glands
Esophagus
Liver
Stomach
Pancreas
Small intestine
Large intestine
Rectum
Anus
1 Your mouth prepares for the food by increasing production of saliva, which aids in chewing and swallowing, and contains an enzyme that begins breaking down some carbohydrates.
2 From the mouth, the food passes down the esophagus, a tube that connects the mouth and stomach.
3 In the stomach, food is mixed by muscular contractions and is broken down with enzymes and stomach acids.
4 Further digestive activity and absorption of nutrients takes place in the small intestine, aided by enzymes from the liver and the pancreas.
5 Water and salts are reabsorbed into the system by the large intestine.
6 Solid waste moves into the rectum and is passed out through the anus.

webphotographeer/iStockphoto

FIGURE 2 **The Digestive Process**
The entire digestive process takes approximately 24 hours.

GREEN GUIDE

Bottled Water Boom: Who Pays the Price?

Globally, factories are churning out bottled water at unprecedented rates. Conservative estimates are that bottled water is now our second most popular drink, right behind soda, with over $100 billion in sales each year. The consumption of bottled water in the United States rose 20 times, or 2,000 percent, between 1978 and 2006. People all over the world have developed a love affair with their special brands of water, many thinking that bottled water is better, safer, and more pure than tap water. It isn't enough that we are spending between 500 to 4,000 times more for bottled than we do for tap water. Most experts argue that all that money is being spent on a product that doesn't really deliver any benefits.

We may imagine that bottled water comes from medicinal mountain streams or aquifers that ensure purity, but the fact is that most of the water sold in bottles comes from municipal water supplies, sometimes with extra minerals being added, or with an extra step in purification. If it was just your money going down the drain and you could afford it, it wouldn't be so worrisome. However, the environmental consequences of bottled water are significant. Consider the following:

- Around the world, factories are using more than 18 million barrels of oil and up to 130 billion gallons of fresh water to quench our bottled water thirst. When you include the resource cost of transporting bottled water, it is estimated that the total amount of energy required to create and transport every bottle is the equivalent of filling the bottle one-quarter full of oil.
- In general, systems such as reverse osmosis purifiers use about 2 liters of fresh water running through a system to realize 1 liter of bottled water.
- In 2006, more than 900,000 tons of plastic were used to package 8 billion gallons of bottled water.
- There is a growing concern about negative health risks from certain chemicals found in plastic bottles that can leach into the water, particularly *bisphenol-A (BPA)*. Research has suggested links between BPA and negative estrogen-related effects, including breast enlargement in young boys, some forms of cancer, early onset of puberty, and increased risk for type 2 diabetes.
- Tap water in the United States is among the safest in the world, largely because community water supplies are subject to strict and constant monitoring required by the Safe Drinking Act, while bottled water is considered a "food" and requires much less frequent monitoring for safety and quality by the Food and Drug Administration (FDA) or individual state oversight.
- Nationwide, less than 15 percent of discarded bottles are recycled.
- Companies taking part in the bottled water boom are buying water supplies throughout the world for financial gain, leaving entire populations vulnerable to water shortages.

You can help to curb the personal and global environmental threats caused by bottled water use:

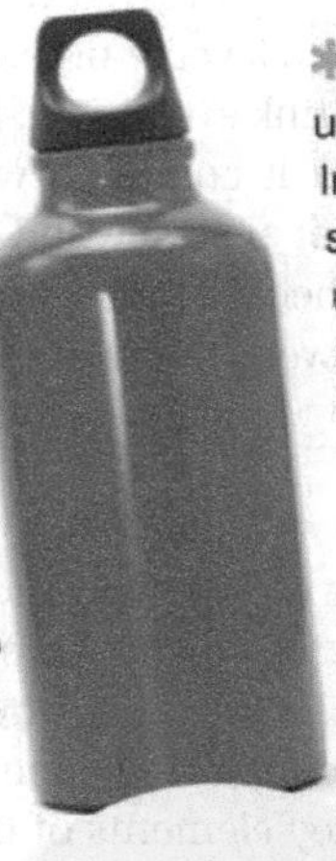

design56/Shutterstock

Purchasing a stainless steel bottle that you can reuse is a better choice than buying plastic bottles every day.

- Don't buy bottled water unless it's absolutely necessary. Instead, purchase a stainless steel or glass container and use it again and again. Look for a container with a wide mouth so that you can wash and dry it regularly.
- When you have parties, use covered pitchers of ice water and recyclable paper cups, rather than serving bottles or using plastic cups.
- Buy an inexpensive water filter to help remove the taste of chlorine from tap water. Refrigerate your water jug as a means of improving taste and clarity.
- Recycle any plastic bottles you use or come across. Many states offer 5 cent deposits on beverage bottles and cans as an incentive to increase recycling efforts.
- Become involved in initiatives to ensure quality tap water in your community. Ask questions about the filters being used, the chemicals and minerals that are removed, and the chemicals and minerals that remain.

Sources: Sierra Club, "Bottled Water: Learning the Facts and Taking Action," 2008, www.sierraclub.org/committees/cac/water/bottled_water/bottled_water.pdf; Oregon State University, "Bottled Water Boom Has Environmental Drawbacks," Media Release, 2007, http://oregonstate.edu/dept/ncs/newsarch/2007/May07/bottledwater.html.

water isn't going to help clear more toxins from your body, cure your headaches, or improve your skin or health. That's not to say that water isn't important to cell functioning and overall health, but we usually get all the fluids that we need per day through the food we eat. In fact, fruits and vegetables are 80 to 95 percent water, meats are more than 50 percent water, and even dry bread and cheese are about 35 percent water. Contrary to popular opinion, caffeinated drinks, including coffee, tea, and soda, also count toward total fluid intake for those who regularly consume them. Caffeinated beverages have not been found to dehydrate people whose bodies are used to caffeine.

Researchers have looked at climates around the world and have concluded that people who live in hot, desertlike places or those who engage in activities where they sweat profusely, such as heavy laborers or athletes, probably need to replenish their lost fluids regularly.[11] In addition, certain diseases, such as diabetes and cystic fibrosis, cause people to lose fluids at a rate necessitating a higher volume of fluid intake. However, for the typical person, if you are thirsty, drink; if you are sweating profusely, drink; and if you have a fever or other illness where there is vomiting and diarrhea, drink even more. Remember that no two people are alike when it comes to water consumption needs. If you are an athlete or are just wondering about general water recommendations, check the guidelines at the American College of Sports Medicine website, www.acsm.org.[12]

Proteins

Next to water, **proteins** are the most abundant substances in the human body. Proteins are major components of nearly every cell and have been called the "body builders" because of their role in developing and repairing bone, muscle, skin, and blood cells. They are the key elements of the antibodies that protect us from disease, of enzymes that control chemical activities in the body, and of hormones that regulate body functions. Proteins help transport iron, oxygen, and nutrients to all body cells and supply another source of energy to cells when fats and carbohydrates are not readily available. In short, adequate amounts of protein in the diet are vital to many body functions and ultimately to survival.

Whenever you consume proteins, your body breaks them down into smaller molecules known as **amino acids,** the building blocks of protein. Nine of the 20 different amino acids are termed **essential amino acids,** which means the body must obtain them from the diet; the other 11 can be produced by the body. Dietary protein that supplies all the essential amino acids is called **complete (high-quality) protein.** Typically, protein from animal products is complete. When we consume foods that are deficient in some of the essential amino acids, the total amount of protein that can be synthesized from the other amino acids is decreased. For proteins to be complete, they also must be present in digestible form and in amounts proportional to body requirements.

What about plant sources of protein? Proteins from plant sources are often **incomplete proteins** in that they may lack one or two of the essential amino acids. Nevertheless, it is relatively easy for the nonmeat eater to combine plant foods effectively and eat complementary sources of plant protein (Figure 3).

proteins The essential constituents of nearly all body cells; necessary for the development and repair of bone, muscle, skin, and blood; the key elements of antibodies, enzymes, and hormones.
amino acids The nitrogen-containing building blocks of protein.
essential amino acids Nine of the basic nitrogen-containing building blocks of protein, which must be obtained from foods to ensure health.
complete (high-quality) proteins Proteins that contain all nine of the essential amino acids.
incomplete proteins Proteins that lack one or more of the essential amino acids.

Eaten in the right combinations, plant-based foods can provide complementary proteins and all essential amino acids.

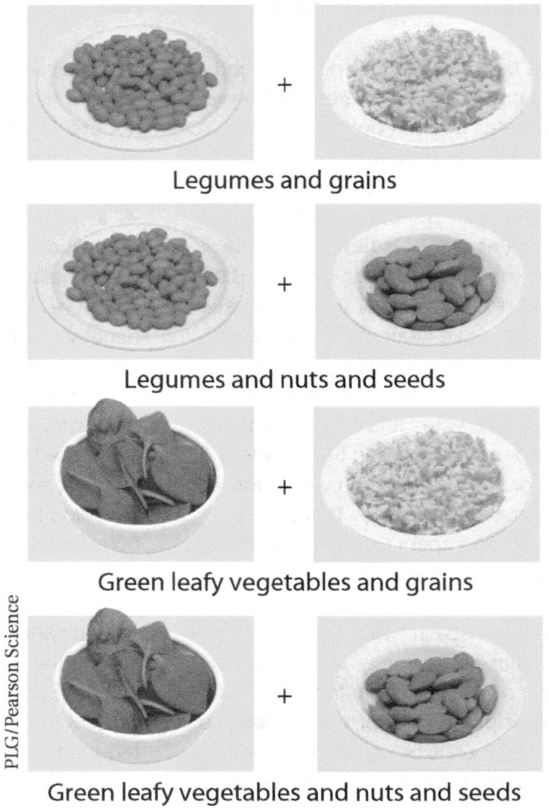

FIGURE 3 **Complementary Proteins**

Plant sources of protein fall into three general categories: *legumes* (beans, peas, peanuts, and soy products), *grains* (e.g., wheat, corn, rice, and oats), and *nuts and seeds.* Certain vegetables, such as leafy green vegetables and broccoli, also contribute valuable plant proteins. Mixing two or more foods from each of these categories during the same meal will provide all the essential amino acids necessary to ensure adequate protein absorption.

Although protein deficiency continues to pose a threat to the global population, few Americans suffer from protein deficiencies. In fact, the average American consumes more than 100 grams of protein daily, and about 70 percent of this comes from high-fat animal flesh and dairy products.[13] The recommended protein intake for adults is only 0.8 gram (g) per kilogram (kg) of body weight per day. The typical recommendation is that in a 2,000-calorie diet, 10 to 35 percent of calories should come from protein, for a total average of 50 to 175 grams per day (a 6-ounce steak contains 53 grams of protein—more than the daily needs of an average-sized woman!).

A person might need to eat extra protein if fighting off a serious infection, recovering from surgery or blood loss, or recovering from burns. In these instances, proteins that are lost to cellular repair need to be replaced. There is considerable controversy over whether someone in high-level physical training needs additional protein to build and repair muscle fibers or whether normal daily requirements should suffice.

Carbohydrates

Although we should not underestimate the importance of water and proteins in the body, it is **carbohydrates** that supply us with the energy needed to sustain normal daily activity. Carbohydrates can actually be metabolized more quickly and efficiently than proteins and are a quick source of energy for the body, being easily converted to glucose, the fuel for the body's cells. These foods also play an important role in the functioning of internal organs, the nervous system, and the muscles. They are the best fuel for endurance athletics because they provide both an immediate and a time-released energy source; they are digested easily and then consistently metabolized in the bloodstream. There are two major types of carbohydrates: **simple carbohydrates** or *simple sugars,* which are found primarily in fruits and many vegetables, and **complex carbohydrates,** which are found in grains, cereals, and vegetables.

Simple Carbohydrates

A typical American diet contains large amounts of simple carbohydrates. The most common form is *glucose.* Eventually, the human body converts all types of simple sugars to glucose to provide energy to cells. *Fructose* (commonly called *fruit sugar*) is another simple sugar found in fruits and berries. Glucose and fructose are **monosaccharides.**

Disaccharides are combinations of two monosaccharides. Perhaps the best-known example is *sucrose* (granulated table sugar). *Lactose* (milk sugar), found in milk and milk products, and *maltose* (malt sugar) are other examples of common disaccharides. These must be broken down into monosaccharides before the body can use them.

Sugar is found in high amounts in a wide range of food products that many people never even think about. Items such as ketchup, barbecue sauce, and flavored coffee creamers derive 30 to 65 percent of their calories from sugar. Read food labels carefully before purchasing. If *sugar* or one of its aliases (including *high fructose corn syrup*) appears near the top of the ingredients list, then that product contains a lot of sugar and is probably not your best nutritional bet. Also, most labels provide the amount of sugar as a percentage of total calories.

Complex Carbohydrates: Starches and Glycogen

Complex carbohydrates, or **polysaccharides,** are formed by long chains of monosaccharides. They must be broken down into simple sugars before the body can use them. *Starches, glycogen,* and *fiber* are the main types of complex carbohydrates.

Starches make up the majority of the complex carbohydrate group and come from flours, breads, pasta, rice, corn, oats, barley, potatoes, and related foods. The body breaks down these complex carbohydrates into glucose, which can be easily absorbed by cells and used as energy. Polysaccharides can also be stored in body muscles and the liver as **glycogen.** When the body requires a sudden burst of energy, it breaks down glycogen into glucose.

Glycemic Index and Glycemic Load

Americans consume far too many refined carbohydrates, which have few health benefits and are a major factor in our growing epidemic of overweight and obesity. Many of these simple sugars come from *added sugars,* sweeteners that are put in during processing to flavor foods, make sodas taste good, and ease our cravings for sweets. A classic example is the amount of added sugar in one can of soda: over 10 teaspoons per can! All that refined sugar can cause tooth decay and put on pounds; however, the greater threats may come from the sudden spike in blood glucose that comes from eating them. In response to an overload of blood glucose, insulin levels also may surge in order to drive blood glucose levels down. Through a typical day, these surges of sugar, bursts of insulin, and resultant dips in blood glucose may cause a cascade of ill health effects.

The **glycemic index (GI)** is a system for rating the potential of foods to raise blood glucose levels. Foods that break down quickly and result in that fast blood glucose surge have a high glycemic index rating. Those that digest slowly and release glucose slowly into the blood tend to have low glycemic index ratings. **Glycemic load (GL)** refers to the amount of carbohydrates in the food you eat multiplied by the glycemic index of that food. In other words, if you eat a tiny amount of a high glycemic index food, the net effect won't be as severe as if you ate a huge serving.

Combining carbohydrates with fats and proteins can lower the overall GI. If, instead of just drinking a glass of orange juice in the morning, you also ate a piece of whole-grain bread with peanut butter, the level of blood glucose surging in your blood would be substantially lower than without that protein and fat combination. Diabetics and others can benefit from eating such combinations of whole grains, proteins, and fats throughout the day as a means of controlling blood glucose levels.[14]

Complex Carbohydrates: Fiber

Fiber, often referred to as "bulk" or "roughage," is the indigestible portion of plant foods that helps move foods through the

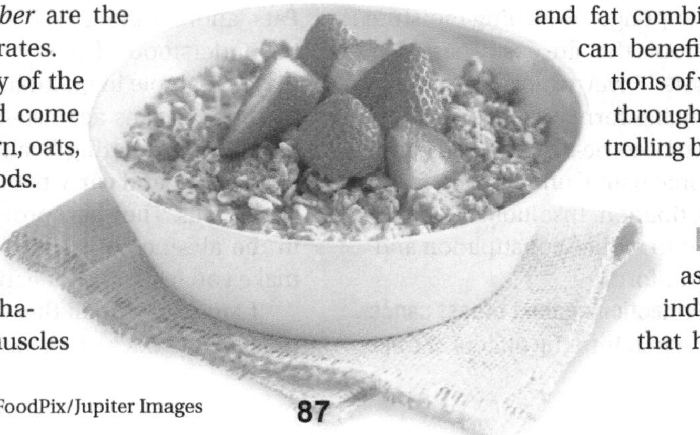

Brian Leatart/FoodPix/Jupiter Images

carbohydrates Basic nutrients that supply the body with glucose, the energy form most commonly used to sustain normal activity.

simple carbohydrates A major type of carbohydrate, which provides short-term energy; also called simple sugars.

complex carbohydrates A major type of carbohydrate, which provides sustained energy.

monosaccharides Simple sugars that contain only one molecule of sugar.

disaccharides Combinations of two monosaccharides.

polysaccharides Complex carbohydrates formed by the combination of long chains of monosaccharides.

starch Polysaccharide that is the storage form of glucose in plants.

glycogen The polysaccharide form in which glucose is stored in the liver and, to a lesser extent, in muscles.

glycemic index (GI) A measure of the effect of particular carbohydrates on blood glucose levels.

glycemic load (GL) A measure of the carbohydrate content of a portion of food multiplied by its glycemic index.

fiber The indigestible portion of plant foods that helps move food through the digestive system and softens stools by absorbing water.

digestive system, delays absorption of cholesterol and other nutrients, and softens stools by absorbing water. Dietary fiber is found only in plant foods, such as fruits, vegetables, nuts, and grains. The Food and Nutrition Board of the Institute of Medicine proposed three fiber distinctions: dietary fiber, functional fiber, and total fiber.[15] *Dietary fiber* is the nondigestible parts of plants that form the structure of leaves, stems, and seeds—the plant's "skeleton." *Functional fiber* consists of nondigestible forms of carbohydrates that may come from plants or are manufactured in the laboratory and have known health benefits. *Total fiber* is the sum of dietary fiber and functional fiber in a person's diet.

A more user-friendly classification of fiber types is either *soluble* or *insoluble*. Soluble fibers, such as pectins, gums, and mucilages, dissolve in water, form gel-like substances, and can be easily digested by bacteria in the colon. Major food sources of soluble fiber include citrus fruits, berries, oat bran, dried beans (such as kidney, garbanzo, pinto, and navy beans), and some vegetables. Insoluble fibers, such as lignins and cellulose, are those that typically do not dissolve in water and that cannot be fermented by bacteria in the colon. They are found in whole grains, such as brown rice, wheat, bran, whole-grain breads and cereals, and most fruits and vegetables.

Research supports many benefits of fiber:

- **Protection against colon and rectal cancer.** One of the leading causes of cancer deaths in the United States, colorectal cancer is much rarer in countries with diets high in fiber and low in animal fat. Several studies have contributed to the theory that fiber-rich diets, particularly those including insoluble fiber, prevent the development of precancerous growths.[16]
- **Protection against constipation.** Insoluble fiber, consumed with adequate fluids, acts like a sponge, absorbing moisture and producing softer, bulkier stools that are easily passed.
- **Protection against diverticulosis.** Diverticulosis is a condition in which tiny bulges or pouches form on the large intestinal wall. These bulges can become irritated and cause chronic pain if under strain from constipation. Insoluble fiber helps to reduce constipation and discomfort.
- **Protection against breast cancer.** Research into the effects of fiber on breast cancer risk is inconclusive. However, some studies indicate that wheat bran (rich in insoluble fiber) reduces blood estrogen levels, which may affect the risk for breast cancer.
- **Protection against heart disease.** Many studies have indicated that soluble fiber helps reduce blood cholesterol, primarily by lowering low-density lipoprotein (LDL: "bad") cholesterol.
- **Protection against type 2 diabetes.** Some studies suggest that soluble fiber improves control of blood sugar and can reduce the need for insulin or medication in people with type 2 diabetes.[17]
- **Protection against obesity.** Because most high-fiber foods are high in carbohydrates and low in fat, they help control caloric intake. Many take longer to chew, which slows you down at the table, and fiber stays in the digestive tract longer than other nutrients, making you feel full sooner.

Mohr Images-Stockfood Munich/Stockfood

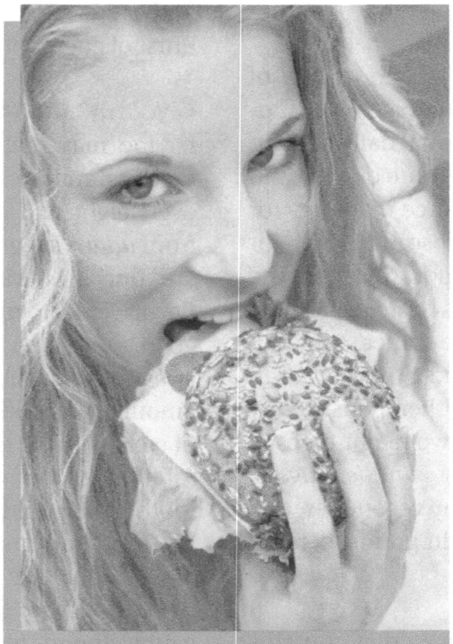

Why are whole grains better than refined ones?

Whole grain foods contain fiber, a crucial form of carbohydrate that protects against some gastrointestinal disorders and reduces risk for certain cancers. Fiber is also associated with lowered blood cholesterol levels; studies have shown that eating 2.5 servings of whole grains per day can reduce cardiovascular disease risk by as much as 21%. But are people getting the message? One nutrition survey showed that only 8% of U.S. adults consume three or more servings of whole grains each day, and 42% ate no whole grains at all on a given day.

In spite of growing evidence supporting the benefits of whole grains and high-fiber diets, intake among the general public remains low. Most experts believe that Americans should double their current consumption of dietary fiber—to 20 to 35 grams per day for most people and perhaps to 40 to 50 grams for others. What's the best way to increase your intake of dietary fiber? Eat more foods high in complex carbohydrates, such as whole grains, fruits, vegetables, legumes (peas and beans), nuts, and seeds. See the **Skills for Behavior Change** box on the next page for more tips to increase your fiber intake. As with most nutritional advice, however, too much of a good thing can pose problems. Sudden increases in dietary fiber may cause flatulence (intestinal gas), cramping, or bloating. Consume plenty of water or other liquids to reduce such side effects.

Fats

Fats, another group of basic nutrients, are perhaps the most misunderstood of the body's required energy sources. Fats play a vital role in maintaining healthy skin and hair, insulating body organs against shock, maintaining body temperature, and promoting healthy cell function. Fats make foods taste better and carry the fat-soluble vitamins A, D, E, and K to the cells. They also provide a concentrated form of energy in the absence of sufficient amounts of carbohydrates and make you feel full after eating.

If fats perform all these functions, why are we constantly urged to cut back on them? Although moderate consumption

fats Basic nutrients composed of carbon and hydrogen atoms; needed for the proper functioning of cells, insulation of body organs against shock, maintenance of body temperature, and healthy skin and hair.

Skills for Behavior Change

Bulk Up Your Fiber Intake!

* Whenever possible, select whole-grain breads, especially those that are low in fat and sugars. Choose breads with three or more grams of fiber per serving. Read labels—just because bread is brown doesn't mean it is better for you.
* Eat whole, unpeeled fruits and vegetables rather than drinking their juices. The fiber in the whole fruit tends to slow blood sugar increases and helps you feel full longer.
* Substitute whole-grain pastas, bagels, and pizza crust for the refined, white flour versions.
* Add wheat crumbs or grains to meat loaf and burgers to increase fiber intake.
* Toast grains to bring out their nutty flavor and make foods more appealing.
* Sprinkle ground flaxseed on cereals, yogurt, and salads, or add to casseroles, burgers, and baked goods. Flaxseeds have a mild flavor and are also high in beneficial fatty acids.

of fats is essential to health, overconsumption can be dangerous. **Triglycerides,** which make up about 95 percent of total body fat, are the most common form of fat circulating in the blood. When we consume too many calories, the liver converts the excess into triglycerides, which are stored throughout our bodies.

The remaining 5 percent of body fat is composed of substances such as **cholesterol,** which can accumulate on the inner walls of arteries and narrow the channels through which blood flows. This buildup, called **plaque,** is a major cause of *atherosclerosis*, a component of cardiovascular disease.

The ratio of total cholesterol to a group of compounds called **high-density lipoproteins (HDLs)** is important to determining risk for heart disease. Lipoproteins facilitate the transport of cholesterol in the blood. High-density lipoproteins are capable of transporting more cholesterol than are **low-density lipoproteins (LDLs).** Whereas LDLs transport cholesterol to the body's cells, HDLs apparently transport circulating cholesterol to the liver for metabolism and elimination from the body. People with a high percentage of HDLs therefore appear to be at lower risk for developing cholesterol-clogged arteries. Regular vigorous exercise plays a part in reducing cholesterol by increasing high-density lipoproteins.

Types of Dietary Fats

Fat molecules consist of chains of carbon and hydrogen atoms. Those that are unable to hold any more hydrogen in their chemical structure are labeled **saturated fats.** They generally come from animal sources, such as meat, poultry, and dairy products, and are solid at room temperature. **Unsaturated fats,** which come from plants and include most vegetable oils, are generally liquid at room temperature and have room for additional hydrogen atoms in their chemical structure.

The terms *monounsaturated fat* (MUFA) and *polyunsaturated fat* (PUFA) refer to the relative number of hydrogen atoms that are missing in an unsaturated fat. Peanut and olive oils are high in monounsaturated fats, whereas corn, sunflower, and safflower oils are high in polyunsaturated fats. There is currently a great deal of controversy about which type of unsaturated fat is most beneficial. Many nutritional researchers believe that PUFAs may decrease levels of beneficial HDLs as well as those of harmful LDLs. PUFAs come in two forms: omega-3 fatty acids and omega-6 fatty acids. MUFAs, such as olive oil, seem to lower LDL levels and increase HDL levels and thus are currently the preferred fats. MUFAs are also resistant to oxidation, a process that leads to cell and tissue damage. For a breakdown of the types of fats in common vegetable oils, see Figure 4 on the next page.

triglycerides The most common form of fat in the body; excess calories consumed are converted into triglycerides and stored as body fat.
cholesterol A form of fat circulating in the blood that can accumulate on the inner walls of arteries, causing a narrowing of the channel through which blood flows.
plaque Cholesterol buildup on the inner walls of arteries; a major cause of atherosclerosis.
high-density lipoproteins (HDLs) Compounds that facilitate the transport of cholesterol in the blood to the liver for metabolism and elimination from the body.
low-density lipoproteins (LDLs) Compounds that facilitate the transport of cholesterol in the blood to the body's cells.
saturated fats Fats that are unable to hold any more hydrogen in their chemical structure; derived mostly from animal sources; solid at room temperature.
unsaturated fats Fats that do have room for more hydrogen in their chemical structure; derived mostly from plants; liquid at room temperature.
***trans* fats (*trans* fatty acids)** Fatty acids that are produced when polyunsaturated oils are hydrogenated to make them more solid.

228,000

deaths related to coronary heart disease could be averted each year by reducing Americans' consumption of *trans* fats, according to some estimates.

Avoiding *Trans* Fatty Acids

For decades, Americans shunned saturated fats found in butter, certain cuts of red meat, and a host of other foods. What they didn't know is that foods low in saturated fat, such as margarine, could be just as bad for us. As early as the 1990s Dutch researchers reported that a form of fat known as *trans* fats increased LDL cholesterol levels while decreasing HDL cholesterol levels. In a more recent study, researchers concluded that just a 2 percent caloric intake of *trans* fats was associated with an increased risk for heart disease of 23 percent and a 47 percent increased chance of sudden cardiac death.[18]

What are ***trans* fats (*trans* fatty acids)**? *Trans* fats are fatty acids that are produced by adding hydrogen molecules to liquid oil to make the oil into a solid. Unlike regular fats and oils, these "partially hydrogenated" fats stay solid or semisolid at room temperature. They change into irregular shapes at the molecular level, priming them to clog up arteries. *Trans* fats

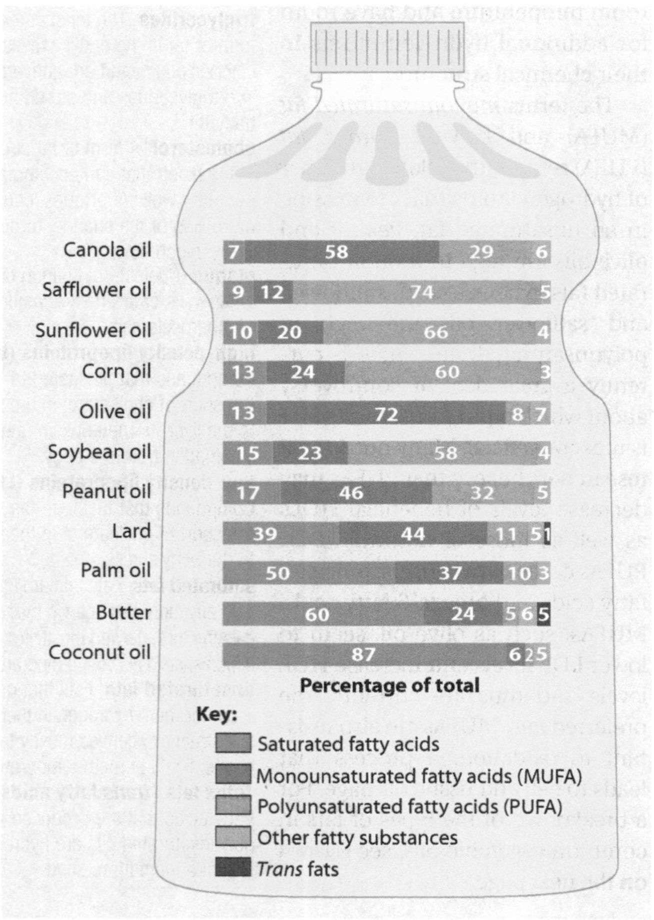

FIGURE 4 **Percentages of Saturated, Monounsaturated, Polyunsaturated, and *Trans* Fats in Common Vegetable Oils**

have been used in margarines, many commercial baked goods, and restaurant deep-fried foods.

In 2006, the Food and Drug Administration began to require labeling that tells consumers how much *trans* fat is in that cookie they are putting in their mouths. In July 2008, California took bold steps toward health by becoming the first state to ban *trans* fats from restaurant food. The American Medical Association (AMA) promptly followed suit in November 2008 by saying that banning *trans* fats would save up to 100,000 lives a year. Today, *trans* fats are being removed from most foods, and, if they *are* present, they must be clearly indicated. If you see the words *partially hydrogenated oils, fractionated oils, shortening, lard,* or *hydrogenation,* then *trans* fats are present.

New Fat Advice: Is More Fat Ever Better? Although most of this section has promoted the long-term recommendation to reduce saturated fat, avoid *trans* fatty acids, and eat more monounsaturated fats, some researchers worry that we have gone too far in our anti-fat frenzy. In fact, according to some experts, our zeal to eat no-fat or low-fat foods may be one of the greatest causes of obesity in America today. According to the American Heart Association, eating fewer than 15 percent of our calories as fat (fewer than 34 g a day on a 2,000-calorie diet) can actually

Skills for Behavior Change

Trimming the Fat for a Healthier You!

Enjoying a healthy intake of dietary fat doesn't have to be difficult or confusing. Follow these guidelines to add more healthy fats to your diet:

- **Eat fatty fish (bluefish, herring, mackerel, salmon, sardines, or tuna) at least twice weekly.**
- **Substitute soy and canola oils for corn, safflower, and sunflower oils. Keep using olive oil, too.**
- **Add healthy doses of green leafy vegetables, walnuts, walnut oil, and ground flaxseed to your diet.**

Follow these guidelines to help reduce your overall intake of less healthy fats:

- **Read the Nutrition Facts Panel on foods to find out how much fat is in your food. Remember that no more than 10 percent of your total calories should come from saturated fat, and no more than 30 percent should come from all forms of fat.**
- **Use olive oil for baking and sautéing.**
- **Chill soups and stews and scrape off any fat that hardens on top, then reheat to serve.**
- **Fill up on fruits and vegetables.**
- **Hold the creams and sauces.**
- **Avoid margarine products with *trans* fatty acids. Whenever possible, opt for other condiments on your bread, such as fresh vegetable spreads, sugar-free jams, fat-free cheese, and other healthy toppings.**
- **Choose lean meats, fish, or skinless poultry. Broil or bake whenever possible. Drain off fat after cooking.**
- **Experiment with eating whole wheat pastas, brown rice, beans, or vegetables as the main dish.**
- **Choose fewer cold cuts, bacon, sausages, hot dogs, and organ meats.**
- **Select nonfat and low-fat dairy products.**
- **When cooking, use substitutes for butter, margarine, oils, sour cream, mayonnaise, and salad dressings. Chicken or beef broth, fresh herbs, wine, vinegar, and low-calorie dressings provide flavor with less fat.**

increase blood triglycerides to levels that promote heart disease while lowering levels of protective HDLs.

The bottom line for fat intake is that moderation is the key. Remember that no more than 7 to 10 percent of your total calories should come from saturated fat and that no more than 30 percent should come from all forms of fat. In general, switching to beneficial fats without increasing total fat intake is a good idea. See the **Skills for Behavior Change** box above for tips on how to include more healthy fats, including the essential fatty acids, in your diet, while reducing your overall fat intake. The **Green Guide** at right provides tips for making healthy and sustainable seafood choices to fulfill your need for omega-3 fatty acids.

GREEN GUIDE

Toward Sustainable Seafood

The USDA recommends consuming fish two or three times per week to reduce saturated fat and cholesterol levels, and to increase omega-3 fatty acid levels. However, there are many environmental concerns surrounding the seafood industry today that call into question the sustainability and safety of such consumption. More than 70 percent of the world's natural fishing grounds have been overfished, and whole stretches of the oceans are, in fact, dead zones, where fish and shellfish can no longer live.

In an effort to counteract the loss of wild fish populations, increasing numbers of fish are being farmed, which poses additional health risks and environmental concerns. Some farmed fish are laden with antibiotics, while highly concentrated levels of parasites and bacteria from fish farm runoff may enter the ocean and river fish populations through adjacent waterways. There are other reasons to think carefully about your farmed fish alternatives. Farmed salmon, for example, are often fed wild fish, resulting in a net loss of fish from the sea.

At the same time that fish populations are threatened, high levels of chemicals, parasites, bacteria, and toxins are also being found in many of the fish available on the market. Mercury, a waste product of many industries, binds to proteins and stays in an animal's body, accumulating as it moves up the food chain; in humans mercury can cause damage to the nervous system and kidneys, and birth defects and developmental problems in fetuses and children. Polychlorinated biphenyls (PCBs), chemicals that can build up in the fatty tissue of fish, are another cause of major concern.

So what is a savvy fish consumer to do? Knowing where your fish are caught and the methods by which they are caught is important. Several major environmental groups have developed guides to inform consumers of safe and sustainable seafood choices. The guide shown here provides general national guidelines for seafood available for purchase in the United States. This guide is also available as a free iPhone application, or can be accessed on other mobile devices at http://mobile.seafoodwatch.org. Another great resource is the FishPhone service offered by the Blue Ocean Institute. Simply send a text message to 30644 with the word FISH and the type of fish you want to know about, and it will send you information about whether it is safe to eat. Remember: Your consumer choices make a difference. Purchasing seafood from environmentally responsible sources will support fisheries and fish farms that are healthier for you and the environment.

BEST CHOICES

- Arctic Char (farmed)
- Barramundi (US farmed)
- Catfish (US farmed)
- Clams (farmed)
- Cobia (US farmed)
- Cod: Pacific (Alaska longline)*
- Crab: Dungeness, Stone
- Halibut: Pacific*
- Lobster: Spiny (US)
- Mussels (farmed)
- Oysters (farmed)
- Pollock (Alaska wild)*
- Salmon (Alaska wild)*
- Scallops: Bay (farmed)
- Striped Bass (farmed or wild*)
- Tilapia (US farmed)
- Trout: Rainbow (farmed)
- Tuna: Albacore (troll/pole, US* or British Columbia)
- Tuna: Skipjack (troll/pole)

GOOD ALTERNATIVES

- Caviar, Sturgeon (US farmed)
- Clams (wild)
- Cod: Pacific (US trawled)
- Crab: Blue*, King (US), Snow
- Crab: Imitation/Surimi
- Flounders, Soles (Pacific)
- Herring: Atlantic
- Lobster: American/Maine
- Mahi mahi/Dolphinfish (US)
- Oysters (wild)*
- Scallops: Sea (wild)
- Shrimp (US, Canada)
- Squid
- Swai, Basa (farmed)
- Swordfish (US)*
- Tilapia (Central America, farmed)
- Tuna: Bigeye, Yellowfin (troll/pole)
- Tuna: Canned Skipjack and Albacore*
- Yellowtail (US farmed)

AVOID

- Caviar, Sturgeon* (imported wild)
- Chilean Seabass/Toothfish*
- Cobia (imported farmed)
- Cod: Atlantic, imported Pacific
- Flounders, Hailbut, Soles (Atlantic)
- Groupers*
- Lobster: Spiny (Caribbean)
- Mahi mahi/Dolphinfish (imported)
- Marlin: Blue*, Striped*
- Monkfish
- Orange Roughy*
- Salmon (farmed, including Atlantic)*
- Sharks*
- Shrimp (imported)
- Snapper: Red
- Swordfish (imported)*
- Tilapia (Asia farmed)
- Tuna: Albacore, Bigeye, Yellowfin (longline)*
- Tuna: Bluefin*, Tongol, Canned (except Albacore and Skipjack)
- Yellowtail (imported, farmed)

Support Ocean-Friendly Seafood

Best Choices are abundant, well-managed and caught or farmed in environmentally friendly ways.

Good Alternatives are an option, but there are concerns with how they're caught or farmed — or with the health of their habitat due to other human impacts.

Avoid for now as these items are caught or farmed in ways that harm other marine life or the environment.

Key

* Limit consumption due to concerns about mercury or other contaminants. Visit www.edf.org/seafood

* Some or all of this fishery is certified as sustainable to the Marine Stewardship Council standard. Visit www.msc.org

Seafood may appear in more than one column

Sustainable Seafood Guide

Source: Monterey Bay Aquarium Seafood Watch, *National Sustainable Seafood Guide, July 2009* Copyright © 2009, Monterey Bay Aquarium Foundation. Used with permission.

Vitamins

Vitamins are potent and essential organic compounds that promote growth and help maintain life and health. Every minute of every day, vitamins help maintain nerves and skin, produce blood cells, build bones and teeth, heal wounds, and convert food energy to body energy—and they do all this without adding any calories to your diet.

Vitamins can be classified as either *fat soluble,* which means they are absorbed through the intestinal tract with the help of fats, or *water soluble,* which means they are dissolved easily in water. Vitamins A, D, E, and K are fat soluble; B-complex vitamins and vitamin C are water soluble. Fat-soluble vitamins tend to be stored in the body, and toxic accumulations in the liver may cause cirrhosis-like symptoms. Water-soluble vitamins generally are excreted and cause few toxicity problems. See Tables 2 and 3 on the following pages for more information on the benefits and dangers of specific vitamins.

Antioxidants The old adage "you are what you eat" is indeed a motto to live by. Beneficial foods are termed **functional foods** based on the ancient belief that eating the right foods not only may prevent disease, but also may actually cure some diseases. This perspective is gaining credibility among the scientific community. Some of the most popular functional foods today are items containing **antioxidants** or other phytochemicals (from the Greek word meaning "plant"). Among the more commonly cited nutrients touted as providing a protective antioxidant effect are vitamin C, vitamin E, and beta-carotene. Although these substances do appear to protect people from the ravages of oxidative stress and resultant tissue damage at the cellular level, you may want to consider all the evidence. First, it is important to understand what damage from *oxidative stress* really is. This damage occurs in a complex process in which *free radicals* (molecules with unpaired electrons that are produced in excess when the body is overly stressed) either damage or kill healthy cells, cell proteins, or genetic material in the cells. Antioxidants produce enzymes that scavenge free radicals, slow their formation, or actually repair oxidative stress damage.

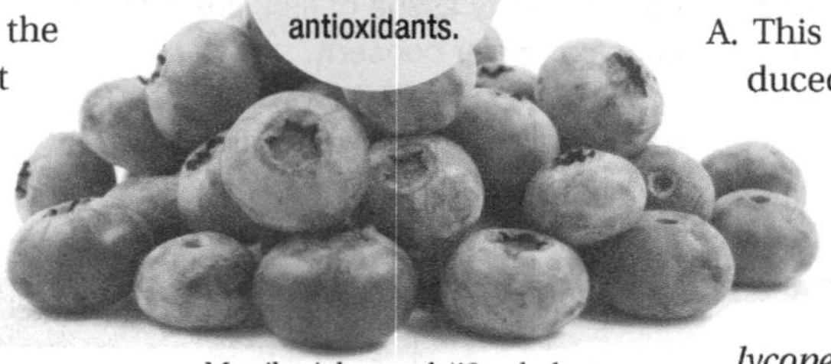

Blueberries are a great source of antioxidants.

Monika Adamczyk/iStockphoto

vitamins Essential organic compounds that promote growth and reproduction and help maintain life and health.

functional foods Foods believed to have specific health benefits and/or to prevent disease.

antioxidants Substances believed to protect against oxidative stress and resultant tissue damage at the cellular level.

carotenoids Fat-soluble plant pigments with antioxidant properties.

To date, many claims about the benefits of antioxidants in reducing the risk of heart disease, improving vision, and slowing the aging process have not been fully investigated, and conclusive statements about their true benefits are difficult to find (see the **Health Headlines** box on soy). Large, longitudinal epidemiological studies support the hypothesis that antioxidants in foods, mostly fruits and vegetables, help protect against cognitive decline and risk of Parkinson's disease.[19] Other studies indicate that these vitamins, particularly when taken as supplements, have no effect on atherosclerosis.[20]

Some studies indicate that when people's diets include foods rich in vitamin C, they seem to develop fewer cancers, but other studies detect no effect from dietary vitamin C.[21] Recent studies indicate that high-dose vitamin C given intravenously, rather than orally, may be effective in treating cancer and protecting from diseases affecting the central nervous system.[22]

Possible effects of vitamin E intake are even more controversial. Researchers have long theorized that because many cancers result from DNA damage, and because vitamin E appears to protect against DNA damage, vitamin E would also reduce cancer risk. Surprisingly, the great majority of studies have demonstrated no effect or, in some cases, a negative effect.[23]

Carotenoids are part of the red, orange, and yellow pigments found in fruits and vegetables. They are fat soluble, transported in the blood by lipoproteins, and stored in the fatty tissues of the body. Beta-carotene, the most researched carotenoid, is a precursor of vitamin A. This means that vitamin A can be produced in the body from beta-carotene; like vitamin A, beta-carotene has antioxidant properties.[24] Although there are over 600 carotenoids in nature, two that have received a great deal of attention are *lycopene* (found in tomatoes, papaya, pink grapefruit, and guava) and *lutein* (found in green leafy vegetables such as spinach, broccoli, kale, and brussels sprouts). Both are believed to be more beneficial than beta-carotene in preventing disease.

The National Cancer Institute and the American Cancer Society have endorsed lycopene as a possible factor in reducing the risk of cancer. A landmark study assessing the effects of tomato-based foods reported that men who ate ten or more servings of lycopene-rich foods per week had a 45 percent lower risk of prostate cancer.[25] However, subsequent research has questioned the benefits of lycopene, and some professional groups are modifying their endorsements of tomato-based products.

Lutein is most often touted as a means of protecting the eyes, particularly from age-related macular degeneration (ARMD), a leading cause of blindness for people aged 65 and older. Although there is considerable controversy over many of the benefits of these nutrients in protecting against selected illnesses, experts generally agree that the best way to obtain these nutrients is through foods, rather than pills.

Folate A form of vitamin B that is needed for DNA production in body cells, folate, is particularly important during fetal development; folate deficiencies during

TABLE 2

A Guide to Water-Soluble Vitamins

Vitamin Name and Recommended Intake	Reliable Food Sources	Primary Functions	Toxicity/Deficiency Symptoms
Thiamin (vitamin B_1) RDA: Men = 1.2 mg/day Women = 1.1 mg/day	Pork, fortified cereals, enriched rice and pasta, peas, tuna, legumes	Required as enzyme cofactor for carbohydrate and amino acid metabolism	*Toxicity:* none known *Deficiency:* beriberi, fatigue, apathy, decreased memory, confusion, irritability, muscle weakness
Riboflavin (vitamin B_2) RDA: Men = 1.3 mg/day Women = 1.1 mg/day	Beef liver, shrimp, milk and dairy foods, fortified cereals, enriched breads and grains	Required as enzyme cofactor for carbohydrate and fat metabolism	*Toxicity:* none known *Deficiency:* ariboflavinosis, swollen mouth and throat, seborrheic dermatitis, anemia
Niacin, nicotinamide, nicotinic acid RDA: Men = 16 mg/day Women = 14 mg/day UL = 35 mg/day	Beef liver, most cuts of meat/fish/poultry, fortified cereals, enriched breads and grains, canned tomato products	Required for carbohydrate and fat metabolism; plays role in DNA replication and repair and cell differentiation	*Toxicity:* flushing, liver damage, glucose intolerance, blurred vision differentiation *Deficiency:* pellagra; vomiting, constipation, or diarrhea; apathy
Vitamin B_6 (pyridoxine, pyridoxal, pyridoxamine) RDA: Men and women 19–50 = 1.3 mg/day Men > 50 = 1.7 mg/day Women > 50 = 1.5 mg/day UL = 100 mg/day	Chickpeas (garbanzo beans), most cuts of meat/fish/poultry, fortified cereals, white potatoes	Required as enzyme cofactor for carbohydrate and amino acid metabolism; assists synthesis of blood cells	*Toxicity:* nerve damage, skin lesions *Deficiency:* anemia; seborrheic dermatitis; depression, confusion, and convulsions
Folate (folic acid) RDA: Men = 400 μg/day Women = 400 μg/day UL = 1,000 μg/day	Fortified cereals, enriched breads and grains, spinach, legumes (lentils, chickpeas, pinto beans), greens (spinach, romaine lettuce), liver	Required as enzyme cofactor for amino acid metabolism; required for DNA synthesis; involved in metabolism of homocysteine	*Toxicity:* masks symptoms of vitamin B_{12} deficiency, specifically signs of nerve damage *Deficiency:* macrocytic anemia; neural tube defects in a developing fetus; elevated homocysteine levels
Vitamin B_{12} (cobalamin) RDA: Men = 2.4 μg/day Women = 2.4 μg/day	Shellfish, all cuts of meat/fish/poultry, milk and dairy foods, fortified cereals	Assists with formation of blood; required for healthy nervous system function; involved as enzyme cofactor in metabolism of homocysteine	*Toxicity:* none known *Deficiency:* pernicious anemia; tingling and numbness of extremities; nerve damage; memory loss, disorientation, and dementia
Pantothenic acid AI: Men = 5 mg/day Women = 5 mg/day	Meat/fish/poultry, shiitake mushrooms, fortified cereals, egg yolk	Assists with fat metabolism	*Toxicity:* none known *Deficiency:* rare
Biotin RDA: Men = 30 μg/day Women = 30 μg/day	Nuts, egg yolk	Involved as enzyme cofactor in carbohydrate, fat, and protein metabolism	*Toxicity:* none known *Deficiency:* rare
Vitamin C (ascorbic acid) RDA: Men = 90 mg/day Women = 75 mg/day Smokers = 35 mg more per day than RDA UL = 2,000 mg	Sweet peppers, citrus fruits and juices, broccoli, strawberries, kiwi	Antioxidant in extracellular fluid and lungs; regenerates oxidized vitamin E; assists with collagen synthesis; enhances immune function; assists in synthesis of hormones, neurotransmitters, and DNA; enhances iron absorption	*Toxicity:* nausea and diarrhea, nose-bleeds, increased oxidative damage, increased formation of kidney stones in people with kidney disease *Deficiency:* scurvy, bone pain and fractures, depression, and anemia

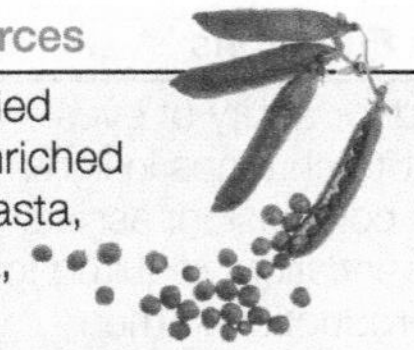
Brand Pictures/AGE Fotostock

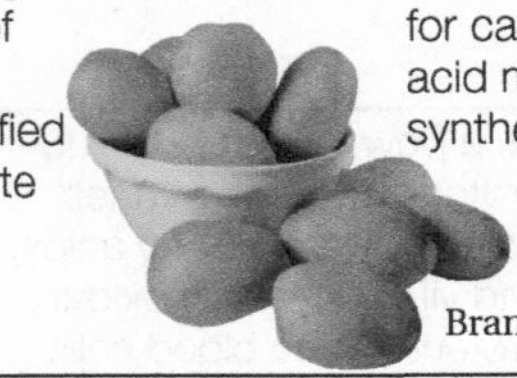
Brand Pictures/AGE Fotostock

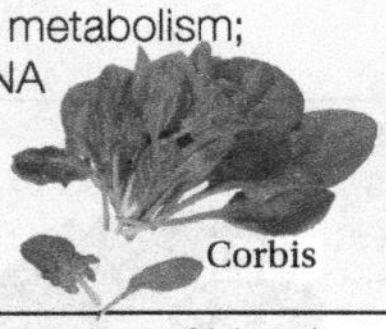
Corbis

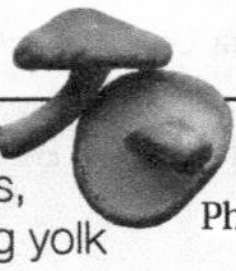
Photodisc/Getty Images

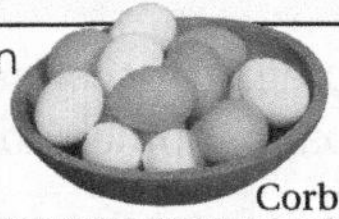
Corbis

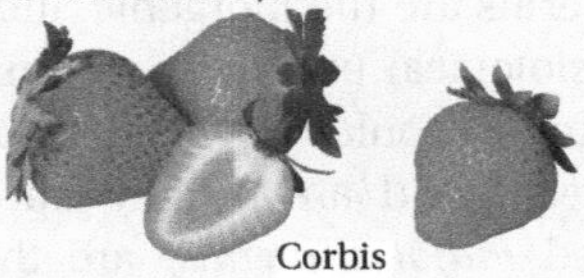
Corbis

Note: RDA = Recommended Daily Allowance; AI = Adequate Intakes; UL = Tolerable Upper Level Intakes. Values are for all adults aged 19 and older, except as noted. Values increase among women who are pregnant or lactating.

Source: From J. Thompson and M. Manore, *Nutrition: An Applied Approach.* 2d ed. (San Francisco: Benjamin Cummings, 2009). Reprinted by permission of Pearson Education.

TABLE 3

A Guide to Fat-Soluble Vitamins

Vitamin Name and Recommended Intake	Reliable Food Sources	Primary Functions	Toxicity/Deficiency Symptoms
Vitamin A (retinol, retinal, retinoic acid) RDA: Men = 900 μg Women = 700 μg UL = 3,000 μg/day 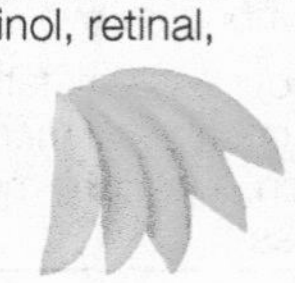 Brand Pictures/AGE Fotostock	Preformed retinol: beef and chicken liver, egg yolks, milk Carotenoid precursors: spinach, carrots, mango, apricots, cantaloupe, pumpkin, yams	Required for ability of eyes to adjust to changes in light; protects color vision; assists cell differentiation; required for sperm production in men and fertilization in women; contributes to healthy bone and healthy immune system	*Toxicity:* fatigue; bone and joint pain; spontaneous abortion and birth defects of fetuses in pregnant women; nausea and diarrhea; liver damage; nervous system damage; blurred vision; hair loss; skin disorders *Deficiency:* night blindness, xerophthalmia; impaired growth, immunity, and reproductive function
Vitamin D (cholecalciferol) AI (assumes that person does not get adequate sun exposure): Adult 19–50 = 5 μg/day Adult 50–70 = 10 μg/day Adult > 70 = 15 μg/day UL = 50 μg/day	Canned salmon and mackerel, milk, fortified cereals 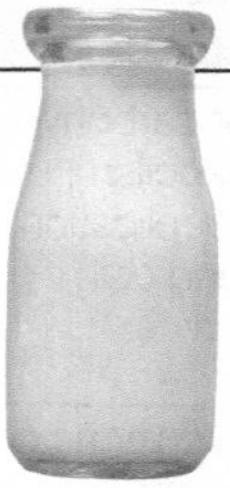 Corbis	Regulates blood calcium levels; maintains bone health; assists cell differentiation	*Toxicity:* hypercalcemia *Deficiency:* rickets in children; osteomalacia and/or osteoporosis in adults
Vitamin E (tocopherol) RDA: Men = 15 mg/day Women = 15 mg/day UL = 1,000 mg/day	Sunflower seeds, almonds, vegetable oils, fortified cereals	As a powerful antioxidant, protects cell membranes, polyunsaturated fatty acids, and vitamin A from oxidation; protects white blood cells; enhances immune function; improves absorption of vitamin A	*Toxicity:* rare *Deficiency:* hemolytic anemia; impairment of nerve, muscle, and immune function 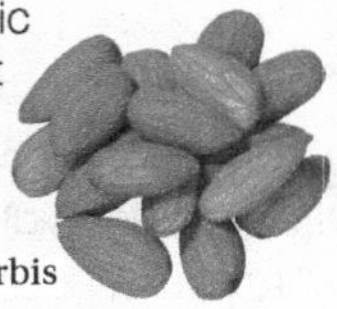 Corbis
Vitamin K (phylloquinone, menaquinone, menadione) AI: Men = 120 μg/day Women = 90 μg/day	Kale, spinach, turnip greens, brussels sprouts 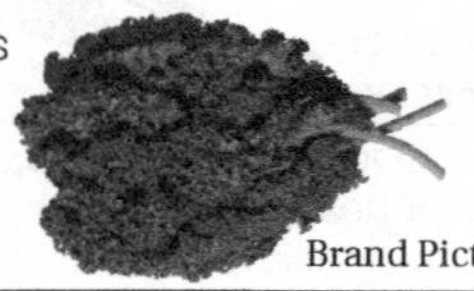 Brand Pictures/AGE Fotostock	Serves as a coenzyme during production of specific proteins that assist in blood coagulation and bone metabolism	*Toxicity:* none known *Deficiency:* impaired blood clotting; possible effect on bone health

Note: RDA = Recommended Daily Allowance; AI = Adequate Intakes; UL = Tolerable Upper Level Intakes. Values are for all adults aged 19 and older, except as noted. Values increase among women who are pregnant or lactating.

Source: From J. Thompson and M. Manore, *Nutrition: An Applied Approach.* 2d ed. (San Francisco: Benjamin Cummings, 2009). Reprinted by permission of Pearson Education.

pregnancy can result in spina bifida, a birth defect in which a baby's spine and spinal cord are not fully developed. In 1998, the FDA began requiring that all bread, cereal, rice, and pasta products sold in the United States be fortified with folic acid, the synthetic form of folate. This practice, which boosts folate intake by an average of 100 micrograms daily, is intended to decrease the number of infants born with spina bifida and other neural tube defects.

minerals Inorganic, indestructible elements that aid physiological processes.
macrominerals Minerals that the body needs in fairly large amounts.
trace minerals Minerals that the body needs in only very small amounts.

Folate was widely studied in the late 1990s for its potential to decrease blood levels of *homocysteine* (an amino acid that has been linked to vascular diseases) and to protect against cardiovascular disease (CVD).[26] More recent research has raised questions about the benefits of the B vitamins in reducing the risks of CVD or stroke, leading researchers to question these earlier results.[27]

Minerals

Minerals are the inorganic, indestructible elements that aid physiological processes within the body. Without minerals, vitamins could not be absorbed. Minerals are readily excreted and are usually not toxic. **Macrominerals** (also called *major minerals*) are those minerals that the body needs in fairly large amounts: sodium, calcium, phosphorus, magnesium, potassium, sulfur, and chloride. **Trace minerals** include iron, zinc, manganese, copper, and iodine. Only very small amounts of trace minerals are needed, and serious problems may result if excesses or deficiencies occur (see Tables 4 and 5).

Health Headlines

SOY WONDER?

Vegetarians and health enthusiasts have long known that foods made from soybeans offer a great alternative to meat, poultry, and other animal-based products. Soy protein is generally lower in calories and fat than animal protein. The FDA, American Heart Association, and others have provided endorsements or support for soy as a staple in the diet, suggesting it is associated with a host of health benefits, including reductions in heart disease, breast cancer, high cholesterol levels, and hot flashes during menopause. But is it all too good to be true?

An increasing number of new studies have failed to support such health claims, and have raised concern over certain components of soy products, particularly specific phytochemicals. In plants, mainly soybeans and other legumes, phytochemicals are biologically active, naturally occurring chemical components that are believed to act as natural defenses for the plant, protecting them from oxidative damage, infection, and microbial invasions. One type of phytochemical, *flavonoids* (a group of over 800 blue, red, and violet plant pigments found in foods ranging from teas and apples to grapes and red wine), have been shown to reduce the risk of heart disease by acting as antioxidants. While soy may have a small effect on reducing lipids, other potential CVD effects need more research. In particular, researchers are looking at the way in which soy is processed, which may reduce its potential effects.

Another phytochemical group, the *isoflavones*, are among those soy components most intensely scrutinized in recent years, particularly in studies focused on their role in reducing cancer. Why the scrutiny? Because some isoflavones are phytoestrogens, that is, plant steroidal versions of estrogens. The simplified theory, based on early research, was that they may be cancer protective and may decrease the hormone-related effects of estrogen-positive breast cancer by blocking carcinogens or suppressing tumors. Newer research calls into question the effect of soy in reducing cancer risk or on survival, particularly at the lower consumption levels typically seen in Western populations. Additional research is needed to assess whether soy consumption that begins during the adult years or earlier affects subsequent risk of cancer development.

The bottom line is that soy foods don't seem to lower cholesterol and triglyceride levels as much as previously thought. If you're supplementing your diet with soy as an alternative to high-fat, high-cholesterol, high-calorie foods or for humane or environmental reasons, you're probably doing the right thing. Most soy products also contain higher fiber and omega-3 fatty acids, which may reduce inflammation and certain health risks. If you are mega-dosing on soy to protect against heart disease, breast cancer, hot flashes, or other chronic diseases, you should take a close look at the research, as more is needed to prove the effectiveness of such actions.

pixhook/iStockphoto

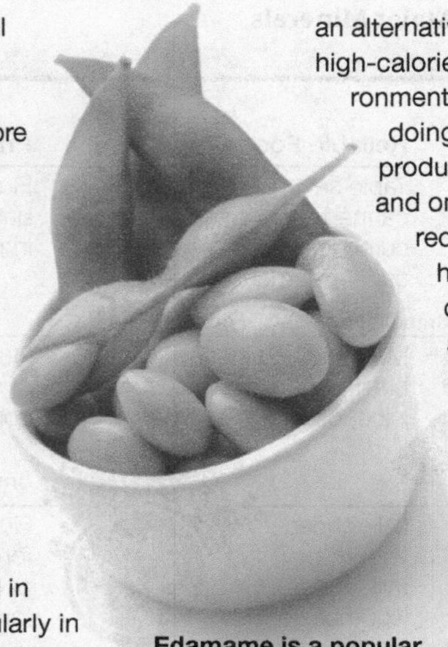

Edamame is a popular and tasty soybean snack.

Sources: C. W. Xiao, "Health Effects of Soy Protein and Isoflavones in Humans," *Journal of Nutrition* 138 (2008): 1244S–49S; E. Balk et al., *Effects of Soy on Health Outcomes*, Evidence Report/Technology Assessment Number 126, AHRQ Publication Number 05-E024-1 (Rockville, MD: Agency for Healthcare Research and Quality, 2005); F. Sacks et al., "Soy Proteins, Isoflavones and Cardiovascular Health: An American Heart Association Science Advisory for Professionals from the Nutrition Committee," *Circulation* 113 (2006): 1034–44; A.C. Yh et al., "Isoflavone Intake in Persons at High Risk of Cardiovascular Events: Implications for Vascular Endothelial Function and the Carotid Atheroschlerotic Burden," *American Journal of Clinical Nutrition* 86, no. 4 (2007): 938–44; M. Gammons, B. Fink, S. Steck, and M. Wolff, "Soy Intake and Breast Cancer: An Elucidation of an Unanswered Question," *British Journal of Cancer* 98 (2008): 2–3; S. Boyapati et al., "Soyfood Intake and Breast Cancer Survival: A Followup of the Shanghai Breast Cancer Study," *Breast Cancer Research and Treatment* 92, no. 1 (2005): 11–17; B. Fink et al., "Dietary Flavonoid Intake and Breast Cancer Risk among Women on Long Island," *American Journal of Epidemiology* 165, no. 5 (2007): 514–23.

Sodium Sodium is necessary for the regulation of blood and body fluids, transmission of nerve impulses, heart activity, and certain metabolic functions. It enhances flavors, balances the bitterness of certain foods, acts as a preservative, and tenderizes meats, so it's often present in high quantities in many of the foods we eat. As a result, most of us consume far too much sodium. Today, the Institute of Medicine, the American Heart Association, the FDA, and the USDA are among the many professional organizations that recommend that healthy people consume fewer than 2,300 milligrams of sodium each day. What does that really mean? For most of us, that means consuming less than 1 teaspoon of table salt per day! Recent studies indicate that, on average, we eat nearly twice that amount each day.[28]

A common misconception is that salt and sodium are the same thing. However, table salt accounts for only 15 percent of sodium intake. The majority of sodium in our diet comes from highly processed foods that are infused with sodium to enhance flavor and preservation. Pickles, salty snack foods, processed cheeses, canned soups, frozen dinners, many breads and bakery products, and smoked meats and sausages often contain several hundred milligrams of sodium per serving.

TABLE 4 **A Guide to Major Minerals**

Mineral Name and Recommended Intake	Reliable Food Sources	Primary Functions	Toxicity/Deficiency Symptoms
Sodium AI: Adults = 1.5 g/day (1,500 mg/day)	Table salt, pickles, most canned soups, snack foods, cured luncheon meats, canned tomato products	Fluid balance; acid–base balance; transmission of nerve impulses; muscle contraction	*Toxicity:* water retention, high blood pressure, loss of calcium *Deficiency:* muscle cramps, dizziness, fatigue, nausea, vomiting, mental confusion
Potassium AI: Adults = 4.7 g/day (4,700 mg/day) 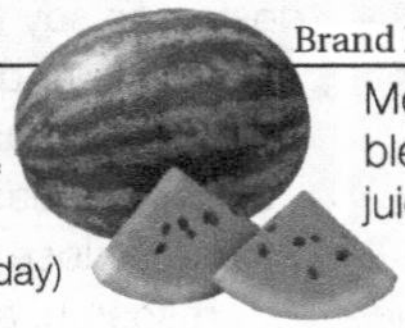 Brand Pictures/AGE Fotostock	Most fresh fruits and vegetables: potato, banana, tomato juice, orange juice, melon	Fluid balance; transmission of nerve impulses; muscle contraction	*Toxicity:* muscle weakness, vomiting, irregular heartbeat *Deficiency:* muscle weakness, paralysis, mental confusion, irregular heartbeat
Phosphorus RDA: Adults = 700 mg/day	Milk/cheese/yogurt, soy milk and tofu, legumes (lentils, black beans), nuts (almonds, peanuts), poultry 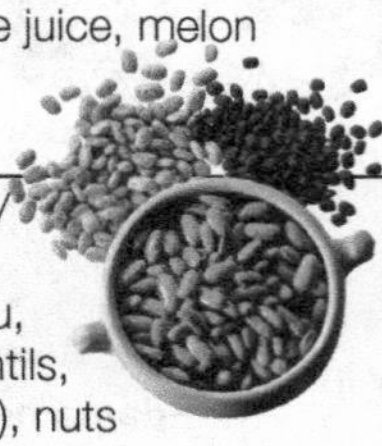 Brand Pictures/AGE Fotostock	Fluid balance; bone formation; component of ATP, which provides energy for our bodies	*Toxicity:* muscle spasms, convulsions, low blood calcium *Deficiency:* muscle weakness, muscle damage, bone pain, dizziness
Chloride AI: Adults = 2.3 g/day (2,300 mg/day)	Table salt	Fluid balance; transmission of nerve impulses; component of stomach acid (HCL); antibacterial	*Toxicity:* none known *Deficiency:* dangerous blood acid–base imbalances, irregular heartbeat
Calcium AI: Adults 19–50 = 1,000 mg/day Adults > 50 = 1,200 mg/day UL = 2,500 mg	Milk/yogurt/cheese (best absorbed form of calcium), sardines, collard greens and spinach, calcium-fortified juices 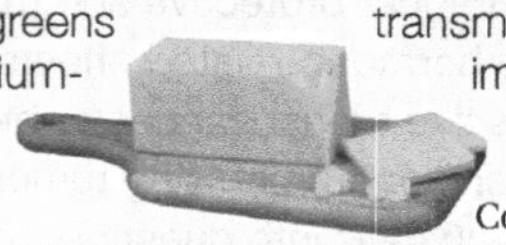 Corbis	Primary component of bone; acid–base balance; transmission of nerve impulses; muscle contraction	*Toxicity:* mineral imbalances, shock, kidney failure, fatigue, mental confusion *Deficiency:* osteoporosis, convulsions, heart failure
Magnesium RDA: Men 19–30 = 400 mg/day Men > 30 = 420 mg/day Women 19–30 = 310 mg/day Women > 30 = 320 mg/day UL = 350 mg/day	Greens (spinach, kale, collards), whole grains, seeds, nuts, legumes (navy and black beans)	Component of bone; muscle contraction; assists more than 300 enzyme systems 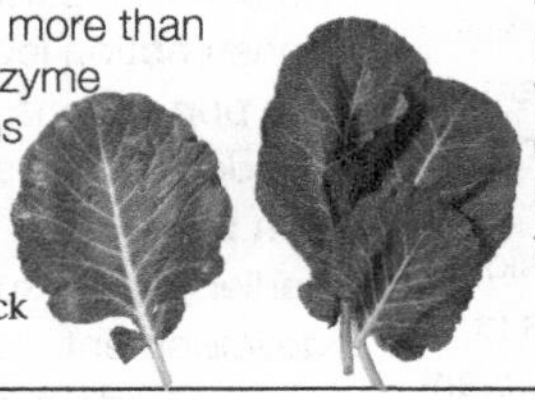 Brand Pictures/AGE Fotostock	*Toxicity:* none known *Deficiency:* low blood calcium; muscle spasms or seizures; nausea; weakness; increased risk of chronic diseases such as heart disease, hypertension, osteoporosis, and type 2 diabetes
Sulfur No DRI	Protein-rich foods	Component of certain B vitamins and amino acids; acid–base balance; detoxification in liver	*Toxicity:* none known *Deficiency:* none known 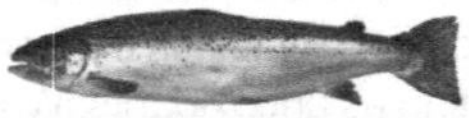 Corbis

Note: RDA = Recommended Daily Allowance; AI = Adequate Intakes; UL = Tolerable Upper Level Intake. Values are for all adults aged 19 and older, except as noted.

Source: From J. Thompson and M. Manore, *Nutrition: An Applied Approach.* 2d ed. (San Francisco: Benjamin Cummings, 2009). Reprinted by permission of Pearson Education.

Why is high sodium intake a concern? Many experts believe that there is a link between excessive sodium intake and hypertension (high blood pressure). Although this theory is controversial, it is recommended that hypertensive Americans cut back on sodium to reduce their risk for cardiovascular disorders including stroke, debilitating bone fractures, and other health problems.[29]

Calcium The issue of calcium consumption has gained national attention with the rising incidence of osteoporosis among older adults. Although calcium plays a vital role in building strong bones and teeth, muscle contraction, blood clotting, nerve impulse transmission, regulating heartbeat, and fluid balance within cells, most Americans do not consume the recommended 1,000–1,200 milligrams of calcium per day.[30]

It is critical to consume the minimum required amount each day. Milk is one of the richest sources of dietary calcium. Calcium-fortified orange juice and soy milk are good alternatives if you do not drink dairy milk. Many green leafy vegetables are good sources of calcium, but some contain oxalic acid,

TABLE 5

A Guide to Trace Minerals

Mineral Name and Recommended Intake	Reliable Food Sources	Primary Functions	Toxicity/Deficiency Symptoms
Selenium RDA: Adults = 55 µg/day UL = 400 µg/day	Nuts, shellfish, meat/fish/poultry, whole grains 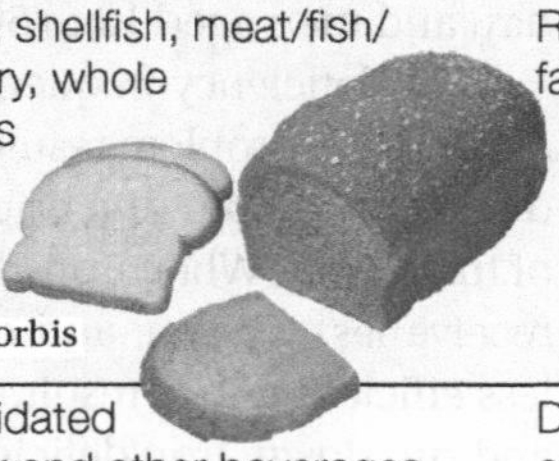 Corbis	Required for carbohydrate and fat metabolism	*Toxicity:* brittle hair and nails, skin rashes, nausea and vomiting, weakness, liver disease *Deficiency:* specific forms of heart disease and arthritis, impaired immune function, muscle pain and wasting, depression, hostility
Fluoride AI: Men = 4 mg/day Women = 3 mg/day UL = 2.2 mg/day for children 4–8 years; children > 8 years = 10 mg/day	Fluoridated water and other beverages made with this water	Development and maintenance of healthy teeth and bones	*Toxicity:* fluorosis of teeth and bones *Deficiency:* dental caries, low bone density
Iodine RDA: Adults = 150 µg/day UL = 1,100 µg/day	Iodized salt and foods processed with iodized salt	Synthesis of thyroid hormones; temperature regulation; reproduction and growth	*Toxicity:* goiter *Deficiency:* goiter, hypothyroidism, cretinism in infant of mother who is iodine deficient
Chromium AI: Men 19–50 = 35 µg/day Men > 50 = 30 µg/day Women 19–50 = 25 µg/day Women > 50 = 20 µg/day	Grains, meat/fish/poultry, some fruits and vegetables	Glucose transport; metabolism of DNA and RNA; immune function and growth	*Toxicity:* none known *Deficiency:* elevated blood glucose and blood lipids, damage to brain and nervous system
Manganese AI: Men = 2.3 mg/day Women = 1.8 mg/day UL = 11 mg/day for adults	Whole grains, nuts, legumes, some fruits and vegetables	Assists many enzyme systems; synthesis of protein found in bone and cartilage	*Toxicity:* impairment of neuromuscular system *Deficiency:* impaired growth and reproductive function, reduced bone density, impaired glucose and lipid metabolism, skin rash
Iron RDA: Men = 8 mg/day Women 19–50 = 18 mg/day Women > 50 = 8 mg/day	Meat/fish/poultry (best absorbed form of iron), fortified cereals, legumes, spinach 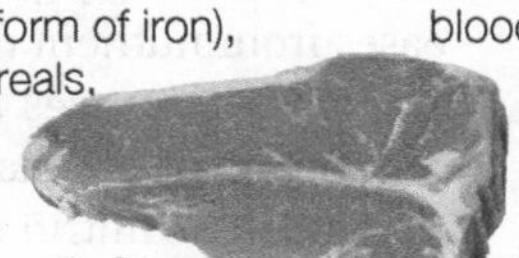 Corbis	Component of hemoglobin in blood cells; component of myoglobin in muscle cells; assists many enzyme systems	*Toxicity:* nausea, vomiting, and diarrhea; dizziness, confusion; rapid heartbeat; organ damage; death *Deficiency:* iron-deficiency microcytic anemia, hypochromic anemia
Zinc RDA: Men 11 mg/day Women = 8 mg/day UL = 40 mg/day 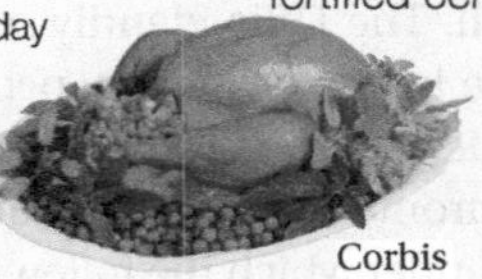 Corbis	Meat/fish/poultry (best absorbed form of zinc), fortified cereals, legumes	Assists more than 100 enzyme systems; immune system function; growth and sexual maturation; gene regulation	*Toxicity:* nausea, vomiting, and diarrhea; headaches; depressed immune function; reduced absorption of copper *Deficiency:* growth retardation, delayed sexual maturation, eye and skin lesions, hair loss, increased incidence of illness and infection
Copper RDA: Adults = 900 µg/day UL = 10 mg/day	Shellfish, organ meats, nuts, legumes	Assists many enzyme systems; iron transport 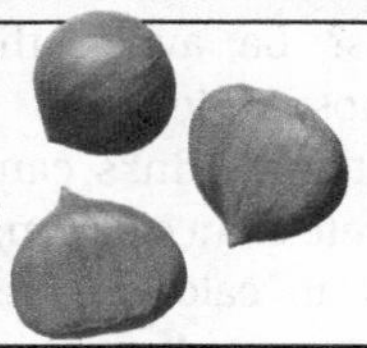 Photodisc/Getty Images	*Toxicity:* nausea, vomiting, and diarrhea; liver damage *Deficiency:* anemia, reduced levels of white blood cells, osteoporosis in infants and growing children

Note: RDA = Recommended Daily Allowance; AI = Adequate Intakes; UL = Tolerable Upper Intake Level. Values are for all adults aged 19 and older, except as noted.

Source: Adapted from J. Thompson and M. Manore, *Nutrition: An Applied Approach.* 2d ed. (San Francisco: Benjamin Cummings, 2009). Reprinted by permission of Pearson Education.

Peter Nicholson/Stone Allstock/Getty Images

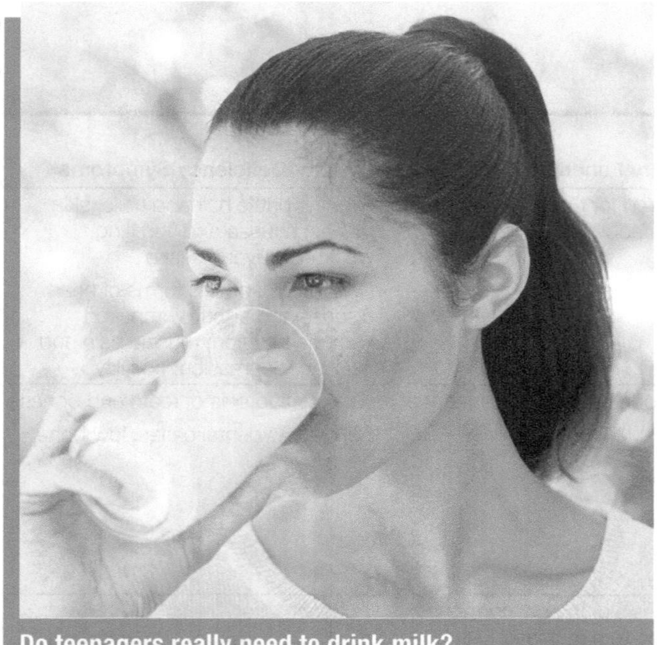

Do teenagers really need to drink milk?

Consumption of calcium, one of the many nutrients in milk, is important for people of all ages. To build healthy bones and teeth, and to prevent bone loss later in life, you need to get enough calcium while you are young; women, in particular, should be sure to obtain adequate amounts. Yet, 85% of adolescent girls do not consume enough calcium, and during the last 25 years, consumption of milk has decreased 36% among teenage girls. If you are one of those who do not drink milk, be sure you are getting enough calcium—at least 1,200 milligrams per day—through other sources.

which makes their calcium harder to absorb. Spinach, chard, and beet greens are not particularly good sources of calcium, whereas broccoli, cauliflower, and many peas and beans offer good supplies.

It is generally best to take calcium throughout the day, consuming it with foods containing protein, vitamin D, and vitamin C for optimal absorption. Many dairy products are fortified with vitamin D, which is known to improve calcium absorption. We also know that sunlight increases the manufacture of vitamin D in the body and is therefore like an extra calcium source.

Do you consume carbonated soft drinks? Be aware that the added phosphoric acid (phosphate) in these drinks can cause you to excrete extra calcium, which may result in calcium loss from your bones. A recent study of 2,500 men and women found that in women who consumed at least three cans of cola per week, even diet cola, bone density of the hip was 4 to 5 percent lower than in women who drank fewer than one cola per month. Colas did not seem to have the same effect on men.[31]

anemia Condition that results from the body's inability to produce hemoglobin.

Recommended Dietary Allowances (RDAs) The average daily intakes of energy and nutrients considered adequate to meet the needs of most healthy people in the United States under usual conditions.

Iron Worldwide, iron deficiency is the most common nutrient deficiency, affecting more than 2 billion people, nearly 30 percent of the world's population. In the United States iron deficiency is less prevalent, but it is still the most common micronutrient deficiency.[32] How much iron do we need? Women aged 19 to 50 need about 18 milligrams per day, and men aged 19 to 50 need about 8 milligrams.

Iron deficiency frequently leads to *iron-deficiency anemia*. **Anemia** is a problem resulting from the body's inability to produce hemoglobin (the bright red oxygen-carrying component of the blood). When iron-deficiency anemia occurs, body cells receive less oxygen, and carbon dioxide wastes are removed less efficiently. As a result, the iron-deficient person feels tired and run down. Iron deficiency in the diet is a common cause, but not the only cause, of anemia; anemia can also result from blood loss, cancer, ulcers, and other conditions.

Iron overload or iron toxicity due to ingesting too many iron-containing supplements remains the leading cause of accidental poisoning in small children in the United States. Symptoms of toxicity include nausea, vomiting, diarrhea, rapid heartbeat, weak pulse, dizziness, shock, and confusion. Excess iron intake has also been associated with other problems: a recent study of over 45,000 men indicated that those who consumed excess heme iron—the kind found in meat, seafood, and poultry—had a 20 percent higher risk of gallstones than those who consumed low-iron foods or got their iron from supplements.[33]

Determining Your Nutritional Needs

Historically, various government and scientific organizations developed dietary guidelines to reduce the public's risk of diseases from nutrient deficiency. Known as the **Recommended Dietary Allowances (RDAs),** these guidelines have provided Americans and Canadians with recommended intake levels that meet the nutritional needs of about 97 percent of healthy individuals. In 1997, the U.S. Food and Nutrition Board replaced and expanded upon the RDAs by creating new *Dietary Reference Intakes (DRIs)*, a list of 26 nutrients essential to maintaining health. The DRIs identify recommended and maximum safe intake levels for healthy people and establish the amount of a nutrient needed to prevent deficiencies or to reduce the risk of chronic disease. DRIs are considered the umbrella guidelines under which the following categories fall:

- *U.S. Recommended Dietary Allowances (USRDAs):* The reference standard for intake levels necessary to meet the nutritional needs of 97 to 98 percent of healthy individuals
- *Adequate Intake (AI):* The recommended average daily nutrient intake level by healthy people when there is not enough research to determine the full RDA
- *Tolerable Upper Intake Level (UL):* The highest amount of a nutrient an individual can consume daily without the risk of adverse health effects

Reading Labels for Health

To help consumers determine the nutritional values of foods, the FDA and the USDA developed the *Reference Daily Intakes (RDIs)* and the *Daily Reference Values (DRVs)*. RDIs are the recommended daily amounts of 19 vitamins and minerals, also known as *micronutrients*, and DRVs are the recommended amounts for macronutrients, such as total fat, saturated fat, cholesterol, total carbohydrates, dietary fiber, sodium, potassium, and protein.

Confused by all of these values? Don't despair—many people are confused by all the numbers, percentages, and serving sizes that make up today's labels. Just remember this: Together, RDIs and DRVs make up the **Daily Values (DVs).** These are the percentages that you will find listed as "% Daily Value" on food and supplement labels (see Figure 5). In addition to the percentage of nutrients found in a serving of food, labels include information on the serving size, calories, calories from fat per serving, and percentage of *trans* fats in a food.

Supplements: Research on the Daily Dose

Dietary supplements are products—usually vitamins and minerals—taken by mouth and intended to supplement existing diets. Ingredients range from vitamins, minerals, and herbs to enzymes, amino acids, fatty acids, and organ tissues. They can come in tablet, capsule, liquid, powder, and other forms. Because of dietary supplements' potential for influencing health, their sales have skyrocketed in the past decades.

Daily Values (DVs) Percentages listed as "% DV" on food and supplement labels; made up of the RDIs and DRVs together.

dietary supplements Vitamins and minerals taken by mouth that are intended to supplement existing diets.

It is important to note that all dietary supplements are not regulated like other food and drug products. The FDA does not evaluate the safety and efficacy of supplements prior to their marketing; it can take action to remove a supplement from the market only after it has been proven harmful. Currently, the United States has no formal

Start here. The size of the serving on the food package influences the number of calories and all the nutrient amounts listed on the top part of the label. Pay attention to the serving size, especially how many servings there are in the food package. Then ask yourself, "How many servings am I consuming"?

Limit these nutrients. The nutrients listed first are the ones Americans generally eat in adequate amounts, or even too much. Eating too much fat, saturated fat, *trans* fat, cholesterol, or sodium may increase your risk of certain chronic diseases, such as heart disease, some cancers, or high blood pressure.

Get enough of these nutrients. Most Americans don't get enough dietary fiber, vitamin A, vitamin C, calcium, and iron in their diets. Eating enough of these nutrients can improve your health and help reduce the risk of some diseases and conditions.

The footnote is not specific to the product. It shows recommended dietary advice for all Americans. The Percent Daily Values are based on a 2,000-calorie diet, but the footnote lists daily values for both a 2,000- and 2,500-calorie diet.

Sample Label for Macaroni and Cheese

Nutrition Facts

Serving size 1 cup (228g)
Servings Per Container 2

Amount Per Serving	
Calories 250	Calories from Fat 110
	% Daily Value*
Total Fat 12g	**18%**
Saturated Fat 3g	**15%**
Trans Fat 1.5g	
Cholesterol 30mg	**10%**
Sodium 470mg	**20%**
Total Carbohydrate 31g	**10%**
Dietary Fiber 0g	**0%**
Sugars 5g	
Protein 5g	
Vitamin A	4%
Vitamin C	2%
Calcium	20%
Iron	4%

* Percent Daily Values are based on a 2,000 calorie diet. Your Daily Values may be higher or lower depending on your calorie needs:

	Calories:	2,000	2,500
Total Fat	Less than	65g	80g
Sat Fat	Less than	20g	25g
Cholesterol	Less than	300mg	300mg
Sodium	Less than	2,400mg	2,400mg
Total Carbohydrate		300g	375g
Dietary Fiber		25g	30g

Pay attention to calories (and calories from fat). Many Americans consume more calories than they need. Remember: The number of servings you consume determines the number of calories you actually eat (your portion amount). Dietary guidelines recommend that no more than 30% of your daily calories consumed come from fat.

5% DV or less is low and 20% DV or more is high. The % DV helps you determine if a serving of food is high or low in a nutrient, whether or not you consume the 2,000-calorie diet they are based on. It also helps you make easy comparisons between products (just make sure the serving sizes are similar).

Note that a few nutrients—*trans* fats, sugars, and protein—do not have a % DV. Experts could not provide a reference value for *trans* fat, but it is recommended that you keep your intake as low as possible. There are no recommendations for the total amount of sugar to eat in one day, but check the ingredient list to see information on added sugars, such as high fructose corn syrup. A % DV for protein is required to be listed if a claim is made (such as "high in protein") or if the food is meant for infants and children under 4 years old. Otherwise, none is needed.

FIGURE 5 **Reading a Food Label**

Source: Center for Food Safety and Applied Nutrition, "How to Understand and Use the Nutrition Facts Label," 2004, www.cfsan.fda.gov/~dms/foodlab.html.

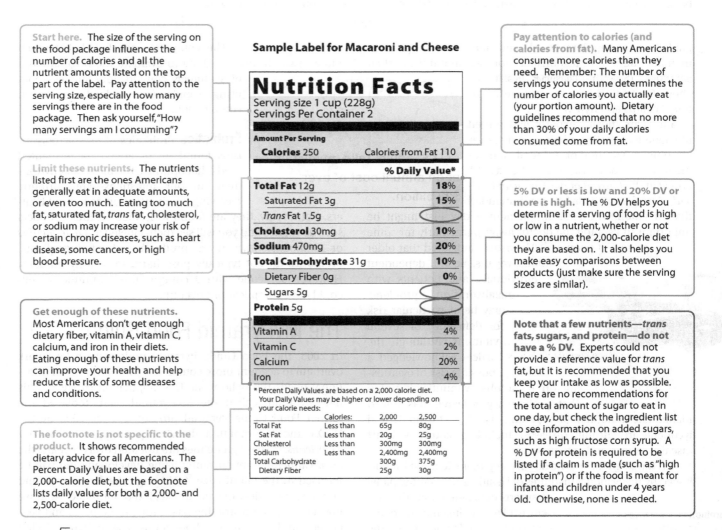

CONSUMER HEALTH

MAKING SENSE OF NUTRITION HYPE

Frustrated by health food discoveries that seem to fizzle as fast as they burst onto the scene? You're not alone. In the past few decades, we've been bombarded with a wide variety of conflicting scientific evidence and claims about dietary choices we can make to reduce the risk of certain diseases and promote health. The good news is that there are positive outcomes in all this research, and positive health effects can be gained from proper nutrition. The bad news? This plethora of studies produces conflicting reports that leave many of us scratching our heads. Here is what you need to consider about reports you hear and read about in the media:

1. Remember that any single study must be viewed with caution. Often there are other, equally reputable, studies that may prove opposite findings.
2. Many of these studies are meta-analyses. This means they summarize the results of many studies, often without regard to population, study design, age of the population studied, confounders (things that could influence effects), dosage, underlying bias of the population, and many other factors.
3. Information gained from studies like the Women's Health Initiative about diet and exercise is largely based on self-reporting. Many people question the validity of some responses. Even randomized, controlled trials have limitations, and results should be viewed in light of potential limitations and the results of previous studies.
4. The best studies will conclude that more research must be done. Though this may seem frustrating and may not give the definitive answers we are looking for, this is the most current and accurate response that researchers can give.

guidelines for supplement sale and safety, and supplement manufacturers are responsible for self-monitoring their activities. (See the **Consumer Health** box above for tips on how to evaluate nutritional claims and hype.)

52% **of U.S. adults take multivitamins, at an annual cost of over $23 billion.**

For years, health experts had touted the benefits of eating a balanced diet over popping a vitamin or mineral supplement, so it came as a surprise when a 2001 article in the *Journal of the American Medical Association (JAMA)* recommended that "a vitamin/mineral supplement a day just might be important in keeping the doctor away, particularly for some groups of people."[34] The article indicated that older adults, vegans, alcohol-dependent individuals, and patients with malabsorption problems may be at particular risk for deficiency of several vitamins. Although the article acknowledged a possible risk of overdosing on fat-soluble vitamins, it noted that preliminary research has linked inadequate amounts of vitamins B_6, B_{12}, D, and E and lycopene to chronic diseases, including coronary heart disease, cancer, and osteoporosis.

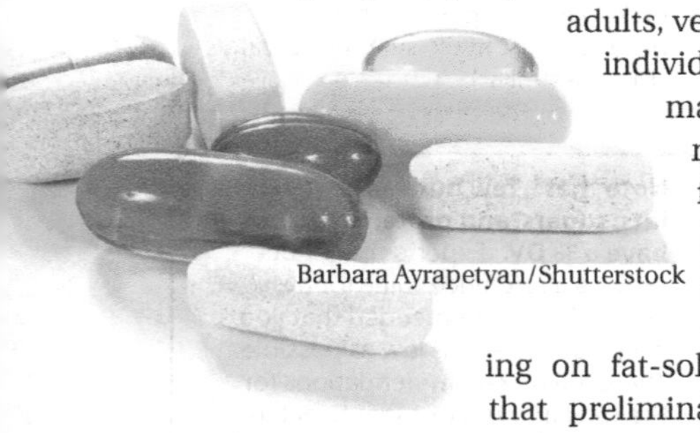
Barbara Ayrapetyan/Shutterstock

Yet, the scientific debate doesn't stop there. In a 2006 report issued by the National Institutes of Health, a 13-member panel of experts concluded that "the present evidence is insufficient to recommend either for or against the use of multivitamins and minerals by the American public to prevent chronic diseases."[35] The committee concluded that much more research must be done to evaluate the huge amount of seemingly contradictory studies about using supplements individually or in combination.

probiotics Live microorganisms found in or added to fermented foods; they are intended to optimize the bacterial environment in our intestines.

Probiotics **Probiotics**—live microorganisms found in, or added to, fermented foods that optimize the bacterial environment in our intestines—are currently receiving much attention as natural healers. Commonly, they are found in fermented milk products such as yogurt, and you will see them labeled as *Lactobacillus* or *Bifidobacterium* in a product's list of ingredients. Probiotics do not typically pose harm to healthy humans. However, someone with a compromised immune system could have complications over time.

The MyPyramid Food Guide

In 2005, the Food Guide Pyramid underwent a landmark overhaul to account more completely for the variety of nutritional needs throughout the U.S. population (Figure 6). This new pyramid, called the MyPyramid Plan, replaced the former Food Guide Pyramid promoted since 1993 by the USDA and incorporated the *2005 Dietary Guidelines for Americans*.[36] These guidelines are updated every 5 years; the *2010 Guidelines* are currently being developed, and will be released in the fall of 2010.[37] Although the former pyramid emphasized variety in daily intake, it did not reflect what we now know about restricting fats, eating more fruits and vegetables, and consuming whole grains. The MyPyramid Plan also takes into consideration the various dietary and caloric needs for a variety of individuals (such as people over age 65,

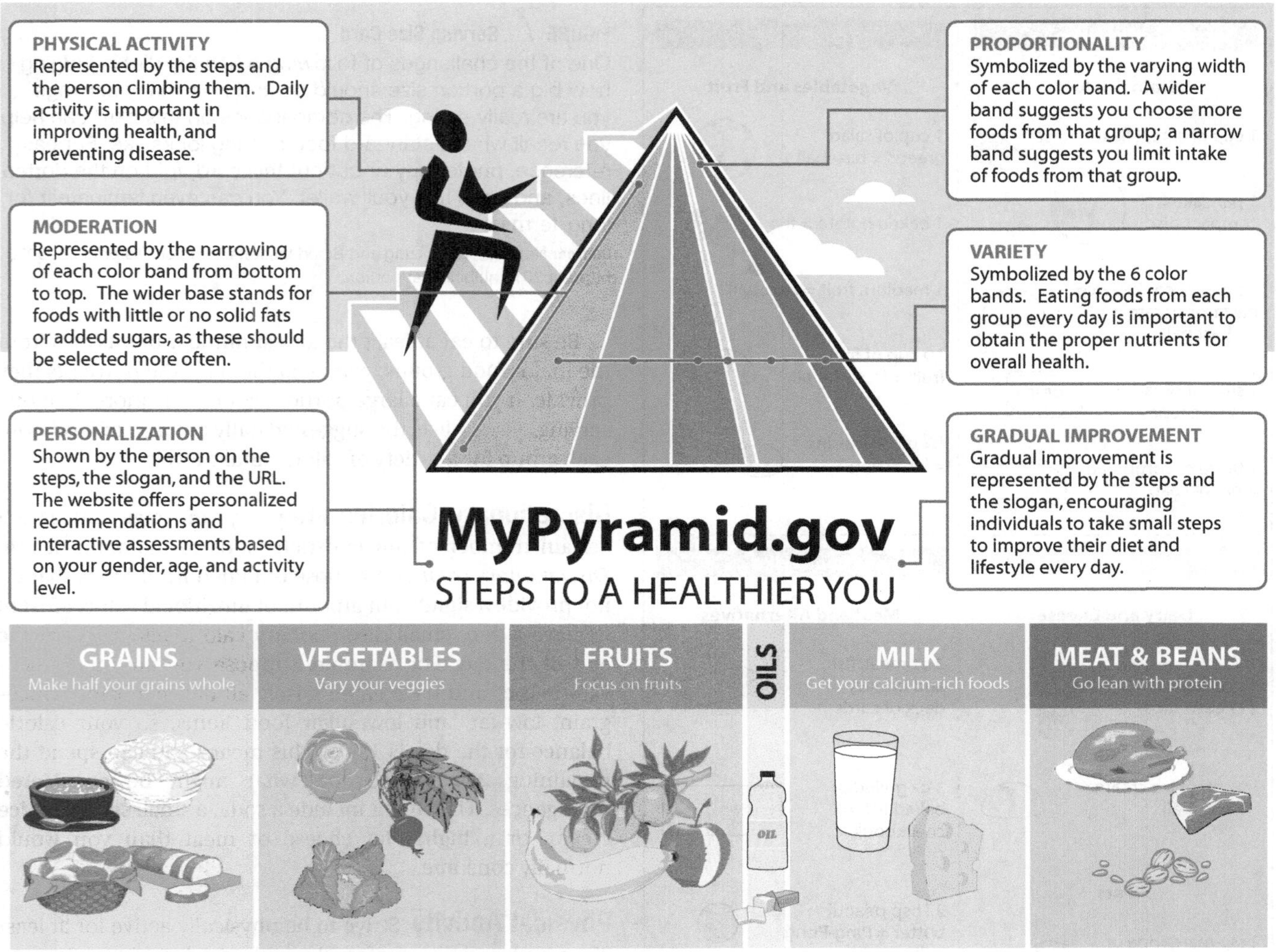

PHYSICAL ACTIVITY
Represented by the steps and the person climbing them. Daily activity is important in improving health, and preventing disease.
MODERATION
Represented by the narrowing of each color band from bottom to top. The wider base stands for foods with little or no solid fats or added sugars, as these should be selected more often.
PERSONALIZATION
Shown by the person on the steps, the slogan, and the URL. The website offers personalized recommendations and interactive assessments based on your gender, age, and activity level.
PROPORTIONALITY
Symbolized by the varying width of each color band. A wider band suggests you choose more foods from that group; a narrow band suggests you limit intake of foods from that group.
VARIETY
Symbolized by the 6 color bands. Eating foods from each group every day is important to obtain the proper nutrients for overall health.
GRADUAL IMPROVEMENT
Gradual improvement is represented by the steps and the slogan, encouraging individuals to take small steps to improve their diet and lifestyle every day.
MyPyramid.gov
STEPS TO A HEALTHIER YOU
GRAINS
Make half your grains whole
VEGETABLES
Vary your veggies
FRUITS
Focus on fruits
OILS
MILK
Get your calcium-rich foods
MEAT & BEANS
Go lean with protein
OIL

FIGURE 6 **MyPyramid Plan**

The USDA MyPyramid Plan takes a new approach to dietary and exercise recommendations. Each colored section of the pyramid represents a food group, with the specific needs of individuals in mind.

Source: U.S. Department of Agriculture, 2005, www.MyPyramid.gov.

children, and active adults) as well as activity levels. (See the **Gender & Health** box for a discussion of men's and women's different nutritional needs.) The MyPyramid Plan promotes personalizing dietary and exercise recommendations based on individual needs.[38]

Using the MyPyramid Plan

Understanding serving sizes, incorporating daily physical activity, and eating a nutritionally balanced diet are key components to using the MyPyramid Plan recommendations successfully. Though these elements are not new to the 2005 pyramid, they have been updated to reflect the latest in nutritional science.

Understanding Serving Sizes How much is one serving? Is it different from a portion? Although these two terms are often used interchangeably, they actually mean very different things. A *serving* is the recommended amount you should consume, whereas a *portion* is the amount you choose to eat at any one time. Most of us select portions that are much bigger than servings. According to a survey conducted by the American Institute for Cancer Research (AICR), respondents were asked to estimate the standard servings defined by the old USDA Food Guide Pyramid for eight different foods. Only 1 percent of those surveyed correctly answered all serving size questions, and nearly 65 percent answered five or more of them incorrectly.[39] See **Figure 7** on the next page for a handy pocket guide with tips on recognizing serving sizes.

Unfortunately, we don't always get a clear picture from food producers and advertisers about what a serving really is. Consider a bottle of soda: The food label may list one serving size as 8 fluid ounces and 100 calories. However, note the size of the entire bottle; the bottle may hold 20 ounces, and drinking the entire bottle serves up a whopping 250 calories.

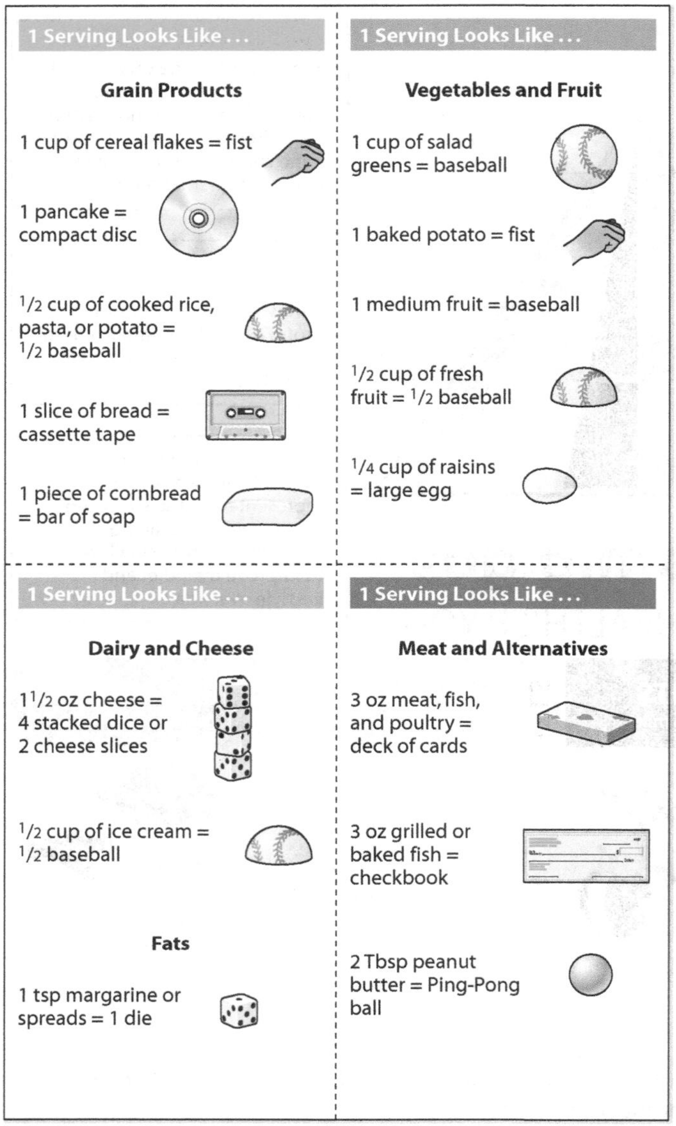
1 Serving Looks Like ...
Grain Products
1 cup of cereal flakes = fist
1 pancake = compact disc
1/2 cup of cooked rice, pasta, or potato = 1/2 baseball
1 slice of bread = cassette tape
1 piece of cornbread = bar of soap
1 Serving Looks Like ...
Vegetables and Fruit
1 cup of salad greens = baseball
1 baked potato = fist
1 medium fruit = baseball
1/2 cup of fresh fruit = 1/2 baseball
1/4 cup of raisins = large egg
1 Serving Looks Like ...
Dairy and Cheese
1 1/2 oz cheese = 4 stacked dice or 2 cheese slices
1/2 cup of ice cream = 1/2 baseball
Fats
1 tsp margarine or spreads = 1 die
1 Serving Looks Like ...
Meat and Alternatives
3 oz meat, fish, and poultry = deck of cards
3 oz grilled or baked fish = checkbook
2 Tbsp peanut butter = Ping-Pong ball

FIGURE 7 **Serving Size Card**

One of the challenges of following a healthy diet is judging how big a portion size should be and how many servings you are really eating. The comparisons on this card can help you recall what a standard food serving looks like. For easy reference, photocopy or cut out this card, fold on the dotted lines, and keep it in your wallet. You can even laminate it for long-term use.

Source: National Heart, Lung and Blood Institute, "Portion Distortion," 2007, http://hp2010.nhlbihin.net/portion.

Be sure to eat at least the lowest number of servings from the major food groups; you need them for the nutrients they provide. If you eat a large portion, count it as more than one serving. Figure 8 lists the suggested daily amount of food from each group for a variety of calorie intake levels.

Discretionary Calories Every day you must consume a certain number of nutrient-rich foods to maintain health. *Discretionary calories* are those obtained from foods that do not provide a significant amount of nutritional value. Most of us have a very small discretionary caloric allowance at the end of the day. For example, suppose you are on a 2,000-calorie diet and have eaten wisely all day, choosing whole-grain, low-fat, and low-sugar food items, so your calorie balance for the day is 1,800. This means you can spend the remaining 200 calories on what might be considered indulgences. This might include a soda, a small serving of ice cream, or a higher fat cheese or meat than you would normally consume.

Physical Activity Strive to be physically active for at least 30 minutes daily, preferably with moderate to vigorous activity levels on most days. Physical activity does not mean you have to go to the gym, jog 3 miles a day, or hire a personal trainer. Any activity that gets your heart pumping (such as

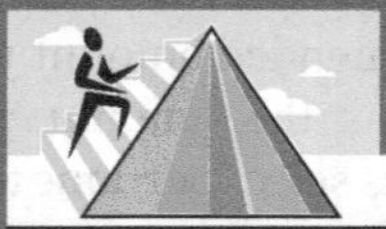

	1,200	1,400	1,600	1,800	2,000	2,200	2,400	2,600	2,800	3,000
Fruits	1 cup	1.5 cups	1.5 cups	1.5 cups	2 cups	2 cups	2 cups	2 cups	2.5 cups	2.5 cups
Vegetables	1.5 cups	1.5 cups	2 cups	2.5 cups	2.5 cups	3 cups	3 cups	3.5 cups	3.5 cups	4 cups
Grains	4 oz-eq.	5 oz-eq.	5 oz-eq.	6 oz-eq.	6 oz-eq.	7 oz-eq.	8 oz-eq.	9 oz-eq.	10 oz-eq.	10 oz-eq.
Meat and Beans	3 oz-eq.	4 oz-eq.	5 oz-eq.	5 oz-eq.	5.5 oz-eq.	6 oz-eq.	6.5 oz-eq.	6.5 oz-eq.	7 oz-eq.	7 oz-eq.
Milk	2 cups	2 cups	3 cups	3 cups	3 cups	3 cups	3 cups	3 cups	3 cups	3 cups
Oils	4 tsp	4 tsp	5 tsp	5 tsp	6 tsp	6 tsp	7 tsp	8 tsp	8 tsp	10 tsp
Discretionary calories	171	171	132	195	267	290	362	410	426	512

FIGURE 8 **Nutritional Needs for People with Different Energy Requirements**

Once you've determined your daily caloric requirements (Table 1), use this chart to determine how many servings of each food group you need per day to maintain good health.

Source: U.S. Department of Agriculture, 2005, www.MyPyramid.gov.

Gender&Health

Different Bodies, Different Needs

Men and women differ in body size, body composition, and overall metabolic rates. They therefore have differing needs for most nutrients throughout their lives (see Tables 2–5 for specifics on vitamin and mineral requirements) and face unique difficulties in keeping on track with their dietary goals. Have you ever wondered why men can eat more than women without gaining weight? Although there are many possible reasons, one factor is that women have a lower ratio of lean body mass to adipose (fatty) tissue at all ages and stages of life. Also, after sexual maturation, men's metabolic rate is higher, meaning that they will burn more calories doing the same activities.

In addition, women have many "milestone" times in the life when their nutritional needs vary significantly. From menarche to menopause, women undergo cyclical physiological changes that can have dramatic effects on metabolism and nutritional needs. For example, during pregnancy and lactation, women's nutritional requirements increase substantially. Those who are unable to follow their doctor's strict dietary recommendations may gain too much weight during pregnancy and retain it afterward. During the menstrual cycle, many women report significant food cravings. Those who experience very heavy menstrual cycles may benefit from increased iron in their diet or by taking a supplement. Later in life, with the advent of menopause, nutritional needs again change rather dramatically. With depletion of the hormone estrogen, the body's need for calcium to ward off bone deterioration becomes pronounced. Women must pay closer attention to exercising and getting enough calcium through diet or dietary supplements, or they run the risk of osteoporosis.

Men and women also tend to have different eating habits. For example, women tend to enjoy more fruits and vegetables than men. The average American male eats fewer than three servings of fruits and vegetables per day although five to nine servings are recommended. Women average three to seven servings per day. Men also tend to consume more red meat than women.

gardening, playing basketball, heavy yard work, and dancing) are all examples of ways to get moving.

Eating Nutrient-Dense Foods Although eating the proper number of servings from MyPyramid is important, it is also important to recognize that there are large caloric, fat, and energy differences among foods within a given food group. For example, fish and hot dogs provide vastly different fat and energy levels per ounce, with fish providing better energy and caloric value per serving. It is important to eat foods that have a high nutritional value for their caloric content. Avoid "empty calories," that is, high-calorie foods that have little nutritional value.

Vegetarianism

According to a new, representative study of over 5,500 U.S. adults, 7.3 million (3.2% of all American adults) are vegetarians and another 22.8 million are "vegetarian inclined" meaning that they are actively choosing to reduce meat consumption in favor of other "faceless" forms of protein.[40] Millions more report being very curious about or contemplating a vegetarian lifestyle. The majority of those who describe themselves as vegetarians are females (59%). Why are so many moving toward meat/dairy reduction and/or elimination in their diets? Of those surveyed, the most common reasons for pursuing a vegetarian lifestyle were:

- Animal welfare (54%)
- Improving health (53%)
- Environmental concerns (47%)
- Natural approaches to wellness (39%)
- Food safety (31%)
- Weight loss (25%)
- Weight maintenance (24%)

Normally, vegetarianism provides a superb alternative to our high-fat, high-calorie, meat-based cuisine. But without proper information and food choices, vegetarians can develop serious dietary problems in much the same way as their meat-eating counterparts.

The term **vegetarian** means different things to different people. Strict vegetarians, or *vegans,* avoid all foods of animal origin, including dairy products and eggs. Far more common are *lacto-vegetarians,* who eat dairy products but avoid flesh foods. *Ovo-vegetarians* add eggs to a vegan diet, and *lacto-ovo-vegetarians* eat both dairy products and eggs. *Pesco-vegetarians* eat fish, dairy products, and eggs, and *semivegetarians* eat chicken, fish, dairy products, and eggs. Some people in the semivegetarian category prefer to call themselves "non-red meat eaters."

Generally, people who follow a balanced vegetarian diet weigh less and have better cholesterol levels, fewer problems with irregular bowel movements (constipation and diarrhea), and a lower risk of heart disease than do nonvegetarians. The benefits of vegetarianism also include a reduced risk of some cancers, particularly colon cancer, and a reduced risk of kidney disease.[41]

vegetarian A person who follows a diet that excludes some or all animal products.

Although in the past vegetarians often suffered from vitamin deficiencies, most vegetarians today are adept at

Brian Hagiwara/Jupiter Images

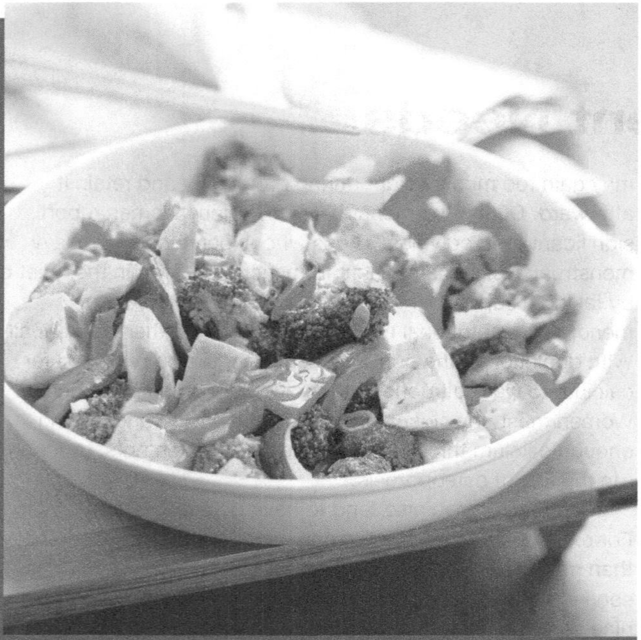

Is vegetarianism healthy?

Adopting a vegan or vegetarian diet can be a very healthy way to eat, as long as you take care to prepare your food healthfully by limiting the use of oils and avoiding added sugars and sodium. Vegetarians also need to ensure that they are getting all the essential amino acids. Meals like this tofu and vegetable stir-fry provide the vegetarian with essential vitamins and protein; adding a whole grain, such as brown rice, would further enhance it by making use of complementary plant proteins.

combining the right types of foods and eating a variety of different foods to ensure proper nutrient intake. Vegan diets may be deficient in vitamins B_2 (riboflavin), B_{12}, and D. Vegans are also at risk for deficiencies of calcium, iron, zinc, and other minerals but can obtain these nutrients from supplements. Strict vegans have to pay much more attention to what they eat than the average person does, but by eating complementary combinations of plant products, they can receive adequate amounts of essential amino acids. In fact, whereas vegans typically get 50 to 60 grams of protein per day, lacto-ovo-vegetarians normally consume between 70 and 90 grams per day, well beyond the RDA. Eating a full variety of grains, legumes, fruits, vegetables, and seeds each day will keep even the strictest vegetarian in excellent health. Pregnant women, older adults, sick people, and children who are vegans need to take special care to ensure that their diets are adequate. In all cases, seek advice from a health care professional if you have questions.

what do you think?

Why are so many people today becoming vegetarians? ● How easy is it to be a vegetarian on your campus? ● What concerns about vegetarianism would you be likely to have, if any?

Improved Eating for the College Student

College students often face a challenge when trying to eat healthy foods. Some students live in dorms and do not have their own cooking or refrigeration facilities. Others live in crowded apartments where everyone forages in the refrigerator for everyone else's food. Still others eat at university food services where food choices may be overwhelming. Nearly all have financial and time constraints that make buying, preparing, and eating healthy food a difficult task. What's a student to do?

When Time and Money Are Short

Many college students may find it hard to fit a well-balanced meal into the day, but eating breakfast and lunch are important to keep energy levels up and get the most out of your classes. If your campus is like many others, you've probably noticed a distinct move toward fast-food restaurants in your student unions. Eating a complete breakfast that includes complex carbohydrates and protein and bringing a small healthy snack (such as carrots, an apple, or even a small sandwich on whole-grain bread) to class are ways to ensure you fit meals into your day. If you must eat fast food, follow the tips below to get more nutritional bang for your buck:

- Ask for nutritional analyses of items. Most fast-food chains now have them.
- Order salads, but be careful about what you add to them. Taco salads and Cobb salads are often high in fat, calories, and sodium. Ask for dressing on the side, and use sparingly. Try the vinaigrette or low-fat alternative dressings. Stay away from eggs and other high-fat add-ons, such as bacon bits, croutons, and crispy noodles.
- If you must have fries, check to see what type of oil is used to cook them. Avoid lard-based or other saturated-fat products and *trans* fats. Some fast-food restaurants offer baked "fries," which may be lower in fat.
- Avoid giant sizes, and refrain from ordering extra sauce, bacon, cheese, dressings, and other extras that add additional calories, sodium, carboydrates, and fat.
- Limit beverages and foods high in added sugars. Common forms of added sugars include sucrose, glucose, fructose, maltose, dextrose, corn syrups, concentrated fruit juices, and honey.
- At least once per week, substitute a vegetable-based meat substitute into your fast-food choices. Most places now offer Gardenburgers, Boca burgers, and similar products, which provide excellent sources of protein and often have considerably less fat and fewer calories.

Maintaining a nutritious diet within the confines of student life can be challenging. However, if you take the time to plan healthy meals, you will find that you are eating better, enjoying it more, and actually saving money. Follow the steps in the **Skills for Behavior Change** box at right for a healthy, affordable diet.

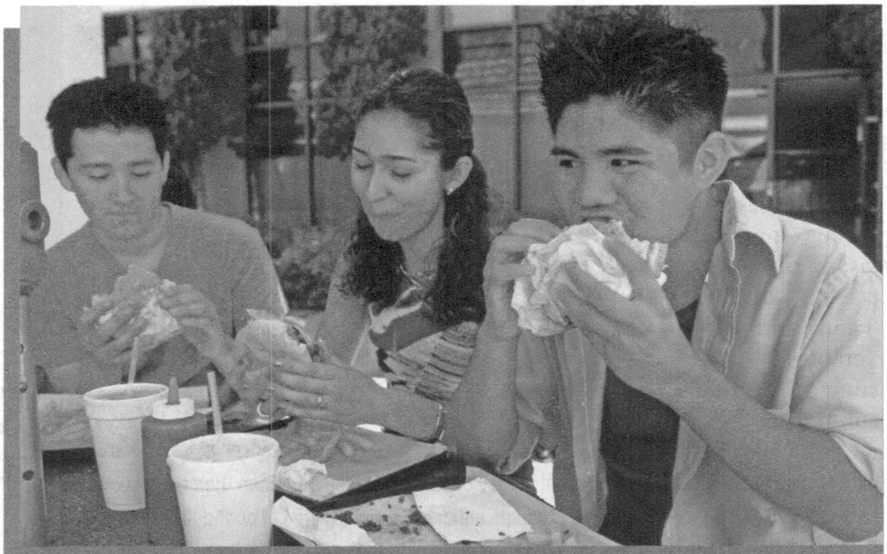

Michael Newman/PhotoEdit

How can I eat well when I'm in a hurry?

Meals like this one may be convenient, but they are high in fat and calories. Even when you are short on time and money, it is possible—and worthwhile—to make healthier choices. Most fast-food restaurants make nutritional analyses of their offerings available to the public. If you are ordering fast food, opt for foods prepared by baking, roasting, or steaming; ask for the leanest meat option; request that sauces, dressings, and gravies be served on the side; and substitute a healthier option for a high-fat one, such as a baked potato or fresh vegetables instead of French fries.

Food Safety: A Growing Concern

Eating unhealthy food is one thing. Eating food that has been contaminated with a pathogen, toxin, or other harmful substance is quite another. You may be surprised to know that more than 200 diseases are transmitted through food. As outbreaks of salmonella in chicken, peanut butter, and vegetables or *Escherichia coli* (a potentially lethal bacterial pathogen) in spinach or beef continue to periodically make the news, the food industry has come under fire. To convince us that their products are safe, some manufacturers have come up with "new and improved" ways of protecting our foods. What are the dangers of contaminated foods, and how well do food manufacturers' new strategies work? Let's find out.

Foodborne Illnesses

Are you concerned that the chicken you are buying doesn't look pleasingly pink or that your "fresh" fish smells a little *too* fishy? You may have good reason to be worried. In increasing numbers, Americans are becoming sick from what they eat, and many of these illnesses are life-threatening. Based on several studies conducted over the past 10 years, scientists estimate that foodborne pathogens sicken over 76 million people and cause some 400,000 hospitalizations and 5,000 deaths in the United States annually. These numbers have remained fairly constant since 2004, in spite of increased attention to prevention in the United States.[42] Because most of us don't go to the doctor every time we feel ill, we may not make a connection between what we eat and later symptoms.

Signs of foodborne illnesses vary and usually include one or several symptoms: diarrhea, nausea, cramping, and vomiting. Depending on the amount and virulence of the pathogen, symptoms may appear as early as 30 minutes after eating contaminated food or as long as several days or weeks later. Most of the time, symptoms occur 5 to 8 hours after eating and last only a day or two. For certain populations, however, including the very young, older adults, and people with severe illnesses such as cancer, diabetes, kidney disease, or AIDS, foodborne diseases can be fatal.

Several factors may be contributing to the increase in foodborne illnesses. The movement away from a traditional meat-and-potato American diet to "heart-healthy" eating—increased consumption of fruits, vegetables, and grains—has spurred

Skills for Behavior Change

Budget Nutrition Tips

- Buy fruits and vegetables in season whenever possible for their lower cost, higher nutrient quality, and greater variety.
- Use coupons and specials to get price reductions. Plan your menu for the week, make a list, and stick to it so you can avoid impulse shopping. No food is cheap if you don't eat it.
- Shop at discount warehouse food chains; capitalize on volume discounts and no-frills products. However, don't buy more than you can reasonably use before the products expire.
- Purchase meats and other products in volume, freeze portions in vacuum-packed bags or freezer bags, put dates on them, and save for future needs. Or purchase small amounts of meat and other expensive proteins and combine them with beans and plant proteins for lower cost, calories, and fat.
- Invest in storage containers that hold up well to microwaving and dishwashing. Cook larger quantities at a time, and freeze leftovers.

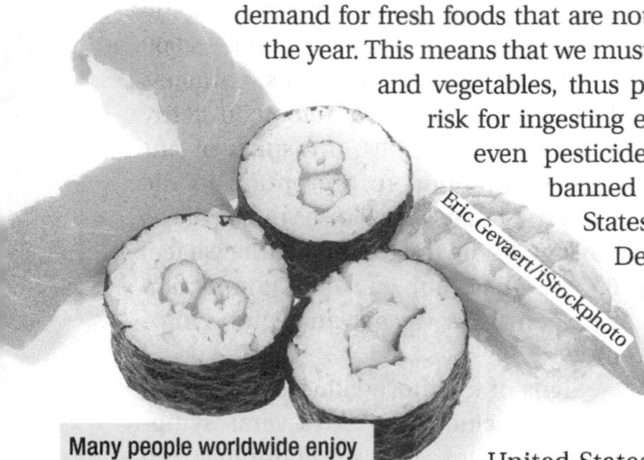
Eric Gevaert/iStockphoto

Many people worldwide enjoy sushi. Use caution when eating it, however, as raw fish can be a breeding ground for dangerous microbes.

demand for fresh foods that are not in season most of the year. This means that we must import fresh fruits and vegetables, thus putting ourselves at risk for ingesting exotic pathogens or even pesticides that have been banned in the United States for safety reasons. Depending on the season, up to 70 percent of the fruits and vegetables consumed in the United States come from Mexico alone. Although we are told when we travel to developing countries, "boil it, peel it, or don't eat it," we bring these foods into our kitchens and eat them, often without even washing them. Food can become contaminated by being watered with contaminated water, being fertilized with animal manure, being picked by people who have not washed their hands properly, or by being exposed to pesticides. To give you an idea of the implications, studies have shown that *E. coli* can survive in cow manure for up to 70 days and can multiply in foods grown with manure unless heat or additives such as salt or preservatives are used to kill the microbes.[43] There are no regulations that prohibit farmers from using animal manure to fertilize crops. Additionally, *E. coli* actually increases in summer months as cows await slaughter in crowded, overheated pens. This increases the chances of meat's coming to market already contaminated.[44]

Other key factors associated with the increasing spread of foodborne diseases include inadvertent introduction of pathogens into new geographic regions and insufficient education about food safety.

Avoiding Risks in the Home

Part of the responsibility for preventing foodborne illness lies with consumers—more than 30 percent of all such illnesses result from unsafe handling of food at home. Fortunately, consumers can take several steps to reduce the likelihood of contaminating their food. Among the most basic precautions are to wash your hands and to wash all produce before eating it. Also, avoid cross-contamination in the kitchen by using separate cutting boards and utensils for meats and produce. Temperature control is also important, and refrigerators must be set at 40 degrees Fahrenheit or less. Hot foods must be kept hot and cold foods kept cold in order to avoid unchecked bacterial growth. Leftovers need to be eaten within 3 days, and if you're unsure how long something has been sitting in the fridge, don't take chances. When in doubt, throw it out. See the **Skills for Behavior Change** box at right for more tips about reducing risk of foodborne illness when shopping for and preparing food.

food irradiation Treating foods with gamma radiation from radioactive cobalt, cesium, or other sources of X rays to kill microorganisms.

Did you Know?

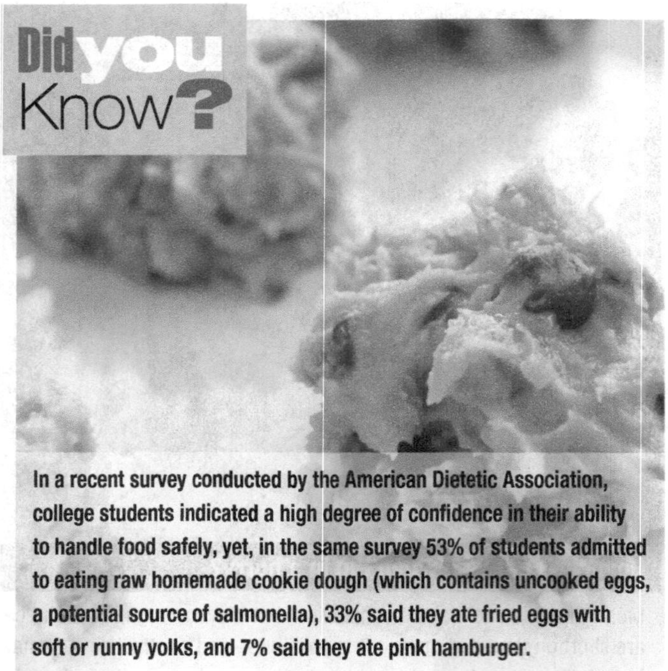
rtyree1/iStockphoto

In a recent survey conducted by the American Dietetic Association, college students indicated a high degree of confidence in their ability to handle food safely, yet, in the same survey 53% of students admitted to eating raw homemade cookie dough (which contains uncooked eggs, a potential source of salmonella), 33% said they ate fried eggs with soft or runny yolks, and 7% said they ate pink hamburger.

Food Irradiation: How Safe Is It?

Food irradiation is a process that involves treating foods with invisible waves of energy that damage microorganisms. These energy waves are actually low doses of radiation, or ionizing energy, which breaks chemical bonds in the DNA of harmful bacteria, destroying the pathogens and keeping them from replicating. The rays essentially pass through the food without leaving any radioactive residue.[45]

U.S. FDA label for irradiated foods

Irradiation lengthens food products' shelf life and prevents the spread of deadly microorganisms, particularly in high-risk foods such as ground beef and pork. Thus, the minimal costs of irradiation should result in lower overall costs to consumers and reduce the need for toxic chemicals now used to preserve foods and prevent contamination from external pathogens. Some environmentalists and consumer groups have raised concerns; however, food irradiation is now common in more than 40 countries. In the United States, foods that have been irradiated are marked with the "radura" logo.

Food Additives

Additives are substances added to food to reduce the risk of foodborne illness, prevent spoilage, and enhance the look and taste of foods. Additives can also enhance nutrient value, especially to benefit the general public. Good examples include the fortification of milk with vitamin D and of grain products with folate. Although the FDA regulates additives according to effectiveness, safety, and ability to detect them in foods, ques-

Skills for Behavior Change

Reduce Your Risk For Foodborne Illness

* When shopping for fish, buy from markets that get their supplies from state-approved sources.
* Check for cleanliness at the salad bar and at the meat and fish counters.
* Keep most cuts of meat, fish, and poultry in the refrigerator no more than 1 or 2 days. Check the shelf life of all products before buying. Use the sniff test—if fish smells really fishy, don't eat it.
* Use a meat thermometer to ensure that meats are completely cooked. Beef and lamb steaks and roasts should be cooked to at least 145°F; ground meat, pork chops, ribs, and egg dishes to 160°F; ground poultry and hot dogs to 165°F; chicken and turkey breasts to 170°F; and chicken and turkey legs, thighs, and whole birds to 180°F. Fish is done when the thickest part becomes opaque and the fish flakes easily when poked with a fork.
* Never leave cooked food standing on the stove or table for more than 2 hours.
* Never thaw frozen foods at room temperature. Put them in the refrigerator for a day to thaw or thaw in cold water, changing the water every 30 minutes.
* Wash your hands and countertop with soap and water when preparing food, particularly after handling meat, fish, or poultry.
* When freezing chicken or other raw foods, make sure juices can't spill over into ice cubes or into other areas of the refrigerator.

tions have been raised about those additives put into foods intentionally and those that get in unintentionally before or after processing. Whenever these substances are added, consumers should take the time to determine what they are and whether there are alternatives. As a general rule, the fewer chemicals, colorants, and preservatives there are, the better. Examples of common additives include the following:

- **Antimicrobial agents.** Substances such as salt, sugar, nitrates, and others that tend to make foods less hospitable for microbes.
- **Antioxidants.** Substances that preserve color and flavor by reducing loss due to exposure to oxygen. Vitamins C and E are among the antioxidants believed to reduce the risk of cancer and cardiovascular disease. The additives BHA and BHT are also antioxidants.
- **Artificial colors, nutrient additives, and flavor enhancers such as MSG (monosodium glutamate).**
- **Sulfites.** Used to preserve vegetable color; some people have severe allergic reactions to them.

Food Allergy or Food Intolerance?

One out of every three people today *think* they have an allergy or avoid a certain food because they think they are allergic to it; however, only 4 percent of the population has a true food allergy. Still, that 4 percent accounts for more than 12 million Americans, and the number may increase in coming years, as rates are on the rise among children under the age of 3.[46]

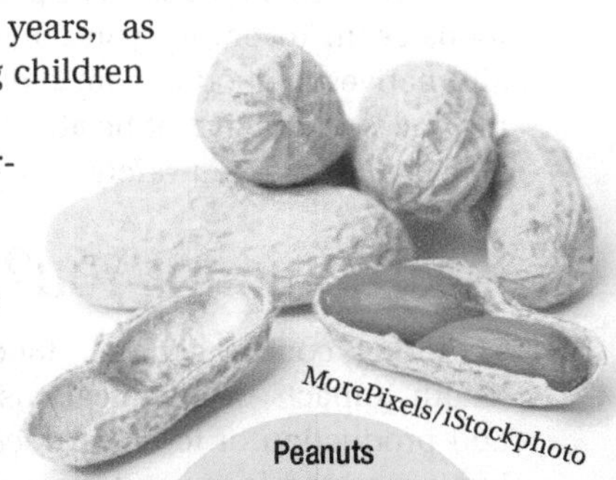

MorePixels/iStockphoto

Peanuts are among the 8 most common food allergens: 0.6% of the general population are allergic to them, with slightly higher rates in children.

A **food allergy,** or hypersensitivity, is an abnormal response to a food that is triggered by the immune system. Symptoms of an allergic reaction vary in severity and may include a tingling sensation in the mouth; swelling of the lips, tongue, and throat; difficulty breathing; hives; vomiting; abdominal cramps; diarrhea; drop in blood pressure; loss of consciousness; and death. Approximately 200 deaths per year occur from the anaphylaxis (the acute systemic immune and inflammatory response) that occurs with allergic reactions. These symptoms may appear within seconds to hours after eating the foods to which one is allergic.[47]

In 2004, Congress passed the Food Allergen Labeling and Consumer Protection Act (FALCPA), which requires food manufacturers to clearly label foods indicating the presence of (or possible contamination by) any of the 8 major food allergens: milk, eggs, peanuts, wheat, soy, tree nuts (walnuts, pecans, etc.), fish, and shellfish. Although over 160 foods have been identified as allergy triggers, these 8 foods account for 90 percent of all food allergies in the United States.[48]

In contrast to allergies, **food intolerance** can cause you to have symptoms of gastric upset, but it is not the result of an immune system response. Probably the best example of a food intolerance is *lactose intolerance,* a problem that affects about one in every ten adults. Lactase is an enzyme in the lining of the gut that degrades lactose, which is in dairy products. If you don't have enough lactase, you cannot digest lactose, and it remains in the gut to be used by bacteria. Gas is formed, and you experience bloating, abdominal pain, and sometimes diarrhea. Food intolerance also occurs in response to some food additives, such as the flavor enhancer MSG, certain dyes, sulfites, gluten, and other substances. In some cases, the food intolerance may have psychological triggers.

food allergy Overreaction by the body to normally harmless proteins, which are perceived as allergens. In response, the body produces antibodies, triggering allergic symptoms.

food intolerance Adverse effects resulting when people who lack the digestive chemicals needed to break down certain substances eat those substances.

If you suspect that you have an actual allergic reaction to food, see an allergist to be tested to determine the source of the problem. Because there are several diseases that share symptoms with food allergies (ulcers and cancers of the gastrointestinal tract can cause vomiting, bloating, diarrhea, nausea, and pain), you should have persistent symptoms checked out as soon as possible. If particular foods seem to bother you consistently, look for alternatives or modify your diet. In true allergic instances, you may not be able to consume even the smallest amount safely.

Is Organic for You?

USDA label for certified organic foods

Mounting concerns about food safety and the health impacts of chemicals used in the growth and production of food have led many people to refuse to buy processed foods and mass-produced agricultural products. Instead, they purchase foods that are **organic**—foods and beverages developed, grown, or raised without the use of synthetic pesticides, chemicals, or hormones.

As of 2002, any food sold in the United States as organic has to meet criteria set by the USDA under the National Organic Rule and can carry a USDA seal verifying products as "certified organic." Under this rule, a product that is certified may carry one of the following terms: "100 percent Organic" (100% compliance with organic criteria), "Organic" (must contain at least 95% organic materials), "Made with Organic Ingredients" (must contain at least 70% organic ingredients), or "Some Organic Ingredients" (contains less than 70% organic ingredients—usually listed individually). To be labeled with any of the above terms, the foods must be produced without hormones, antibiotics, herbicides, insecticides, chemical fertilizers, genetic modification, or germ-killing radiation. However, reliable monitoring systems to ensure credibility are still under development.

organic Grown without use of pesticides, chemicals, or hormones.
locavore A person who primarily eats food grown or produced locally.

Is buying organic really better for you? Perhaps if we could put a group of people in a pristine environment and ensure that they never ate, drank, or were exposed to chemicals, we could test this hypothesis. In real life, however, it is almost impossible to assess the health impact of organic versus nonorganic foods. Nevertheless, the market for organics has been increasing by more than 20 percent per year—five times faster than food sales in general. Nearly 40 percent of U.S. consumers now reach occasionally for something labeled organic; as of 2010, annual organic food sales are estimated to be about $23.8 billion.[49]

In 2007, several reports by consumer groups questioned the nutrient value of organic foods. Some sources have actually indicated that smaller organic farmers may have more trouble getting their produce to market in the proper climate-controlled vehicles. As such, their foods might lose valuable nutrients while sitting in warm trucks or at a roadside stand as compared to the refrigerated section of a local supermarket; or, more important, increased bacterial growth may be noted. In general, the closer to the field you can purchase produce and the faster you can get it home and into the refrigerator, the more nutritious foods will be.

Today, the new word **locavore** has been coined to describe people who eat only food grown or produced locally, usually within close proximity to their homes. Farmers' markets or home-grown foods or those grown by independent farmers are thought to be fresher, more environmentally friendly, and requiring far fewer resources to get them to market and keep them fresh for longer periods of time. Locavores believe that locally grown organic food is preferable to large corporation or supermarket-based organic foods, as they have a smaller impact on the environment. Although there are many reasons why organic farming is better for the environment, the fact that pesticides, herbicides, and other products are not used is perhaps the greatest benefit. Other benefits of locally grown organic products include the fact that they can often be harvested and brought to market with minimal fossil-fuel usage and are more likely to be grown on independent, small farms rather than on huge corporate farms.

Assess yourself

How Healthy Are Your Eating Habits?

PEARSON myhealthlab

Fill out this assessment online at www.pearsonhighered.com/myhealthlab or www.pearsonhighered.com/donatelle.

1 Keep Track of Your Food Intake

Keep a food diary for 5 days, writing down everything you eat or drink. Be sure to include the approximate amount or portion size. Add up the number of servings from each of the major food groups on each day and enter them into the chart below.

Number of Servings of:	Day 1	Day 2	Day 3	Day 4	Day 5	Average
Fruits						
Vegetables						
Grains						
Protein Foods						
Dairy						
Fats and Oils						
Sweets						

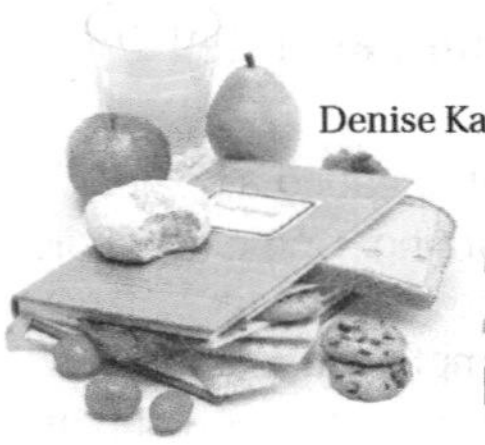

Denise Kappa/iStockphoto

2A Does your diet have proportionality?

	Yes	No
1. Are grains the main food choice at all your meals?	◯	◯
2. Do you often forget to eat vegetables?	◯	◯
3. Do you typically eat fewer than three pieces of fruit daily?	◯	◯
4. Do you often have fewer than 3 cups of milk daily?	◯	◯
5. Is the portion of meat, chicken, or fish the largest item on your dinner plate?	◯	◯

Scoring 2A

If you answered yes to three or more of these questions, your diet probably lacks proportionality. Review the recommendations in this chapter, particularly the MyPyramid guidelines, to learn how to balance your diet.

2 Evaluate Your Food Intake

Now compare your consumption patterns to the MyPyramid recommendations. Look at Table 1 and Figure 8 or visit www.mypyramid.gov/mypyramid/index.aspx to evaluate your daily caloric needs and the recommended consumption rates for the different food groups. How does your diet match up?

	Less than the recommended amount	About equal to the recommended amount	More than the recommended amount
1. How does your daily fruit consumption compare to the recommendation for your age and activity level?	◯	◯	◯
2. How does your daily vegetable consumption compare to the recommendation for your age and activity level?	◯	◯	◯
3. How does your daily grain consumption compare to the recommendation for your age and activity level?	◯	◯	◯
4. How does your daily protein food consumption compare to the recommendation for your age and activity level?	◯	◯	◯
5. How does your daily fats and oils consumption compare to the recommendation for your age and activity level?	◯	◯	◯
6. How does your daily consumption of discretionary calories compare to the recommendation for your age and activity level?	◯	◯	◯

Scoring

If you found that your food intake is consistent with the MyPyramid recommendations, congratulations! If, on the other hand, you are falling short in a major food group or are overdoing it in certain categories, consider taking steps to adopt healthier eating habits. There are some additional assessments at left and on the next page to help you figure out where your diet is lacking.

2B Are you getting enough fat-soluble vitamins in your diet?

	Yes	No
1. Do you eat at least 1 cup of deep yellow or orange vegetables, such as carrots and sweet potatoes, or dark green vegetables, such as spinach, every day?	◯	◯
2. Do you consume at least two glasses (8 ounces each) of milk daily?	◯	◯
3. Do you eat a tablespoon of vegetable oil, such as corn or olive oil, daily (tip: salad dressings, unless they are fat free, count!)?	◯	◯
4. Do you eat at least 1 cup of leafy green vegetables in your salad and/or put lettuce in your sandwich every day?	◯	◯

Scoring 2B

If you answered yes to all four questions, you are on your way to acing your fat-soluble vitamin needs! If you answered no to any of the questions, your diet needs some fine-tuning. Deep orange and dark green vegetables are excellent sources of vitamin A, and milk is an excellent choice for vitamin D. Vegetable oils provide vitamin E, and if you put them on top of your vitamin K-rich leafy green salad, you'll hit the vitamin jackpot.

2C Are you getting enough water-soluble vitamins in your diet?

	Yes	No
1. Do you consume at least 1/2 cup of rice or pasta daily?	◯	◯
2. Do you eat at least 1 cup of a ready-to-eat cereal or hot cereal every day?	◯	◯
3. Do you have at least one slice of bread, a bagel, or a muffin daily?	◯	◯
4. Do you enjoy a citrus fruit or fruit juice, such as an orange, a grapefruit, or orange juice every day?	◯	◯
5. Do you have at least 1 cup of vegetables throughout your day?	◯	◯

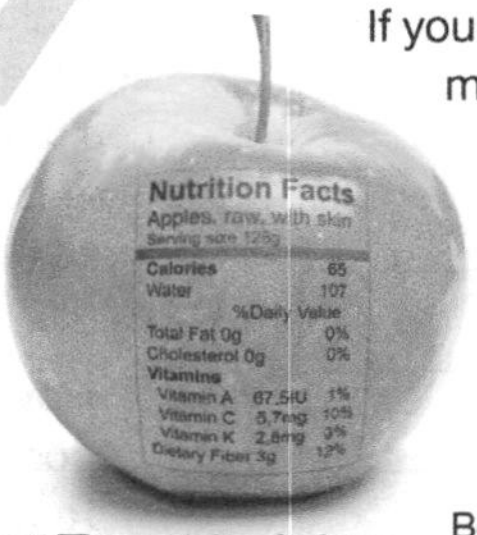

Алексей Пинчу/iStockphoto

Scoring 2C

If you answered yes to all of these questions, you are a vitamin B and C superstar! If you answered no to any of the questions, your diet could use some refinement. Rice, pasta, cereals, bread, and bread products are all excellent sources of B vitamins. Citrus fruits are a ringer for vitamin C. In fact, all vegetables can contribute to meeting your vitamin C needs daily.

Source: Adapted from J. Blake, *Nutrition and You* (San Francisco: Benjamin Cummings, 2008).

YOUR PLAN FOR CHANGE

The Assess yourself activity gave you the chance to evaluate your current nutritional habits. Now that you have considered these results, you can decide whether you need to make changes in your daily eating for long-term health.

Today, you can:

◯ Start keeping a more detailed food log. Take note of the nutritional information of the various foods you eat and write down particulars about the number of calories, grams of fat, grams of sugar, milligrams of sodium, and so on of each food. Try to find specific weak spots: Are you consuming too many calories or too much salt or sugar? Do you eat too little calcium or iron?

◯ Take a field trip to the grocery store. Forgo your fast-food dinner and instead spend some time in the produce section of the supermarket. Purchase your favorite fruits and vegetables, and try something new to expand your tastes.

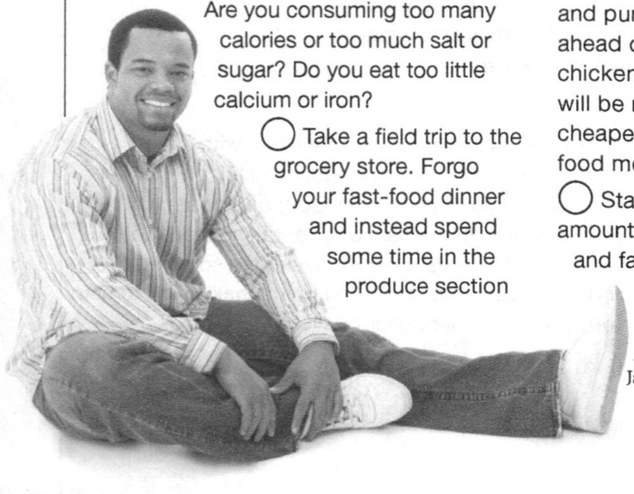
Jaimie Duplass/iStockphoto

Within the next 2 weeks, you can:

◯ Plan at least three meals that you can make at home or in your dorm room, and purchase the ingredients you'll need ahead of time. Something as simple as a chicken sandwich on whole-grain bread will be more nutritious, and probably cheaper, than heading out for a fast-food meal.

◯ Start reading labels. Be aware of the amounts of calories, sodium, sugars, and fats in prepared foods; aim to buy and consume those that are lower in all of these and are higher in calcium and fiber.

By the end of the semester, you can:

◯ Get in the habit of eating a healthy breakfast every morning. Combine whole grains, proteins, and fruit in your breakfast—for example, eat a bowl of cereal with milk and bananas or a cup of yogurt combined with granola and berries. Eating a healthy breakfast will jump-start your metabolism, prevent drops in blood glucose levels, and keep your brain and body performing at their best through those morning classes.

◯ Commit to one or two healthful changes to your eating patterns for the rest of the semester. You might resolve to eat five servings of fruits and vegetables every day, to switch to low-fat or nonfat dairy products, to stop drinking soft drinks, or to use only olive oil in your cooking. Use your food diary to help you spot places where you can make healthier choices on a daily basis.

Summary

* Recognizing that we eat for more reasons than just survival is the first step toward changing our nutritional habits.
* The essential nutrients include water, proteins, carbohydrates, fats, vitamins, and minerals. Water makes up 50 to 60 percent of our body weight and is necessary for nearly all life processes. Proteins are major components of our cells and are key elements of antibodies, enzymes, and hormones. Carbohydrates are our primary sources of energy. Fats play important roles in maintaining body temperature and cushioning and protecting organs. Vitamins are organic compounds, and minerals are inorganic compounds. We need both in relatively small amounts to maintain healthy body function.
* Food labels provide information on the serving size, number of calories in a food, as well as the amounts of various nutrients and the percentage of recommended daily values those amounts represent.
* MyPyramid provides guidelines for healthy eating. These recommendations, developed by the USDA, place emphasis on personalization, proportionality, moderation, variety, physical activity, and gradual improvement.
* Vegetarianism can provide a healthy alternative for people wishing to reduce animal consumption from their diets.
* College students face unique challenges in eating healthfully. Learning to make better choices at fast-food restaurants, to eat healthfully when funds are short, and to eat nutritionally in the dorm are all possible when you use the information in this chapter.
* Foodborne illnesses, food irradiation, food allergies, and other food safety and health concerns are becoming increasingly important to health-wise consumers. Recognizing potential risks and taking steps to prevent problems are part of a sound nutritional plan.
* Organic foods are grown and produced without the use of synthetic pesticides, chemicals, or hormones. The USDA offers certification of organics. These foods have become increasingly available and popular, as people take a greater interest in eating healthfully and sustainably.

Pop Quiz

1. What type of carbohydrates is found primarily in fruits?
   a. glucose
   b. dextrose
   c. simple carbohydrates
   d. complex carbohydrates

2. Which of the following foods would be considered a healthy, *nutrient-dense* food?
   a. nonfat milk
   b. cheddar cheese
   c. soft drink
   d. potato chips

3. What is the most crucial nutrient?
   a. water
   b. fiber
   c. minerals
   d. starch

4. Which of the following nutrients moves food through the digestive tract?
   a. water
   b. fiber
   c. minerals
   d. starch

5. Which of the following nutrients are required for the repair and growth of body tissue?
   a. carbohydrates
   b. proteins
   c. vitamins
   d. fats

6. What substance plays a vital role in maintaining healthy skin and hair, insulating body organs against shock, maintaining body temperature, and promoting healthy cell function?
   a. fats
   b. fibers
   c. proteins
   d. carbohydrates

7. What substance supplies us with the energy needed to sustain normal daily activity?
   a. fats
   b. fibers
   c. proteins
   d. carbohydrates

8. What is the most common nutrient deficiency worldwide?
   a. fat deficiency
   b. iron deficiency
   c. fiber deficiency
   d. calcium deficiency

9. Carrie eats fish, dairy products, and eggs, but she does not eat red meat. Carrie is considered a(n)
   a. vegan.
   b. lacto-vegetarian.
   c. ovo-vegetarian.
   d. pesco-vegetarian.

10. Which of the following fats is a healthier fat to include in the diet?
    a. *trans* fats
    b. saturated fats
    c. unsaturated fats
    d. hydrogenated fats

Answers to Chapter Review Questions
1. c; 2. a; 3. a; 4. b; 5. b;
6. a; 7. d; 8. b; 9. d; 10. c

Think about It!

1. Which factors influence a person's dietary patterns and behaviors? What factors have been the greatest influences on your eating behaviors?
2. What are the six major food groups in MyPyramid? From which groups do you eat too few servings? What can you do to increase or decrease your intake of selected food groups?

3. What are the major types of nutrients that you need to obtain from the foods you eat? What happens if you fail to get enough of some of them? Are there significant differences between men and women in particular areas of nutrition?
4. Distinguish between the different types of vegetarianism. Which types are most likely to lead to nutrient deficiencies? What can be done to ensure that even the most strict vegetarian receives enough of the major nutrients?
5. What are the major problems that many college students face when trying to eat the right foods? List five actions that you and your classmates could take immediately to improve your eating.
6. What are the major risks for foodborne illnesses, and what can you do to protect yourself? How do food illnesses differ from food allergies?

Accessing Your Health on the Internet

The following websites explore further topics and issues related to personal health. For links to the websites below, visit the Companion Website for *Health: The Basics,* Green Edition at www.pearsonhighered.com/donatelle.

1. *American Dietetic Association (ADA).* Provides information on a full range of dietary topics, including sports nutrition, healthful cooking, and nutritional eating. Links to scientific publications and information on scholarships and public meetings. www.eatright.org
2. *U.S. Food and Drug Administration (FDA).* Provides information for consumers and professionals in the areas of food safety, supplements, and medical devices. Links to other sources of information about nutrition and food. www.fda.gov
3. *Food and Nutrition Information Center.* Offers a wide variety of information related to food and nutrition. http://fnic.nal.usda.gov
4. *National Institutes of Health: Office of Dietary Supplements.* Site of the International Bibliographic Information on Dietary Supplements (IBIDS), updated quarterly. http://dietary-supplements.info.nih.gov
5. *U.S. Department of Agriculture (USDA).* Offers a full discussion of the USDA Dietary Guidelines for Americans. www.usda.gov
6. *Linus Pauling Institute.* Key U.S. research center for studies on macro- and micronutrients; leaders in antioxidant research. http://lpi.oregonstate.edu

References

1. D. Mackinson, A. Anderson, and W. Wriden, "A Review of Consumers' Use and Understanding of Nutrition Information on Food Labels," *Proceedings of the Nutrition Society* 67 (2008): E215; G. Cowburn and L. Stockly, "Consumer Understanding and Use of Consumer Labeling: A Systematic Review," *Public Health Nutrition* 8 (2007): 21–28; R. Eckel et al., "Americans' Awareness, Knowledge, and Behaviors Regarding Fats: 2006–2007," *Journal of the American Dietetic Association* 109, no. 2 (2009): 288–96.
2. K. Flegal et al., "Cause-Specific Excess Deaths Associated with Underweight, Overweight, and Obesity," *Journal of the American Medical Association* 298 (2007): 2020–37.
3. American Institute of Cancer Research, *Food, Nutrition and the Prevention of Cancer: A Global Perspective* (Washington, DC: American Institute of Cancer Research, 1997).
4. F. Sofi et al., "Adherence to Mediterranean Diet and Health Status: Meta-Analysis," *BMJ* 337 (2008): a1344; M. Streppel et al., "Dietary Fiber Intake in Relation to Coronary Heart Disease and All Cause Mortality over 40," *American Journal of Clinical Nutrition* 88, no. 4 (2008): 1119–25; D. A. Timm and J. Slavin, "Dietary Fiber and the Relationship to Chronic Diseases," *American Journal of Lifestyle Medicine* 2, no. 3 (2008): 233–40.
5. World Health Organization, "Nutrition for Health and Development: Challenges," 2009, www.who.int/nutrition/challenges/en/index.html.
6. J. Thompson, M. Manore, and L. Vaughn, *The Science of Nutrition* (San Francisco: Benjamin Cummings, 2008).
7. U.S. Department of Agriculture, "Food Consumption Patterns: How We've Changed, 1970–2005," December 2005, www.usda.gov.
8. U.S. Department of Agriculture, "Economic Research Services," March 2008, www.ers.usda.gov.
9. J. Thompson and M. Manore, *Nutrition: An Applied Approach.* 2d ed. (San Francisco: Benjamin Cummings, 2009).
10. G. Block, "Foods Contributing to Energy Intake in the U.S.: Data from NHANES III and NHANES 1999–2000," *Journal of Food Composition and Analysis* 17, nos. 3–4 (2004): 439–47.
11. S. Goldfarb and D. Negoianu, "Just Add Water," *Journal of the American Society of Nephrology* 19 (2008): 1–3.
12. American College of Sports Medicine, "Exercise and Fluid Replacement," *Medicine and Science in Sports and Exercise* 39, no. 2 (2007): 377–90.
13. U.S. Department of Agriculture, Center for Nutrition Policy and Promotion. "Food Availability (Per Capita) Data System," 2009, www.ers.usda.gov.
14. J. E. Miltonal et al., "Relationship of Glycemic Index with Cardiovascular Risk Factors: Analysis of the National Diet and Nutrition Survey for People Aged 65 and Older," *Public Health Nutrition* 10, no. 11 (2007): 1321–35.
15. Institute of Medicine of the National Academies, "Dietary, Functional, and Total Fiber," in *Dietary Reference Intakes for Energy, Carbohydrate, Fiber, Fat, Fatty Acids, Cholesterol, Protein, and Amino Acids* (Washington, DC: The National Academies Press, 2002) pp. 7-1–7-2.
16. E. T. Jacobs et al., "Fiber, Sex, and Colorectal Adenoma: Results of a Pooled Analysis," *American Journal of Clinical Nutrition* 83 (2006): 343–49; American Institute for Cancer Research, "Colorectal Cancer Called 'Most Preventable,'" News Release, March 10, 2008, www.aicr.org; A. Millen et al., "Fruit and Vegetable Intake and Prevalence of Colorectal Adenoma in Cancer Screening Trial," *American Journal of Clinical Nutrition* 86, no. 6 (2007) 1754–64; P. "Newby et al., "Intake of Whole Grains, Refined Grains and Cereal Fiber Measured with 7-d Diet Records and Associations with Risk Factors for Chronic Disease," *American Journal of Clinical Nutrition* 86, no. 6 (2007): 1745–53.
17. E. J. Brunner et al., "Dietary Patterns and 15 Year Risks of Major Coronary Events, Diabetes and Mortality," *American Journal of Clinical Nutrition* 87, no. 5 (2008): 1414–21; P. Newby et al., "Intake of

Whole Grains, Refined Grains and Cereal Fiber," 2007.
18. D. Mozaffarian et al., "Trans Fatty Acids and Cardiovascular Disease," *New England Journal of Medicine* 354 (2006): 1601–13.
19. G. Bjelakovic et al., "Mortality in Randomized Trials of Antioxidant Supplements for Primary and Secondary Prevention: Systematic Review and Meta-Analysis," *Journal of the American Medical Association* 297, no. 8 (2007): 842–57; J. H. Kang and F. Grodstein, "Plasma Carotenoids and Tocopherols and Cognitive Function: A Prospective Study," *Neurobiological Aging* 29, no. 9 (2008): 1394–1403.
20. J. May, "Ascorbic Acid Transporters in Health and Disease," Paper presented at the Linus Pauling Diet and Optimum Health Annual Conference (Portland, OR: May 2007).
21. D. Albanes, "Vitamin Supplements and Cancer Prevention: Where Do Randomized Controlled Trials Stand?" *Journal of the National Cancer Institute* 101, no. 1 (2009): 2–4; J. Lin, et al., "Vitamins C and E and Beta Carotene Supplementation and Cancer Risk: A Randomized Controlled Trial," *Journal of the National Cancer Institute* 101, no. 1 (2009): 14–23.
22. M. Levine, "Pharmacologic Ascorbate Concentrations Selectively Kill Cancer Cells: Ascorbic Acid as a Pro-Drug for Ascorbate Radical and/or H_2O_2 Delivery to Tissues," Paper presented at the Linus Pauling Diet and Optimum Health Annual Conference (Portland, OR: May 2007); J. May, "Ascorbic Acid Transporters in Health and Disease," 2007.
23. C. M. Hasler et al., "Position Statement of the American Dietetic Association: Functional Foods," *Journal of the American Dietetic Association* 104, no. 5 (2004): 814–18; Linus Pauling Institute, Oregon State University, 2009, http://lpi.oregonstate.edu/infocenter.
24. M. Manore and J. Thompson, *Sport Nutrition for Health and Performance* (Champaign, IL: Human Kinetics, 2000), 283.
25. J. Chan and E. Giovannucci, "Vegetables, Fruits, Associated Micronutrients and Risk of Prostate Cancer," *Epidemiology Review* 23, no. 1 (2001): 82–86.
26. A. Chait et al., "Increased Dietary Micronutrients Decrease Serum Homocysteine Concentrations in Patients at High Risk of Cardiovascular Disease," *American Journal of Clinical Nutrition* 70, no. 5 (1999): 881–87.
27. J. Manson et al., "A Randomized Trial of Folic Acid and B-Vitamins in the Secondary Prevention of Cardiovascular Events in Women: Results from the Women's Antioxidant and Folic Acid Cardiovascular Study (WAFACS)," *Circulation* 114, no. 22 (2006): 2424; J. Manson et al., "A Randomized Factorial Trial of Vitamins C, E, and Beta-Carotene in the Secondary Prevention of Cardiovascular Events in Women: Results from the Women's Antioxidant Cardiovascular Study (WACS)," *Circulation* 114, no. 22 (2006): 2424.
28. Institute of Medicine, *Dietary Reference Intake for Water, Potassium, Sodium, Chloride, and Sulfate* (Washington, DC: The National Academies Press, 2004); H. Cohen et al., "Sodium Intake and Mortality in the NHANES II Follow-Up Study," *American Journal of Medicine* 119, no. 275 (2006): e7–e14.
29. H. Cohen et al., "Sodium Intake," (2006); J. Feng et al., "Salt Intake and Cardiovascular Mortality," *American Journal of Medicine* 120, no. 1 (2007): e5–e7; H. Harpannen and E. Mervaala, "Sodium Intake and Hypertension," *Progress in Cardiovascular Diseases* 49, no. 2 (2006): 59–75.
30. J. Ma, R. Johns, and R. Stafford, "Americans Are Not Meeting Current Calcium Recommendations," *American Journal of Clinical Nutrition* 85 (2007): 1361–66.
31. K. Tucker et al., "Colas, but Not Other Carbonated Beverages, Are Associated with Low Bone Mineral Density in Older Women: The Framingham Osteoporosis Study," *American Journal of Clinical Nutrition* 84 (2006): 936–42.
32. World Health Organization, "Miconutrient Deficiencies," www.who.int/nutrition/topics/ida/en/index.html. Accessed June 2008.
33. C. Tsai et al., "Heme and Non-Heme Iron Consumption and Risk of Gallstone Disease in Men," *American Journal of Clinical Nutrition* 85 (2007): 518–22.
34. K. M. Fairfield and R. H. Fletcher, "Vitamins for Chronic Disease Prevention in Adults: Scientific Review," *Journal of the American Medical Association* 287, no. 23 (2001): 3116–26.
35. "NIH State-of-the-Science Conference Statement on Multivitamin/Mineral Supplements and Chronic Disease Prevention," *Annals of Internal Medicine* 145 (2006): 364–71.
36. U.S. Department of Health and Human Services and U.S. Department of Agriculture, *Dietary Guidelines for Americans, 2005* (Washington, DC: Government Printing Office, 2005).
37. U.S. Department of Agriculture, Center for Nutrition Policy and Promotion, 2009, www.cnpp.usda.gov/DietaryGuidelines.htm.
38. U.S. Department of Agriculture, "Johanns Reveals USDA's Steps to a Healthier You," Press Release, April 19, 2005.
39. B. Black, "Health Library: Just How Much Food Is on That Plate? Understanding Portion Control," Last reviewed February 2009, EBSCO Publishing, www.ebscohost.com/healthLibrary.
40. "*Vegetarian Times* Study Shows 7.3 Million Americans Are Vegetarians" *Vegetarian Times*, Press Release, April 15, 2008, www.vegetariantimes.com/features/667.
41. J. Thompson and M. Manore, *Nutrition: An Applied Approach* (San Francisco: Benjamin Cummings, 2005).
42. Centers for Disease Control and Prevention, "Preliminary FoodNet Data on the Incidence of Infection with Pathogens Transmitted Commonly Through Food—10 States, 2007," *Morbidity and Mortality Weekly Report* 57, no. 14 (April 11, 2008): 366–70.
43. National Center for Infectious Diseases, Division of Bacterial and Mycotic Diseases, "*E. Coli*," Updated 2007, www.cdc.gov/ecoli; Centers for Disease Control and Prevention, "Preliminary FoodNet Data," April, 11, 2008.
44. Ibid.
45. Iowa State University, "Food Irradiation: What Is It?" *Iowa State University Extension Newsletter*, www.extension.iastate.edu/foodsafety/irradiation. Revised August 2006.
46. Food Allergy and Anaphylaxis Network, "Food Allergy Facts and Statistics," 2008, www.foodallergy.org.
47. Ibid.
48. Food Allergy and Anaphylaxis Network, "Advocacy: Food Labeling," 2008, www.foodallergy.org.
49. U.S. Department of Agriculture, Economic Research Services, "Diet Quality and Food Consumption," 2006, www.ers.usda.gov/briefing/DietQuality.

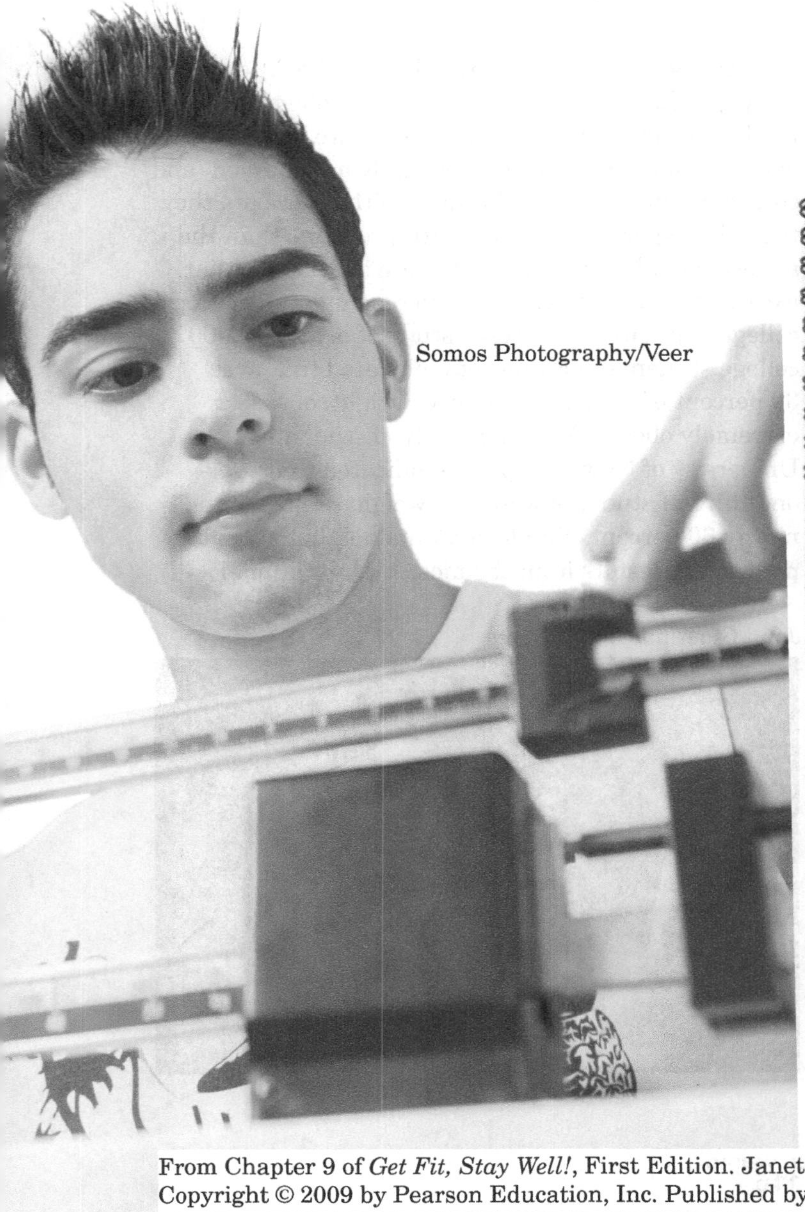

Somos Photography/Veer

Managing Your Weight

OBJECTIVES

Explain why obesity is both a worldwide trend and a serious concern in America.

Discuss the effects of body weight on wellness.

Acquire effective tools for successful weight management.

List reasons why some diets work but most fail.

Describe the major eating disorders.

Choose a realistic target weight based on your metabolic rate, activity level, eating habits, and environment.

Create a behavior change plan for long-term weight management.

From Chapter 9 of *Get Fit, Stay Well!*, First Edition. Janet L. Hopson, Rebecca J. Donatelle, Tanya R. Littrell.

CASE STUDY

Maria

"My name is Maria. I'm 25 and am a full-time student in southern Florida, finishing a BA in child development. I was halfway through college when my daughter, Anna, was born. Now that she's in school, I'm back to taking a full load of classes and hope to finish college in two more years. Overall, I am pretty happy with my life—the only thing I'd really like to change is my weight! Ever since Anna was born, I've been trying to get back my old figure. I'm 5'3"and used to weigh 120 pounds; now I weigh 155. I've tried lots of ways to lose the extra pounds—diet pills, liquid diets, Atkins, South Beach—you name it, I've tried it! Sometimes it works for a while, but eventually the weight always comes back. I'm willing to try again, but how do I find a plan that will stick?"

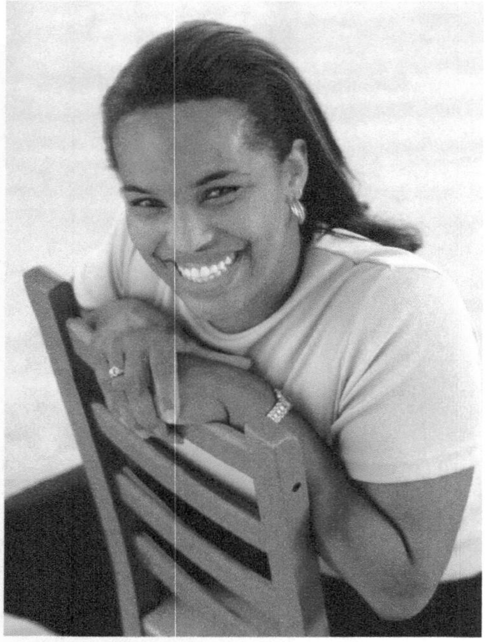

Photodisc/Getty Images

Weight has become a serious issue in America. About two-thirds of American adults are **overweight,** meaning that their body weight is more than 10 percent over the recommended range (see Figure 1) and their body mass index, or BMI, is over 25. Nearly one-third of adults are **obese,** with a BMI of 30 or above, or a body weight more than 20 percent above recommended range. Only about 2 percent of American adults are **underweight,** with a BMI below 18.5 or a weight 10 percent below recommended range.

College students have historically been in better shape than other adult populations. Until fairly recently, only about 25 percent of college students were overweight or obese, a much smaller percentage than the 66 percent of overweight and obese people in the population as a whole.[1, 2] Because college students tend to be younger, more educated, more likely to exercise, and more socioeconomically advantaged (and thus more likely to have better health coverage), they typically experience fewer health problems than the general population. However, there is evidence that excess weight is becoming an increasing problem for college populations. A recent study of nearly 10,000 college students in Minnesota indicated that over 39 percent of students were overweight, obese, or extremely obese.[3] A similar study of students at the University of New Hampshire indicated that over one-third of students were overweight or obese, and nearly 60 percent of male students had high blood pressure.[4] Results from the most recent national

overweight In an adult, having a BMI of 25 to 29. Also defined as having a body weight more than 10 percent above recommended levels

obese In an adult, having a BMI of 30 or more, or a body weight more than 20 percent above recommended levels

underweight In an adult, having a BMI below 18.5, or a body weight more than 10 percent below recommended levels

John Giustina/Getty Images

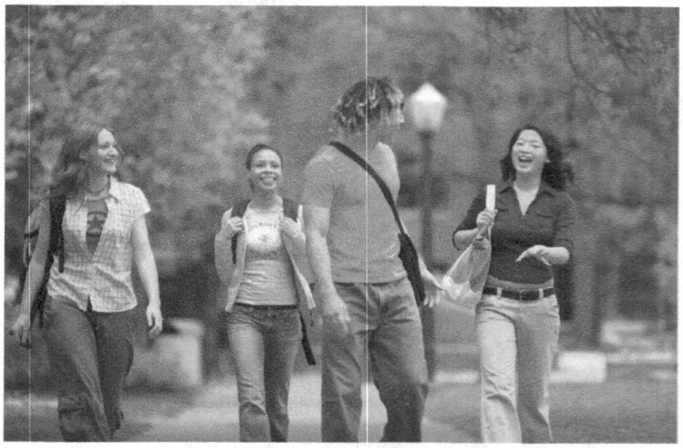

BMI	19	20	21	22	23	24	25	26	27	28	29	30	31	32	33	34	35
Height							**Weight in pounds**										
4'10"	91	96	100	105	110	115	119	124	129	134	138	143	148	153	158	162	167
4'11"	94	99	104	109	114	119	124	128	133	138	143	148	153	158	163	168	173
5'	97	102	107	112	118	123	128	133	138	143	148	153	158	163	158	174	179
5'1"	100	106	111	116	122	127	132	137	143	148	153	158	164	169	174	180	185
5'2"	104	109	115	120	126	131	136	142	147	153	158	164	169	175	180	186	191
5'3"	107	113	118	124	130	135	141	146	152	158	163	169	175	180	186	191	197
5'4"	110	116	122	128	134	140	145	151	157	163	169	174	180	186	192	197	204
5'5"	114	120	126	132	138	144	150	156	162	168	174	180	186	192	198	204	210
5'6"	118	124	130	136	142	148	155	161	167	173	179	186	192	198	204	210	216
5'7"	121	127	134	140	146	153	159	166	172	178	185	191	198	204	211	217	223
5'8"	125	131	138	144	151	158	164	171	177	184	190	197	203	210	216	223	230
5'9"	128	135	142	149	155	162	169	176	182	189	196	203	209	216	223	230	236
5'10"	132	139	146	153	160	167	174	181	188	195	202	209	216	222	229	236	243
5'11"	136	143	150	157	165	172	179	186	193	200	208	215	222	229	236	243	250
6'	140	147	154	162	169	177	184	191	199	206	213	221	228	235	242	250	258
6'1"	144	151	159	166	174	182	189	197	204	212	219	227	235	242	250	257	265
6'2"	148	155	163	171	179	186	194	202	210	218	225	233	241	249	256	264	272
6'3"	152	160	168	176	184	193	200	208	216	224	232	240	248	256	264	272	279
	Healthy weight						**Overweight**					**Obese**					

FIGURE 1

Locate your height. Read across to find your weight. Then read up to determine your BMI.

Source: NIH/National Heart, Lung, and Blood Institute (NHLBI). *Evidence Report of Clinical Guidelines on the Identification, Evaluation, and Treatment of Overweight and Obesity in Adults,* 1998.

survey by the National College Health Association also indicate increasing trends of overweight and obesity, as well as increasing indicators of disordered eating.[5]

Regardless of your age and stage of life, several key principles are important to consider as you assess your own dietary, exercise, and weight management strategies:

- Recognize that no diet program, product, or service will magically make weight melt away. Successful weight loss takes time, effort, and motivation. The changes you make in your diet and exercise habits need to become a new way of life, rather than be regarded as short-term fixes.

- Recognize that weight loss, per se, is far less important than your overall percentage of body fat. A high body fat percentage is correlated with numerous health risks. Reducing body fat through resistance exercise, aerobic exercise, and sound nutrition can help lower your risk, improve energy levels, and make you feel better. "Healthy weight loss" means the slow, sustained loss of fat, coupled with increases in muscle mass and the preservation and maintenance of lean body mass.
- Learn how long-term weight management balances calories consumed in foods with calories expended through metabolism, activity, and exercise—an equation called **energy balance.** If you expend more calories than you consume over time, you'll lose weight due to a **negative caloric balance** (Figure 2). Consume more calories than you expend and you'll gain weight due to a **positive caloric balance.** Consume and expend approximately the same number of calories over a period of time and you'll reach an **isocaloric balance**—and with it, be able to maintain your weight.

This chapter presents the tools and techniques you need to determine a healthy target weight and create a sound plan for reaching and maintaining it. Incorporating **weight management** into your ongoing wellness program will allow you to realize the significant benefits—physiological, social, and emotional—of sustaining your body mass and body composition within recommended ranges throughout adult life.

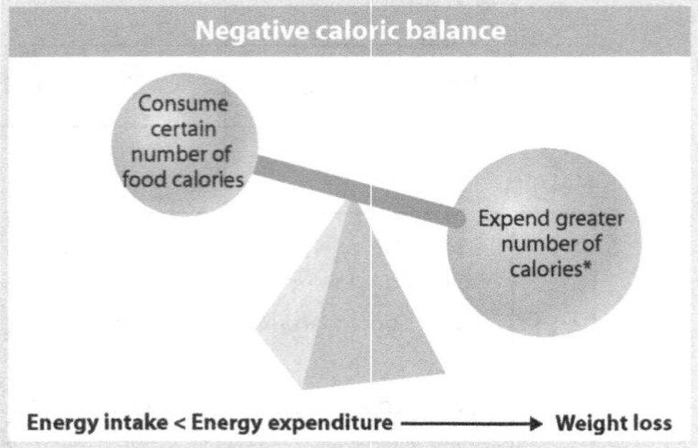

(a)

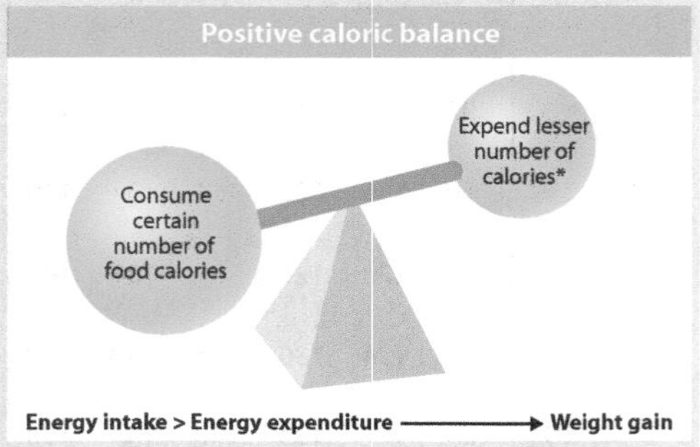

(b)

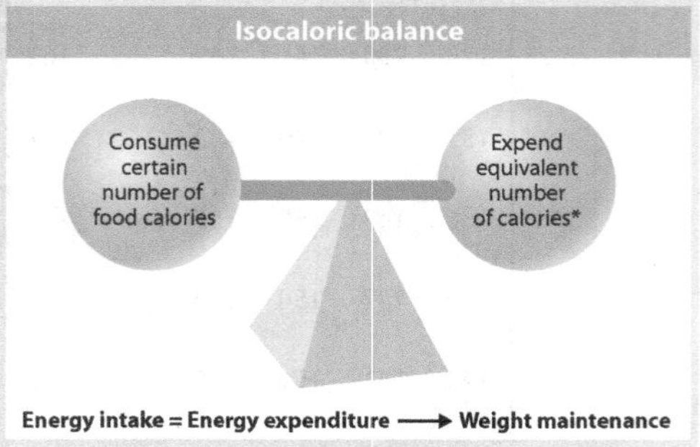

(c)

* Calories are expended through metabolism, activity and exercise

FIGURE 2
On any given day, each of us has a personal energy equation with either a negative caloric balance, a positive caloric balance, or an isocaloric balance. Over time, this equation helps determine our body weight.

energy balance The relationship between the amount of calories consumed in food with the amount of calories expended through metabolism and physical activity

negative caloric balance A state in which the amount of calories consumed in food falls short of the amount of calories expended through metabolism and physical activity

positive caloric balance A state in which the amount of calories consumed in food exceeds the amount of calories expended through metabolism and physical activity

isocaloric balance A state in which the amount of calories consumed in food is approximately the same as the amount of calories expended through metabolism and physical activity

weight management A lifelong balancing of calories consumed and calories expended through exercise and activity to control body fat and weight

WHY IS OBESITY ON THE RISE?

In recent decades, people all over the world have been getting heavier and heavier. What's behind this trend? And why does it matter?

"GLOBESITY" IS A WORLDWIDE TREND

In 2006, the World Health Organization (WHO) estimated that 1.6 billion of the world's people are overweight and that the number could increase to 2.3 billion by 2015. Obese adults number over 400 million worldwide and are a problem in high-income industrialized countries as well as in low- and middle-income developing countries.[6]

Epidemic rates of obesity in the global population, or "globesity," results from energy imbalance. Diets high in processed fats, meats, sugars, and refined starches provide excess calories while labor-saving devices and sedentary lifestyles reduce energy expenditure. In developing countries, entire cultures are moving away from traditional diets—rich in fruits, vegetables, grains, and low-fat proteins—as well as from manual labor. As a result, residents in developing countries are experiencing the same upward shift in body fat percentages and weight that Americans began to show three decades ago. Only the poorest countries of sub-Saharan Africa do not reflect this worldwide trend.[7]

ENERGY IMBALANCE IS COMMON IN AMERICA

In the last quarter century, the percentage of overweight Americans rose 40 percent while the percentage of obese adults more than doubled. The maps in Figure 3 reveal that the rapid increase is distributed unevenly, with the southern and upper Midwestern states now showing the highest rates of obesity in the nation.

American children are getting heavier, too. More than 37 percent of American children are overweight or obese. That represents twice as many heavy preschoolers and teens today as in the 1970s, and three times as many children aged 6 to 11.[8] What's behind this widespread energy imbalance?

Overconsumption

Americans consume 250 to 500 calories more per day now than they did 30 years ago. Without additional exercise, this imbalance in energy input can lead to considerable yearly weight gain. Many societal factors encourage overeating: portion distortion, the constant availability of food, advertising, and price.

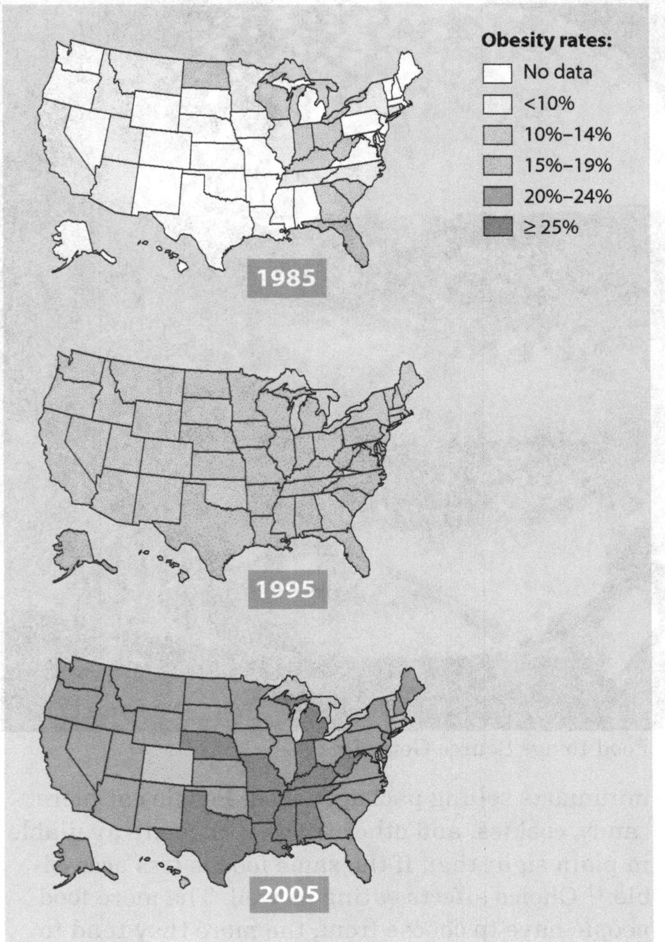

FIGURE 3
Obesity rates have risen dramatically over recent decades. Rates are highest in the upper Midwest and in the South.
Source: Centers for Disease Control, 2006.

Food portions in restaurants and supermarkets have grown steadily over the past half-century, along with consumers' preferences and expectations. In 1954, a Burger King hamburger weighed 3.9 ounces. Today, it weighs 4.4 ounces—a 13 percent increase. Most people, however, don't order the regular-sized hamburger, choosing instead the much larger Whopper with 9 ounces of meat, or the Double Whopper with 12.6 ounces.[9] In addition, researchers have found that people don't read their own "fullness signals," or feelings of *satiety,* very well. As a result, the bigger the portions (and the more food available), the more they will eat overall.[10]

Easy access to food also encourages overeating. Today, most drugstores, gas stations, schools, and public buildings have vending machines and

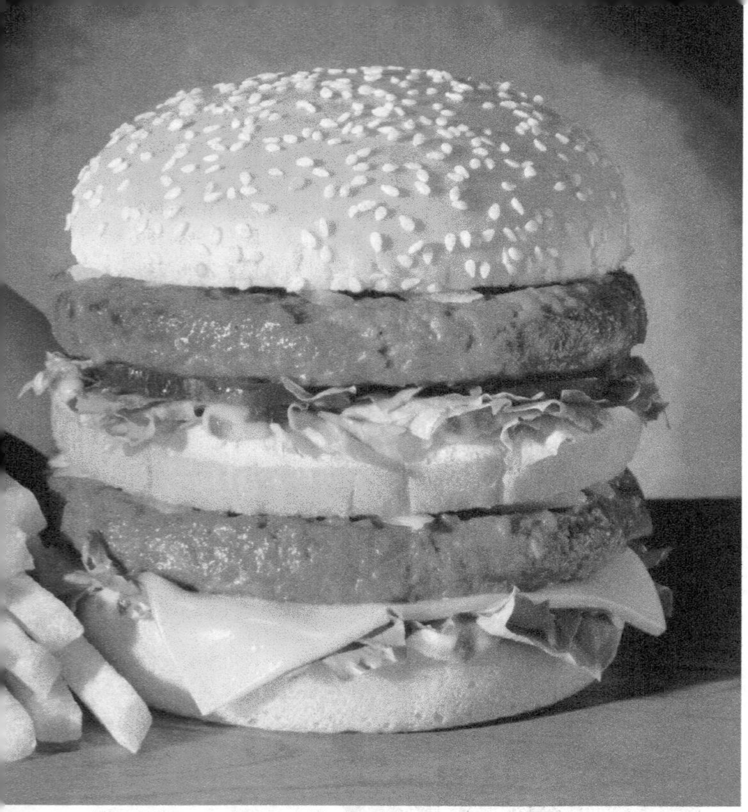

Food Image Source/Getty Images

minimarts selling packaged food. People eat more candy, cookies, and other treats if they are available in plain sight than if the same food is less accessible.[11] Choice affects eating as well. The more food people have to choose from, the more they tend to eat. People will eat more total food at a four-course meal than at a two-course meal—and even more at a buffet.

The persuasiveness of product advertising also contributes to overeating. An amazing one-third of our daily calories come from just a few categories of highly advertised foods that contribute little more than empty calories: sweets, sodas and fruit drinks, alcoholic beverages, and salty snacks.[12]

The relatively low price of food in America is yet another environmental influence on overconsumption. When experimenters lowered the price of snacks in vending machines, the discount stimulated sales immediately—regardless of whether a snack food had any nutritional value.[13]

Too Little Exercise Do you plant and harvest your own food? Carry your own water from a well? Hand-deliver letters to people when you want to communicate? Probably not! The ease of our modern life is an improvement over the hard physical labor of past generations. The exertion we are spared, however, amounts to hundreds of calories per day that we *don't* burn off as we sit at our desks, drive our cars, and change channels with a remote control.

Even the layout of modern towns and cities contributes to reduced energy expenditure. The majority of Americans live in suburbs—an environment designed and built around automotive transportation. Suburban living is strongly linked to decreased activity, and this, in turn, contributes to a number of medical conditions. The greater the sprawl, the less people walk, the more they weigh, and the more likely they are to have high blood pressure,[14] heart disease, cancer, diabetes, and other diseases.

Biological Factors Our modern food supply, culture, and environment clearly encourage overconsumption and underexercise. But why, then, isn't *everyone* overweight or obese? The answer lies mostly in heredity, demographics, and personal choice.

If most of your relatives—parents, siblings, and others—are overweight or obese, you will be more likely to gain weight during adulthood yourself. Researchers have learned that dozens—perhaps hundreds—of genes help determine your weight.[15] Genes control whether our metabolism is fast and tends to burn off most of our excess calories, or is slow and tends to conserve food energy. Genes also control appetite, fullness, fat storage, fat utilization, and activity levels.

Our natural tendencies to conserve or use energy during rest and activity also influence our weight. Some people tend to save energy by sitting quietly for long stretches and being generally less active all day. Others tend to use energy by being fidgety, jiggling their head, hands, and feet, and getting up to walk around every few minutes. James Levine and colleagues at the Mayo Clinic have demonstrated that lean people burn 279 to 477 more calories per day than obese people through this type of **non-exercise activity**—an expenditure that can significantly affect fat storage and body weight.[16]

The box **Understanding Diversity: Race/Ethnicity, Gender, and Weight** examines how ethnicity and gender can also be factors in an individual's propensity toward weight gain.

non-exercise activity Routine daily activities like standing up and walking around that use energy but are not part of deliberate exercise

UNDERSTANDING DIVERSITY

RACE/ETHNICITY, GENDER, AND WEIGHT

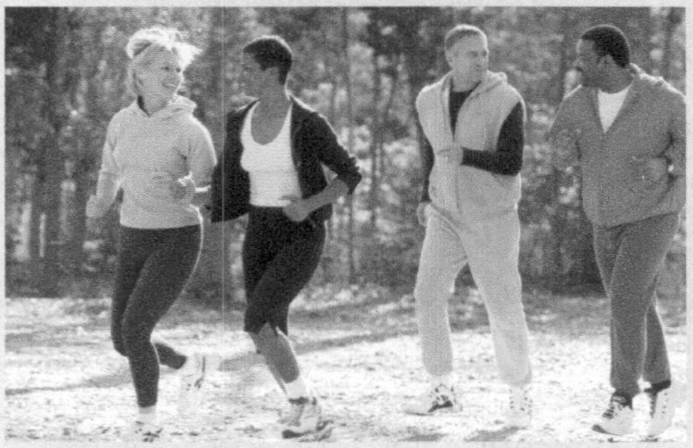

Ariel Skelley/Corbis

Body weight varies by racial/ethnic groups to some degree, based on genes as well as on cultural preferences for food and exercise. Hispanic males, African American males and females, and white males have the highest percentages of overweight (60 and 70 percent of adults in these groups). Hispanic females and white females have somewhat lower rates of overweight (45 to 55 percent). Asian Americans have the lowest percentages of overweight (men 35 percent, women 25 percent).[1]

Some ethnic groups appear to have "thrifty genes" that helped their ancestors survive during extended periods of famine by slowing down metabolism to conserve food energy. In a modern environment of plentiful food, widespread mechanization, and diminished activity, however, "thrifty genes" can lead to easy weight gain. This helps explain, for example, why 90 percent of Pima Indians are overweight and 75 percent are obese.[2]

Women have a tendency to burn fewer calories than men due to their higher level of essential body fat and lower ratio of lean body mass to fat mass. Because muscle cells burn more energy, and because men usually have more muscle tissue than women, men burn 10 to 20 percent more calories than women do, even at rest. Monthly hormonal cycles and pregnancy also increase the likelihood of weight fluctuation and gain. Significantly, though, adult men are more likely to be overweight than adult women.

Sources:

1. Charlotte. A. Schoenborn and others, "Body Weight Status of Adults: United States, 1997–1998." Advance Data from *Vital and Health Statistics,* no. 330 (September 6, 2002). U.S. Centers for Disease Control and Prevention.
2. P. Jaret, "The Way to Lose Weight," *Health* (January-February 1995): 52–59.

Lifestyle Factors For most people, exercise, activity, nutrition, and other personal choices impact body weight as much or more than do inherited tendencies. For example, 25 percent of Americans do not engage in exercise, sports, or other physical activity during their leisure time.[17] Education is also a factor in both weight and exercise. The more education a person attains, and the more money he or she makes, the less likely he or she is to be overweight or obese. And the higher a person's educational attainment, the more likely he or she is to be physically active.

CASE STUDY

Maria

"I was never overweight as a kid, and I gained a normal amount of weight during my pregnancy, but now I'm considered overweight. My parents, grandparents, and two older sisters are all kind of on the heavy side, so I wonder if my "heavy" gene just decided to kick in! While I was pregnant, I got used to eating more food than I used to, and after giving birth to Anna, I guess I just didn't cut back. I spend a lot of time running around after Anna, but otherwise, I drive everywhere and don't set aside special time to exercise. Meanwhile, it seems like Anna will eat only three things—macaroni and cheese, chicken strips, and pizza—so that's what we eat most nights. My husband and I joke that all three of us eat like stereotypical college students."

1. **List three factors that probably contributed to Maria's becoming overweight.**
2. **Do you share any of Maria's habits? Is she like any of your friends?**
3. **Are you satisfied with your current weight? If not, are there aspects of your lifestyle that may have led to your current dissatisfaction?**

HOW DOES BODY WEIGHT AFFECT YOUR WELLNESS?

A leading nutritionist has written that "weight sits like a spider at the center of an intricate, tangled web of health and disease."[18] Indeed, research shows that three weight-related factors impact your long-term health: your BMI, increases in BMI over time, and body fat stored in the abdominal regions. You are more likely to remain healthy throughout life if (1) your BMI is between 21 and 23 for women and 22 and 24 for men; (2) you maintain approximately the same BMI and the same waist size throughout your adult life; and (3) your body's fat deposits tend to occur around the hips and thighs rather than the abdomen. High BMIs and abdominal fat (indicated by a large waist size) are associated with higher risk for several chronic diseases.[19]

Being underweight is an important but far less common problem. Fewer than 5 percent of Americans have a BMI under 18.5. Underweight carries its own significant health risks and can be the result of an unusually fast metabolism, excessive dieting, extreme levels of exercise, eating disorders, smoking, or illness.

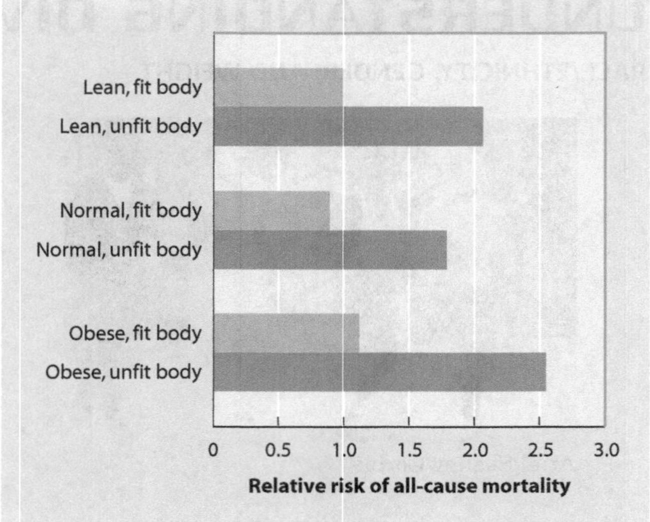

FIGURE 4

Being fit significantly reduces your mortality risk in any given year, regardless of your degree of body fat.

Source: Chong Do Lee, Steven N. Blair, and Andrew S. Jackson, "Cardiorespiratory Fitness, Body Composition, and All-Cause and Cardiovascular Disease Mortality in Men," *American Journal of Clinical Nutrition* 69, no. 3 (March 1999): 373–80.

BODY WEIGHT CAN AFFECT LIFE EXPECTANCY

People who maintain a weight and BMI within recommended ranges generally have longer life expectancies than people who are obese or underweight. As Figure 4 shows, being fit significantly reduces mortality risk, especially when combined with healthy weight. Being obese (having a BMI of 30 or above) cuts an average of 6 to 7 years from the life of a nonsmoker and 13 to 14 years from a smoker.[20] Research indicates that America's 200-year rise in life expectancy may begin to decline because obesity is so prevalent and can shorten life so dramatically.[21]

Underweight people have a higher death rate than normal-weight or overweight people.[22] In fact, some studies indicate that underweight people may have more than 18 times the risk of dying of cancer, and four times the risk of CVD death.[23] Only obese people have a shorter life expectancy. The statistics for early deaths among the underweight reflect the fact that a low BMI is characteristic of patients with illnesses such as cancer, uncontrolled diabetes, and disordered eating. People who are underweight but *not* ill and who are careful to get complete daily nutrition may actually realize greater longevity.[24] Underweight associated with poor nutrition, however, can lead to life-shortening conditions such as anemia, susceptibility to disease and infection, slower recovery from illness, muscle wasting and weakness, and osteoporosis and bone fractures.

BODY WEIGHT CAN PROMOTE OR DIMINISH FITNESS

A stable, healthy-range BMI goes hand in hand with regular exercise. Maintaining weight and BMI within recommended ranges leads to increased energy and reduced likelihood of injury during fitness activities. Safety and comfort, in turn, encourage continued exercise and the many wellness benefits it produces.

Over- and underweight can contribute to poor fitness. The reverse is also true: Low fitness can contribute to unhealthy weight levels. Overweight can lead to a downward fitness spiral: An over-accumulation of body fat leads to strain on the bones, joints, and muscles that makes exercising harder and injury more likely. Stiffness and pain in

CASE STUDY

Maria

"Here's the funny thing: My husband, Tim, is extremely skinny. He's 5'9" and weighs only 130 pounds. We eat the same foods, but he has the metabolism of a hummingbird. I don't know where it all goes. His whole family is thin, so I guess that is part of it. He's just as out of shape as I am, though. We moved to a new apartment recently and need to walk up one flight of stairs—both of us get so out of breath by the time we make it to the door. Just because he's skinnier doesn't mean he's any more fit! What a pair: I want to lose weight, while he wants to gain weight."

1. **What chronic health problems is Maria at risk for if she remains overweight?**
2. **Maria must now walk up and down a flight of stairs every day to leave/return to her apartment. Do you see this as a good or bad thing? Explain your answer.**
3. **Do you think Tim faces fewer chronic health risks than Maria? What else would you want to know about Tim's and Maria's habits that would help you answer this question?**
4. **Which of the benefits of maintaining a healthy weight are most important to you?**

the hands, feet, knees, and back, in turn, make exercising more difficult. They also make work, employment, and activities of daily living—walking up stairs, carrying books or grocery bags, shoveling snow, getting in and out of automobiles, and so on—harder. With lower levels of exercise, fitness and wellness decline.

Below-normal body weight can lead to muscle wasting as the body breaks down muscle tissue for energy when fat stores are low. Muscle wasting, in turn, can lead to weakness and declining ability to exercise and accomplish daily tasks. These inevitably reduce both fitness and wellness unless the underweight individual works hard to maintain strength and endurance.

BODY WEIGHT CAN INFLUENCE THE RISKS FOR CHRONIC DISEASES

Researchers have confirmed that people with excess body fat have higher levels of several serious chronic diseases, including high blood pressure, stroke, heart disease, certain cancers, type 2 diabetes, and metabolic syndrome.[25] Specific cancers linked to high BMI include prostate, colon, rectum, esophagus, pancreas, kidney, gallbladder, ovary, cervix, liver, breast, uterus, and stomach.[26]

Fat accumulation around the waist (a 40-inch waistline or higher for a man, or a 35-inch waistline or higher for a woman) increases the risk for developing **metabolic syndrome.** This serious medical condition is a combination of high blood cholesterol, high blood pressure, abdominal fat deposits, and insulin resistance or full-fledged type 2 diabetes.

Gaining weight may increase the risk for cardiovascular disease, diabetes, and other chronic diseases because of *inflammation,* a primitive immune reaction. Fat tissue may be giving off chemicals that trigger inflammation, and inflammation may aggravate heart disease, diabetes, and other conditions.[27] Losing weight, on the other hand, may diminish inflammation and is known to decrease levels of blood cholesterol and triglycerides, and lower blood pressure and diabetes risk.[28] A weight loss of just 10 to 15 pounds can bring measurable health benefits, even to an obese individual.[29]

WHAT ARE EFFECTIVE TOOLS FOR WEIGHT MANAGEMENT?

Understanding role of metabolic rates, setting realistic goals, recognizing your body's set point, and taking lessons from successful weight maintainers will help you achieve your weight goals.

metabolic syndrome A medical condition characterized by a combination of high blood cholesterol, high blood pressure, abdominal fat deposits and large waist circumference, and insulin resistance or type 2 diabetes

FACTS AND FALLACIES

DO DIET DRUGS WORK?

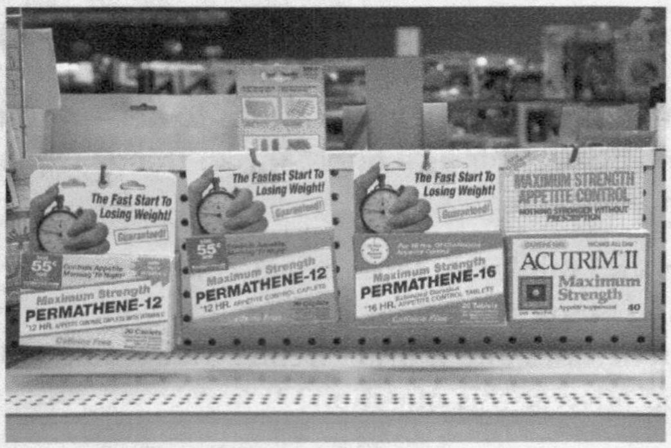

Michael Newman/PhotoEdit Inc.

Millions of people think to themselves, "I hate diets and exercise, and they don't work for me, anyway. Why can't I just take a pill to get thin?" Unfortunately, prescription diet drugs can cost over $100 per month and have significant side effects, and even the most effective among them don't bring about much weight loss. What's more, without modified diet and increased exercise, any lost weight comes right back as soon as a person stops taking the pills.[1]

Currently on the market is Meridia (sibutramine), a drug that keeps levels of the neurotransmitter serotonin high and helps to cut hunger. Users average a 10- to 14-pound weight loss over 6 months, or about one-half pound per week. However, the drug can cause headaches, insomnia, high blood pressure, and other symptoms, and can interfere with antidepressant drugs.

Another currently prescribed drug called Xenical (orlistat) partially blocks digestion of fats. Users lose an average of 13 pounds in a year (about 4 ounces per week) with side effects that include oily stools and spotting, gas with fecal discharge, and urgent elimination. A lower-dose over-the-counter version called Alli is being marketed now.

Several prescription drugs suppress appetite, including Phentride (phentermine), and Tenuate (diethylpropion). These drugs are addictive, cause tolerance, and can only be used in the short-term. A French drug called Acomplia (rimonabant) blocks appetites and helps users lose an average of 19 pounds per year (a little over one-third pound per week), but it has undergone limited human testing and is currently unavailable in the United States.

The FDA has banned many other drugs and supplements (for example, drugs containing ephedra or phenylpropanolamine, also called *fen-phen*) because of elevated blood pressure, stroke risk, and other harmful side effects.[2]

You will also find many supplements in the vitamin section of drug and food stores, despite a lack of proof that they are effective or safe. One such product, bitter orange, contains a stimulant similar to ephedra. There have been no conclusive human studies proving either the safety or effectiveness of bitter orange. Claims for several other supplements await supporting evidence. These include herbal laxatives; the heavy metals chromium and vanadium; ginseng and ginkgo; green tea extracts; and an extract from shrimp and crab shells called *chitosan*. Until someone invents a truly effective, low-risk weight-loss drug, the best options are improved diet and increased exercise, perhaps in conjunction with a prescription.

Sources:

1. S. B. Moyers, "Medications as an Adjunct Therapy for Weight Loss: Approved and Off-Label Agents in Use," *Journal of the American Dietetic Association* 10, no. 6 (June 2005): 948–59.
2. B. F. McBride and others, "Electrocardiographic and Hemodynamic Effects of a Multicomponent Dietary Supplement Containing Ephedra and Caffeine: A Randomized Controlled Trial," *Journal of the American Medical Association* 291, no. 2 (January 14, 2004): 216–21.

RECOGNIZE THE ROLE OF METABOLIC RATE

Lifelong weight maintenance requires deliberately balancing calories consumed and calories expended. Just to stay at roughly the same weight as the years pass and metabolism slows bit by bit, most people must gradually decrease their food intake as they gradually increase their physical activity. Fully 60 to 70 percent of your daily calorie intake—typically between 900 and 1,800 food Calories per day—is consumed as your body sustains functions like heartbeat, breathing, and maintaining body temperature. The rate at which your body consumes food energy to sustain these basic functions is your **basal metabolic rate** (BMR). Your **resting metabolic rate** (RMR) is slightly higher, because it also includes the energy expended as you digest food. BMR has genetic underpinnings but can be influenced by your activity level and your body composition. Since muscle tissue is highly active, the more lean tissue you have, the greater your basal metabolic rate; the more fat tissue you have, the lower your BMR. This explains

basal metabolic rate Your baseline rate of energy use, dictated by your body's collective metabolic activities

resting metabolic rate Basal metabolic rate plus the energy expended in digesting food

Try it NOW! Is your current weight in the healthy weight range for your height? If not, what is a realistic target weight for you?

why both your activity level and your fitness influence your BMR; the higher your fitness level, the greater your ratio of lean tissue to fat mass is likely to be, and the more energy you will burn while exercising and at rest. Cardiovascular and strength-building exercises contribute most directly to speeding up BMR.

ASSESS YOUR CURRENT WEIGHT AND CHOOSE A REALISTIC GOAL

Figure 1 shows healthy weight and BMI ranges based on height. In using weight and BMI charts, people often wonder if their ideal weight should be on the high or low end of the range. If your body fat percentage is low and your muscle development is high, your healthy weight (including your BMI) will be on the higher end of the range. The same is also true if your frame size is large (as judged by a measure such as wrist circumference). If your body fat percentage is high and your muscle development is low, your healthy weight will be in the middle-to-low end of the range. This is also true if your frame size is medium or small. Knowing these factors will help you calculate a realistic weight goal.

RECOGNIZE YOUR BODY'S SET POINT

Perhaps you've noticed that your body is programmed around a certain weight or **set point** that it returns to fairly easily when you gain or lose a few pounds. Many dieters reach a plateau after a certain amount of weight loss and can't seem to trim off more pounds. This plateau is due, in part, to a downshifted metabolism balancing out lower calorie intake: the person's energy balance is now at a weight-maintenance, not a weight-loss, level.

To "outsmart" and reset one's set point, a dieter must lose weight slowly and increase exercise. Physiologists have known for some time that exercise both speeds resting metabolism and preserves lean body mass so more muscle tissue remains to continue burning extra calories.[31]

TAKE LESSONS FROM *SUCCESSFUL* WEIGHT MAINTAINERS

People who sustain a normal, healthy weight over years or decades tend to do some of the same kinds of things. Successful weight maintainers engage in a physically active lifestyle, averaging an hour per day of moderate to vigorous physical activity.[32]

Successful weight maintainers also tend to have a regular eating pattern. They don't skip meals, they eat breakfast every day, and they don't "cheat" over the weekends by indulging in junk food. They eat a nutritious diet that is low in fats, high in complex carbohydrates, has moderate levels of protein, and has a high volume but a low calorie density. They avoid sodas and juice drinks sweetened with sugar or corn syrup.

Successful weight maintainers also stay conscious of situations that trigger overeating, and they apply strategies to prevent overeating. They are motivated to stay at a healthy weight, and they respond quickly by cutting back calories and increasing activity as soon as their weight starts to creep up.[33]

People who are successful at maintaining a healthy weight typically have tools for coping with problems and handling life stresses. They assume responsibility for their lifestyle behaviors, know where to seek help, and tend to be self-reliant. They have a good social support system, both for their weight maintenance and their lives in general. They are more likely to maintain weight loss if they are satisfied with their new weight.[34]

BALANCE YOUR ENERGY EQUATION

Long-term weight management relies on balancing your energy equation—that is, attaining an isocaloric balance so that the calories you consume are equivalent over time to the calories you burn.

set point A preprogrammed weight that your body returns to easily when you gain or lose a few pounds

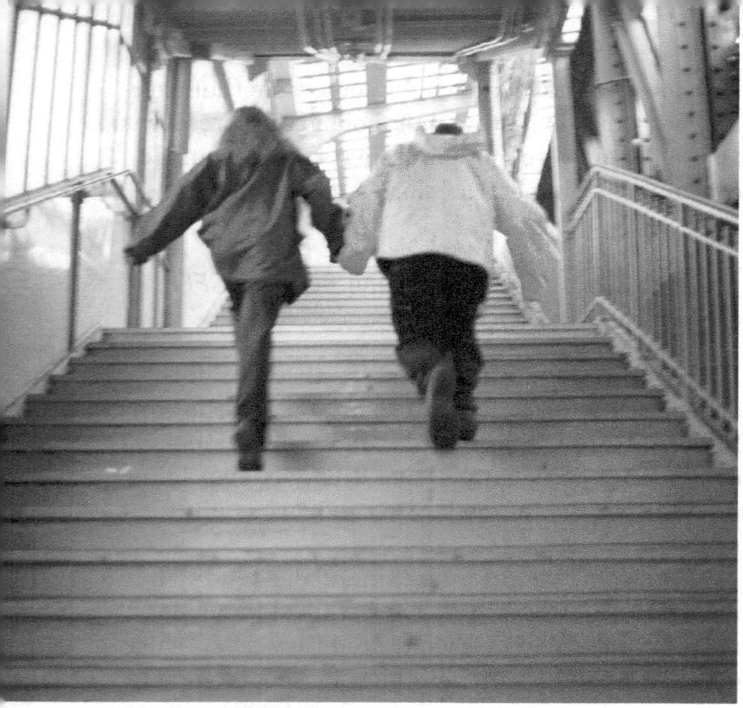

P. Sheandell/AGE Fotostock

To lose or gain weight, you must deliberately "unbalance" that equation for a while: negative caloric balance for loss, positive caloric balance for gain.

There are several ways to determine your approximate daily calorie consumption and expenditure. Try logging on to the MyPyramid.gov website to get a target number for calorie consumption based on your age, sex, and level of daily moderate or vigorous activity.

Websites like MyPyramid.gov also provide calorie counts for specific foods and portions so you can keep track of how many calories you consume each day. You can get calorie-counting programs for small handheld computer devices, or find them online at websites like www.caloriecontrol.org. MyPyramid.gov also supplies calorie expenditure information from various activities, as does Table 1.

If you follow good nutritional and eating habits and establish and stick with a regular exercise program, weight maintenance can become second nature to you and a habit you keep throughout adult life.

Try it NOW! Log on to www.MyPyramid.gov and click on "MyPyramid Tracker." • Set up your own user login and password. • Enter your daily activity level. • Then click "Energy Balance"—how many calories do you need, given your activity level?

ESTABLISH A REGULAR EXERCISE PROGRAM

Along with monitored and controlled eating, exercise is essential both to weight change (loss or gain) and to weight maintenance. Exercise burns calories directly, pumps up your metabolic rate to burn additional calories, and builds muscle tissue that burns still more energy. Many people find that in addition to a healthy diet, they need to be active for more than an hour per day in order to lose weight, while 60 minutes per day will sustain weight at current levels. These figures are cumulative: Add 7 minutes of stair-climbing here, plus 11 minutes of brisk walking across campus there, plus 20 minutes of stationary biking, and so on. Aerobic exercise, of course, is the best calorie burner.

The greater the frequency, intensity, and time spent on an activity, the more energy you use and the more calories you burn. There are other considerations for choosing types of fitness exercise as well. The larger the muscle groups you use, for example, the more you boost your metabolism, and in turn, your calorie expenditure. Your baseline physiological activities—heartbeat, breathing, generating body heat, and so on—also consume calories while you are contracting arm, leg, abdomen, and other body muscles. Table 1 lists the caloric expenditures for several popular activities, sports, and exercises for adults of three different weight levels.

MODIFY YOUR BEHAVIOR FOR LONG-TERM WEIGHT CHANGE

Weight loss is hard work, but in some ways, it's the easy part of weight management. Most people can lose some weight, but relatively few—perhaps 20 percent—can maintain that lower weight for more than a few months. In one study, more than half of successful dieters thought dieting was easier than weight maintenance. Nevertheless, with the right basic approach, weight loss or gain can simply be phases of lifelong weight stabilization that use very similar tools and techniques.

TABLE 1

Calories Burned through Activity

Activity, Sport, or Exercise	Calories Expended/Min in 110 lb Person	Calories Expended/Min in 150 lb Person	Calories Expended/Min in 190 lb Person
Aerobics, 10" step	7.0	9.5	12.0
Basketball, pick-up	7.0	9.5	12.0
Biking, slow	5.3	7.1	9.0
Bowling	2.6	3.6	4.5
Dancing, moderate pace	4.2	5.7	9.0
Downhill skiing, moderate pace	5.5	7.5	9.5
Driving	1.8	2.4	3.0
Frisbee, casual	2.6	3.6	4.5
Golf, walking, and pulling clubs	4.4	6.0	7.5
Grocery shopping	3.1	4.2	5.3
Hiking, hills	5.3	7.1	9.0
Jogging, moderate pace	5.3	7.1	9.0
Kickboxing	8.8	12.0	14.7
Office work	1.3	1.8	2.3
Ping-Pong	3.5	4.8	6.0
Reading	0.9	1.2	1.5
Soccer, noncompetitive	6.1	8.3	10.5
Softball	4.4	6.0	7.5
StairMaster: 40 stairs/minute	6.1	8.3	10.2
Stretching	3.5	4.8	5.8
Swimming	~8	~10	~13
Tennis, singles, recreational	7.0	9.5	12.0
Watching TV	1.0	1.4	1.8

Source: Adapted from *Calorie Expenditure Charts*, by Frank I. Katch, Victor L. Katch, and William D. McArdle (Ann Arbor, Michigan: Fitness Technologies Press, 1996).

Readiness requires motivation, commitment, goals, and attitudes.

You must be motivated to change your long-term eating and exercise habits, and you must be willing to work to accomplish those changes. Talking with friends, learning about the benefits of healthy BMI, and writing in a journal about your current eating and exercise habits can all help motivate you to set and reach body goals. Work on your attitude, too. Accept the fact that only through permanently controlled eating and a long-term commitment to activity and exercise can you maintain desired weight, BMI, and body composition over the long-term.

You also need realistic goals in order to change your weight and then maintain the new desired level. Weight and nutrition experts recommend that

CASE STUDY

Maria

"After living in our new apartment for a month, I've noticed something interesting: It's gotten easier to climb up and down the flight of stairs. I guess I'm getting used to it! Of course, that alone is not going to make me lose weight, but it's become the unofficial kickoff to my plan to get more active. One of the things I'm realizing is that I need to stop this idea of 'going on a diet' and instead try to figure out how to change my habits in a way that feels manageable to me. If I just 'go on a diet,' I'll regain everything I lose as soon as I go *off* of it, right? So what I need to do is figure out how to get more active and change my habits in a way that feels natural.

"I weigh 155 right now. I need to lose 35 pounds to get back to my old prepregnancy weight of 120. For now, I'm just going to try losing 10 pounds, at least to start off with. I've heard about weight-loss groups that help you with meal planning, portion control, and regular exercise. I think that might be a good approach for me."

1. **Just by climbing a flight of stairs every day, Maria has increased her daily activity level and is expending more calories than she used to. What other small things could she do to increase her daily physical activity?**
2. **You've just learned about several tools for effective weight management. Which tools do you see Maria using?**
3. **Do you have a regular exercise program? If not, what are some steps you can take to begin establishing one?**

people set a goal of losing no more than 10 percent of their body weight at a rate of one-half to 2 pounds per week. This requires expending 300 to 500 more calories per day than you consume. Once you have lost 10 percent of your body weight, you should maintain that level for a few months. Then you can set a new weight-loss goal of 10 percent of this new, lower body weight, and so on.

WHY DON'T MOST DIETS SUCCEED?

Many people are convinced that dieting success depends on simply finding the right diet. They bounce from one highly publicized diet to another: low-fat, high carbohydrate; low carbohydrate, high protein and so on. Most experts tend to agree that any calorie-cutting diet can produce weight loss in the short-term, often through water-weight loss. But without improved nutrition and sustained exercise and activity, lost weight will return and the overall dieting process will have failed. Let's look more closely at the reasons why.

DIETS OFTEN LEAD TO WEIGHT CYCLING

Nearly three-quarters of dieters regain their weight within 2 years (or sooner) after a major diet. Most begin a process called **weight cycling**—a pattern of repeatedly losing and regaining weight.

Marketers of diet plans and foods often promise quick weight loss with no hunger and very little effort, but these usually backfire. People on rigid diets tend to have higher fat-to-lean ratios than people on more flexible plans based on energy balancing of calories eaten and burned.[35] The followers of rigid diets tend to exhibit more depression, anxiety, and binge eating as well. Taken alone, even prescription diet drugs don't work very well unless the patient also makes long-term changes in diet and exercise that produce a favorable energy balance.[36] Research reveals that four-fifths of dieters fail to both cut calories *and* increase exercise.[37] Three-quarters also eat too few fruits and vegetables despite their appetite-satisfying volume.

Rigid and flexible diets are distinctly different. **Rigid diets** specify rules like "eat only 1,200 Calories per day," or "eat only cabbage soup and grapefruit," or "never eat after 6:00 PM." Because

weight cycling The pattern of repeatedly losing and gaining weight, from illness or dieting

rigid diets Weight-loss regimens that specify strict rules on calorie consumption, types of foods, and eating patterns

rigid diets are unpleasant and restrictive, people seldom stick with them. **Flexible diets** focus on portion size and make allowances for variations in daily routine, appetite, and food availability. For example, if you go to a party and overeat, a flexible diet allows you to cut extra calories tomorrow and increase your exercise regimen to compensate. As a result, people tend to stay on flexible diets longer and in the process, learn better long-term eating habits.

Weight experts refer to a series of diets, each followed by eventual weight gain, as **yo-yo dieting.** Yo-yo dieting can have significant health consequences. As a person regains lost body fat and weight, blood lipids, blood pressure, and diabetes risk rise once again, and with them, the risk of heart disease and other serious illnesses.[38]

MANY DIET PRODUCTS AND PLANS ARE INEFFECTIVE

Dieting is a $30 billion annual industry. Most of the over-the-counter products—"fat burners," "starch blockers," muscle stimulators, diet supplements, weight-loss program memberships, meal replacements, and other diet aids—are ineffective, and some are even dangerous. For example, in 2004, the U.S. Food and Drug Administration banned the popular supplement ephedra (also called *ma huang*) after it caused heart attacks, seizures, and strokes in over 16,000 people and precipitated more than 100 deaths.

What about commercial diet plans and programs? One comprehensive study revealed that most of the best-known diet programs are only minimally effective. A 2005 study revealed that none of the nationally known programs—Weight Watchers, Jenny Craig, Optifast, eDiets.com, and Overeaters Anonymous—really deliver.[39] After 2 years, people who joined Weight Watchers had lost an average of just 6.4 pounds. Nearly half of those who took Optifast dropped out within 6 months, and those who continued did no better than people dieting at home on their own. Those on eDiets.com lost only about 1 percent of their body weight after a year.

Of the many consumer diet products and approaches, low-cost support groups are probably the best alternative for most people and do succeed in providing one very important component of every diet: encouragement and support, either in person, through weekly groups, or online. Campus health centers can usually help students find group support for dieting. It's also important to enlist the personal encouragement of friends, roommates, and family members. If people try tempting you with fattening foods or undermine your diet efforts in other ways, tell them firmly that you need a different approach.

CASE STUDY

Maria

"I joined a campus weight management group that emphasizes portion control and nutrition instead of special diet foods and calorie counting. They also have organized activities that promote fitness for the whole family. I'm excited about their approach, because I can still eat what my family eats—though we're all going to try eating less pizza! Mainly, I am going to pay more attention to monitoring how *much* I eat. The group is helping me with ideas for bringing more fruits and vegetables into our daily meals. And they have a weekend family bike ride coming up that sounds really fun. If I can stick with this, it will help not only me, but Tim and Anna, too."

1. **How does Maria's new weight management program differ from other approaches she has tried in the past?**
2. **What successful strategies can you identify in Maria's new approach? How will they help her achieve an appropriate energy balance?**
3. **Knowing what you know now about basal metabolic rate, calories, and energy balance, what strategies should you use to achieve or maintain a healthy weight?**

WHAT ARE EATING DISORDERS?

Skipping meals, going on diet after diet, and binging on junk food are all forms of **disordered eating:** atypical, abnormal food consumption that is very common in the general public and diminishes your wellness but is usually neither long-lived nor

flexible diets Weight-loss regimens that focus on portion size and make allowances for variations in daily routine, appetite, and food availability

yo-yo dieting A series of diets followed by eventual weight gain. Yo-yo dieting can lead to weight cycling.

disordered eating Atypical, abnormal food consumption that diminishes your wellness but is usually neither long-lived nor disruptive to everyday life

Eating disordered	Disruptive eating patterns	Food preoccupied/ obsessed	Concerned well	Food is not an issue
• I regularly stuff myself and then exercise, vomit, use diet pills or laxatives to get rid of the food or calories. • My friends/family tell me I am too thin. • I am terrified of eating fat. • When I let myself eat, I have a hard time controlling the amount of food I eat. • I am afraid to eat in front of others.	• I have tried diet pills, laxatives, vomiting or extra time exercising in order to lose or maintain my weight. • I have fasted or avoided eating for long periods of time in order to lose or maintain my weight. • I feel strong when I can restrict how much I eat. • Eating more than I wanted to makes me feel out of control.	• I think about food a lot. • I feel I don't eat well most of the time. • It's hard for me to enjoy eating with others. • I feel ashamed when I eat more than others or more than what I feel I should be eating. • I am afraid of getting fat. • I wish I could change how much I want to eat and what I am hungry for.	• I pay attention to what I eat in order to maintain a healthy body. • I may weigh more than what I like, but I enjoy eating and balance my pleasure with eating with my concern for a healthy body. • I am moderate and flexible in goals for eating well. • I try to follow Dietary Guidelines for healthy eating.	• I am not concerned about what others think regarding what and how much I eat. • When I am upset or depressed I eat whatever I am hungry for without any guilt or shame. • Food is an important part of my life but only occupies a small part of my time.

Body hate/ dissociation	Distorted body image	Body preoccupied/ obsessed	Body Acceptance	Body ownership
• I often feel separated and distant from my body—as if it belongs to someone else. • I don't see anything positive or even neutral about my body shape and size. • I don't believe others when they tell me I look OK. • I hate the way I look in the mirror and often isolate myself from others.	• I spend a significant amount of time exercising and dieting to change my body. • My body shape and size keeps me from dating or finding someone who will treat me the way I want to be treated. • I have considered changing or have changed my body shape and size through surgical means so I can accept myself.	• I spend a significant time viewing my body in the mirror. • I spend a significant time comparing my body to others. • I have days when I feel fat. • I am preoccupied with my body. • I accept society's ideal body shape and size as the best body shape and size.	• I base my body image equally on social norms and my own self-concept. • I pay attention to my body and my appearance because it is important to me, but it only occupies a small part of my day. • I nourish my body so it has the strength and energy to achieve my physical goals.	• My body is beautiful to me. • My feelings about my body are not influenced by society's concept of an ideal body shape. • I know that the significant others in my life will always find me attractive.

FIGURE 5

The continuums of thought associated with healthy eating and positive body image to thoughts associated with disordered eating and poor body image. Adapted from Smiley/King/Avery: Campus Health Service. Original continuum, C. Schislak: *Preventive Medicine and Public Health.* Copyright 1997 Arizona Board of Regents. Used with permission.

disruptive to everyday life. Less common but still disturbingly prevalent are **eating disorders,** which are long-lasting, disturbed patterns of eating, dieting, and perceptions of body image that have psychological, environmental, and possibly genetic underpinnings. Eating disorders can disrupt relationships, emotions, and concentration, and can lead to physical injury, hospitalization, and even death. They require diagnosis and treatment from a psychiatrist or other physician.

Recognizing an eating disorder in yourself or a loved one can lead to treatment that improves or stops the spiral. The statements in Figure 5 can help you recognize when thoughts about food and body image verge from normal to abnormal and disordered. People with eating disorders often believe they look fat even when they are rail thin. This unrealistic and negative self-perception can be part of a

eating disorders Disturbed patterns of eating, dieting, and perceptions of body image that have psychological, environmental, and possibly genetic underpinnings, and that lead to consequent medical issues

related syndrome called **body dysmorphic disorder** (BDD), in which a person becomes obsessed with a physical "defect" such as nose size or body shape. It often requires a professional to sort out the symptoms of an eating disorder from BDD since a person can have either or both conditions.

The three common types of eating disorders are anorexia nervosa, bulimia nervosa, and binge eating disorder. About 10 million Americans—9 million of whom are young women—meet the criteria for one of these disorders.[40]

EATING DISORDERS HAVE DISTINCTIVE SYMPTOMS

Anorexia nervosa is a persistent, chronic eating disorder characterized by deliberate food restriction and severe, life-threatening weight loss. People with anorexia first restrict their intake of high-calorie foods, then of almost all foods and purge what they do eat through vomiting or using laxatives. They sometimes fast or exercise compulsively as well. The symptoms of anorexia include refusal to maintain a BMI of 18.5 or more; intense fear of gaining weight; disturbed body perception; and in teenage girls and women, amenorrhea (cessation of menstruation) for 3 months or more. Five to 20 percent of anorexics eventually die from medical conditions brought on by vitamin or mineral deficiencies or physiological results of starvation.

Bulimia nervosa is characterized by frequent bouts of binge eating, followed by purging (self-induced vomiting), laxative abuse, or excessive exercise. Bulimics tend to consume much more food than most people would during a given time period and feel a loss of control over it. Binging and purging are often done secretly. A medical diagnosis includes binging and purging at least twice a week for 3 months. People with bulimia are also obsessed with their bodies, weight gain, and how they appear to others. Unlike those with anorexia, however, people with bulimia are often normal weight. Also, treatment appears to be more effective for bulimia than for anorexia.

Binge eating disorder (BED), a variation of bulimia, involves binge eating but usually no purging, laxatives, exercise, or fasting. Individuals with BED often wind up significantly overweight or obese but tend to binge much more often than does the typical obese person.

EATING DISORDERS CAN BE TREATED

Because eating disorders have complex physical, psychological, and social causes that unfold over many years, there are no quick or simple solutions for them. That said, eating disorders *are* treatable. The primary goal of treatment is usually to reduce the threat to the patient's life posed by his or her eating behaviors and the physical damage they can cause to the bones, teeth, throat, esophagus, stomach, intestines, heart, and other organs. Once the patient is stabilized medically, long-term therapy can begin. Oftentimes, the affected individual comes from a family that places undue emphasis on achievement, body weight, and appearance. Genetic susceptibility can also play a role.[41] Therapy involves family, friends, and other significant people in the individual's life and focuses on the psychological, social, environmental, and physiological factors that have contributed. Therapy is aimed at helping

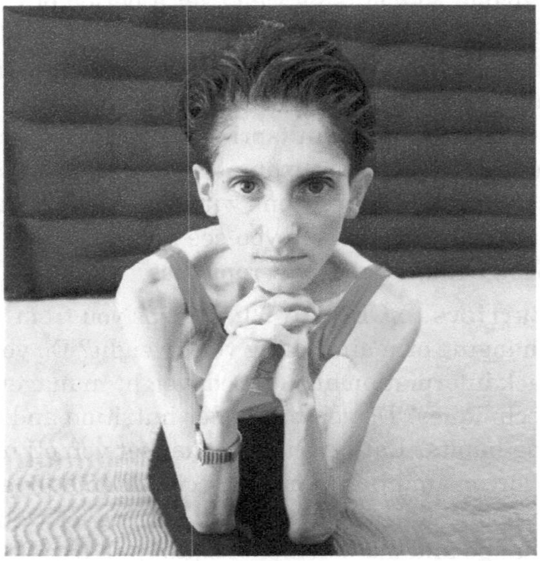

Express Newspapers/Liaison/Getty Images

body dysmorphic disorder A psychological syndrome characterized by unrealistic and negative self-perception focusing on a physical defect such as nose size

anorexia nervosa A persistent, chronic eating disorder characterized by deliberate food restriction and severe, life-threatening weight loss

bulimia nervosa An eating disorder characterized by frequent bouts of binge eating followed by purging (self-induced vomiting), laxative abuse, or excessive exercise

binge eating disorder A variation of bulimia that involves binge eating but usually no purging, laxatives, exercise, or fasting

the patient develop new eating behaviors, build self-confidence, deal with depression, and find constructive ways of dealing with life's problems. Eating disorder support groups can be pivotal as well.

HOW CAN YOU CREATE A BEHAVIOR CHANGE PLAN FOR WEIGHT MANAGEMENT?

Let's look at the kinds of attitudes, decisions, and activities you can apply to creating a behavioral change plan for weight management.

CONTEMPLATE WEIGHT MANAGEMENT

The tools and tips in this chapter are designed for direct application in a personal plan. If you are part of the minority of students who are satisfied with your current weight, you can simply pursue and refine your application of good nutritional principles and regular exercise. If you are in the dissatisfied majority, you will need to assess your current weight and BMI using Figure 1 to determine whether you truly need to lose or gain weight. You will also need to choose a realistic weight goal based on no more than a 10 percent initial loss or gain. Even if you don't need weight change now, keep in mind that most normal-weight students will become overweight during the postcollege years. The specifics in this section are useful for weight change now or in the future, as well as for stabilizing your current weight and maintaining it for the next few decades.

PREPARE FOR BETTER WEIGHT MANAGEMENT

The steps of the behavioral change model we've discussed in every chapter apply equally well to weight change and weight management.

- **Beliefs and Attitudes** The concepts of self-efficacy and locus of control are central to successful weight management. Do you see yourself as a hopeless victim of "bad genes," overwork, and low budget, or perhaps as too young to worry about nutrition, exercise programs, or deliberate weight management? Or do you believe that you can take effective control of your body composition and weight largely through eating intelligently, limiting your calorie intake, and establishing a program of regular exercise? Talk with others to clarify your own attitudes in preparation for making an effective weight management plan.
- **Consider Your Motivations** What is motivating you to change or maintain your weight? The best motivations are usually personal and extended, such as looking good, feeling fit and capable, and staying well over a period of years. People sometimes have very short-term goals that can lead to little more than weight cycling and yo-yo dieting. If one of your reasons is a specific upcoming event (spring break in Florida or a sports match, for example) try identifying some additional reasons with long time frames. Long-term goals help you see beyond poorly designed quick-fix diet remedies.
- **Barriers to Change** What keeps you from changing or maintaining your weight? Do you lack information about good weight management techniques? Do you have poor nutrition and eating habits? Eating triggers that set you off into overconsumption? Lack of social or emotional support? Lack of exercise? Preparing for weight change and management requires that you

CASE STUDY

Maria

"I've never had an eating disorder, but I admit that at times, I've been desperate enough to be tempted to binge and purge. There's so much pressure from all sides. You go to a family party and everyone tells you to eat, eat, eat. At the same time, all you see on TV are super-thin people. How can you please everyone—and yourself?

"Meanwhile, my daughter, Anna, is still very young, but I worry about the pressures she'll feel when she gets older. I hear so many stories about adolescents and high school students with eating disorders. Although I want to lose weight, I don't want Anna to get the message that being thin matters above everything else. There's a big difference between wanting to lose excess weight to become healthier, and feeling a need to lose weight when you are already at a healthy weight."

1. **What signs of eating disorders or disordered eating should Maria watch for as Anna gets older?**
2. **If you recognize symptoms of an eating disorder in yourself or a friend, how should you address the problem?**

identify your own particular barriers and brainstorm solutions to them.

- **Visualizing New Behaviors** What specific new behaviors can you adopt that will allow you to change your BMI and body composition to within the recommended ranges? Here are some positive ones:

  Choosing only nutritious foods

  Avoiding foods filled with saturated fats, sweeteners, or sodium

  Tracking the numbers of servings you eat from each food group

  Tracking the calories you consume

  Planning for exercise most days of the week

  Keeping a log of your daily and weekly exercise

  Asking friends for support

  From this list, target one or a few behaviors, concentrate on them first, then move on to other behaviors later. Make a short priority list of the two or three most important behaviors.

- **Write Out Your Specific Goals** Lab 3 provides spaces for recording your body fat and body weight goals and the time frame for reaching them.
- **Commit to Your Goals** Behavior change requires commitment. Thinking and talking about your commitment with friends is helpful; so is writing it down and showing it to someone.
- **Set up Support** Solicit the help of people you can trust to support your efforts. Let's say it is 9:30 PM, you've finished studying, you're hungry, but you've already eaten the 1,800 calories on your day's food plan. You call a supportive friend and he or she might say, "Well, you can always have a diet soda and some raw vegetables to fill up. You'll be glad you stuck with your program. Just think, once you've lost weight, you can add back some extra calories each day—and that won't be so long from now!"

> ***Try it NOW!*** **Healthy substitutions at mealtime are the key to weight maintenance success! The next time you make dinner, look at the proportions on your plate. • Veggies and whole grains should take up most of the space; if not, substitute 1 cup of the meat, pasta, or cheese on your plate with 1 cup of legumes, salad greens, or a favorite vegetable. • You'll reduce the number of calories in your meal while eating the same amount of food!**

TAKE ACTION

Now that you have calculated your target weight and goals for daily calorie consumption and energy expenditure, set your plan in motion and keep track of the results. The box **Tools for Change: Tips for Weight Loss** provides some tips.

ACHIEVE WEIGHT MAINTENANCE

Weight management and weight change are very similar in principle. The tools are the same; your daily calorie goal for weight management will simply be isocaloric while your daily goal for weight loss or gain will have a negative or positive caloric balance. Some degree of calorie-tracking is usually involved in both maintenance and change, and a weekly weigh-in is important. If you have lost or gained 10 percent of your body weight, you will need to maintain that level for a few months before resuming more weight change. The skills you employ during an interim phase of weight maintenance will be excellent practice for the indefinite postchange period: translation, for the rest of your life. Once weight management skills become second nature and you've mastered good nutrition and daily exercise and activity, both change and maintenance become relatively easy for most people.

As for the termination stage, there *is* none for weight management. Maintaining recommended weight and BMI confer so many benefits upon your appearance, energy level, and overall wellness that once you master the needed skill set, you'll rarely miss the junk food you used to eat, nor will you miss the few minutes it will take each day to track energy consumed and expended. The rewards in lifelong wellness are fully worth the trade-off!

TOOLS FOR CHANGE

TIPS FOR WEIGHT LOSS

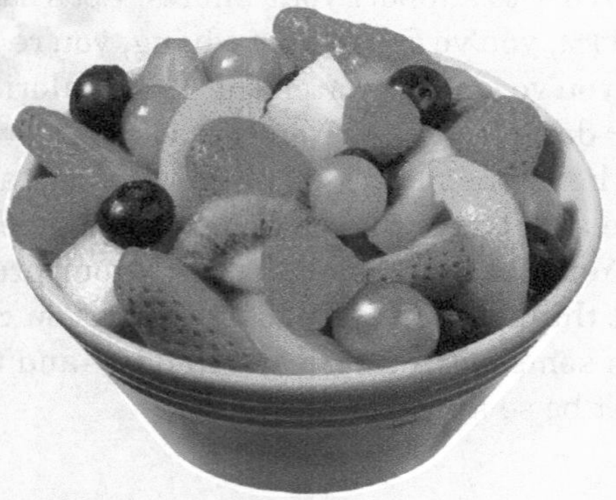

Burke/Triolo Productions/Foodpix/Jupiter Images.

Try these ideas for reframing weight loss in your mind, rather than jumping right in to a diet regimen unprepared:

- Think substitution. Instead of cookies, pie, candy, cake, or ice cream at snack time, substitute fresh fruit. Instead of tortilla chips or French fries, substitute unbuttered popcorn, nuts, or vegetable sticks and low-fat dip.
- Consider yourself successful if you lose 1/2 to 1 pound per week. Faster weight loss stimulates too much hunger, slows metabolism, and loses lean tissue.
- Avoid feeling famished by choosing high-volume, nutrient-dense foods. Items such as clear soups, light salads, whole grains, fruits, vegetables, and beans fill you more quickly and control hunger, at least for a while.
- Avoid rigid dieting. Strictly limiting calorie counts or forbidding yourself certain foods can trigger binging and weight gain, not loss. Flexible dieting works better and emphasizes portion control and lower-calorie, higher-volume foods.
- Don't drink "empty" calories. Drinks sweetened with sugar or corn syrup contribute disproportionately to weight gain.[1] Alcoholic drinks pack a lot of calories and stimulate the appetite.
- Sleep well. Get 7 to 9 hours of sleep each night. Sleep deprivation triggers greater levels of hunger and eating.
- Join a support group. Support groups help most people lose at least a small amount of weight and keep it off.[2]

Sources:

1. G. A. Bray, S. J. Nielsen, and B. M. Popkin, "Consumption of High-Fructose Corn Syrup in Beverages May Play a Role in the Epidemic of Obesity," *American Journal of Clinical Nutrition* 79, no. 4 (April 2004): 537–43.
2. A. G. Tsai and T. A. Wadden, "Systematic Review: An Evaluation of Major Commercial Weight Loss Programs in the United States," *Annals of Internal Medicine* 142, no. 1 (January 2005): 56–66.

CHAPTER IN REVIEW

REVIEW QUESTIONS

1. At more than 20 percent above the recommended weight range for 5′8″ tall, a person is
   a. overweight.
   b. obese.
   c. ideal weight.
   d. at his/her set point.
2. A BMI of 16 in a woman indicates
   a. overweight.
   b. underweight.
   c. normal weight.
   d. obesity.
3. Getting up, walking around, and jiggling your feet when seated are all examples of
   a. energy conservation.
   b. appetite control.
   c. non-exercise activity.
   d. depression.
4. To lose weight, you must establish a(n)
   a. negative caloric balance.
   b. isocaloric balance.
   c. positive caloric balance.
   d. set point.
5. Which of these is not considered an eating disorder?
   a. Anorexia nervosa
   b. Bulimia nervosa
   c. Amenorrhea
   d. Binge eating disorder
6. Metabolic syndrome is characterized by all of the following except
   a. high blood cholesterol.
   b. high blood pressure.
   c. insulin resistance.
   d. small waist circumference.

7. The rate at which your body consumes food energy to sustain basic functions is your
   a. basal metabolic rate.
   b. resting metabolic rate.
   c. BMI.
   d. set point.
8. Successful weight maintainers are most likely to do which of the following?
   a. Indulge in junk food on weekends
   b. Skip meals
   c. Drink diet sodas
   d. Eat a nutritious diet that is low in fats, with high volume but low calorie density
9. Weight cycling is
   a. a pattern of repeatedly losing and regaining weight.
   b. characterized by rigid diets.
   c. characterized by flexible diets.
   d. uncommon.
10. Anorexia nervosa is characterized by
    a. frequent bouts of binge eating followed by self-induced vomiting.
    b. deliberate food restriction and severe, life-threatening weight loss.
    c. the use of laxatives.
    d. obesity.

CRITICAL THINKING QUESTIONS

1. How do height, physical build, and musculature affect recommended weight and BMI?
2. Discuss the chronic disease risks of obesity.
3. What do you see as the greatest contributor to "globesity"? Defend your answer.

ONLINE RESOURCES

Please visit this book's website at **www.aw-bc.com/hopson** to access links related to topics in this chapter.

REFERENCES

1. American College Health Association, "National College Health Assessment. Reference Group Executive Summary Fall 2006" (Baltimore: American College Health Association, 2007).
2. Charlotte A. Schoenborn and others, "Body Weight Status of Adults: United States, 1997–1998." Advance Data from *Vital and Health Statistics* no. 330 (September. 6, 2002).
3. University of Minnesota, Boynton Health Service, "First Ever Comprehensive Report on the Health of Minnesota College Students Looks at Mental Health, Obesity, Financial Health, Sexual Health and More," November 15, 2007.
4. University of New Hampshire, "College Students Face Obesity, High Blood Pressure, Metabolic Syndrome." *ScienceDaily* (June 18, 2007), www.sciencedaily.com.
5. See note 1.
6. World Health Organization, "Obesity and Overweight Factsheet," September 2006.
7. International Union of Nutritional Sciences, "The Global Challenge of Obesity and the International Obesity Task Force," September 2002, www.iuns.org/features/obesity/obesity.htm (accessed August 12, 2007).
8. "Preventing Childhood Obesity: Health in the Balance," Institute of Medicine, National Academies of Science, Washington, D.C., 2005.
9. Erica Goode, "The Gorge Yourself Environment," *New York Times* (July 3, 2003): D1.
10. B. Wamsink, J. E. Painter, and J. North, "Bottomless Bowls: Why Visual Cues of Portion Size May Influence Intake," *Obesity Research* 13, no. 1 (January 2005): 93–100.
11. G. Wamsink, "Environmental Factors that Increase the Food Intake and Consumption Volume of Unknowing Customers," *Annual Review of Nutrition* 24 (2004): 455–79.
12. G. Block and others, "Foods Contributing to Energy Intake in the U.S.: Data from NHANES III and NHANES 1999–2000," *Journal of Food Chemistry and Analysis* 17 (June 2004): 439–47.
13. S. A. French, "Public Health Strategies for Dietary Change: Schools and Workplaces," *Journal of Nutrition* 135, no. 4 (April 2005): 91–92.
14. M. Papas and others, "The Built Environment and Obesity," *Epidemiological Reviews* 29, no. 1 (2007): 129–43. Also M. Rao and others, "The Built Environment and Health," *The Lancet* 370, no, 9593 (2007): 1111–13; and E. M. Berke and others, "Association of the Built Environment with Physical Activity and Obesity in Older Persons," *American Journal of Public Health* (2007).
15. I. S. Farooqi and S. O'Rahilly, "Genetic Factors in Human Obesity," *Obesity Reviews* 8, Suppl 1 (2007): 37–40. Also University of Cambridge, "New Insight into the Link Between Genetics and Obesity," *Science Daily,* www.sciencedaily.com.

16. James A. Levine and others, "Interindividual Variation in Posture Allocation: Possible Role in Human Obesity," *Science* 307, no. 4 (January 28, 2005): 584–86.

17. Centers for Disease Control and Prevention: U.S. Physical Activity Statistics, "1988–2005 No Leisure-Time Physical Activity Trend Chart," www.cdc.gov/nccdphp/dnpa/physical/stats/leisure_time.htm (accessed August 12, 2007).

18. Walter Willett, *Eat, Drink, and Be Healthy: The Harvard Medical School Guide to Healthy Eating* (New York: Free Press, 2003), 35.

19. American Heart Association, "Abdominal Fat Distribution Predicts Heart Disease, Study Shows," *ScienceDaily* (December 11, 2007), www.sciencedaily.com.

20. Charles Mann, "Provocative Study Says Obesity May Reduce U.S. Life Expectancy," *Science* 307 (March 18, 2005): 1717.

21. S. J. Olshansky and others, "A Potential Decline in Life Expectancy in the United States in the 21st Century," *New England Journal of Medicine* 352, no. 11 (March 17, 2005): 1135–37.

22. Katherine Flegal and others, "Excess Deaths Associated with Underweight, Overweight, and Obesity," *Journal of the American Medical Association* 293, no. 15 (April 20, 2005) 1861–67.

23. Y. Takata and others, "Association Between Body Mass Index and Mortality in an 80-Year-Old Population," *Journal of the American Geriatric Society* 55, no. 6 (2007): 913–17.

24. Luigi Fontana and others, "Long-Term Calorie Restriction Is Highly Effective in Reducing the Risk for Atherosclerosis in Humans," Proceedings of the National Academy of Sciences, 101, no. 17 (April 27, 2004): 6659–63.

25. Carol O'Neil and Theresa Nicklas, "State of the Art Reviews: Relationship Between Diet/Physical Activity and Health," *American Journal of Lifestyle Medicine,* Vol.1 (December 2007): 457–81.

26. Eugenia Calle and others, "Overweight, Obesity, and Mortality from Cancer in a Prospectively Studied Cohort of U.S. Adults," *New England Journal of Medicine* 348 (April 24, 2003): 1625–38.

27. Stuart P. Weisberg, "Obesity Is Associated with Macrophage Accumulation in Adipose Tissue," *Journal of Clinical Investigation* 112 (2003): 1796–1808.

28. USDA, "Popular Weight Loss Diets," U.S. Department of Agriculture White Paper (January 10, 2001).

29. Mayo Clinic, "Lose a Little: It Helps a Lot," Mayo Clinic, Consumer Health Tips and Products (January 6, 2005). www.mayoclinic.org.

30. M. A. Pelleymounter and others, "Effects of the Obese Gene Product on Body Weight Regulation in Ob/Ob Mice," *Science* 269, no. 5223 (July 28, 1995): 540–43.

31. P. A. Mole, "Exercise Reverses Depressed Metabolic Rate Produced by Severe Caloric Restriction," *Medical Science and Sports Exercise* 21, no. 1 (February 1989): 29–33. Also P. A. Mole, "Impact of Energy Intake and Exercise on Resting Metabolic Rate," *Sports Medicine* 10, no. 2 (August 1991): 72–87.

32. R. R. Wing and S. Phelan, "Long-Term Weight Loss Maintenance," *American Journal of Clinical Nutrition* 82, no. 1 (July 2005): 222S–25S.

33. K. Elfhag and S. Rossner, "Who Succeeds in Maintaining Weight Loss?" *Obesity Review* 6, no. 1 (February 2005): 67–85.

34. Ibid.

35. C. F. Smith and others, "Flexible versus Rigid Dieting Strategies: Relationship with Adverse Behavioral Outcomes," *Appetite* 32, no. 3 (June 1999): 295–305.

36. S. B. Moyers, "Medications as Adjunct Therapy for Weight Loss: Approved and Off-label Agents in Use," *Journal of the American Dietetic Association,* 105, no. 6 (June 2005): 948–59.

37. J. Kruger and others, "Weight Specific Practices Among U.S. Adults," *American Journal of Preventative Medicine* 26, no. 5 (June 2004): 402–6. Also J. Kruger and others, "Attempting to Lose Weight: Specific Practices Among U.S. Adults," *American Journal of Preventative Medicine* 26, no. 5 (January 2004): 402–6.

38. M. Schulz and others, "Weight Cycling and Hypertension," *Current Hypertension Reports* 7 (2005): 9–10.

39. A. Tsai and T. Wadden, "Systematic Review: An Evaluation of Major Commercial Weight Loss Programs in the U.S.," *Annals of Internal Medicine* 142, no. 1 (January 4, 2005): 56–66.

40. Sutter Health, "Eating Disorders," April 1, 2003.

41. R. Bachner-Melman and others, "Association Between a Vasopressin Receptor AVPR1A Promoter Region Microsatellite and Eating Behavior Measured by a Self-Report Questionnaire (Eating Attitudes Test) in a Family-Based Study of a Non-Clinical Population," *International Journal of Eating Disorders* 36, no. 4 (December 2004): 451–60.

ANSWERS TO END-OF-CHAPTER QUESTIONS

1.a; 2.b; 3.c; 4.a; 5.c; 6.d; 7.a; 8.d.; 9.a; 10.b

Comstock Images/Jupiter Images

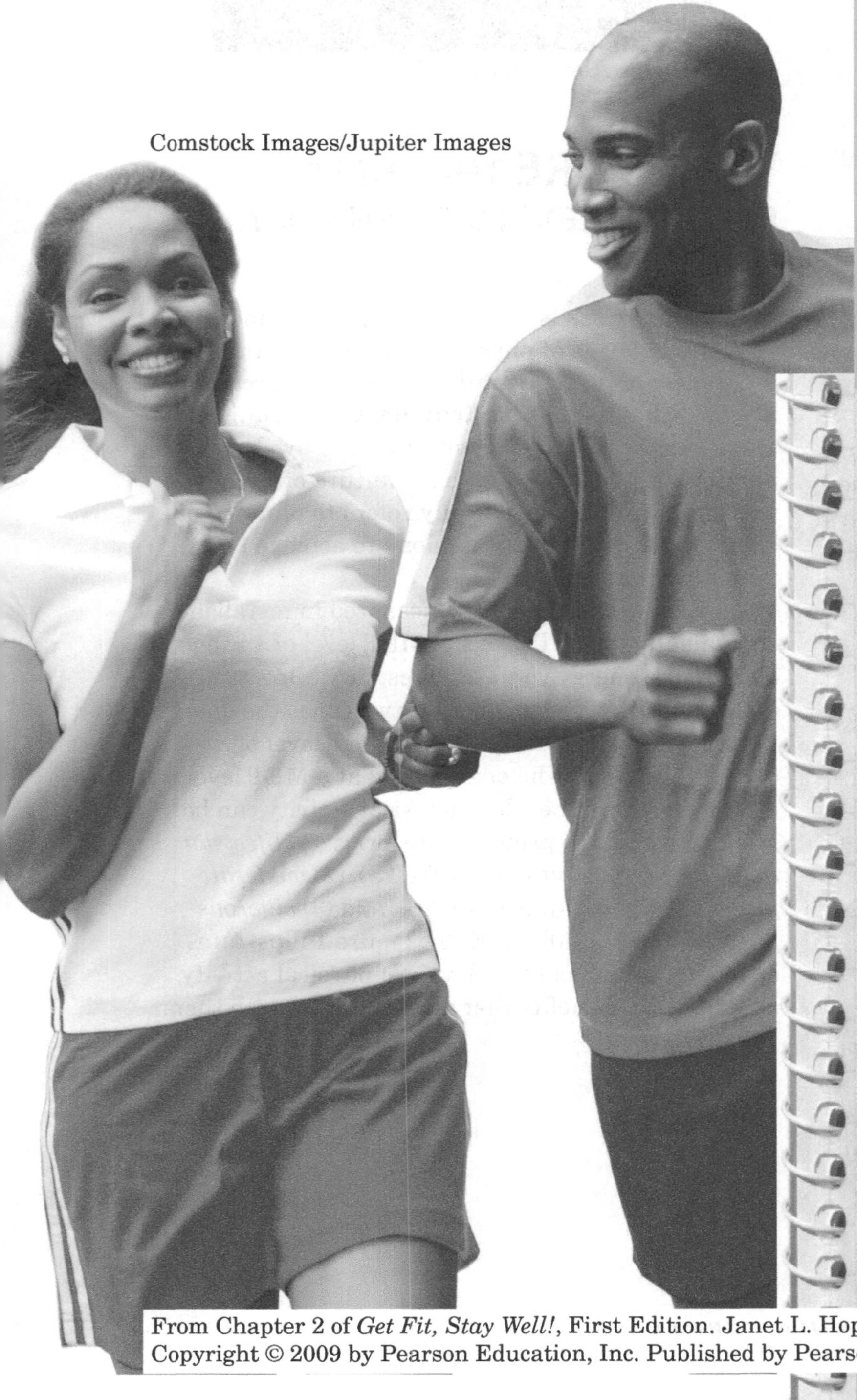

Understanding Fitness Principles

OBJECTIVES

Identify the three primary levels of physical activity and describe the benefits of each.

Describe the five health-related components of fitness.

Identify the six skill-related components of fitness.

Explain the principles of overload, progression, specificity, reversibility, individuality, and recovery.

Describe how much physical activity is recommended for optimal health and wellness.

Describe general strategies for exercising safely.

Identify individual attributes that should be taken into account before beginning a fitness program.

Discuss strategies for beginning to design your own individualized fitness program.

From Chapter 2 of *Get Fit, Stay Well!*, First Edition. Janet L. Hopson, Rebecca J. Donatelle, Tanya R. Littrell.

CASE STUDY

Lily

"Hi, I'm Lily. I just started my junior year, and after a summer of lazing around, I want to get back into shape. I'm ready to put some serious time and energy into it, but the last time I started exercising, I tried to do too much and ended up getting injured. How do I keep from doing the same thing this time? How much exercise do I really need? And what does it actually mean to be fit, anyway—does it just mean being able to run a certain distance, or is there more to it than that?"

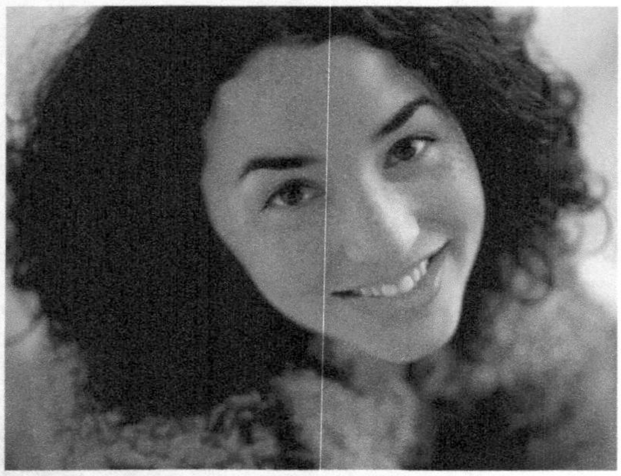

Photodisc/Getty Images

Fitness is a critical component of overall wellness. The benefits of physical fitness are almost too numerous to list. Being physically fit can improve your mood, give you more energy for daily activities, help you maintain a healthy weight, and lessen your risk of developing chronic diseases. All of these benefits can, in turn, help you live a longer, healthier life.

In this chapter, we will cover the basic principles of fitness, address the question of how much exercise you need, introduce general guidelines for exercising safely, and discuss individual factors that should be taken into account when you design a personal fitness program.

physical fitness A set of attributes that relate to one's ability to perform moderate to vigorous levels of physical activity without undue fatigue

physical activity Any bodily movement produced by skeletal muscles that results in an expenditure of energy

exercise Physical activity that is planned or structured and involves repetitive bodily movement, done to improve or maintain one or more of the components of fitness

MET The standard metabolic equivalent used to estimate the amount of energy (oxygen) used by the body during physical activity; 1 MET = resting or sitting quietly

WHAT ARE THE THREE PRIMARY LEVELS OF PHYSICAL ACTIVITY?

Physical fitness is the ability to perform moderate to vigorous levels of physical activity without undue fatigue. Note that *physical activity* and *exercise* are not the same thing: **physical activity** technically means any bodily movement produced by skeletal muscles that results in an expenditure of energy, whereas **exercise** specifically refers to planned or structured physical activity done to achieve and maintain fitness.

Physical activity is often measured in metabolic equivalents, or **MET** levels. A MET level of 1 is equivalent to the energy you use at rest or while sitting quietly. A MET level of 2 equals two times the energy used at a MET level of 1, while a MET level of 3 equals three times the energy used at a MET level of 1, and so forth. Levels of physical activity can be grouped into three primary categories: (1) *lifestyle/light physical activities* (< 3 METS), (2) *moderate physical activities* (3 to 6 METS), and (3) *vigorous physical activities* (6+ METS). Figure 1 illustrates examples of each of these levels of physical activity, as well as the benefits that are associated with them.

Lifestyle/ Light Physical Activities (< 3 METS)

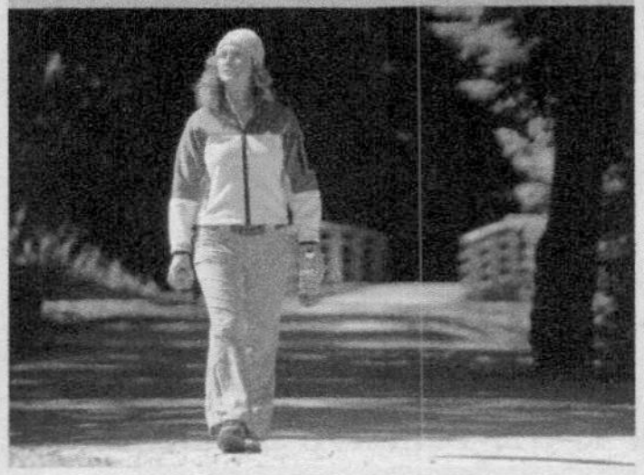

Richard Smith/Masterfile

Examples:

Light yard work and housework, leisurely walking, self-care and bathing, light stretching, light occupational activity

Benefits:

A moderate increase in health and wellness in those who are completely sedentary; reduced risk of some chronic diseases

Moderate Physical Activities (3–6 METS)

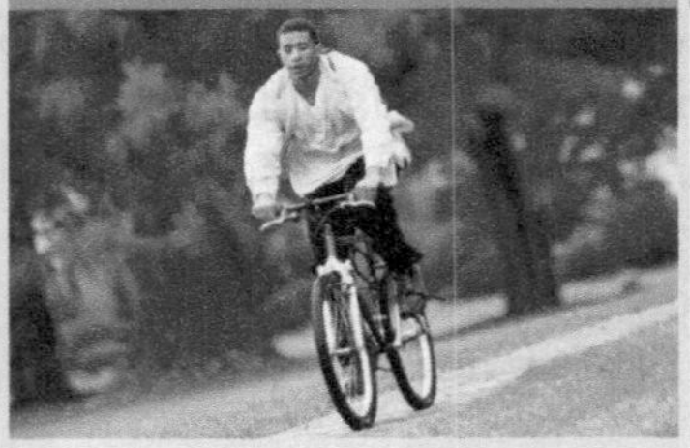

Doug Menuez/Getty Images

Examples:

Walking 3–4.5 mph on a level surface, weight training, hiking, climbing stairs, bicycling 5–9 mph on a level surface, dancing, softball, recreational swimming, moderate yard work and housework

Benefits:

Increased cardiorespiratory endurance, lower body fat levels, improved blood cholesterol and pressure, better blood glucose management, decreased risk of disease, increased overall physical fitness

Vigorous Physical Activities (6+ METS)

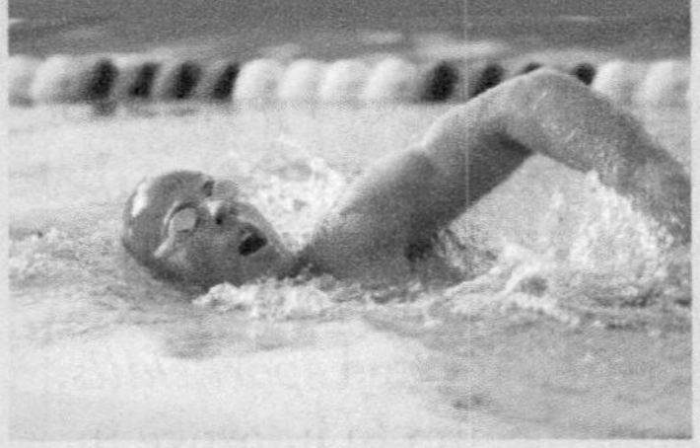

Stockbyte/Getty Images

Examples:

Jogging, running, circuit training, backpacking, aerobic classes, competitive sports, swimming laps, heavy yard work or housework, hard physical labor/ construction, bicycling over 10 mph up steep terrain

Benefits:

Increased overall physical fitness, decreased risk of disease, further improvements in overall strength and endurance

FIGURE 1

Examples and benefits of lifestyle/light physical activity, moderate physical activity, and vigorous physical activity.

WHAT ARE THE HEALTH-RELATED COMPONENTS OF PHYSICAL FITNESS?

The five **health-related components of physical fitness** are *cardiorespiratory endurance, muscular strength, muscular endurance, flexibility,* and *body composition.* Minimal competence in each of these areas is necessary for you to carry out daily activities, lower your risk of developing chronic diseases, and optimize your health and well-being.

CARDIORESPIRATORY ENDURANCE

Cardiorespiratory endurance (also called *cardiovascular fitness/endurance, aerobic fitness,* and *cardiorespiratory fitness*) is the ability of the cardiovascular and respiratory systems to provide oxygen to working muscles during sustained exercise.

health-related components of physical fitness Components of physical fitness that have a relationship with good health

Achieving adequate cardiorespiratory endurance decreases your risk of diabetes, heart disease, obesity, and other chronic diseases.[1] Increased cardiorespiratory endurance also improves your ability to enjoy recreational activities, such as bicycling and hiking, and to participate in them for extended periods of time. Your cardiorespiratory endurance level is determined by measuring your oxygen consumption during exercise, your heart rate response to exercise, and your rate of recovery after exercise.

MUSCULAR STRENGTH

Muscular strength is the ability of your muscles to exert force. You may think of it as your ability to lift a heavy weight. Improved muscular strength decreases your risk of low bone density and musculoskeletal injuries.[2] In order to improve muscular strength, you need to tax your muscles in a controlled setting. This typically involves a weight room, as well as supervision to avoid injury.

MUSCULAR ENDURANCE

Muscular endurance is the ability of your muscles to contract repeatedly over time. Along with cardiorespiratory endurance, muscular endurance allows you to participate in recreational sports without undue fatigue. For example, in order to play a continuous game of basketball, you need to have good cardiorespiratory endurance to move up and down the court for the entire 90 minutes—and you need to have good lower-body muscular endurance to keep guarding, blocking, and shooting the ball effectively. You can improve your muscular endurance with resistance exercises or by participating in certain sports and activities.

FLEXIBILITY

Flexibility is the ability to move your joints in a full range of motion. This component of fitness is often overlooked but is crucial for successful exercise and sports performance. A minimal level of flexibility in your working muscles helps prevent injuries. Maintaining that minimal level also increases your ability to train and work toward specific fitness goals. Having adequate flexibility can be especially important to prevent lower back pain and the decreased range of motion that often occurs with aging.[3]

BODY COMPOSITION

Body composition refers to the relative amounts of fat and lean tissue in your body. Lean tissue consists of muscle, bone, organs, and fluids. A healthy body composition has adequate muscle tissue with moderate to low amounts of fat tissue. The recommendations for fat percentages will vary based upon your gender and age. Increased levels of fat will put you at risk for diabetes, heart disease, and certain cancers. Working toward (and maintaining) a healthy body composition should be one of the cornerstones of all health, fitness, and diet programs.

WHAT ARE THE SKILL-RELATED COMPONENTS OF PHYSICAL FITNESS?

In addition to the five health-related components of fitness, physical fitness also involves attributes that improve your ability to perform athletic and exercise tasks. These attributes are called the **skill-related components of fitness.** Often termed *sport skills,* these are qualities that athletes aim to improve in order to gain a competitive edge. Recreational athletes and general exercisers can also benefit from improving these skills, because doing so can improve their enjoyment of their chosen sports. The six skill-related components of fitness are:

- Agility: The ability to rapidly change the position of your body with speed and accuracy
- Balance: The maintenance of equilibrium while you are stationary or moving
- Coordination: The ability to use both your senses and your body to perform motor tasks smoothly and accurately

skill-related components of fitness Components of physical fitness that have a relationship with enhanced motor skills and performance in sports

- Power: The ability to perform work or contract muscles with high force quickly
- Speed: The ability to perform a movement in a short period of time
- Reaction time: The time between a stimulus and the initiation of your physical reaction to that stimulus

Although skill-related fitness is largely determined by heredity,[4] regular training can result in significant improvements. In order to improve skill-related components of fitness, athletes and exercisers first need to target the skills that will be important to their specific sport or exercise. For instance, a runner can benefit from increasing power for hill running and speed for winning races, whereas a tennis player can benefit from increased agility and reaction time.

Improving your sport skills can be as easy as simply participating regularly in any sport or activity. Playing football will increase reaction time and power, while dancing will increase balance, agility, and coordination. Another way to increase sport skills is to perform drills that mimic a sport-specific skill, or work specifically on any of the skill-related components of fitness. You can practice drills in group exercise classes that incorporate sport skills, or you can work with a personal trainer. Specialized equipment is often used in such drills: for example, exercises utilizing obstacles such as ladders, hurdles, and cones can help you improve your speed, agility, and coordination, while working on balance boards or with exercise balls can help you improve your balance.

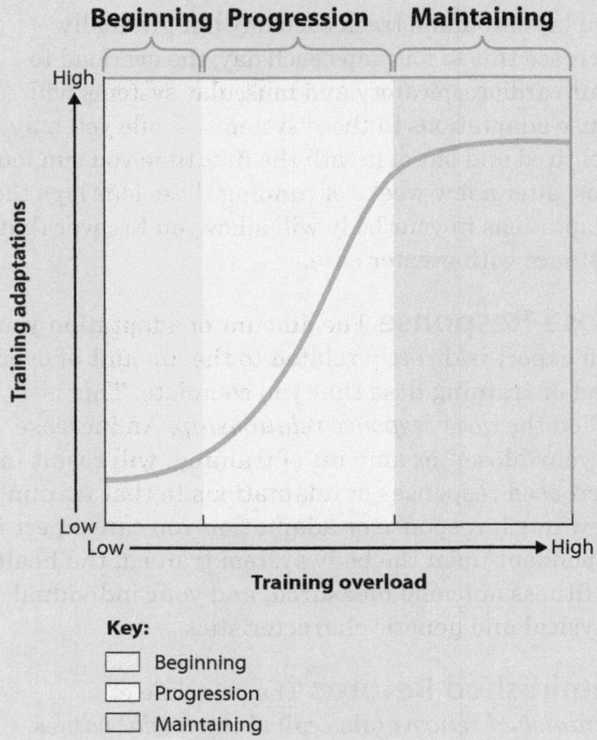

FIGURE 2

After adjusting to new training overloads at the beginning of your exercise program, you will see larger adaptations and improvements during the progression phase. As you approach your goal or genetic limits, your increases in overload will not result in further adaptations. This is a sign that you have reached a plateau and should maintain (if satisfied) or adjust your program for further improvement.

WHAT ARE THE PRINCIPLES OF FITNESS?

In order to design an effective fitness program, you need to take into account the basic **principles of fitness** (also called *principles of exercise training*). These guiding principles explain how the body responds or adapts to exercise training and inform the best methods of training to reach your fitness goals.

OVERLOAD

The principle of **overload** states that in order to see improvements in your physical fitness, the amount or dose of training you undertake must be more than your body or specific body system is used to. This applies to any of the components of physical fitness (health- or skill-related) discussed earlier. For example, in order to increase your flexibility, you must stretch a little farther than you are used to. If you have had the same fitness routine for years, you are *maintaining* your current level of fitness but are probably no longer seeing any improvements. To improve your current level of fitness, you must increase the frequency or intensity of your exercise.

Training Effects Consistent overloads or stresses on a body system will cause an **adaptation** to occur (Figure 2). An adaptation is a change in the body as a result of an overload. In exercise training this is called

principles of fitness General principles of exercise adaptation that guide fitness programming

overload Subjecting the body or body system to more physical activity than it is used to

adaptation A change in a body system as a result of physical training

a **training effect.** For example, if you normally run two laps around a track each day but gradually increase this to four laps each day, the overload to your cardiorespiratory and muscular systems will cause adaptations in those systems. While you may feel tired and out of breath the first time you run four laps, after a few weeks of running those four laps the adaptations in your body will allow you to cover that distance with greater ease.

Dose-Response The amount of adaptation you can expect is directly related to the amount of overload or training dose that you complete. This is called the *dose-response relationship.* An increase in your "dose," or amount of training, will result in increased responses or adaptations to that training. How much response or adaptation you can expect is dependent upon the body system trained, the health or fitness outcome measured, and your individual physical and genetic characteristics.

Diminished Returns The principle of *diminished returns* (also called the *initial values principle*) states that the rate of fitness improvement diminishes over time as fitness levels approach genetic limits. Initial fitness levels determine the amount of improvement that you can achieve from exercise training overloads. If you are sedentary and far from your genetic limits, you might experience large increases in fitness levels from moderate amounts of training. If you are active and closer to your genetic limits already, you may gain only small increases in fitness from larger amounts of training.

Diminished returns in overall health may occur from excessively high levels of physical activity. It is possible to be very fit while not being very healthy! Increasing physical activity only results in greater health gains to a certain point or *threshold.* After that threshold, extremely high levels of activity may actually start to harm you (see Figure 3). So, the goal is to design a fitness program that is vigorous enough to result in health benefits—but not one that is so hard on your body that you end up injuring yourself.

training effect An increase in physical fitness as a result of overload adaptations in body systems

progression A gradual increase in a training program's intensity, frequency, and/or time

specificity The concept that only the body systems worked during training will show adaptations

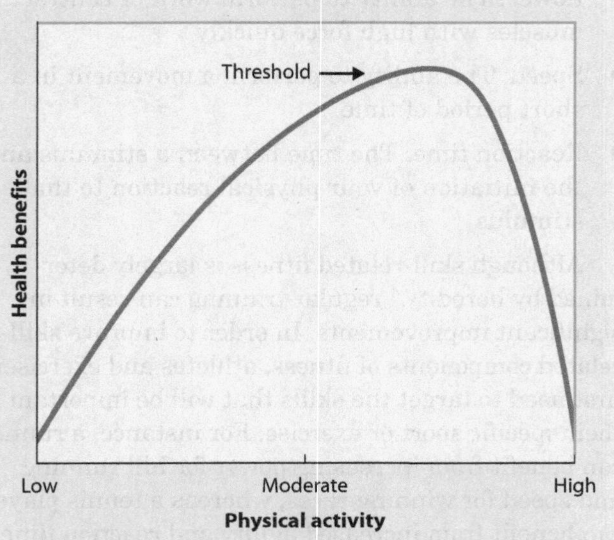

FIGURE 3

Increases in physical activity will result in greater health benefits until a threshold is reached; afterward, higher levels of physical activity will result in fewer overall health benefits.

PROGRESSION

The principle of **progression** states that in order to effectively and safely increase fitness, you need to apply an optimal level of overload to the body within a certain time period. Simply stated, you need to increase your workout levels enough to see results, but not so much that you increase your risk of injury. Your body will then progressively adapt to the overloads presented to it. To make sure that you are not progressing too quickly, follow the "10 percent rule": increase your program frequency, intensity, or duration by no more than 10 percent per week.

SPECIFICITY

The principle of **specificity** states that improvements in a body system will occur only if that specific body system is stressed or progressively overloaded by the physical activity. To follow this principle, make sure that you are training targeted muscle groups specific to your sport or that your program is specifically designed to meet your goals. For instance, if you are planning to walk a marathon, you should primarily *walk* during your training. If, instead, you decide to do lap swimming as your training, you may increase your cardiorespiratory fitness levels, but you will not be specifically training your lower body muscles to walk 26 miles.

REVERSIBILITY

All fitness gains are reversible, according to the principle of **reversibility.** This is the "use it or lose it" principle. If you do not maintain a minimal level of physical activity and exercise, your fitness levels will slip. Unfortunately, you cannot accumulate fitness or workout sessions in a "bank" for later. Doing a great deal of exercise during one week will not compensate for a subsequent month of doing no exercise. Whenever you stop exercising, it only takes about half the time that you spent exercising to lose any fitness gains you may have made while training.[5] For example, if you spent 4 months running 4 miles three times a week, you could lose any fitness gains from those 4 months within 2 months of *no* training.

INDIVIDUALITY

The principle of **individuality** states that adaptations to a training overload may vary greatly from person to person. Two people participate in the same training program but have very different responses. A person who responds well to a training program is considered a *responder.* One who does not respond well is considered a *nonresponder.* Of those individuals who show improvements, some may respond better to increases in total amount of physical activity, while others may show more improvement with increases in exercise intensity.

Genetics greatly influence all individual differences in training adaptations. While you cannot control your genetic makeup, understanding how you respond to exercise is important in designing your personal fitness plan. In most cases, figuring out your individual response to certain exercise programs is a trial-and-error process. By completing regular fitness or performance assessments (and keeping a training log), you can track your individual response and adjust your program accordingly to meet your goals.

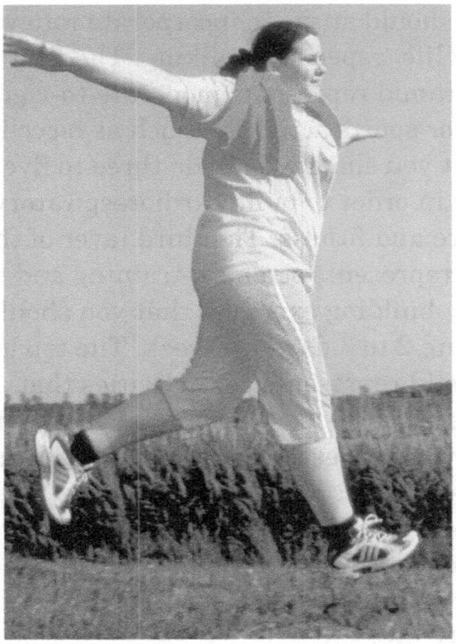

Marija Kasalo/vario images GmbH & Co.KG/Alamy

CASE STUDY

Lily

"The last time I decided to start exercising, I started off slowly, jogging about half an hour twice a week. That went well. Then I got busy with school and stopped jogging for a whole month. To make up for it, I decided to run a 10k. It was a gorgeous day, and there were tons of other people running it. There were kids, and older people, and people who looked way more out of shape than I was—so even though I hadn't trained for it, I thought it'd be no problem. Well, 3 miles into it, my knees started to hurt. The pain came and went, and I managed to finish the race, but my knees hurt for 2 weeks afterward. That was the end of my big exercise plans."

1. **What principles of fitness would you advise Lily to keep in mind before she attempts a new exercise routine? What mistakes did Lily make?**
2. **Think about your own past experiences with exercise. Did you exercise in a way that puts the principles of fitness into practice? If not, how might you adjust your exercise plans?**

REST AND RECOVERY

The principle of rest and recovery (also called the *principle of recuperation*) is critical to ensuring continued progress toward your fitness goals. As you will recall, the overload principle states that you must subject your body to more exercise than it is used to doing. However, your body also needs time to recover from the increased physiological and structural training stresses that you place

reversibility The concept that training adaptations will revert toward initial levels when training is stopped

individuality Refers to the variable nature of physical activity dose-response or adaptations in different persons

TOOLS FOR CHANGE

SIX EASY WAYS TO GET MORE ACTIVE

You can improve your fitness level simply by adding more physical activity to your daily life. Below are a few ways you can incorporate more physical activity into your daily life:

- Instead of driving your car to campus, ride your bike or walk.
- If you must drive to campus, park your car farther from your destination than usual.
- If you have a dog, walk it daily. If you already do that, add a second daily walk—your dog will love you for it!
- While grocery shopping, carry a handbasket instead of pushing a cart (assuming your grocery list is not very long).
- If you have children, actively play with them.
- If you have a desk job, get up, stretch, and walk around often.

Source: U.S. Department of Health and Human Services, "Choices." Small Step Program. www.smallstep.gov/ga/choices.html.

on it. In resistance training (also called *weight training*) in particular, most of the training adaptations actually take place during the rest periods between workouts.

Constant training day after day with insufficient rest periods can result in reduced health benefits and can eventually lead to **overtraining.** If you are exercising consistently and start feeling more fatigue and muscle soreness than usual during and after exercise, you could be doing too much. Reduce the duration or intensity of your exercise and rest for a day or two. To prevent overtraining and to gain optimal benefits from your training program, schedule regular rest days (1 to 3 per week) in any cardiorespiratory endurance program and every other day for any strength-training program. Another important tip to avoid overtraining and injury is to alternate hard workout days with easier workout days during your weekly plan.

overtraining Excessive volume and intensity of physical training leading to diminished health, fitness, and performance

HOW MUCH EXERCISE IS ENOUGH?

How much exercise or physical activity do you really need? The answers will vary, depending on which sources you turn to and on your individual fitness goals.

VARIOUS ORGANIZATIONS RECOMMEND MINIMAL ACTIVITY LEVELS

The best sources of information rely on credible scientific research in developing their recommendations. These sources can be *government agencies* (such as the President's Council on Physical Fitness and Sports), *professional organizations* (such as the American College of Sports Medicine), or *private organizations* (such as the American Heart Association). Table 1 compares the major physical activity guidelines from various organizations. Notice that, for adults, most organizations recommend at least 30 minutes of moderate exercise per day, for most days of the week.

THE PHYSICAL ACTIVITY PYRAMID SUMMARIZES GENERAL GUIDELINES

The Physical Activity Pyramid (Figure 4) visually summarizes minimal physical activity and exercise guidelines. Similar in concept to the USDA's Food Guide Pyramid, the Physical Activity Pyramid presents recommended levels of activity for optimal health and wellness. The pyramid's bottom layer represents light recreational "lifestyle" activities that you should strive to incorporate into your everyday life, especially walking. The next layer of the pyramid represents moderate-to-vigorous aerobic and/or sports activities (such as bicycling or jogging) that you should try to do three to five times per week in order to build cardiorespiratory endurance and fitness. The third layer of the pyramid represents strength-training and flexibility-building exercises that you should try to incorporate 2 to 3 days per week. The top layer of the pyramid represents the activities that should ideally receive the least amount of your time—sedentary activities such as watching TV or surfing the Web—in favor of more active pursuits.

The box **Tools for Change: Six Easy Ways to Get More Active** provides suggestions for how to incorporate more physical activity into your daily life.

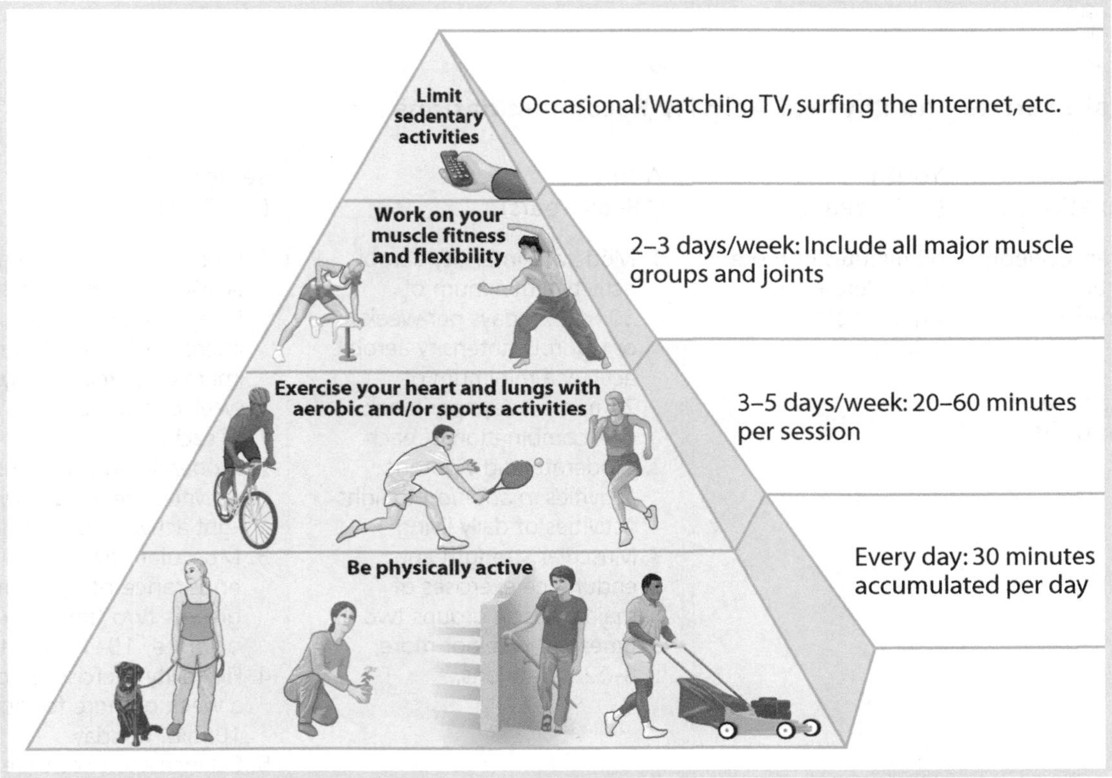

FIGURE 4
The Physical Activity Pyramid presents recommended levels of activity for optimal health and wellness. Adapted from The Activity Pyramid. Pyramids of Health, Park Nicollet Health Source.

> **Try it NOW!** Examine the Physical Activity Pyramid. • How does your weekly physical activity match up to its recommendations? • In which areas of the pyramid should you try to improve?

THE FITT FORMULA CAN HELP YOU PLAN YOUR PROGRAM

The **FITT formula** stands for *frequency, intensity, time,* and *type.* These are all factors that you should consider when planning your personal exercise program.

- *Frequency* is the number of times per week that you will perform an exercise.
- *Intensity* refers to how "hard" you will exercise. For aerobic activities, intensity is often measured in terms of how much the given activity increases the heart rate. For resistance activities, intensity is represented in the amount of resistance or weight lifted and the number of repetitions.
- *Time* is the amount of time that you will devote to a given exercise. It can be the total amount of time you spend on an aerobic or sport activity or the amount of time you spend holding a stretch for a flexibility exercise.
- *Type* refers to the kind of exercise you will do. Within each of the exercise components of fitness (cardiorespiratory endurance, muscular

FITT formula A formula for designing a safe and effective exercise program that specifies frequency, intensity, time, and type

TABLE 1

General Exercise and Physical Activity Recommendations

Title & Organization(s)	Youth (< 18 Years)	Adults (18–65 Years)	Seniors (> 65 Years)
American College of Sports Medicine[1,2] and American Heart Association[1,2]	60 minutes or more of moderate to vigorous physical activity.	1. Moderate-intensity aerobic activity a minimum of 30 min., 5 days per week or vigorous-intensity aerobic activity a minimum of 20 min., 3 days per week or a combination of each. 2. Moderate and vigorous activities *in addition* to light activities of daily living. 3. Muscular strength and endurance exercises of major muscle groups two times per week or more, 8–12 repetitions.	1. Moderate-intensity aerobic activity a minimum of 30 min., 5 days per week or vigorous-intensity aerobic activity a minimum of 20 min., 3 days per week or a combination of each. 2. Moderate and vigorous activities are *in addition* to light activities of daily living. 3. Muscular strength and endurance of major muscle groups two times per week or more, 10–15 repetitions. 4. Flexibility exercises two days a week or more for at least 10 min. per day. 5. Balance exercises to reduce the risk of injury from falls.
U. S. Department of Agriculture[3] and U. S. Department of Health[3] and Human Services	At least 60 min. of physical activity on most, preferably all, days of the week.	1. *Reduce chronic disease*—At least 30 min. of moderate-intensity activity, above usual activity, on most days of the week. 2. *Prevent weight gain*—60 min. of moderate- to vigorous-intensity activity on most days of the week while not exceeding caloric intake. 3. *Sustain weight loss*—60–90 min. of moderate-intensity physical activity while not exceeding caloric intake.	Participate in regular physical activity to reduce functional declines associated with aging and to achieve the other benefits of physical activity identified for all adults.
World Health Organization[4]	N/A	At least 30 min. of regular, moderate-intensity physical activity on most days reduces the risk of cardiovascular disease and diabetes, colon cancer, and breast cancer. More activity may be required for weight control.	Muscle strengthening and balance training can reduce falls and increase functional status among older adults.

strength and endurance, and flexibility), there are many types of exercises that will increase fitness levels. Your type, or **mode,** of exercise will be determined by your preferences, physical abilities, environment, and personal goals.

mode The specific type of exercise performed

If you are beginning a fitness program for the first time, you may want to start with the Physical Activity Pyramid recommendations, and then customize your program using the FITT formula concepts to suit your personal goals.

TABLE 1 *continued*

Title & Organization(s)	Youth (< 18 Years)	Adults (18–65 Years)	Seniors (> 65 Years)
Institute of Medicine[5]	An average of 60 min. of daily moderate physical activity.	An average of 60 min. of daily moderate physical activity (e.g., walking/jogging at 3–4 miles/hr) or shorter periods of more vigorous exertion (e.g., jogging for 30 min. at 5.5 miles/hr)	N/A
Office of the Surgeon General[6] and U. S. Department of Health[6] and Human Services	1. Parents can help their children maintain a physically active lifestyle by providing encouragement and opportunities for physical activity. Family events can include opportunities for everyone in the family to be active. 2. Teenagers—regular physical activity improves strength, builds lean muscle, and decreases body fat. It can build stronger bones to last a lifetime.	Minimum of 30 min. of moderate physical activity (150 calories) on most, if not all, days of the week.	Muscle-strengthening exercises can reduce the risk of falling and fracturing bones and can improve the ability to live independently.

Sources:

1. Haskell, W.L. et.al. "Physical Activity and Public Health: Updated Recommendation for Adults from the American College of Sports Medicine and the American Heart Association." *Medicine & Science in Sports and Exercise,* 2007; *39*(8): 1423–34. www.acsm-msse.org
2. Nelson, M.E. et.al. "Physical Activity and Public Health in Older Adults: Recommendation from the American College of Sports Medicine and the American Heart Association." *Medicine & Science in Sports and Exercise,* 2007; *39*(8): 1435–45. www.acsm-msse.org
3. U.S. Department of Health and Human Services and U.S. Department of Agriculture. *Dietary Guidelines for Americans,* 2005. 6th Edition, Washington, DC: U.S. Government Printing Office, January 2005.
4. World Health Organization. *Global Strategy on Diet, Physical Activity and Health.* Geneva, Switzerland: Marketing and Dissemination, World Health Organization, 2004.
5. Institute of Medicine of the National Academies. *Dietary Reference Intakes for Energy, Carbohydrate, Fiber, Fat, Fatty Acids, Cholesterol, Protein, and Amino Acids.* Food and Nutrition Board, Washington, DC: The National Academies Press, September 2002.
6. U.S. Department of Health and Human Services. *Physical Activity and Health: A Report of the Surgeon General.* Atlanta. U.S. Department of Health and Human Services, Centers for Disease Control and Prevention, National Center for Chronic Disease Prevention and Health Promotion, 1996.

WHAT DOES IT TAKE TO EXERCISE SAFELY?

Exercise-related injuries have risen in recent decades. Over 7 million Americans receive medical attention for sports-related injuries each year, with the greatest numbers of injuries affecting 5- to 24-year-olds.[6] To reduce your risk of exercise injury, follow the guidelines below.

WARM UP PROPERLY BEFORE YOUR WORKOUT

A proper warm-up consists of two phases: a general warm-up and a specific warm-up. In a *general warm-up,* your goal is to warm up the body by doing 3 to 10 minutes of light physical activity similar to the activities you will be performing during exercise. During this period of time (called the *rest-to-exercise*

FACTS AND FALLACIES

SHOULD YOU STRETCH WHILE WARMING UP?

Many people incorrectly think that a good warm-up consists primarily of stretching. While stretching can be a component of an effective warm-up, it is not the most important. In fact, in power athletes, too much stretching can actually decrease muscle power output during an athletic event.[1] If you enjoy stretching during your warm-up, limit it to 10-to-15-second stretches of the major muscle groups used during the activity, and stretch during the end of your specific warm-up.

Source: Young W. B., and Behm D. G. "Effects of Running, Static Stretching and Practice Jumps on Explosive Force Production and Jumping Performance," *The Journal of Sports Medicine and Physical Fitness* 2003; *43*(1): 21–7.

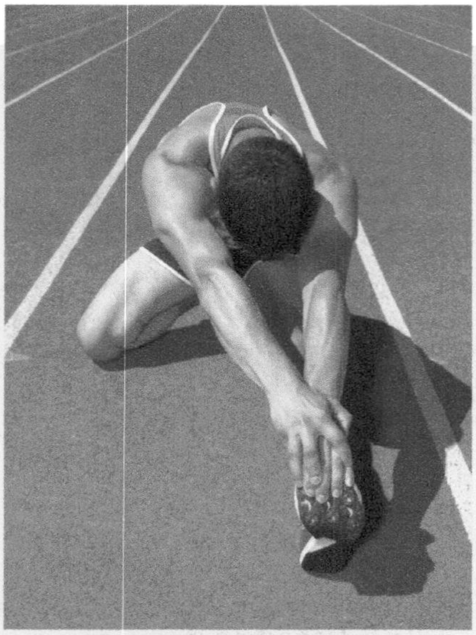

John Lund/Drew Kelly/Getty Images

transition), you are preparing your body to withstand the more vigorous exercise to come. Your core body temperature should rise a few degrees, and you should break a slight sweat. This movement and temperature rise will increase your overall blood flow, ready the joint fluid and structures, and improve muscle elasticity.

During a *specific warm-up,* your goal is to focus on the particular muscle groups and joints that you will be using during the activity set. This part of the warm-up should consist of 3 to 5 minutes of **range-of-motion** movements. You should move the joints involved in your exercise through the range of motion that they will experience during the activity. Move joints through a full range of motion in a relaxed and controlled manner. If you want to add light stretching to your warm-up, do so at the end of your specific warm-up. The box **Facts and Fallacies: Should You Stretch While Warming Up?** addresses the misconceptions about stretching before a workout.

COOL DOWN PROPERLY AFTER YOUR WORKOUT

After you finish your workout, cool down in a manner that is appropriate to the activity that you performed. This *exercise-to-rest transition* should last anywhere from 5 to 15 minutes. If your heart rate and temperature rose during your workout, you should perform a *general cool-down* in which your goal is to bring your heart rate, breathing rate, and temperature closer to resting levels. This cool-down is usually a less vigorous version of the activity you just performed. For example, if you jogged for 25 minutes, your general cool-down may consist of 10 minutes of walking.

If you have just finished a resistance-training program and your heart rate is not elevated, you should perform a *specific cool-down* for the joints and muscles you have exercised. A specific cool-down can be performed after a general cool-down for aerobic activities and right after exercise for resistance-training activities. During a specific cool-down, you should stretch the muscle groups worked during the activity.

TAKE THE TIME TO PROPERLY LEARN THE SKILLS FOR YOUR CHOSEN ACTIVITY

There are hundreds of different activities that you can do to increase your health and fitness, each with a specific set of physical skills required for participation. You might choose simple activities like walking or jogging, which require little skill and have short learning curves, or you might focus on activities that require more complex skills, such as fencing or hockey. Whatever you choose, *properly learn the*

range of motion The movement limits that limbs have around a specific joint

physical skills required for the activity to enhance your enjoyment and to avoid injury. If you are just beginning a sport for the first time—for example, skiing—do not immediately approach the sport the way a more experienced athlete would. Take lessons, start on the beginner slopes, and give yourself time to safely perform your chosen activity.

CONSUME ENOUGH ENERGY AND WATER FOR EXERCISE

Deciding how much to eat and drink prior to exercise can be tricky. You need enough energy to work out, but you should not exercise on a full stomach. Eating a small meal 1 1/2 to 2 hours before exercise is a good way to make sure that you have energy (but not an upset stomach) during the workout. A *light* snack 30 to 60 minutes before your workout is acceptable as well.

Dehydration is more likely than food intake to affect your exercise performance. During the hours before your workout, be sure to drink enough water so that you do not feel thirsty as you go into your exercise session. Guidelines for drinking before, during, and after exercising should be tailored to the individual and the exercise session.[7] General guidelines are 17 to 20 oz. of fluid 2 to 3 hours before exercise and 7 to 10 oz. 10 to 20 minutes prior to exercise.[8] During your workout, hydrate when you feel thirsty, and increase the amount of water you consume as you start to sweat more profusely.

SELECT APPROPRIATE FOOTWEAR AND CLOTHING

Consider this: Your feet will typically strike the ground 1,000 times during 1 mile of running. Over weeks of training, that translates to a great deal of wear and tear on your feet and lower body. Needless to say, proper footwear is critical to a safe and successful training program—regardless of the activity you choose.

While some sports require specialized footwear, most beginning exercisers just need one pair of good, all-around cross-trainers or running shoes. The most important aspect of footwear is proper fit and cushioning. Always try on shoes before purchasing them, and if possible, spend a few minutes mimicking the activity you will be doing in them. The best shoes are not always the most expensive ones, but you should aim to purchase the highest quality footwear you can afford. Ask for assistance from a knowledgeable salesperson—let him or her know what activities you are planning to pursue, and ask which shoes would be most appropriate for your plans.

Clothing for exercise can be very simple (e.g., shorts and a T-shirt) or very technical (e.g., clothing with wicking fibers or special treatments for protection against harsh weather). The most important thing is to *dress appropriately for your chosen activity.* Make sure that your clothing is comfortable and does not restrict your range of motion. Women may wish to wear supportive athletic bras, and men may want to consider wearing supportive compression shorts or undergarments. If you are planning to exercise outdoors, take temperature into consideration and dress accordingly. The longer you plan to exercise, the more carefully you should think about what kind of attire will be most conducive to a successful workout.

WHAT INDIVIDUAL FACTORS SHOULD YOU CONSIDER WHEN DESIGNING A FITNESS PROGRAM?

There is no such thing as a "one-size-fits-all" physical fitness program. Different individuals have different needs, and general recommendations often need to be adapted to fit those individual needs. Your age, weight, current fitness level, and any disabilities and special health concerns are all factors that should be considered in order to design a safe and effective exercise routine.

AGE

Older adults may require additional precautions in order to prevent injury while exercising. Men over age 45 and women over age 55 should obtain medical clearance before beginning an exercise program.[9] Moderate aerobic activity, muscle-strengthening exercises, and flexibility work are all recommended activities for older adults. In addition, balance exercises should be included to help prevent the risk of falls and injury.

WEIGHT

Overweight individuals are at higher risk of musculoskeletal injuries due to increased stress on their muscles and joints, and they should take precautions to ensure safe workouts. If you are overweight,

UNDERSTANDING DIVERSITY

GETTING ACTIVE DESPITE DISABILITY

In the documentary film *Murderball,* muscular, aggressive rugby players compete in fierce, international competitions alongside other world-class athletes—all of them in wheelchairs. Their stories are an inspiration to disabled and nondisabled people alike, and demonstrate that while disability does pose undeniable obstacles, it does not have to hinder the achievement of even the highest levels of physical fitness.

With personal motivation, support from friends and family, and assistance from medical and fitness professionals, persons with disability can make exercise part of their daily routine and live physically active lives. For example, most strength-training machines are used from a seated position and can be operated by people in wheelchairs. Rubber exercise bands, meanwhile, can serve as alternative strength-building aids.[1] Many companies also offer modified sports equipment for people with disabilities: Handcycles allow people to ride bikes using arm power, and wakeboards and flotation devices enable waterskiing and swimming activities. Several kinds of seated skis make downhill skiing accessible to those with physical handicaps.

And disabled people can play a long list of sports—with modified rules and equipment—including volleyball, tennis, golf, soccer, basketball, bowling, bocci, archery, tai chi, and karate.

If you have a physical disability, consult with your doctor or physical therapist about what kinds of activities will best meet your goals and needs.

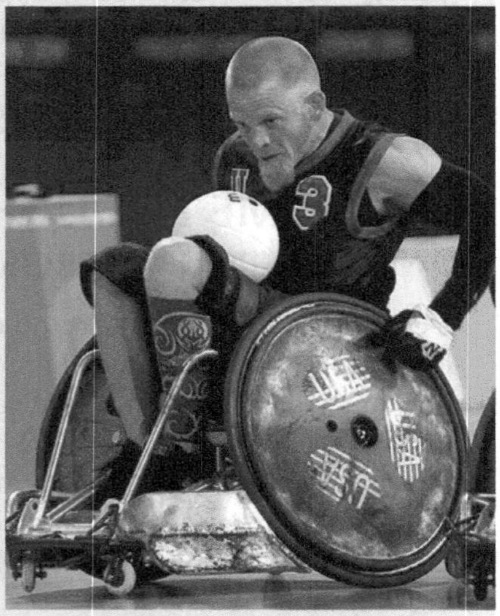

Murderball/The Kobal Collection

Source: Mayo Clinic, "Exercise and Disability: Physical Activity Is Within Your Reach." Mayo Clinic, June 22, 2006, www.mayoclinic.com/health/exercise/SM00042.

consider a cross-training routine with a mix of moderate weight-bearing (e.g., walking, stair-climbing) and non-weight-bearing (e.g., bicycling, water exercise) activities. If you feel pain in your lower-body joints during exercise, shift to more non-weight-bearing activities during your workout.

Underweight individuals, on the other hand, should perform more strength-training and weight-bearing activities to ensure proper muscle and bone maintenance.

CURRENT FITNESS LEVEL

Design a program that is appropriate to your current fitness level. If you already exercise regularly, consider gradually increasing the frequency or intensity of your workouts to realize more fitness gains. If you are currently sedentary and are just beginning to think about starting an exercise routine, do not just suddenly attempt to participate in a triathlon! Pick an activity that you find enjoyable, start at a level that is comfortable for you, and proceed from there.

DISABILITIES

If you have mobility restrictions, poor balance, dizziness, or other conditions that are physically limiting, you can still incorporate fitness into your daily life with alternative or adaptive exercises. Many colleges, community centers, parks and recreation facilities, and fitness centers offer adaptive courses, equipment, and instructors who are specially trained to help you meet your fitness goals. After obtaining medical clearance, seek out such facilities; your physician or a physical therapist may have good recommendations. The box **Understanding Diversity: Getting Active Despite Disability** provides additional suggestions.

SPECIAL HEALTH CONCERNS

Certain medical conditions may require you to exercise under medical supervision. Individuals with asthma, heart disease, hypertension, and diabetes all need medical clearance prior to beginning exercise and may need to be monitored by medical personnel during exercise. If you have special health concerns, seek out the advice of a qualified medical professional on how to exercise safely.

Individuals with significant bone or joint problems can benefit from selecting lower-impact activities such as swimming, water exercise, bicycling, walking, or low-impact aerobics. They can also benefit from resistance-training exercises that can strengthen

SPOTLIGHT

CAN YOU EXERCISE WHILE PREGNANT?

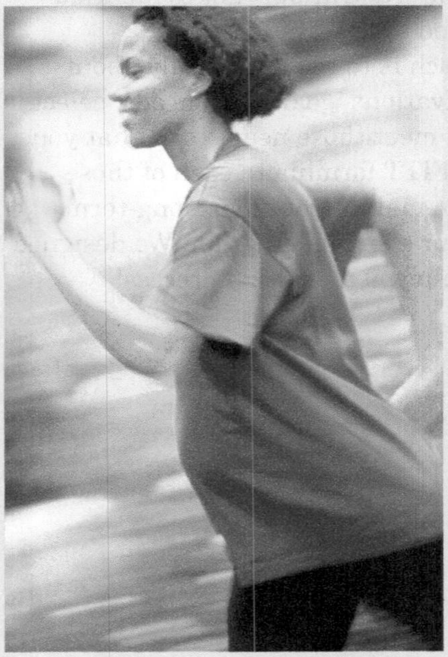

Leland Bobbe/Getty Images

Although pregnancy is not the time to start an intense fitness or weight-loss program, most pregnant women can maintain pre-pregnancy activities with just a few modifications. The American College of Obstetrics and Gynecology recommends the following guidelines:

- First, be sure to get medical clearance for the particular exercise that you intend to do. Your physician may have some specific recommendations for your fitness program.
- If you are relatively new to exercising, seek out a pregnancy fitness exercise program where qualified instructors lead safe exercise sessions. These programs can also provide a good social support network for mothers-to-be.
- Choose fitness activities that do not increase risk of injury to you or the fetus. Avoid high-intensity sports, activities with the potential for falls or abdominal injury, and environmental extremes (such as temperature or barometric pressure—no scuba diving, in particular). Pay attention to your body temperature and avoid getting too hot during exercise, especially during the first trimester. Choose low-impact activities like swimming, water exercise, indoor cycling, yoga, and walking.
- In the absence of medical complications, perform 30 minutes or more of moderate exercise on most, if not all, days of the week.
- Monitor your exercise intensity levels by determining how you feel during exercise.
- In the third trimester, avoid supine exercises (i.e., exercises that require you to lie on your back), because these may restrict blood flow to the fetus. Also, exercise moderately and avoid higher-intensity workouts during this time.
- Add pelvic floor exercises to your fitness routine. These exercises, called *kegels,* involve tightening the pelvic floor muscles for 5 to15 seconds at a time and will help with pregnancy-induced incontinence and delivery recovery. Add three to five sets of 10 to your daily routine.

Pregnancy can be both a wonder-filled and scary time. Maintaining a minimum level of fitness can help you cope with the stresses coming your way. Consult your physician and other pregnancy fitness resources to get started.

Source: American College of Obstetrics and Gynecology, "Exercise During Pregnancy and the Postpartum Period." *Obstetrics & Gynecology* 2002; *99*(1): 171–173.

CASE STUDY

Lily

"I've started jogging again! I'm back to jogging 30 minutes twice a week and thinking of bumping things up to three times a week. I'm hoping to eventually work my way up to jogging for 45 minutes straight, each time I go out. I'm not tempted to run a 10k again any time soon, but if I can keep this new routine going, maybe I will be ready for a 5k—without hurting my knees this time."

1. **Describe Lily's exercise routine, using the FITT formula.**
2. **What kinds of things would you advise Lily to do, in order to reduce her chances of injury?**
3. **Think back to Lily's question at the beginning of the chapter about what it means to be fit. Given what you have learned in this chapter, how would you answer that question?**

muscles and joint structures, and contribute to bone-density maintenance and improvement (if their joint limitations will allow it).

If you are taking any prescription medications, ask your doctor if there are side effects that you should consider before exercising. In addition, beware of over-the-counter medications and other products that may cause drowsiness (such as antihistamines, certain cough/cold medicines, and alcohol), as this will decrease your reaction time, coordination, and balance during exercise.

If you are pregnant, read the box **Spotlight: Can You Exercise While Pregnant?** for advice on exercising safely while expecting.

HOW CAN YOU GET STARTED?

Preparing to exercise for the first time (or after a long sedentary period) can be daunting. Most people are unsure how to start, what to do, and how much to exercise. This often leads people to just jump right in, do something their friends are doing, or try something they saw on TV or in a magazine. This haphazard, impulsive approach often leads to disappointment and frustration—not to mention muscle soreness and even injury.

A better approach is to think carefully about your exercise motivations, goals, and needs, select activities that will meet those needs (and that you enjoy!), apply the FITT formula to each of those activities, and then make a conscious long-term commitment to your exercise program. We designed this textbook to help you along this process!

REVIEW QUESTIONS

1. Moderate physical activity is best defined as activity that is:
   a. Less than 3 METS
   b. 3–6 METS
   c. 7–9 METS
   d. Over 10 METS
2. Which health-related component of fitness involves moving your joints through a full range of motion?
   a. Cardiorespiratory fitness
   b. Muscular endurance
   c. Flexibility
   d. Body composition
3. Which skill-related component of fitness is most involved in braking quickly when a car in front of you stops suddenly?
   a. Agility
   b. Power
   c. Coordination
   d. Reaction time
4. Which principle of fitness relies on the idea that the rate of improvement in a fitness program depends upon your initial fitness level?
   a. Progression
   b. Overload
   c. Diminished returns
   d. Specificity
5. The principle of individuality states that:
   a. Adaptations to training overload may vary widely from person to person
   b. All individuals respond the same way to exercise
   c. Genetic makeup has nothing to do with individual responses to exercise
   d. *Nonresponders* are individuals who do not benefit from exercise
6. The Physical Activity Pyramid recommends which of the following?
   a. Two to 3 days/week of cardiorespiratory activity, 3 to 5 days/week of strength-training and flexibility activities
   b. Two to 3 days/week of strength-training and flexibility exercises, 3 to 5 days/week of cardiorespiratory activity
   c. Constant sedentary activity every day
   d. Limiting the amount of time you spend walking
7. The F in the FITT formula stands for what?
   a. Family
   b. Friends
   c. Frequency
   d. Fitness
8. A proper warm-up consists of how many phases?
   a. One
   b. Two
   c. Three
   d. Four
9. If you are learning a sport for the first time, you should:
   a. Challenge yourself by immediately attempting to perform the exercise the way an experienced athlete would
   b. Not care about clothing and footwear
   c. Do whatever your friends are doing
   d. Take the time to properly acquire the physical skills necessary for your chosen activity
10. When designing your own fitness program, it is important to consider all of the following factors EXCEPT:
    a. Your weight
    b. Your current fitness level
    c. Any special health concerns
    d. A one-size-fits-all approach

CRITICAL THINKING QUESTIONS

1. Give an example of how a training overload can lead to adaptations and training effects.
2. Describe the similarities and differences between the principle of diminished returns and the principle of progression.
3. Imagine you are about to begin a fitness program centered around bicycling. Apply the FITT formula to describe how you might set up your program.

ONLINE RESOURCES

1. **Centers for Disease Control and Prevention: Physical Activity for Everyone**
   www.cdc.gov/nccdphp/dnpa/physical/everyone.htm
   Information about the importance of physical activity, measuring physical activity, getting started, incorporating lifestyle physical activity, resources, and more.
2. **Medline Plus**
   www.medlineplus.gov
   Health information from the U.S. National Library of Medicine and the National Institute for Health.
3. **MyPyramid.gov**
   www.mypyramid.gov
   USDA site with personal planning and tracking programs for diet and physical activity.
4. **National Institutes of Health (NIH)**
   www.health.nih.gov/result.asp/245
   Health information about exercise and physical fitness from various member institutions.

Web addresses are subject to change. Please visit this book's website at **www.aw-bc.com/hopson** for updates and additional Web resources.

REFERENCES

1. M.R. Carnethon and others. "Prevalence and Cardiovascular Disease Correlates of Low Cardiorespiratory Fitness in Adolescents and Adults." *The Journal of the American Medical Association.* 2005; 294(23): 2981–88.
2. H. Suominen, "Muscle Training for Bone Strength." *Aging, Clinical and Experimental Research.* 2006; *18*(2): 85–93.
3. M.A. Jones and others. "Biological Risk Indicators for Recurrent Non-Specific Low Back Pain in Adolescents." *British Journal of Sports Medicine.* 2005; *39*(3): 137–40.
4. T.D. Brutsaert and E.J. Parra. "What Makes a Champion? Explaining Variation in Human Athletic Performance." *Respiratory Physiology and Neurobiology.* 2006; 151: 109–23.
5. W.D. McArdle and others. *Exercise Physiology: Energy, Nutrition, and Human Performance.* 6th Edition. Lippincott Williams & Wilkins, Baltimore, MD, 2007.
6. J.M. Conn and others. "Sports and Recreation Related Injury Episodes in the U.S. Population, 1997–99." *Injury Prevention.* 2003; *9*(2): 117–23.
7. M.N. Sawka and others. "American College of Sports Medicine Position Stand: Exercise and Fluid Replacement." *Medicine and Science in Sports and Exercise.* 2007; *39*(2): 377–90.
8. F.H. Fink and others. *Practical Applications in Sports Nutrition.* Jones and Bartlett Publishers, Inc, Sudbury, MA, 2006.
9. American College of Sports Medicine. *ACSM's Guidelines for Exercise Testing and Prescription.* 7th Edition. Lippincott Williams & Wilkins, Baltimore, MD, 2006.

ANSWERS TO END-OF-CHAPTER QUESTIONS

1.b; 2.c; 3.d; 4.c; 5.a; 6.b; 7.c; 8.b; 9.d; 10.d

Cardiovascular Disease and Cancer

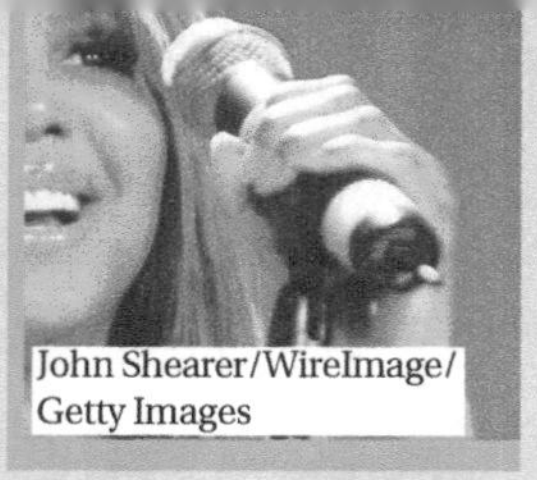
John Shearer/WireImage/Getty Images

Why should I worry about cardiovascular disease?

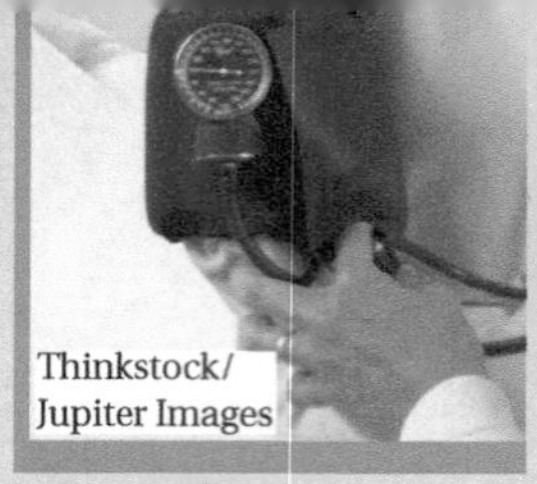
Thinkstock/Jupiter Images

Is heart disease hereditary?

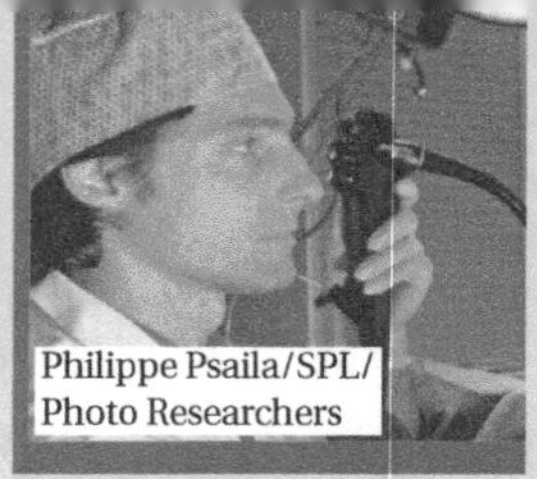
Philippe Psaila/SPL/Photo Researchers

What does it mean for a tumor to be malignant?

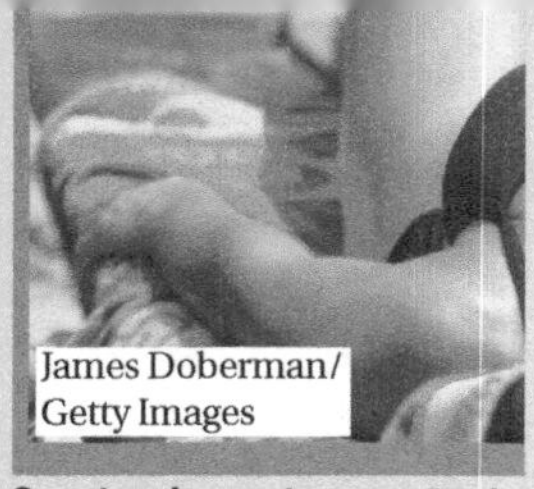
James Doberman/Getty Images

Can having a tan protect me from skin cancer?

Cardiovascular Disease and Cancer

Objectives

* Discuss the incidence, prevalence, and outcomes of cardiovascular disease in the United States, including its impact on society.
* Review major types of cardiovascular disease, controllable and uncontrollable risk factors, methods of prevention, and current strategies for diagnosis and treatment.
* Explain what cancer is, and describe the different types of cancer, including the risks they pose to people at different ages and stages of life.
* Discuss cancer's risk factors, and outline strategies and recommendations for prevention, screening, and treatment.

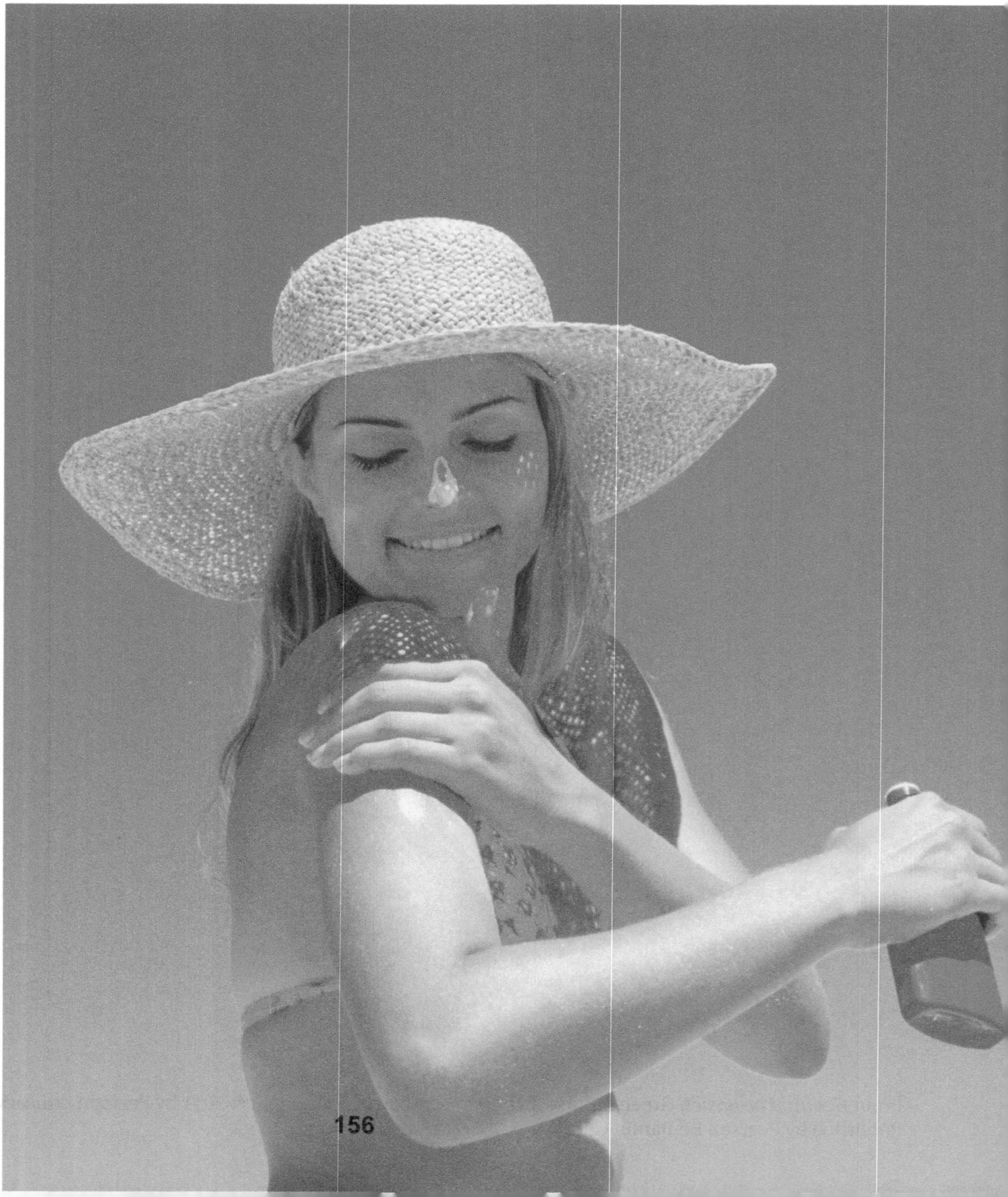
Purestock/Getty Images

In this chapter, we focus on two groups of chronic diseases that contribute to the greatest global burden of death, illness, and disability of the past century: *cardiovascular diseases* and *cancer*. Cardiovascular diseases are the number one cause of death globally, with over 17.5 million deaths each year (30% of all deaths). Cancer is another leading cause of death globally, with nearly 7.5 million deaths each year (around 13% of all deaths).[1] More than half of all Americans suffer from one or more chronic diseases, with cardiovascular disease and cancer being the most likely.[2]

What do we mean when we say a disease is chronic? Essentially, **chronic diseases** are defined as illnesses that are prolonged, do not resolve spontaneously, and are rarely cured completely. As such, they are responsible for significant rates of disability, lost productivity, pain, and suffering, not to mention soaring health care costs. Cardiovascular diseases, in particular, and cancer, to a lesser extent, are closely related to lifestyle factors such as obesity, sedentary behavior, poor nutrition, stress, lack of sleep, tobacco use, and excessive alcohol use. The good news is that in many cases, these lifestyle factors can be changed or modified and disease risks will then decrease.

Cardiovascular Disease: An Epidemiological Overview

More than 80 million Americans—one out of every three adults—suffer from one or more types of **cardiovascular disease (CVD),** the broad term used to describe diseases of the heart and blood vessels.[3] Although numbers continue to increase, it's important to note that CVD has been the leading killer of U.S. adults in every year since 1900, with the exception of 1918, when a pandemic flu killed more people. Put into perspective, CVD claims more lives each year than the next four leading causes of death combined (cancer, chronic lower respiratory diseases, accidents, and diabetes), accounting for nearly 37 percent of all deaths in the United States.[4] Although we've made advances in diagnosis and in pharmaceutical and surgical treatments, CVD continues to pose a serious threat to the health of all Americans, no matter their age, socioeconomic status, or gender (Figure 1). Consider the following facts: [5]

- Over 150,000 Americans killed by CVD are under age 65, and nearly one third of these deaths are premature (meaning that the person doesn't live to full life expectancy).
- The probability at birth of eventually dying of CVD is 47 percent; of dying from cancer, 22 percent; from accidents, 3 percent; from diabetes, 2 percent; and from HIV, 0.7 percent.

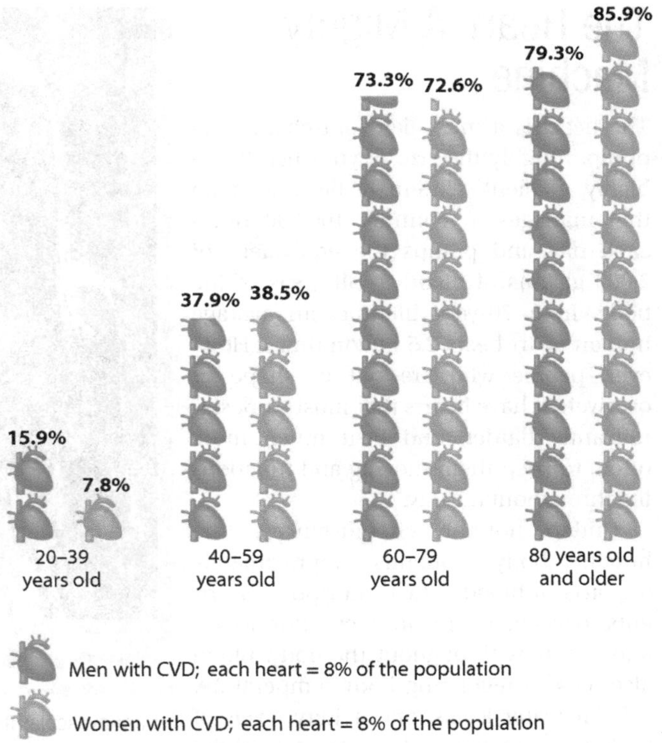

FIGURE 1 **Prevalence of Cardiovascular Diseases (CVDs) in Adults Aged 20 and Older by Age and Sex**

Source: Data are from American Heart Association, *Heart Disease and Stroke Statistics—2009 Update* (Dallas: American Heart Association, 2009).

- Lifetime risk for CVD is two in three for men and more than one in two for women at 40 years of age.
- If all forms of major CVD were eliminated, life expectancy would rise by almost 7 years; if all forms of cancer were eliminated, the gain would be 3 years.

chronic disease An illness that is prolonged, does not resolve spontaneously, and is rarely cured.
cardiovascular disease (CVD) Disease of the heart and blood vessels.
cardiovascular system Organ system, consisting of the heart and blood vessels, that transports nutrients, oxygen, hormones, metabolic wastes, and enzymes throughout the body.

The best defense against CVD is to prevent it from developing in the first place. Understanding how your cardiovascular system works and the factors that can impair its functioning will help you understand your risk and how to reduce it.

Understanding the Cardiovascular System

The **cardiovascular system** is the network of organs and vessels through which blood flows as it carries oxygen and nutrients to all parts of the body. It includes the *heart, arteries, arterioles* (small arteries), *veins, venules* (small veins), and *capillaries* (minute blood vessels).

The Heart: A Mighty Machine

The heart is a muscular, four-chambered pump, roughly the size of your fist. It is a highly efficient, extremely flexible organ that manages to contract 100,000 times each day and pumps the equivalent of 2,000 gallons of blood to all areas of the body. In a 70-year lifetime, an average human heart beats 2.5 billion times. However, people who are out of shape or overweight have hearts that must work significantly harder, and beat much more often, to keep them moving and functioning throughout the day.

Under normal circumstances, the human body contains approximately 6 quarts of blood, which transports nutrients, oxygen, waste products, hormones, and enzymes throughout the body. Blood also aids in regulating body temperature, cellular water levels, and acidity levels of body components, and it helps defend the body against toxins and harmful microorganisms. An adequate blood supply is essential to health and well-being.

The heart has four chambers that work together to circulate blood constantly throughout the body. The two upper chambers of the heart, called **atria,** are large collecting chambers that receive blood from the rest of the body. The two lower chambers, known as **ventricles,** pump the blood out again. Small valves regulate the steady, rhythmic flow of blood between chambers and prevent leakage or backflow between chambers.

atria (singular: *atrium*) The heart's two upper chambers, which receive blood.
ventricles The heart's two lower chambers, which pump blood through the blood vessels.
arteries Vessels that carry blood away from the heart to other regions of the body.
arterioles Branches of the arteries.
capillaries Minute blood vessels that branch out from the arterioles and venules; their thin walls permit exchange of oxygen, carbon dioxide, nutrients, and waste products among body cells.
veins Vessels that carry blood back to the heart from other regions of the body.
venules Branches of the veins.
sinoatrial node (SA node) Cluster of electric pulse–generating cells that serves as a natural pacemaker for the heart.

John Shearer/WireImage/Getty Images

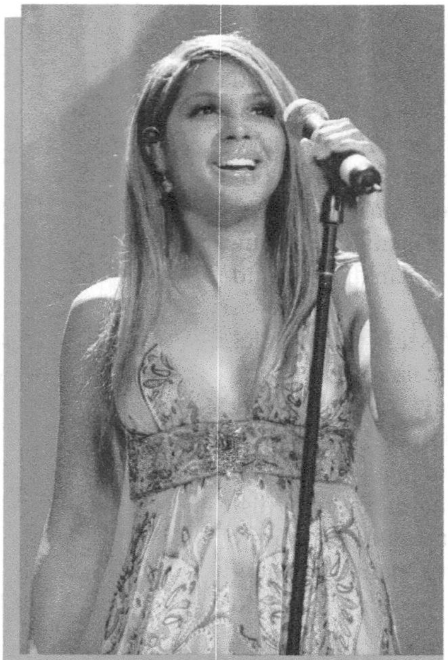

Why should I worry about cardiovascular disease?

Cardiovascular disease can affect even the youngest and most fit people. Grammy-winning singer Toni Braxton was first diagnosed with heart disease in 2003, at the age of 34. At that time she had pericarditis (an inflammation of the lining of the heart) and since then she has been diagnosed with high blood pressure, and briefly hospitalized for microvascular angina. In recent years, Braxton has been a vocal spokesperson for the American Heart Association, urging women not to ignore signs of possible heart disease or to assume that it won't affect them because they are too young and because it is a "men's disease." In fact, heart disease is the number one killer for both men and women.

Heart Function Heart activity depends on a complex interaction of biochemical, physical, and neurological signals. Here are the basic steps involved in heart function (Figure 2):

1. Deoxygenated blood enters the right atrium after having been circulated through the body.
2. From the right atrium, blood moves to the right ventricle and is pumped through the pulmonary artery to the lungs, where it receives oxygen.
3. Oxygenated blood from the lungs then returns to the left atrium of the heart.
4. Blood from the left atrium moves into the left ventricle. The left ventricle pumps blood through the aorta to all body parts.

Various types of blood vessels are required for different parts of this process. **Arteries** carry blood away from the heart; all arteries carry oxygenated blood, *except* for pulmonary arteries, which carry deoxygenated blood to the lungs, where the blood picks up oxygen and gives off carbon dioxide. As the arteries branch off from the heart, they branch into smaller blood vessels called **arterioles,** and then into even smaller blood vessels known as **capillaries.** Capillaries have thin walls that permit the exchange of oxygen, carbon dioxide, nutrients, and waste products with body cells. Carbon dioxide and other waste products are transported to the lungs and kidneys through **veins** and **venules** (small veins).

For the heart to function properly, the four chambers must beat in an organized manner. Your heartbeat is governed by an electrical impulse that directs the heart muscle to move when the impulse travels across it, which results in a sequential contraction of the four chambers. This signal starts in a small bundle of highly specialized cells, the **sinoatrial node (SA node),** located in the right atrium. The SA node serves as a natural pacemaker for the heart. People with a damaged SA node must often have a mechanical pacemaker implanted to ensure the smooth passage of blood through the sequential phases of the heartbeat.

The average adult heart at rest beats 70 to 80 times per minute, although a well-conditioned heart may beat only 50 to 60 times per minute to achieve the same results. If your resting heart rate is routinely in the high 80s or 90s, it may indicate that you are out of shape or suffering from some underlying illness. When overly stressed, a heart may beat more than 200 times per minute. A healthy heart functions more efficiently and is less likely to suffer damage from overwork.

Cardiovascular Disease

There are several types of cardiovascular disease, including atherosclerosis, coronary heart disease (CHD), angina pectoris, arrhythmia, congestive heart failure (CHF), and stroke.

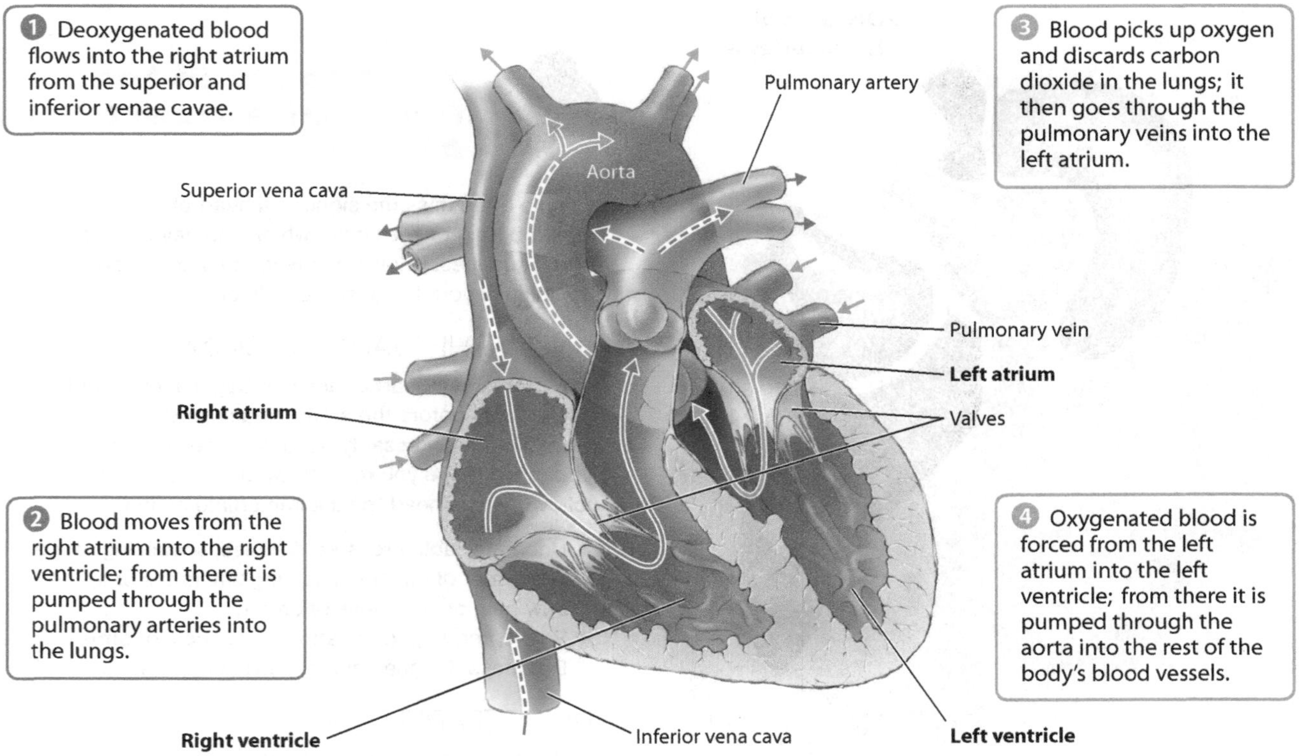
1 Deoxygenated blood flows into the right atrium from the superior and inferior venae cavae.
Pulmonary artery
3 Blood picks up oxygen and discards carbon dioxide in the lungs; it then goes through the pulmonary veins into the left atrium.
Aorta
Superior vena cava
Pulmonary vein
Left atrium
Right atrium
Valves
2 Blood moves from the right atrium into the right ventricle; from there it is pumped through the pulmonary arteries into the lungs.
4 Oxygenated blood is forced from the left atrium into the left ventricle; from there it is pumped through the aorta into the rest of the body's blood vessels.
Right ventricle
Inferior vena cava
Left ventricle

FIGURE 2 **Blood Flow within the Heart**

Many forms of CVD are potentially fatal; Figure 3 on the next page presents the percentage breakdown of deaths from these different diseases in the United States.

Atherosclerosis

Arteriosclerosis, thickening and hardening of arteries, is a condition that underlies many cardiovascular health problems and is believed to be the biggest contributor to disease burden globally. **Atherosclerosis** is a type of arteriosclerosis and is characterized by deposits of fatty substances, cholesterol, cellular waste products, calcium, and fibrin (a clotting material in the blood) in the inner lining of an artery. *Hyperlipidemia* (an abnormally high blood lipid level) is a key factor in this process, and the resulting buildup is referred to as **plaque.**

As plaque accumulates, vessel walls become narrow and may eventually block blood flow or cause vessels to rupture. This is similar to putting your thumb over the end of a hose while water is running through it. Pressure builds within arteries just as pressure builds in the hose. If vessels are weakened and pressure persists, the artery may become weak and eventually burst. Fluctuation in the blood pressure levels within arteries may actually damage their internal walls, making it even more likely that plaque will accumulate.

Atherosclerosis is often called *coronary artery disease (CAD)* because of the resultant damage done to the body's main coronary arteries on the outer surface of the heart. These are the arteries that provide blood supply to the heart muscle itself. Most heart attacks result from blockage of these arteries.

When atherosclerosis occurs in the lower extremities, such as in the feet, calves, or legs, or in the arms, it is called *peripheral artery disease (PAD)*. In recent years, increased attention has been drawn to PAD's role in subsequent blood clots and resultant heart attacks. In June 2008, when Tim Russert, a well-known NBC news correspondent, died suddenly of a heart attack after a long flight to Italy, there was speculation that he might have had a blood clot form in his legs from sitting for a prolonged period. This theory has not been confirmed; however, people are routinely advised to get up and walk around and flex or extend their legs to keep blood from pooling during long airplane flights or when sitting at a desk for long periods.

arteriosclerosis A general term for thickening and hardening of the arteries.
atherosclerosis Condition characterized by deposits of fatty substances (plaque) on the inner lining of an artery.
plaque Buildup of deposits in the arteries.

Whether from CAD or PAD, damage to vessels and threats to health can be severe. According to current thinking, four factors discussed later in this chapter are responsible for this damage: inflammation, elevated levels of cholesterol and triglycerides in the blood, high blood pressure, and tobacco smoke.

Coronary Heart Disease

Of all the major cardiovascular diseases, coronary heart disease (CHD) is the greatest killer, accounting for nearly one in

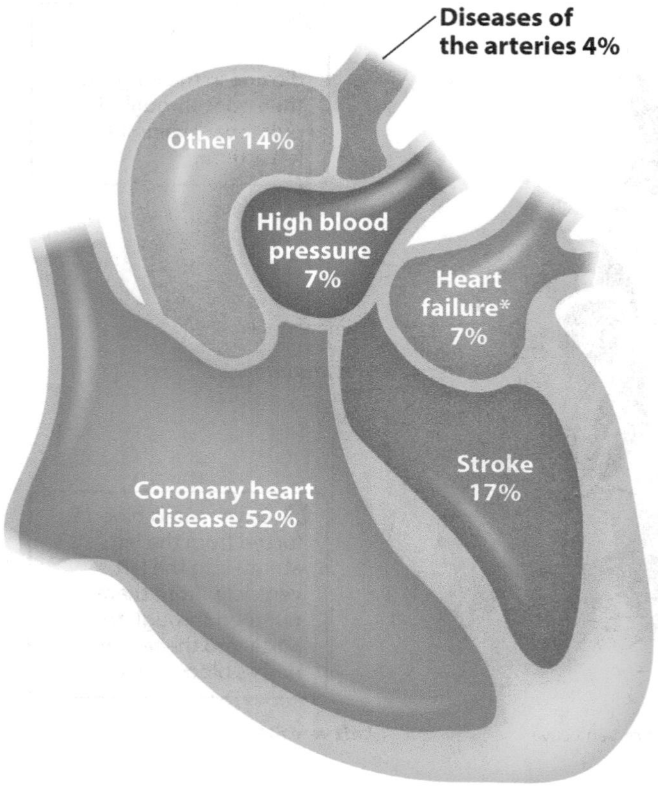

FIGURE 3 **Percentage Breakdown of Deaths from Cardiovascular Disease in the United States**
Totals may not add up to 100% due to rounding.

*Not a true underlying cause.

Source: Data are from *Heart Disease and Stroke Statistics—2009 Update.* (Dallas: American Heart Association, 2009).

five deaths in the United States. Of the nearly 785,000 people who suffer a heart attack each year, over 37 percent will die because of it.[6] A **myocardial infarction (MI),** or **heart attack,** involves an area of the heart that suffers permanent damage because its normal blood supply has been blocked. This condition is often brought on by a blood clot in a coronary artery or an atherosclerotic narrowing that blocks an artery (see Figure 4). When blood does not flow readily, there is a corresponding decrease in oxygen flow. If the blockage is extremely minor, an otherwise healthy heart will adapt over time by enlarging existing blood vessels and growing new ones to reroute blood through other areas.

myocardial infarction (MI; heart attack) A blockage of normal blood supply to an area in the heart.
ischemia Reduced oxygen supply to a body part or organ.
angina pectoris Chest pain occurring as a result of reduced oxygen flow to the heart.

40% of heart attack victims die within the first hour following the heart attack.

Skills for Behavior Change

What to Do in the Event of a Heart Attack

People often miss the signs of a heart attack, or they wait too long to seek help, which can have deadly consequences. Knowing how to act in an emergency could save your life or somebody else's.

KNOW THE WARNING SIGNS

Symptoms of a heart attack can begin a few minutes or a few hours before the actual attack, and all warning signs do not necessarily occur with every episode. If you or someone you're with experiences any of the following, you need to take immediate action:

* Uncomfortable pressure, fullness, squeezing, or pain in the center of the chest, lasting 2 minutes or longer
* Jaw pain or shortness of breath
* Pain spreading to the shoulders, neck, or arms
* Dizziness, fatigue, fainting, sweating, or nausea

BE PREPARED

* Keep a list of emergency rescue service numbers next to your telephone and in your pocket, wallet, or purse. Be aware of whether your local area has a 9-1-1 emergency service.
* It's normal for someone to deny the possibility of anything as serious as a heart attack, particularly if they are young and appear to be in good health. If you're with someone who appears to be having a heart attack, don't take no for an answer; insist on taking prompt action.
* If you are with someone who suddenly collapses, perform cardiopulmonary resuscitation (CPR). See www.americanheart.org for information on the new chest-compression-only techniques recommended by the American Heart Association. If you're trained and willing, use conventional CPR methods.

Sources: American Heart Association, "Heart Attack, Stroke and Cardiac Arrest Warning Signs," 2009, www.americanheart.org/presenter.jhtml?identifier=3053.

When heart blockage is more severe, however, the body is unable to adapt on its own, and outside lifesaving support is critical. See the Skills for Behavior Change box above to learn what to do in case of a heart attack.

Angina Pectoris

Atherosclerosis and other circulatory impairments often reduce the heart's blood and oxygen supply, a condition known as **ischemia.** People with ischemia often suffer from varying degrees of **angina pectoris,** or chest pain and pressure. In fact, an estimated 4.3 million men and 5.5 million women suffer

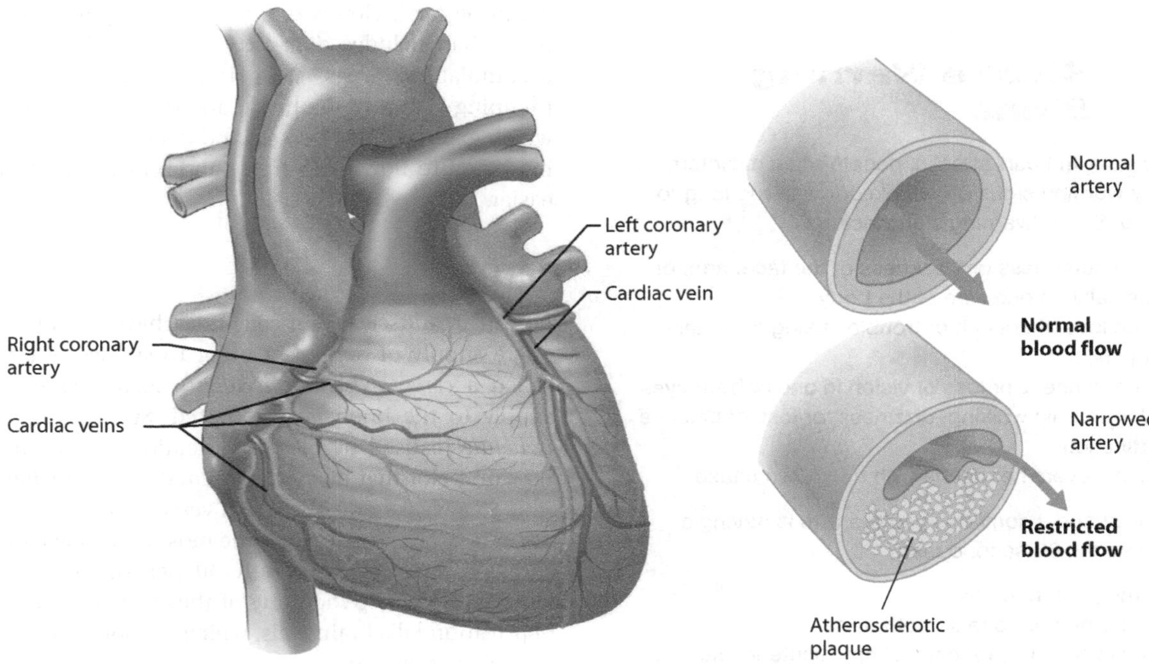

FIGURE 4 **Atherosclerosis and Coronary Heart Disease**
The coronary arteries are located on the exterior of the heart and supply blood and oxygen to the heart muscle itself. In atherosclerosis, arteries become clogged by a buildup of plaque. When atherosclerosis occurs in coronary arteries, blood flow to the heart muscle is restricted and a heart attack may occur.

Sources: Adapted from Joan Salge Blake, *Nutrition & You*, p. 152; and Michael D. Johnson, *Human: Biology: Concepts and Current Issues*, 4th ed., p. 172. Both copyright © 2008 Pearson Education, Inc., publishing as Benjamin Cummings. Reprinted by permission.

mild to crushing forms of chest pain each day, many of whom take powerful medications to control their symptoms.[7] Symptoms may range from slight indigestion, to pain upon slight exertion, to a feeling that the heart is being crushed. Generally, the more serious the oxygen deprivation, the more severe the pain. Although angina pectoris is not a heart attack, it does indicate underlying heart disease.

Currently, there are several methods of treating angina. In mild cases, rest is critical. The most common treatments for more severe cases involve drugs that affect either the supply of blood to the heart muscle or the heart's demand for oxygen. Pain and discomfort are often relieved with *nitroglycerin,* a drug used to relax (dilate) veins, thereby reducing the amount of blood returning to the heart and thus lessening its workload. Patients whose angina is caused by spasms of the coronary arteries are often given drugs called *calcium channel blockers,* which prevent calcium atoms from passing through coronary arteries and causing heart contractions. They also appear to reduce blood pressure and slow heart rate. *Beta-blockers,* the other major type of drugs used to treat angina, control potential overactivity of the heart muscle.

Arrhythmias

Over 4 million Americans have experienced some type of **arrhythmia,** an irregularity in heart rhythm.[8] A person who complains of a racing heart in the absence of exercise or anxiety may be experiencing *tachycardia,* the medical term for abnormally fast heartbeat. On the other end of the continuum is *bradycardia,* or abnormally slow heartbeat. When a heart goes into **fibrillation,** it beats in a sporadic, quivering pattern that results in extreme inefficiency in moving blood through the cardiovascular system. If untreated, fibrillation may be fatal.

Not all arrhythmias are life threatening. In many instances, excessive caffeine or nicotine consumption can trigger an arrhythmia episode. However, severe cases may require drug therapy or external electrical stimulus to prevent serious complications.

arrhythmia An irregularity in heartbeat.

fibrillation A sporadic, quivering pattern of heartbeat that results in extreme inefficiency in moving blood through the cardiovascular system.

congestive heart failure (CHF) An abnormal cardiovascular condition that reflects impaired cardiac pumping and blood flow; pooling blood leads to congestion in body tissues.

Congestive Heart Failure

When the heart muscle is damaged or overworked and lacks the strength to keep blood circulating normally through the body, its chambers are often taxed to the limit. **Congestive heart failure** (CHF) affects over 5 million Americans and dramatically increases risk of premature death.[9] The heart muscle may be injured by a number of health conditions, including rheumatic fever, pneumonia, heart attack, or other cardiovascular problems. In some cases, the damage is due to

Skills for Behavior Change

Stroke Warning Signs

As they do with heart attacks, people often misinterpret the early warning signs of a stroke, or wait too long to seek help. Stroke warning signs include:

* Sudden numbness or weakness of the face, arm, or leg, especially on one side of the body
* Sudden loss of speech or trouble talking or understanding speech
* Sudden dimness or loss of vision in one or both eyes
* Sudden trouble walking, dizziness, or loss of balance or coordination
* Sudden, severe headache with no known cause

If you suspect someone you are with is having a stroke, use the 60-second test:

1. Ask the person to smile.
2. Ask the person to raise both arms.
3. Ask him or her to repeat a simple sentence such as "It is sunny out today."

If you or someone with you has one or more of the signs above or has difficulty performing any of the tasks in the 60-second test, don't delay! Immediately call 9-1-1 or the emergency medical service (EMS) number so an ambulance (ideally with advanced life support) can be dispatched. Also, note the time so that you'll know when the first symptoms appeared. If given within 3 hours of the start of symptoms, a clot-busting drug called *tissue plasminogen activator* (tPA) can reduce long-term disability from ischemic strokes, the most common type of stroke.

Sources: American Heart Association, "Heart Attack, Stroke and Cardiac Arrest Warning Signs," 2009, www.americanheart.org/presenter.jhtml?identifier=3053; American Stroke Foundation, "How to Recognize a Stroke," 2009, www.americanstroke.org/content/view/17/46.

radiation or chemotherapy treatments for cancer. These weakened muscles respond poorly, impairing blood flow out of the heart through the arteries. The return flow of blood through the veins begins to back up, causing congestion in body tissues. This pooling of blood enlarges the heart, makes it less efficient, and decreases the amount of blood that can be circulated. Fluid begins to accumulate in other body areas, such as the vessels in the legs, ankles, or lungs, where it can leak into surrounding tissues and cause swelling or difficulty in breathing.

Today, CHF is the single most frequent cause of hospitalization in the United States.[10] If untreated, it can be fatal. However, most cases respond well to treatment that includes *diuretics* ("water pills") to relieve fluid accumulation; drugs, such as *digitalis,* that increase the pumping action of the heart; and drugs called *vasodilators,* which expand blood vessels and decrease resistance, allowing blood to flow more freely and making the heart's work easier.

stroke A condition occurring when the brain is damaged by disrupted blood supply; also called *cerebrovascular accident.*

aneurysm A weakened blood vessel that may bulge under pressure and, in severe cases, burst.

transient ischemic attacks (TIAs) Brief interruption of the blood supply to the brain that causes only temporary impairment; often an indicator of impending major stroke.

Stroke

Like heart muscle, brain cells must have a continuous adequate supply of oxygen in order to survive. A **stroke** (also called a *cerebrovascular accident*) occurs when the blood supply to the brain is interrupted. Strokes may be either *ischemic* (caused by plaque formation that narrows blood flow or a clot that obstructs a blood vessel) or *hemorrhagic* (due to a weakening of a blood vessel that causes it to bulge or rupture). An **aneurysm** is the most well known of the hemorrhagic strokes, with nearly 40 percent of victims dying within 30 days.[11] When any of these events occurs, oxygen deprivation kills brain cells, which do not have the capacity to heal or regenerate.

Some strokes are mild and cause only temporary dizziness or slight weakness or numbness. More serious interruptions in blood flow may impair speech, memory, or motor control. Other strokes affect parts of the brain that regulate heart and lung function and kill within minutes. According to the American Heart Association's latest statistics, every year more than 6.5 million Americans suffer strokes, 150,000 of whom die as a result. Strokes cause countless levels of disability and suffering, and account for 1 in 15 deaths each year, surpassed only by CHD and cancer.[12]

About 15 percent of all major strokes are preceded days, weeks, or months earlier by **transient ischemic attacks (TIAs),** brief interruptions of the blood supply to the brain that cause only temporary impairment. Symptoms of TIAs include dizziness, particularly when first rising in the morning, weakness, temporary paralysis or numbness in the face or other regions, temporary memory loss, blurred vision, nausea, headache, slurred speech, or other unusual physiological reactions. Some people may actually experience unexpected falls or have blackouts; however, others may have no obvious symptoms. TIAs often indicate an impending major stroke. The earlier a stroke is recognized and treatment started, the more effective that treatment will be. See the **Skills for Behavior Change** box at left for tips on recognizing a stroke.

One of the greatest medical successes in recent years has been the decline in the fatality rate from strokes, which has dropped by one-third in the United States since the 1980s and continues to fall. Improved diagnostic procedures, better surgical options, clot-busting drugs injected soon after a stroke has occurred, and acute care centers specializing in stroke treatment and rehabilitation have all been factors.

Unfortunately, like many victims of other forms of CVD, stroke survivors do not always make a full recovery. Some 50 to 70 percent of stroke survivors regain functional independence, but 15 to 30 percent are permanently disabled and require assistance. Today stroke is a leading cause of serious long-term disability and contributes a significant amount to Medicaid and Medicare expenses for older Americans, particularly women.

Reducing Your Risks

Scientific evidence has shown a large cluster of factors related to a person's being at a higher risk for developing cardiovascular diseases over the lifespan. Obesity, lack of physical activity, high cholesterol, and high blood pressure have all shown strong associations with subsequent CVD problems.[13] Interestingly, although selected factors increase risks specific to CVD, the combination of these and other risk factors appears also to increase risks for insulin resistance and type 2 diabetes.[14] The term **cardiometabolic risks** refers to these combined risks that indicate physical and biochemical changes that can lead to these major diseases. Some of these risks result from choices and behaviors, and so are modifiable, whereas others are inherited or are intrinsic to you (such as your age and gender) and therefore cannot be modified.

Metabolic Syndrome: Quick Risk Profile

Over the past decade, different health professionals have attempted to establish diagnostic cutoff points for a cluster of combined cardiometabolic risks, variably labeled as *syndrome X, insulin resistance syndrome,* and, most recently, **metabolic syndrome.** Historically, metabolic syndrome is believed to increase the risk for atherosclerotic heart disease by as much as three times the normal rates. It has captured international attention, as an estimated 50 million people potentially classify as having this syndrome. Typically, for a diagnosis of metabolic syndrome, a person would have three or more of the following risks:

- Abdominal obesity (waist measurement of more than 40 inches in men or 35 inches in women)
- Elevated blood fat (triglycerides greater than 150)
- Low levels of HDL ("good") cholesterol (less than 40 in men and less than 50 in women)
- Elevated blood pressure greater than 130/85
- Elevated fasting glucose greater than 100 mg/dL (a sign of insulin resistance or glucose intolerance)
- High levels of C-reactive proteins, indicating inflammation is present

The use of the metabolic syndrome classification and other, similar terms has been important in highlighting the relationship between the number of risks a person possesses and that person's likelihood of developing CVD and diabetes. Critics have questioned the usefulness of this risk profile, saying that the way data are collected makes it impossible to determine whether additional and compounded risk factors really contribute more to total risk. In addition, these classifications have not been as useful in telling patients and health care providers which risk factors might be more important and which ones should be given the highest priority when taking action to reduce risks.

Modifiable Risks

Although younger adults often think of heart attacks and strokes as something that happens to "old" people, the reality is that you may already be on course to have significant risks. The lifestyle choices you have made and continue making play a significant role in your likelihood for developing CVD well before you hit the golden years. In fact, hypertension, prediabetes, high cholesterol, and other risks have increased significantly among elementary, high school, and college students in the United States and globally. Blacks, Mexican American males, and white females are among the highest risk groups for both obesity and hypertension in children and adolescents, while male college students have higher rates of obesity, hypertension, and triglycerides than do female students.[15] Behaviors you choose today and over the coming decades can actively reduce or promote your risk for CVD. Among the most important behaviors you can adopt are choosing not to smoke, following a healthy diet, staying physically active, controlling blood pressure, and managing stress.

Avoid Tobacco In spite of massive campaigns to educate us about the dangers of smoking, and in spite of increasing numbers of states and municipalities that have enacted policies to go "smoke free," cigarette smoking remains the leading cause of preventable death in the United States, accounting for approximately one of every five deaths. These statistics are particularly surprising given the fact that smoking rates have declined by 49 percent among people aged 18 and older since 1965.[16] The risk for cardiovascular disease is 70 percent greater for smokers than it is for nonsmokers. Smokers who have a heart attack are more likely to die suddenly (within 1 hour) than are nonsmokers. Evidence also indicates that chronic exposure to environmental tobacco smoke (ETS, or secondhand smoke) increases the risk of heart disease by as much as 30 percent, with over 35,000 nonsmokers dying from ETS exposure each year.[17]

cardiometabolic risks Risk factors that impact both the cardiovascular system and the body's biochemical metabolic processes.

metabolic syndrome A group of metabolic conditions occurring together that increases a person's risk of heart disease, stroke, and diabetes.

How does smoking damage the heart? There are two plausible explanations. One is that nicotine increases heart rate, heart output, blood pressure, and oxygen use by heart muscles. The heart is forced to work harder to obtain sufficient oxygen. The other explanation is that chemicals in smoke damage and inflame the lining of the coronary arteries, allowing cholesterol and plaque to accumulate more easily, increasing blood pressure and forcing the heart to work harder.

When people stop smoking, regardless of how long or how much they've smoked, their risk of heart disease declines rapidly. By 3 years after they quit, the risk of death from heart disease and stroke for people who had smoked a pack a day or less is almost the same as for people who have never smoked.

Cut Back on Saturated Fat and Cholesterol Cholesterol is a soft, fatty, waxy substance found in the bloodstream and in your body cells. Although we hear only the bad things about it, in truth cholesterol plays an important role in the production of cell membranes and hormones and in other body functions. However, when blood levels of it get too high, risks for CVD escalate. Nearly 36 percent of adults in the United States aged 18 and above have been told they have high cholesterol, and vast numbers of others have never been tested yet probably have higher than normal levels. Less than half of the people who should be on cholesterol-reducing medications are on them, and many who are on them are unable to reach their cholesterol level goals.

You get cholesterol from two primary sources: from your body (which involves genetic predisposition) and from food. Much of your cholesterol level is predetermined: 75 percent of blood cholesterol is produced by your liver and other cells, and the other 25 percent comes from the foods you eat. The good news is that the 25 percent you get from foods is the part where you can make real improvements in overall cholesterol profiles, even if you have a high genetic risk.

Diets high in saturated fat and *trans* fats are known to raise cholesterol levels, send the body's blood-clotting system into high gear, and make the blood more viscous in just a few hours, increasing the risk of heart attack or stroke. Increased blood levels of cholesterol also contribute to atherosclerosis. Switching to a low-fat diet lowers the risk of clotting; even a 10 percent decrease in total cholesterol levels may result in an estimated 30 percent reduction in the incidence of heart disease.[18]

Total cholesterol level isn't the only level to be concerned about; the type of cholesterol also matters. As discussed in earlier, the two major types of blood cholesterol are *low-density lipoprotein (LDL)* and *high-density lipoprotein (HDL)*. Low-density lipoprotein, often referred to as "bad" cholesterol, is believed to build up on artery walls. In contrast, high-density lipoprotein, or "good" cholesterol, appears to remove cholesterol from artery walls, thus serving as a protector. In theory, if LDL levels get too high or HDL levels too low, cholesterol will accumulate inside arteries and lead to cardiovascular problems. Scientists now believe that there are other blood lipid factors that may also increase CVD risk, such as lipoprotein-associated phospholipase A_2 (Lp-PLA_2), an enzyme that circulates in the blood and attaches to LDL. Lp-PLA_2 plays an important role in plaque accumulation and increased risk for stroke and coronary events, particularly in men. Studies suggest that the higher the Lp-PLA_2 level, the higher the risk of developing CVD.[19] One relatively new consideration in the saturated fat dietary menace is apolipoprotein B (apo B), a primary component of LDL that is essential for cholesterol delivery to cells. Although the mechanism is unclear, some researchers believe that apo B levels may be more important to heart disease risk than total cholesterol or LDL levels.[20]

The most common types of lipids in your body are *triglycerides*, a major energy source that comes from food, and that is manufactured by the body. High levels of blood triglycerides are often found in people who have high cholesterol levels, heart problems or diabetes, or who are overweight. As people get older, heavier, or both, their triglyceride and cholesterol levels tend to rise. It is recommended that a baseline cholesterol test (known as a lipid panel or lipid profile) be taken at age 20, with follow-ups every 5 years. This test, which measures triglyceride levels as well as HDL, LDL, and total cholesterol levels, requires that you fast for 12 hours prior to the test, are well hydrated, and avoid coffee and tea prior to testing. Men over the age of 35 and women over the age of 45 should have their lipid profile checked annually, with more frequent tests for those at high risk. See Table 1 for recommended levels of cholesterol and trigylcerides.

TABLE 1 **Recommended Cholesterol Levels for Adults**

Total Cholesterol Level (lower numbers are better)	
Less than 200 mg/dL	Desirable level that puts you at lower risk for coronary heart disease.
200 to 239 mg/dL	Borderline high
240 mg/dL and above	High blood cholesterol. A person with this level has more than twice the risk of coronary heart disease as someone whose cholesterol is below 200 mg/dL.
HDL Cholesterol Level (higher numbers are better)	
Less than 40 mg/dL (for men) Less than 50 mg/dL (for women)	Low HDL cholesterol. A major risk factor for heart disease.
60 mg/dL and above	High HDL cholesterol. An HDL of 60 mg/dL and above is considered to be protective against heart disease.
LDL Cholesterol Level (lower numbers are better)	
Less than 100 mg/dL	Optimal
100 to 129 mg/dL	Near or above optimal
130 to 159 mg/dL	Borderline high
160 to 189 mg/dL	High
190 mg/dL and above	Very high
Triglyceride Level (lower numbers are better)	
Less than 150 mg/dL	Normal
150–199 mg/dL	Borderline high
200–499 mg/dL	High
500 mg/dL and above	Very high

Source: American Heart Association, "Cholesterol Levels," 2009, www.americanheart.org/presenter.jhtml?identifier=4500.

Health Headlines

HEART-HEALTHY SUPER FOODS

Although there are countless recommendations for reducing your chances of heart disease through exercise, sleep, stress reduction, and so on, the foods you eat also play a major role in your risk by affecting the levels of triglycerides, LDL, and HDL in your bloodstream. Several foods have been shown to reduce the chances that cholesterol will be absorbed in the cells, reduce levels of LDL cholesterol, or enhance the protective effects of HDL cholesterol. To protect your heart, include the following in your diet:

✱ **Fish high in omega-3 fatty acids.** Consumption of fish such as salmon, sardines, and herring helps reduce blood pressure and the risk associated with blood clots as well as lowering cholesterol.

✱ **Olive oil.** Using any of a number of monounsaturated fats in cooking, particularly extra virgin olive oil, helps lower total cholesterol and raise your HDL levels. Canola oil; margarine labeled "*trans* fat free"; and cholesterol-lowering margarines such as Benecol, Promise Activ, or Smart Balance are also excellent choices.

✱ **Whole grains and fiber.** Getting enough fiber each day in the form of 100 percent whole wheat, steel cut oats, oat bran, flaxseed, fruits, and vegetables helps lower LDL or "bad" cholesterol. Soluble fiber, in particular, seems to keep cholesterol from being absorbed in the intestines.

✱ **Plant sterols and stanols.** Although these sound like substances derived in the lab, they are actually essential components of plant membranes and are found naturally in vegetables, fruits, and legumes. In addition, many food products, including juices and yogurt, are now fortified with them. These compounds are believed to benefit your heart health by blocking cholesterol absorption in the bloodstream, thus reducing LDL levels.

✱ **Nuts.** Long maligned for being high in calories, walnuts, almonds, and other nuts are naturally high in omega-3 fatty acids, which are important in lowering cholesterol and good for the blood vessels themselves.

✱ **Chocolate, red wine, and green tea.** Could it really be true? Are dark chocolate, red wine, green tea, and other foods really protecting us from cardiovascular diseases? Over the past decade, several major studies have indicated that dark chocolate appears to significantly reduce blood pressure, whereas green tea seems to reduce LDL cholesterol. The flavonoids in chocolate and green tea act as powerful antioxidants that protect the cells of the heart and blood vessels. Red wine also contains flavonoids and research initially seemed to support beneficial effects; however, newer research has been conflicting. Much more research on all of these foods must be done to say definitively how beneficial they might be, and what dosage is recommended.

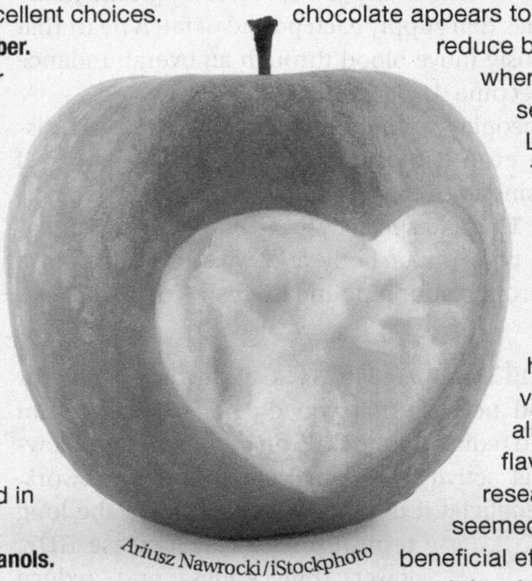
Ariusz Nawrocki/iStockphoto

Sources: A. Mente, L. deKoning, M. Shannon, and S. Anand, "A Systematic Review of the Evidence Supporting a Causal Link between Dietary Factors and Coronary Heart Disease," *Archives of Internal Medicine* 169, no. 7 (2009): 659–69; L. Hooper, P. Kroon, et al., "Flavonoids, Flavonoid-Rich Foods, and Cardiovascular Risk: A Meta-Analysis of Randomized Controlled Trials," *American Journal of Clinical Nutrition* 88, no. 1 (2008): 38–50; E. Corti et al., "Cocoa and Cardiovascular Health," *Circulation* 119, no. 10 (2009):1433–41; M. Corder, "Red Wine, Chocolate and Vascular Health: Developing the Evidence Base," *Heart* 94, no. 7 (2008): 821–23; N. Tanabe et al., "Consumption of Green and Roasted Teas and the Risk of Stroke Incidence: Results from the Tokamachi-Nakasato Cohort Study in Japan," *International Journal of Epidemiology* 37, no. 5 (2008): 1030–40.

In general, LDL is more closely associated with cardiovascular risk than is total cholesterol. However, most authorities agree that looking only at LDL ignores the positive effects of HDL. Perhaps the best method of evaluating risk is to examine the ratio of HDL to total cholesterol, or the percentage of HDL in total cholesterol. If the level of HDL is lower than 35 Mg/dL, the risk increases dramatically. To reduce risk, the goal is to manage the ratio of HDL to total cholesterol by lowering LDL levels, raising HDL, or both. Regular exercise and a healthy diet low in saturated fat continue to be the best methods for maintaining healthy ratios. See the **Health Headlines** box above for information about foods and dietary practices that can help maintain healthy cholesterol levels.

Of the more than 100 million Americans who have high cholesterol levels, almost half, particularly those at the low to moderate risk levels, should be able to reach their LDL and HDL goals through lifestyle changes alone. People who are at higher risk or those for whom lifestyle modifications are not effective may need to take cholesterol-lowering drugs while they continue modifying their lifestyle.

Maintain a Healthy Weight No question about it—body weight plays a role in CVD. Researchers are not sure whether high-fat, high-sugar, high-calorie diets are a direct risk for CVD or whether they invite risk by causing obesity, which strains the heart, forcing it to push blood through the many miles of capillaries that supply each pound of fat. A heart that has to continuously move blood through an overabundance of vessels may become damaged.

Overweight people are more likely to develop heart disease and stroke even if they have no other risk factors. If you're heavy, losing even 5 to 10 pounds can make a significant difference. This is especially true if you're an "apple" (thicker around your upper body and waist) rather than a "pear" (thicker around your hips and thighs).

Exercise Regularly Inactivity is a clear risk factor for CVD.[21] The good news is that you do not have to be an exercise fanatic to reduce your risk. Even modest levels of low-intensity physical activity—walking, gardening, housework, dancing—are beneficial if done regularly and over the long term. Exercise can increase HDL, lower triglycerides, and reduce coronary risks in several ways.

hypertension Sustained elevated blood pressure.
systolic pressure The upper number in the fraction that measures blood pressure, indicating pressure on the walls of the arteries when the heart contracts.
diastolic pressure The lower number in the fraction that measures blood pressure, indicating pressure on the walls of the arteries during the relaxation phase of heart activity.

Control Diabetes Research underscores the unique CVD risks for people with diabetes.[22] Diabetics who have taken insulin for a number of years have a greater chance of developing CVD. In fact, CVD is the leading cause of death among diabetic patients. Because overweight people have a higher risk for diabetes, distinguishing between the effects of the two conditions is difficult. People with diabetes also tend to have elevated blood fat levels, increased atherosclerosis, and a tendency toward deterioration of small blood vessels, particularly in the eyes and extremities. However, through a prescribed regimen of diet, exercise, and medication, they can control much of their increased risk for CVD.

Did you Know? At an international conference on the health benefits of cocoa, researchers revealed that cocoa flavonol molecules found in chocolate may reduce the risk of blood clotting and improve blood flow in the brain!

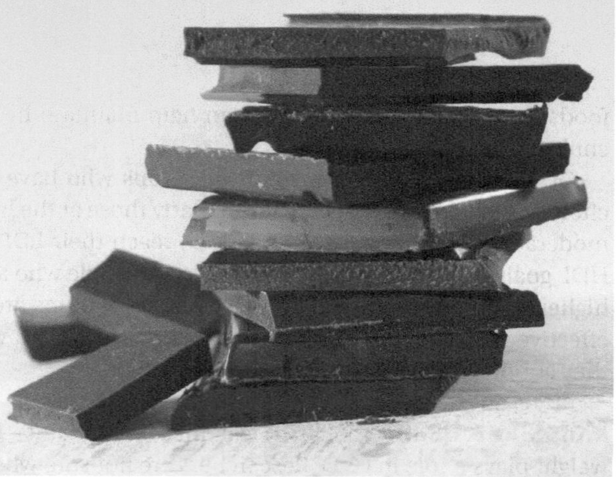

Petros Tsonis/iStockphoto

Control Your Blood Pressure **Hypertension** refers to sustained high blood pressure. In general, the higher your blood pressure is, the greater your risk will be for CVD. Hypertension is known as the silent killer because it usually has no symptoms. Its prevalence has increased by over 30 percent in the past 10 years; today one in three adults in the United States has blood pressure above the recommended level.[23] The prevalence of high blood pressure in Blacks in the United States is among the highest in the world and it's increasing. More than 44 percent of Black women have HBP, compared to 28 percent among white women.

Blood pressure is measured in two parts and is expressed as a fraction—for example, 110/80, or "110 over 80." Both values are measured in *millimeters of mercury* (mm Hg). The first number refers to **systolic pressure,** or the pressure being applied to the walls of the arteries when the heart contracts, pumping blood to the rest of the body. The second value is **diastolic pressure,** or the pressure applied to the walls of the arteries during the heart's relaxation phase. During this phase, blood is reentering the chambers of the heart, preparing for the next heartbeat.

Normal blood pressure varies depending on weight; age; physical condition; and for different groups of people, such as women and minorities. Systolic blood pressure tends to increase with age, whereas diastolic blood pressure increases until age 55 and then declines. As a rule, men have a greater risk for high blood pressure than do women until age 55, when their risks become about equal. After age 75, women are more likely to have high blood pressure than men.[24]

For the average person, 110/80 is a healthy blood pressure level. High blood pressure is usually diagnosed when systolic pressure is 140 or above. Diastolic pressure does not have to be high to indicate high blood pressure. When only systolic pressure is high, the condition is known as *isolated systolic hypertension (ISH),* the most common form of high blood pressure in older Americans. See Table 2 for a summary of blood pressure values and what they mean.

Treatment of hypertension can involve dietary changes (reducing sodium and calorie intake), weight loss (when appropriate), the use of diuretics and other medications (only when prescribed by a physician), regular exercise, treatment of sleep disorders such as sleep apnea, and the practice of relaxation techniques and effective coping and communication skills.

Manage Stress Some scientists have noted a relationship between CVD risk and a person's stress level, behavior habits, and socioeconomic status. These factors may influence established risk factors. For example, people under stress may start smoking or smoke more than they otherwise

TABLE 2 **Blood Pressure Classifications**

Classification	Systolic Reading (mm Hg)		Diastolic Reading (mm Hg)
Normal	<120	and	<80
Prehypertension	120–139	or	80–89
Hypertension			
Stage 1	140–159	or	90–99
Stage 2	≥160	or	≥100

Note: If systolic and diastolic readings fall into different categories, treatment is determined by the highest category. Readings are based on the average of two or more properly measured, seated readings on each of two or more health care provider visits.

Source: National Heart, Lung, and Blood Institute, *The Seventh Report of the Joint National Committee on Prevention, Detection, Evaluation, and Treatment of High Blood Pressure* (NIH Publication no. 03-5233) (Bethesda, MD: National Institutes of Health, revised June 2005).

would. A large study funded by the National Heart, Lung, and Blood Institute found that impatience and hostility, two key components of the Type A behavior pattern, increase young adults' risk of developing high blood pressure. Other related factors, such as competitiveness, depression, and anxiety, did not appear to increase risk. In recent years, scientists have tended to agree that unresolved stress—whether real or perceived, personal, work related, or from a combination of factors—appears to increase risk for hypertension, heart disease, and stroke. Although the exact mechanism is unknown, scientists are closer to discovering why stress can affect us so negatively. Newer studies indicate that chronic stress may result in three times the risk of hypertension, CHD, and sudden cardiac death and that there is a link between anxiety, depression, and negative cardiovascular effects.[25]

Nonmodifiable Risks

There are, unfortunately, some risk factors for CVD that we cannot prevent or control. The most important are these:

- **Race and ethnicity.** African Americans are at 45 percent greater risk for hypertension and heart disease and tend to have more severe levels of high blood pressure than Caucasians. The rate of high blood pressure in African Americans is among the highest in the world. Heart disease risk is also higher among Mexican Americans, Native Americans, and native Hawaiians (partly due to higher rates of obesity and diabetes).
- **Heredity.** A family history of heart disease appears to increase risk significantly.[26] In fact, as stated previously, the amount of cholesterol you produce, tendencies to form plaque, and a host of other factors seem to have genetic links. If you have close relatives with CVD, your risk may be double that of others. The younger these relatives are, and the closer their relationship to you (parents or siblings, in particular), the greater your risk will be. The difficulty comes in sorting out genetic influences from the multiple confounders common among family members that may also influence risk, including environment, stress, dietary habits, and so on. Newer research has focused on studying the interactions between nutrition and genes (nutrigenetics) and the role that diet may play in increasing or decreasing risks among certain genetic profiles.[27]
- **Age.** Although cardiovascular disease can affect people of any age, 75 percent of all heart attacks occur in people over age 65. The rate of CVD increases with age for both sexes.
- **Gender.** Men are at greater risk for CVD until about age 60. Women under age 35 have a fairly low risk unless they have high blood pressure, kidney problems, or diabetes. Using oral contraceptives and smoking also increase the risk. Hormonal factors appear to reduce risk for women, although after menopause or after estrogen levels are otherwise reduced (e.g., because of hysterectomy), women's LDL levels tend to go up, which increases their chances for CVD.

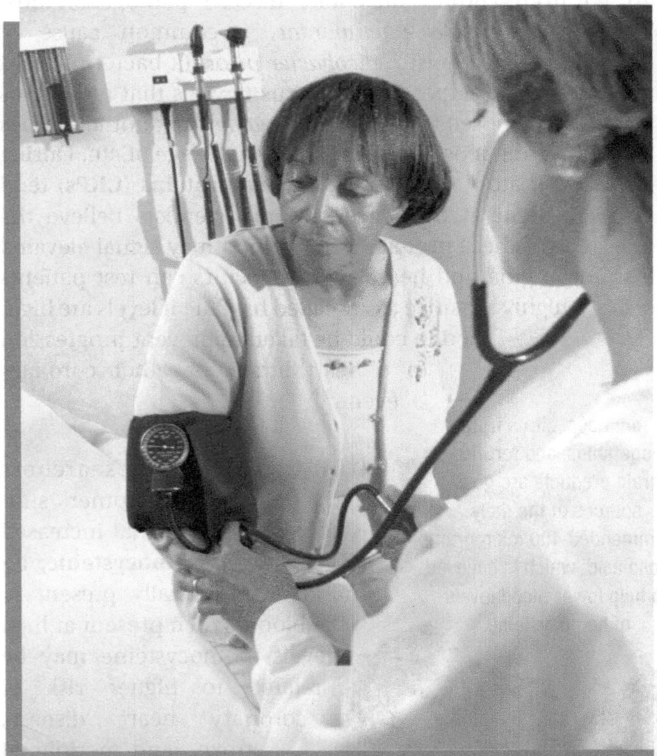

Thinkstock/Jupiter Images

Is heart disease hereditary?

Many behavioral and environmental factors contribute to a person's risk for cardiovascular diseases, but research suggests that there are hereditary aspects as well. If there is a history of CVD in your family or your racial or ethnic background indicates a propensity for CVD, it is all the more important for you to have regular blood pressure and blood cholesterol screenings, and for you to avoid lifestyle risks including tobacco use, physical inactivity, and poor nutrition.

Other Risk Factors Being Studied

Several other factors and indicators have been linked to CVD risk, including inflammation and homocysteine levels.

Inflammation and C-Reactive Protein Recent research has prompted many experts to believe that inflammation may play a major role in atherosclerosis development. Inflammation occurs when tissues are injured by bacteria, trauma, toxins, or heat, among others. Injured vessel walls are more prone to plaque formation. To date, several factors, including cigarette smoke, high blood pressure, high LDL cholesterol, diabetes mellitus, certain forms of arthritis, and exposure to toxic substances, have all been linked to increased risk of inflammation. However, the greatest risk appears to be from certain infectious disease pathogens, most notably *Chlamydia pneumoniae,* a common cause of respiratory infections; *Helicobacter pylori* (a bacterium that causes ulcers); herpes simplex virus (a virus that most of us have been exposed to); and *Cytomegalovirus* (another herpes virus infecting most Americans before the age of 40). During an inflammatory reaction, **C-reactive proteins (CRPs)** tend to be present at high levels. Many scientists believe the presence of these proteins in the blood may signal elevated risk for angina and heart attack. Doctors can test patients using a highly sensitive assay called hs-CRP; if levels are high, action could be taken to prevent progression to a heart attack or other coronary event.[28]

C-reactive protein (CRP) A protein whose blood levels rise in response to inflammation.
homocysteine An amino acid normally present in the blood that, when found at high levels, may be related to higher risk of cardiovascular disease.
electrocardiogram (ECG) A record of the electrical activity of the heart; may be measured during a stress test.
angiography A technique for examining blockages in heart arteries.

Homocysteine Researchers have discovered another substance that may signal increased risk for CVD: **homocysteine,** an amino acid normally present in the blood. When present at high levels, homocysteine may be related to higher risk of coronary heart disease, stroke, and peripheral vascular disease. Although research is still in its infancy in this area, scientists hypothesize that homocysteine works in much the same way as CRP, inflaming the inner lining of the arterial walls and promoting fat deposits on the damaged walls and development of blood clots.[29] Folic acid and other B vitamins may help break down homocysteine in the body; however, conclusive evidence of risk reduction from folic acid is not available, and authorities such as the American Heart Association do not currently recommend taking folic acid supplements to lower homocysteine levels and prevent CVD.[30] For now, a healthy, balanced diet that includes at least five servings of fruits and vegetables a day is the best preventive action.

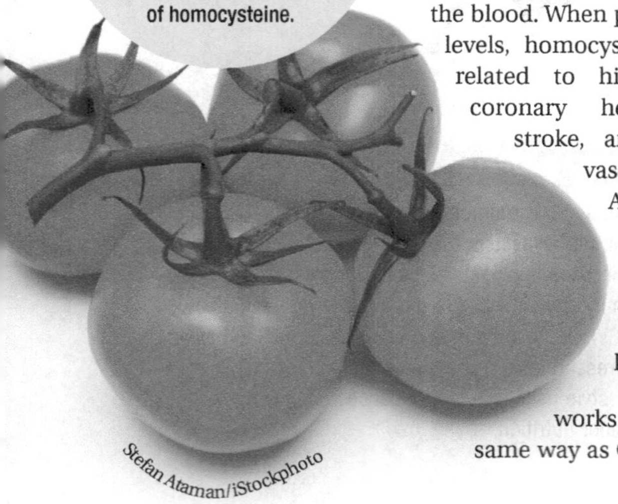

Tomatoes, citrus fruit, vegetables, and fortified grain products are good sources of the daily recommended 400 micrograms of folic acid, which is believed to help lower blood levels of homocysteine.

Stefan Ataman/iStockphoto

Weapons against Cardiovascular Disease

Today, CVD patients have many diagnostic, treatment, prevention, and rehabilitation options that were not available a generation ago. Medications can strengthen heartbeat, control arrhythmias, remove fluids (in the case of congestive heart failure), reduce blood pressure, improve heart function, and reduce pain. Among the most common groups of drugs are the following: s*tatins*, chemicals used to lower blood cholesterol levels; *ace-inhibitors*, which cause the muscles surrounding blood vessels to contract, thereby lowering blood pressure; and *beta-blockers*, which reduce blood pressure by blocking the effects of the hormone epinephrine. New diagnostic procedures, surgical techniques, and devices are saving countless lives. Even long-standing methods of CPR have been changed recently to focus primarily on chest compressions rather than mouth-to-mouth procedures. The thinking behind this is that people will be more likely to do CPR if the risk for exchange of body fluids is reduced—any effort to save a person in trouble is better than inaction.

Techniques for Diagnosing Cardiovascular Disease

Several techniques are used to diagnose CVD, including electrocardiogram, angiography, and positron emission tomography scans. An **electrocardiogram (ECG)** is a record of the electrical activity of the heart. Patients may undergo a *stress test*—standard exercise on a stationary bike or treadmill with an electrocardiogram and no injections—or a *nuclear stress test,* which involves injecting a radioactive dye and taking images of the heart to reveal problems with blood flow. While these tests provide a good indicator of potential heart blockage or blood flow abnormalities, a more accurate method of testing for heart disease is **angiography** (often referred to as *cardiac catheterization*). In this procedure, a needle-thin tube called a *catheter* is threaded through heart arteries, a dye is injected, and an X-ray image is taken to discover which areas are blocked. A more recent and even more effective method of measuring heart activity is *positron emission tomography (PET),* which produces three-dimensional images of the heart as blood flows through it. Other tests include the following:

- **Magnetic resonance imaging (MRI).** This test uses powerful magnets to look inside the body. Computer-generated pictures can show the heart muscle and help physicians identify damage from a heart attack and evaluate disease of larger blood vessels such as the aorta.
- **Ultrafast computed tomography (CT).** This is an especially fast form of X-ray imaging of the heart designed to evaluate bypass grafts, diagnose ventricular function, and measure calcium deposits.

One of the newest forms of CT scans is used to assess your *cardiac calcium score,* an indicator of the level of calcium in the plaque in your coronary arteries: The greater amount of calcium, the higher your calcium score and the greater your risk of heart attack. Although some people ask for this as a noninvasive measure of risk (compared to angiograms), recent reports of high radiation levels from some machines have caused many to rethink this procedure.

Bypass Surgery and Angioplasty

Coronary bypass surgery has helped many patients who suffered coronary blockages or heart attacks. In a coronary artery bypass graft (CABG, referred to as a "cabbage"), a blood vessel is taken from another site in the patient's body (usually the saphenous vein in the leg or the internal thoracic artery in the chest) and implanted to "bypass" blocked coronary arteries and transport blood to heart tissue.

Another procedure, **angioplasty** (sometimes called *balloon angioplasty*), carries fewer risks and may be more effective than bypass surgery in selected cases. As in angiography, a thin catheter is threaded through blocked heart arteries. The catheter has a balloon at the tip, which is inflated to flatten fatty deposits against the artery walls, allowing blood to flow more freely. A *stent* (a meshlike tube) may be inserted to prop open the artery. In about 30 percent of patients, the treated arteries become clogged again within 6 months. Some surgeons argue that given this high rate of recurrence, bypass may be a more effective treatment. Today, newer forms of laser angioplasty and *atherectomy,* a procedure that removes plaque, are being done in several clinics.

Can Aspirin Help Heart Disease?

Today, over 50 million people (36% of all adults) pop an aspirin everyday, believing that this will prevent a heart attack.[31] Research indicates that low doses of aspirin (75–81 mg daily or every other day) are beneficial to heart patients because of the drug's blood-thinning properties. Higher levels do not provide significantly more protection. Aspirin has even been advised as a preventive strategy for people with no current heart disease symptoms. Major problems associated with chronic aspirin use are gastrointestinal intolerance and a tendency for some people to have difficulty with blood clotting, and these factors may outweigh aspirin's benefits in some cases.

An Overview of Cancer

Although heart disease is the number one cause of death in the United States, cancer continues to be the second leading cause of death for all age groups, even though cancer-related mortality rates have declined over the past decade.[32] **Five-year survival rates** (the relative rates for survival in persons who are living 5 years after diagnosis) are up dramatically from the virtual death sentences of many cancers in the early 1900s and the 40 to 50 percent survival rates of the 1960s and 1970s. Today, of the approximately 1.5 million people diagnosed each year, about 66 percent will still be alive 5 years from now.[33] Many will be considered "cured," meaning that they have no subsequent cancer in their bodies and can expect to live a long and productive life. Improvements in diagnosis and treatment mean that cancers that used to present a very poor outlook are often cured today.

coronary bypass surgery A surgical technique whereby a blood vessel taken from another part of the body is implanted to bypass a clogged coronary artery.

angioplasty A technique in which a catheter with a balloon at the tip is inserted into a clogged artery; the balloon is inflated to flatten fatty deposits against artery walls and a stent is typically inserted to keep the artery open.

five-year survival rates The percentage of people in a study or treatment group who are alive 5 years after they were diagnosed with or treated for cancer.

cancer A large group of diseases characterized by the uncontrolled growth and spread of abnormal cells.

25% of all deaths that occur on a given day are from some form of cancer.

During 2009, approximately 562,340 Americans died of cancer, and nearly 1.5 million new cases were diagnosed.[34] Of these, one-third of the cancers were related to poor nutrition, physical inactivity, and obesity, which means they could have been prevented. Certain other cancers are related to exposure to infectious organisms such as hepatitis B virus (HBV), human papillomavirus (HPV; also the cause of genital warts), HIV (the virus that causes AIDS), *Helicobacter pylori* (the bacterium responsible for most peptic ulcers), and others, and could be prevented through behavioral changes, vaccines, or antibiotics.

What Is Cancer?

Cancer is the name given to a large group of diseases characterized by the uncontrolled growth and spread of abnormal cells. If these cells aren't stopped, they can impair vital functions of the body and lead to death. Think of a healthy cell as a small computer, programmed to operate in a particular fashion. When something interrupts normal cell programming, uncontrolled growth and abnormal cellular development result in a **neoplasm,** a new growth of tissue serving no physiological function. This neoplasmic mass often forms a clumping of cells known as a **tumor.**

Not all tumors are **malignant** (cancerous); in fact, most are **benign** (noncancerous). Benign tumors are generally harmless unless they grow to obstruct or crowd out normal tissues. A benign tumor of the brain, for instance, is life threatening when it grows enough to restrict blood flow and cause a stroke. The only way to determine whether a tumor is malignant is through **biopsy,** or microscopic examination of cell development.

neoplasm A new growth of tissue that serves no physiological function and results from uncontrolled, abnormal cellular development.
tumor A neoplasmic mass that grows more rapidly than surrounding tissue.
malignant Very dangerous or harmful; refers to a cancerous tumor.
benign Harmless; refers to a noncancerous tumor.
biopsy Microscopic examination of tissue to determine whether a cancer is present.
metastasis Process by which cancer spreads from one area to different areas of the body.
mutant cells Cells that differ in form, quality, or function from normal cells.
carcinogens Cancer-causing agents.

Benign and malignant tumors differ in several key ways. Benign tumors generally consist of ordinary-looking cells enclosed in a fibrous shell or capsule that prevents their spreading to other body areas. Malignant tumors are usually not enclosed in a protective capsule and can therefore spread to other organs (Figure 5). This process, known as **metastasis,** makes some forms of cancer particularly aggressive in their ability to overcome bodily defenses. By the time they are diagnosed, malignant tumors have frequently metastasized throughout the body, making treatment extremely difficult. Unlike benign tumors, which merely expand to take over a given space, malignant cells invade surrounding tissue, emitting clawlike protrusions that disturb the RNA and DNA within normal cells. Disrupting these substances, which control cellular metabolism and reproduction, produces **mutant cells** that differ in form, quality, and function from normal cells.

What Causes Cancer?

After decades of research, scientists and epidemiologists believe that most cancers are, at least in theory, preventable. Many specific causes of cancer are well documented, the most important of which are represented by two major classes of factors: hereditary risk and acquired (environmental) risk. Heredity factors cannot be modified. Environmental factors are potentially modifiable. In this context they include the macrophysical environment and personal lifestyle factors and situations, such as tobacco use; poor nutrition; physical inactivity; obesity; certain infectious agents; certain medical treatments; drug and alcohol consumption; excessive sun exposure; and exposures to **carcinogens** (cancer-causing agents), such as chemicals in our foods, the air we breathe, the water we drink, and the homes we live in. Several of these hereditary and environmental factors may interact to make cancer more likely, accelerate cancer progression, or increase individual susceptibility during certain periods of life, but the mechanisms are not fully understood. We do not know why some people have malignant cells in their

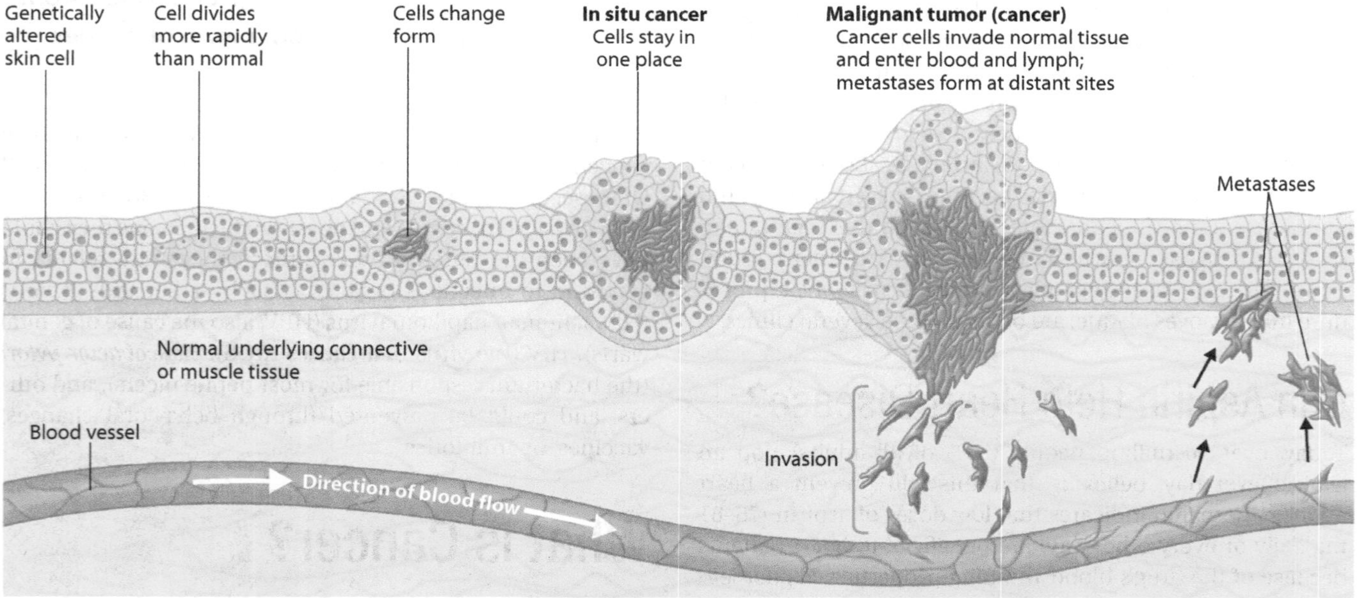

FIGURE 5 **Metastasis**
A mutation to the genetic material of a skin cell triggers abnormal cell division and changes cell formation, resulting in a cancerous tumor. If the tumor remains localized, it is considered *in situ* cancer. If the tumor spreads, it is considered a malignant cancer.

Philippe Psaila/SPL/Photo Researchers

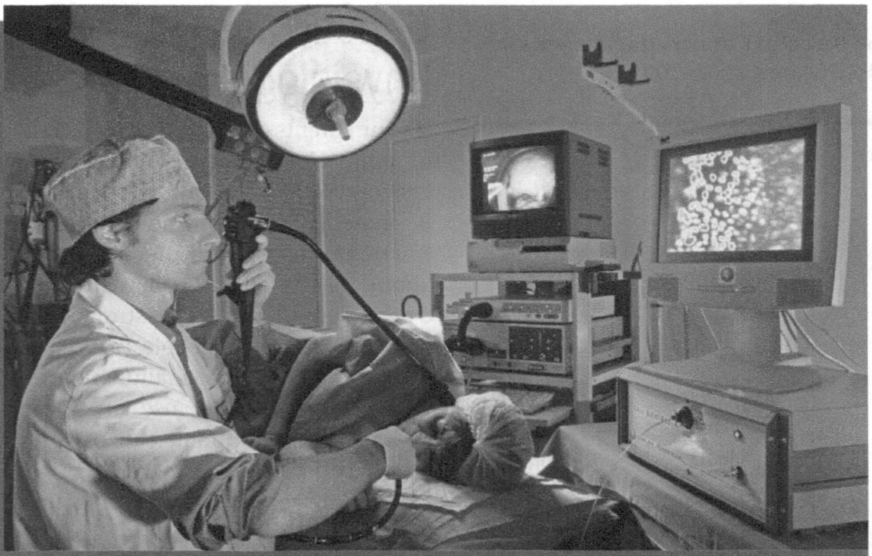

What does it mean for a tumor to be malignant?

A malignant tumor is one whose cells are cancerous. Malignant tumors are generally more dangerous than benign tumors because cancer cells divide quickly and can spread, or metastasize, from the original tumor to other parts of the body. Physicians usually order biopsies of tumors, in which sample cells are taken from the tumor and studied under a microscope to determine whether they are cancerous. Newer techniques, like the minimally invasive "optical biopsy" shown here, allow for the microscopic examination of tissue without doing a physical biopsy.

body and never develop cancer, whereas others may eventually develop the disease.

Lifestyle Risks

Anyone can develop cancer; however, most cases affect adults beginning in middle age. In fact, nearly 76 percent of cancers are diagnosed at age 55 and above. Cancer researchers refer to one's cancer risk when they assess risk factors. *Lifetime risk* refers to the probability that an individual, over the course of a lifetime, will develop cancer or die from it. In the United States, men have a lifetime risk of about one in two; women have a lower risk, at one in three.[35] See Table 3 on the next page for an overview of the probability of developing cancer by age and sex.

Relative risk is a measure of the strength of the relationship between risk factors and a particular cancer. Basically, relative risk compares your risk if you engage in certain known risk behaviors with that of someone who does not engage in such behaviors. For example, if you are a man and smoke, your relative risk of getting lung cancer is about 23 times greater than that of a male nonsmoker.[36]

Over the years, researchers have found that diet, a sedentary lifestyle (and resultant obesity), overconsumption of alcohol, tobacco use, stress, and other lifestyle factors seem to play a role in the incidence of cancer. Keep in mind that a high relative risk does not guarantee cause and effect. It merely indicates the likelihood of a particular risk factor being related to a particular outcome.

Alamy

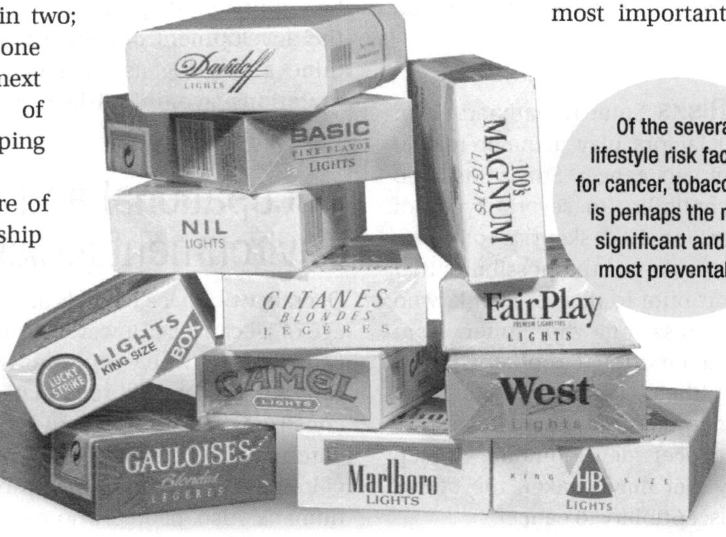

Of the several lifestyle risk factors for cancer, tobacco use is perhaps the most significant and the most preventable.

Tobacco Use Of all the potential risk factors for cancer, smoking is among the greatest. In the United States, tobacco is responsible for nearly one in five deaths annually, accounting for at least 30 percent of all cancer deaths and 87 percent of all lung cancer deaths.[37] In fact, by all accounts, smoking is the leading cause of preventable death in the United States and around the world today.[38] Smoking is associated with increased risk of at least 15 different cancers, including those of the nasopharynx, nasal cavity, paranasal sinuses, lip, oral cavity, pharynx, larynx, lung, esophagus, pancreas, uterine cervix, kidney, bladder, and stomach, and acute myeloid leukemia.

Poor Nutrition, Physical Inactivity, and Obesity Mounting scientific evidence suggests that about one-third of the cancer deaths that occur in the United States each year may be due to lifestyle factors such as overweight or obesity, physical inactivity, and poor nutrition—cancers that can be prevented! Dietary choices and physical activity are the most important modifiable determinants of cancer risk (besides not smoking). Several studies indicate a relationship between a high body mass index (BMI) and death rates from cancers of the esophagus, colon, rectum, liver, stomach, kidney, and pancreas. Newer studies point to differences in risks by gender and race.[39]

Women with a high BMI have a higher mortality rate from breast,

TABLE 3 **Probability of Developing Invasive Cancers during Selected Age Intervals by Sex, United States, 2003–2005***

Site	Sex	Birth to age 39	Ages 40 to 59	Lifetime
All types†	Male	1 in 70	1 in 12	1 in 2
	Female	1 in 48	1 in 11	1 in 3
Breast	Female	1 in 208	1 in 26	1 in 8
Colon and	Male	1 in 1,296	1 in 109	1 in 18
rectum	Female	1 in 1,343	1 in 138	1 in 20
Lung and	Male	1 in 3,398	1 in 101	1 in 13
bronchus	Female	1 in 2,997	1 in 124	1 in 16
Melanoma of	Male	1 in 645	1 in 157	1 in 39
the skin§	Female	1 in 370	1 in 189	1 in 58
Prostate	Male	1 in 10,002	1 in 41	1 in 6
Uterine cervix	Female	1 in 651	1 in 368	1 in 145
Uterine corpus	Female	1 in 1,499	1 in 140	1 in 40

*For people free of cancer at beginning of age interval.
†Excludes basal and squamous cell skin cancers and in situ cancers except in the urinary bladder.
§Statistic is for whites only.

Sources: DevCan: Probability of Developing or Dying of Cancer 6.3.0. Statistical Research and Applications Branch, National Cancer Institute, 2008, http://srab.cancer.gov/devcan; American Cancer Society, Surveillance and Health Policy Research, 2009.

uterine, cervical, and ovarian cancers; men with a high BMI have higher death rates from prostate and stomach cancers. In a study of over 900,000 U.S. adults, 34 percent of all cancer deaths were attributable to overweight and obesity. The relative risk of breast cancer in postmenopausal women is 50 percent higher for obese women than it is for nonobese women, whereas the relative risk of colon cancer in men is 40 percent higher for obese men than it is for nonobese men. The relative risks of gallbladder and endometrial cancers are five times higher in obese individuals than they are in individuals of healthy weight. Numerous other studies support the link between cancer and obesity.[40]

oncogenes Suspected cancer-causing genes.

Stress and Psychosocial Risks Some researchers claim that social and psychological factors play a major role in determining whether a person gets cancer. Stress has been implicated in increased susceptibility to several types of cancers. Although medical personnel are skeptical of overly simplistic solutions, we cannot rule out the possibility that negative emotional states contribute to illness. People who are under chronic, severe stress or who suffer from depression or other persistent emotional problems show higher rates of cancer than their healthy counterparts. Several newer studies appear to support the premise that stress can play a role in cancer development.[41] Sleep disturbances or an unhealthy diet may weaken the body's immune system, increasing susceptibility to cancer.

Genetic and Physiological Risks

If your parents, aunts and uncles, siblings, or other close family members develop cancer, does it mean that you have a genetic predisposition toward it? Although there is still much uncertainty about this, scientists believe that about 5 percent of all cancers are strongly hereditary, in that some people may be more predisposed to the malfunctioning of genes that ultimately cause cancer.[42]

Cancer development can be affected by suspected cancer-causing genes called **oncogenes.** While these genes are typically dormant, certain conditions such as age, stress, and exposure to carcinogens, viruses, and radiation may activate them. Once activated, they cause cells to grow and reproduce uncontrollably. Scientists are uncertain whether only people who develop cancer have oncogenes, or whether we all have genes that can become oncogenes under certain conditions.

Certain cancers, particularly those of the breast, stomach, colon, prostate, uterus, ovaries, and lungs, appear to run in families. For example, a woman runs a much higher risk of breast cancer if her mother or sisters (primary relatives) have had the disease, particularly at a young age. Hodgkin's disease and certain leukemias show similar familial patterns. Can we attribute these familial patterns to genetic susceptibility or to the fact that people in the same families experience similar environmental risks? To date, the research in this area is inconclusive. It is possible that we can inherit a tendency toward a cancer-prone, weak immune system or, conversely, that we can inherit a cancer-fighting potential. But the complex interaction of hereditary predisposition, lifestyle, and environment on the development of cancer makes it a challenge to determine a single cause. Even among those predisposed to mutations, avoiding risks may decrease chances of cancer development.

Occupational and Environmental Risks

Overall, workplace hazards account for only a small percentage of all cancers. However, various substances are known to cause cancer when exposure levels are high or prolonged. One is asbestos, a fibrous material once widely used in the construction, insulation, and automobile industries. Nickel, chromate, and chemicals such as benzene, arsenic, and vinyl chloride have been shown definitively to be carcinogens for humans. Also, people who routinely work with certain dyes

GREEN GUIDE

Go Green against Cancer

We live in an environment that is filled with potential cancer-causing agents. Some of them are natural, but many are created by humans, or increased by human activities. There are many things you can do to help reduce the number of carcinogens in the environment and to limit your exposure to those that are there. The following are just a few ideas:

1. Leave the car at home. Try commuting by bicycle or by foot instead of driving a vehicle. This will reduce your daily carbon emissions and your risk for cancer by increasing your physical activity.
2. Choose organic foods when possible. Conventional produce is often sprayed with chemicals and pesticides. When we eat these chemicals, our risk for cancer can be elevated.
3. When shopping for home furnishings, explore ecofriendly furniture, upholstery, and home textiles. Many furnishings are manufactured with toxic chemicals that are released into the air. This can dramatically reduce indoor air quality and increase your risk for cancer. Select products that have not been treated with stain-resistant chemicals and look for ecofriendly flooring, carpets, and other products to ensure the best possible indoor air quality and minimize carcinogenic exposures. Such ecofriendly products include bamboo (which is really a grass and not a wood), recycled glass tiles, recycled metal tiles, cork flooring, and flooring made from reclaimed wood products.
4. Turn off your lights. According to sleep experts and others, artificial light decreases the production of melatonin, a hormone manufactured in the brain that is produced during sleep cycles. This hormone is being shown to have a protective effect against some forms of cancer.
5. Use "green" paper. By purchasing ecofriendly paper products that are bleach free, we reduce the amount of dioxins released into the atmosphere. Dioxins are carcinogenic, and fewer of them in the atmosphere will reduce everyone's risk for cancer.
6. Buy ecofriendly hygiene products. When purchasing personal hygiene products or cosmetics, select items that are environmentally responsible. Many products contain petroleum and plastics, agents that are not good for your skin or the environment. Consider avoiding the following:
   * Diethanolamine (DEA), commonly found in shampoos, is thought to be carcinogenic.
   * Formaldehyde, commonly found in eye shadows, is well known as a carcinogenic agent.
   * Phthalates, found in many hygiene and cosmetic products such as nail polish and perfumes, are thought to be carcinogenic.
   * Parabens, used as preservatives in food and cosmetic products such as makeup, lotion, shampoo, and soap, have been found in breast tumors and are being researched as potential carcinogens.
7. Avoid dry cleaning. Try to avoid buying clothes that require dry cleaning. Conventional dry cleaning uses a chemical called *perchloroethylene* (PERC), an agent known to increase the risk for cancer and harm the environment. If dry cleaning is unavoidable, explore local dry cleaners using ecofriendly alternatives such as "wet cleaning," which includes biodegradable soaps or silicone-based solvents and special machinery used to reduce shrinkage.

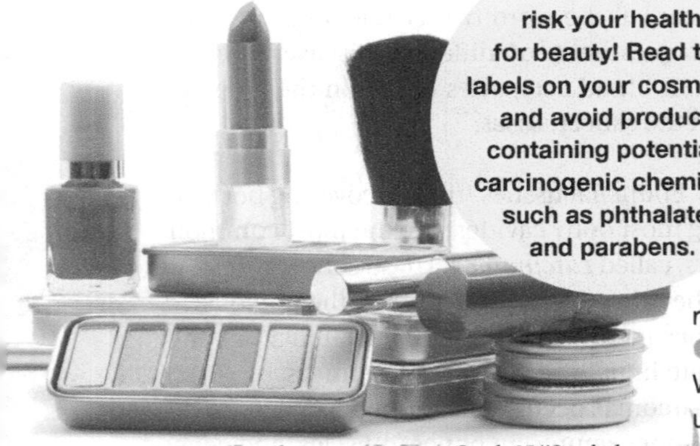

Don't risk your health for beauty! Read the labels on your cosmetics and avoid products containing potentially carcinogenic chemicals such as phthalates and parabens.

Gordo25/iStockphoto

and radioactive substances may have increased risks for cancer. Working with coal tars, as in the mining profession, or with inhalants, as in the auto-painting business, is hazardous. So is working with herbicides and pesticides, although the evidence is inconclusive for low-dose exposures. Several federal and state agencies are responsible for monitoring such exposures and ensuring that businesses comply with standards designed to protect workers.

You don't have to work in one of these industries to come in contact with environmental carcinogens. See the **Green Guide** above to explore some ways you can avoid carcinogens in the products you buy and use every day.

Radiation Ionizing radiation (IR)—radiation from X rays, radon, cosmic rays, and ultraviolet radiation (primarily ultraviolet B, or UVB radiation)—is the only form of radiation proven to cause human cancer. Evidence that high-dose IR causes cancer comes from studies of atomic bomb survivors, patients receiving radiotherapy, and certain occupational groups (e.g., uranium miners). Virtually any part of the body can be affected by IR, but bone marrow and the thyroid are particularly susceptible. Radon exposure in homes can increase lung cancer risk, especially in cigarette smokers. To reduce the risk of harmful effects, diagnostic medical and dental X rays are set at the lowest dose levels possible.

Nonionizing radiation produced by radio waves, cell phones, microwaves, computer screens, televisions, electric blankets, and other products has been a topic of great concern in recent years, but research has not proven excess risk to date. Although highly controversial, some suggest that cell phones beam radio frequency energy that can penetrate the brain, raising concerns about cancers of the head and neck, brain tumors, or leukemia. Most research, including the biggest study of cancer and cell phone risk to date, indicate that having a cell phone glued to your ear for hours causes little more than a sore ear and a hefty bill.[43]

Chemicals in Foods Among the food additives suspected of causing cancer is *sodium nitrate,* a chemical used to preserve and give color to red meat. The actual carcinogen is not sodium nitrate but *nitrosamines,* substances formed when the body digests sodium nitrate. Sodium nitrate has not been banned, primarily because it kills *Clostridium botulinum,* the bacterium that causes the highly virulent foodborne disease botulism. It should also be noted that the bacteria found in the human intestinal tract may contain more nitrates than a person could ever take in from eating cured meats or other nitrate-containing food products. Nonetheless, concern about the carcinogenic properties of nitrates has led to the introduction of meats that are free of nitrates or contain reduced levels of the substance.

Much of the concern about chemicals in foods centers on the possible harm caused by pesticide and herbicide residues. Although some of these chemicals cause cancer at high doses in experimental animals, the very low concentrations found in some foods are well within established government safety levels. Continued research regarding pesticide and herbicide use is essential, and scientists and consumer groups stress the importance of a balance between chemical use and the production of high-quality food products. Prevention efforts should focus on policies to protect consumers, develop low-chemical pesticides and herbicides, and reduce environmental pollution.

Infectious Diseases and Cancer

According to recent estimates, 15 percent of new cancers worldwide in 2007 were attributable to infection. Rates of cancers related to infections are about three times higher in developing countries than in developed countries (26% vs. 8%).[44] Infections are thought to influence cancer development in several ways, most commonly through chronic inflammation, suppression of the immune system, or chronic stimulation.

Hepatitis B, Hepatitis C, and Liver Cancer Viruses such as hepatitis B (HBV) and C (HCV) are believed to stimulate the growth of cancer cells in the liver because they are chronic diseases that inflame liver tissue. This may prime the liver for cancer or make it more hospitable for cancer development. Global increases in hepatitis B and C rates and concurrent rises in liver cancer rates seem to provide evidence of such an association.

Human Papillomavirus and Cervical Cancer Nearly 100 percent of women with cervical cancer have evidence of human papillomavirus (HPV) infection, believed to be a major cause of cervical cancer. Fortunately, only a small percentage of HPV cases progress to cervical cancer.[45] Today, a new vaccine is available to help protect young women from becoming infected with HPV and developing cervical cancer. However, as of this writing, preliminary questions have been raised about the safety and potential minor adverse effects of this vaccine.

what do you think?

How do we determine whether a behavior or substance is a risk factor for a disease? ● Although a direct causal relationship between lung cancer and smoking has not been proved, the evidence supporting such a relationship is strong. Must a clearly established causal link exist before consumers are warned about risk? ● How does the consumer know what to believe?

Types of Cancers

As mentioned earlier, the word *cancer* refers not to a single disease, but to hundreds of different diseases. They are grouped into four broad categories based on the type of tissue from which the cancer arises:

- **Carcinomas.** Epithelial tissues (tissues covering body surfaces and lining most body cavities) are the most common sites for cancers, called *carcinomas.* These cancers affect the outer layer of the skin and mouth as well as the mucous membranes. They metastasize through the circulatory or lymphatic system initially and form solid tumors.
- **Sarcomas.** Sarcomas occur in the mesodermal, or middle, layers of tissue—for example, in bones, muscles, and general connective tissue. They metastasize primarily via the blood in the early stages of disease. These cancers are less common but generally more virulent than carcinomas. They also form solid tumors.
- **Lymphomas.** Lymphomas develop in the lymphatic system—the infection-fighting regions of the body—and metastasize through the lymphatic system. Hodgkin's disease is an example. Lymphomas also form solid tumors.
- **Leukemias.** Cancer of the blood-forming parts of the body, particularly the bone marrow and spleen, is called leukemia. A nonsolid tumor, leukemia is characterized by an abnormal increase in the number of white blood cells.

Figure 6 shows the most common sites of cancer and the number of new cases and deaths from each type in 2009. A comprehensive discussion of the many different forms of

Estimated New Cases of Cancer *

Male	Female
Prostate 192,280 (25%)	**Breast** 192,370 (27%)
Lung & bronchus 116,090 (15%)	**Lung & bronchus** 103,350 (14%)
Colon & rectum 75,590 (10%)	**Colon & rectum** 71,380 (10%)
Urinary bladder 52,810 (7%)	**Uterine corpus** 42,160 (6%)
Melanoma of the skin 39,080 (5%)	**Non-Hodgkin lymphoma** 29,990 (4%)
Non-Hodgkin lymphoma 35,990 (5%)	**Melanoma of the skin** 29,640 (4%)
Kidney & renal pelvis 35,430 (5%)	**Thyroid** 27,200 (4%)
Leukemia 25,630 (3%)	**Kidney & renal pelvis** 22,330 (3%)
Oral cavity & pharynx 25,240 (3%)	**Ovary** 21,550 (3%)
Pancreas 21,050 (3%)	**Pancreas** 21,420 (3%)
All Sites 766,130 (100%)	**All Sites** 713,220 (100%)

Estimated Deaths from Cancer *

Male	Female
Lung & bronchus 88,900 (30%)	**Lung & bronchus** 70,490 (26%)
Prostate 27,360 (9%)	**Breast** 40,170 (15%)
Colon & rectum 25,240 (9%)	**Colon & rectum** 24,680 (9%)
Pancreas 18,030 (6%)	**Pancreas** 17,210 (6%)
Leukemia 12,590 (4%)	**Ovary** 14,600 (5%)
Liver & intrahepatic bile duct 12,090 (4%)	**Non-Hodgkin lymphoma** 9,670 (4%)
Esophagus 11,490 (4%)	**Leukemia** 9,280 (3%)
Urinary bladder 10,180 (3%)	**Uterine corpus** 7,780 (3%)
Non-Hodgkin lymphoma 9,830 (3%)	**Liver & intrahepatic bile duct** 6,070 (2%)
Kidney & renal pelvis 8,160 (3%)	**Brain & other nervous system** 5,590 (2%)
All Sites 292,540 (100%)	**All Sites** 269,800 (100%)

*Excludes basal and squamous cell skin cancers and in situ carcinoma except urinary bladder. Percentages may not total 100% due to rounding.

FIGURE 6 **Leading Sites of New Cancer Cases and Deaths, 2009 Estimates**

Source: *Cancer Facts and Figures 2009*. Copyright © 2009, American Cancer Society. Used with permission from American Cancer Society, Atlanta, GA.

cancer is beyond the scope of this text, but we will discuss the most common types in the next sections.

90% of all lung cancers could be avoided if people did not smoke.

Lung Cancer

Lung cancer is the leading cause of cancer deaths for both men and women in the United States, killing an estimated 159,390 Americans in 2009, even as rates for men and women have decreased in recent decades due to declines in smoking and policies that prohibit smoking in public places.[46] Since 1987, more women have died each year from lung cancer than from breast cancer, which over the previous 40 years had been the major cause of cancer deaths in women. Although past reductions in smoking rates have boded well for cancer and CVD statistics, there is growing concern about the number of youth, particularly young women and persons of low income and low educational level, who continue to pick up the habit.

Detection, Symptoms, and Treatment Symptoms of lung cancer include a persistent cough, blood-streaked sputum, chest pain, and recurrent attacks of pneumonia or bronchitis. Treatment depends on the type and stage of the cancer. Surgery, radiation therapy, and chemotherapy are all options. If the cancer is localized, surgery is usually the treatment of choice. If it has spread, surgery is combined with radiation and chemotherapy. Unfortunately, despite advances in medical technology, survival rates 1 year after diagnosis are low, at only 41 percent overall. Newer tests, such as low-dose computerized tomography (CT) scans, molecular markers in sputum, and improved biopsy techniques, have helped improve diagnosis, but we still have a long way to go.

Risk Factors and Prevention Smokers, especially those who have smoked for more than 20 years, and people who have been exposed to industrial substances such as arsenic and asbestos or to radiation are at the highest risk for lung cancer. Exposure to secondhand cigarette smoke increases the risk for nonsmokers. Apparent increases in lung cancer among nonsmokers have caused increasing concern about the hazards of secondhand smoke, leading health advocates to argue vigorously for smoking bans.[47]

Breast Cancer

In 2009, approximately 192,370 women and 1,910 men in the United States were diagnosed with invasive breast cancer for the first time. In addition, 62,280 new cases of in situ breast cancer, a more localized cancer, were diagnosed. About 40,170 women (and 440 men) died, making breast cancer the

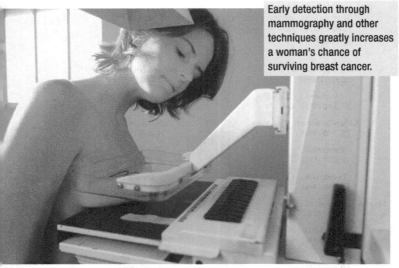

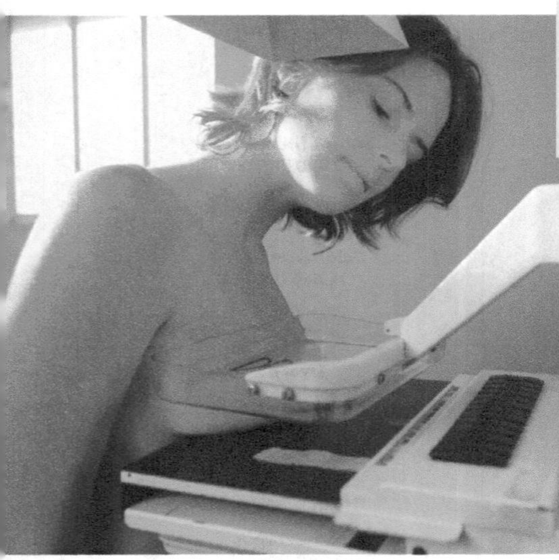

Early detection through mammography and other techniques greatly increases a woman's chance of surviving breast cancer.

Garo.Photo Researchers

second leading cause of cancer death for women, even as rates continue to level off.[48]

Detection, Symptoms, and Treatment The earliest signs of breast cancer are usually observable on mammograms, often before lumps can be felt. However, mammograms are not foolproof. Hence, regular breast self-examination (BSE) is also important (see the **Gender & Health** box on the next page). Although mammograms detect between 80 and 90 percent of breast cancers in women without symptoms, a newer form of magnetic resonance imaging (MRI) appears to be more accurate, particularly in women with genetic risks for tumors.

Once breast cancer has grown enough that it can be felt by palpating the area, many women will recognize the threat and seek medical care. Symptoms may include persistent breast changes, such as a lump in the breast or surrounding lymph nodes, thickening, dimpling, skin irritation, distortion, retraction or scaliness of the nipple, nipple discharge, or tenderness.

Treatments range from a lumpectomy to radical mastectomy to various combinations of radiation or chemotherapy. Among nonsurgical options, promising results have been noted among women using *selective estrogen-receptor modulators (SERMs)* such as tamoxifen and raloxifene, particularly among women whose cancers appear to grow in response to estrogen. These drugs, as well as new *aromatase inhibitors,* work by blocking estrogen. The 5-year survival rate for people with localized breast cancer (which includes all people living 5 years after diagnosis, whether they are in remission, disease free, or under treatment) has risen from 80 percent in the 1950s to 98 percent today. However, these statistics vary dramatically, based on the stage of the cancer when it is first detected and whether it has spread. As with most cancers, the earlier the stage in which it is caught, the greater the chances will be for a full recovery.

Risk Factors and Prevention The incidence of breast cancer increases with age. Although there are many possible risk factors, those that are well supported by research include family history of breast cancer, menstrual periods that started early and ended late in life, obesity after menopause, recent use of oral contraceptives or postmenopausal hormone therapy, never having children or having a first child after age 30, consuming two or more drinks of alcohol per day, and physical inactivity.[49] Genes appear to account for approximately 5 to 10 percent of all cases of breast cancer. Screening for mutations in the *BRCA1* and *BRCA2* genes is recommended for women with a family history of breast cancer.

International differences in breast cancer incidence correlate with variations in diet, especially fat intake, although a causal role for these dietary factors has not been firmly established. Sudden weight gain has also been implicated. Research also shows that regular exercise, even some forms of recreational exercise, can reduce risk.[50]

Colon and Rectal Cancers

Colorectal cancers (cancers of the colon and rectum) continue to be the third most common cancer in both men and women, with over 146,970 cases diagnosed in the United States in 2009.[51] Although colon cancer rates have increased steadily in recent decades, many people are unaware of their risk.

Detection, Symptoms, and Treatment In its early stages, colorectal cancer has no symptoms. Bleeding from the rectum, blood in the stool, and changes in bowel habits are the major warning signals. Because colorectal cancer tends to spread slowly, the prognosis is quite good if it is caught in the early stages. However, only 21 percent of all Americans over age 50 have had the most basic screening test—the fecal occult blood test—in the past 5 years, and only 33 percent have had a colonoscopy during the same time period. Colonoscopy or barium enemas are recommended screening tests for at-risk populations and everybody over age 50. Treatment often consists of radiation or surgery. Chemotherapy, although not used extensively in the past, is today a possibility.

Risk Factors and Prevention Anyone can get colorectal cancer, but people who are over age 50, who are obese, who have a family history of colon and rectal cancer, a personal or family history of polyps (benign growths) in the colon or rectum, or who have inflammatory bowel problems such as colitis run an increased risk. Other possible risk factors include diets high in fat or low in fiber, smoking, sedentary lifestyle, high alcohol consumption, and low intake of fruits and vegetables. Indeed, approximately 90 percent of all colorectal cancers are preventable.

Regular exercise, a diet with lots of fruits and other plant foods, a healthy weight, and moderation in alcohol consumption appear to be among the most promising prevention strategies. Consumption of milk and calcium appears to decrease risks. New research suggests that aspirin-like drugs,

Gender&Health

Breast Awareness and Self-Exam

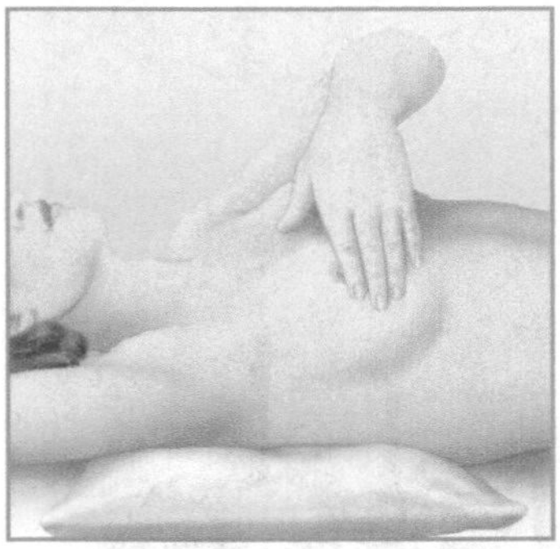

1 Perform exam lying down.

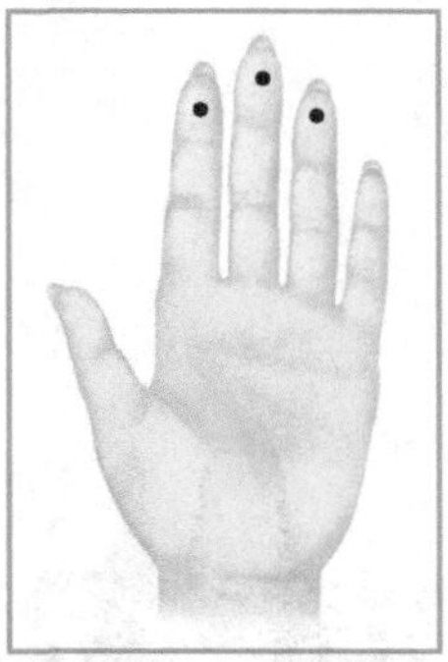

2 Use pads of the 3 middle fingers.

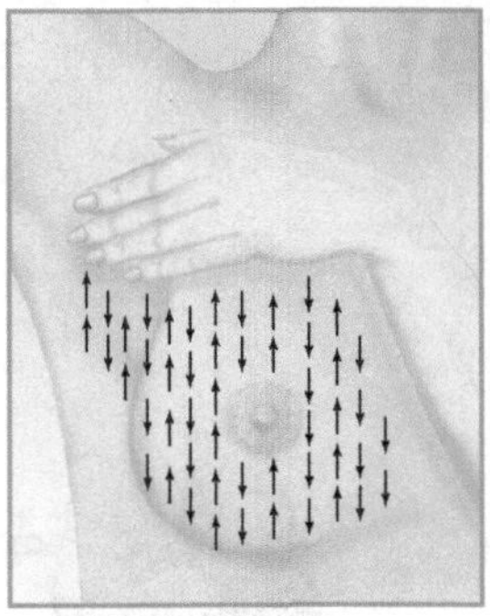

3 Follow an up-and-down pattern.

Women should know how their breasts normally look and feel and report any new breast changes to a health professional as soon as these changes are noted. Finding a breast change does not necessarily mean there is a cancer. A woman can notice changes by being aware of how her breasts normally look and feel and by feeling her breasts for changes (breast awareness), or by choosing to use a step-by-step approach (see below) and using a specific schedule to examine her breasts.

The best time for a woman to examine her breasts is when the breasts are not tender or swollen. Women who examine their breasts should have their technique reviewed during their periodic health exams by their health care professional. Note that the American Cancer Society recommends the use of mammography and clinical breast exam in addition to self-examination.

HOW TO EXAMINE YOUR BREASTS

* Lie down and place your right arm behind your head (1). When you are lying down, the breast tissue spreads evenly over the chest wall and is as thin as possible, making it much easier to feel all the breast tissue.
* Use the finger pads of the three middle fingers on your left hand to feel for lumps in the right breast (2). Use overlapping dime-sized circular motions of the finger pads to feel the tissue.
* Use three different levels of pressure to feel all the breast tissue. Light pressure is needed to feel the tissue closest to the skin; medium pressure to feel a little deeper; and firm pressure to feel the tissue closest to the chest and ribs. A firm ridge in the lower curve of each breast is normal. If you're not sure how hard to press, talk with your doctor or nurse. Use each pressure level to feel the breast tissue before moving on to the next spot.
* Move around the breast in an up-and-down pattern starting at an imaginary line drawn straight down your side from the underarm and moving across the breast to the middle of the chest bone (sternum or breastbone) (3). Be sure to check the entire breast area going down until you feel only ribs and up to the neck or collarbone (clavicle).
* Repeat the exam on your left breast, using the finger pads of the right hand.
* While standing in front of a mirror with your hands pressing firmly down on your hips, look at your breasts for any changes of size, shape, contour, or dimpling, or redness or scaliness of the nipple or breast skin. (The pressing down on the hips position contracts the chest wall muscles and enhances any breast changes.)
* Examine each underarm while sitting up or standing and with your arm only slightly raised so you can easily feel in this area. Raising your arm straight up tightens the tissue in this area and makes it harder to examine.

Source: American Cancer Society, "Breast Awareness and Self-Examination," Revised May 13, 2009, www.cancer.org/docroot/CRI/content/CRI_2_4_3X_Can_breast_cancer_be_found_early_5.asp. Reprinted by the permission of the American Cancer Society, Inc. from www.cancer.org.

postmenopausal hormones, folic acid, calcium supplements, selenium, and vitamin E may also help.

Skin Cancer

Skin cancer is the most common form of cancer in the United States today, affecting over 1 million people every year (one in five of all adults). In 2009, an estimated 11,590 people died of skin cancer (8,420 from melanoma and 2,940 from other forms of skin cancer).[52] **Malignant melanoma,** the deadliest form of skin cancer, is beginning to occur at a much higher rate in women under age 40. In fact, the highly virulent malignant melanoma has become the most frequent cancer in women aged 25 to 29 and runs second only to breast cancer in women aged 30 to 34.

Detection, Symptoms, and Treatment Many people do not know what to look for when examining themselves for skin cancer. Fortunately, potentially cancerous growths are often visible as abnormalities on the skin. Basal and squamous cell carcinomas can be a recurrent annoyance, showing up most commonly on the face, ears, neck, arms, hands, and legs as warty bumps, colored spots, or scaly patches. Bleeding, itchiness, pain, or oozing are other symptoms that warrant

malignant melanoma A virulent cancer of the melanocytes (pigment-producing cells) of the skin.

James Doberman/Getty Images

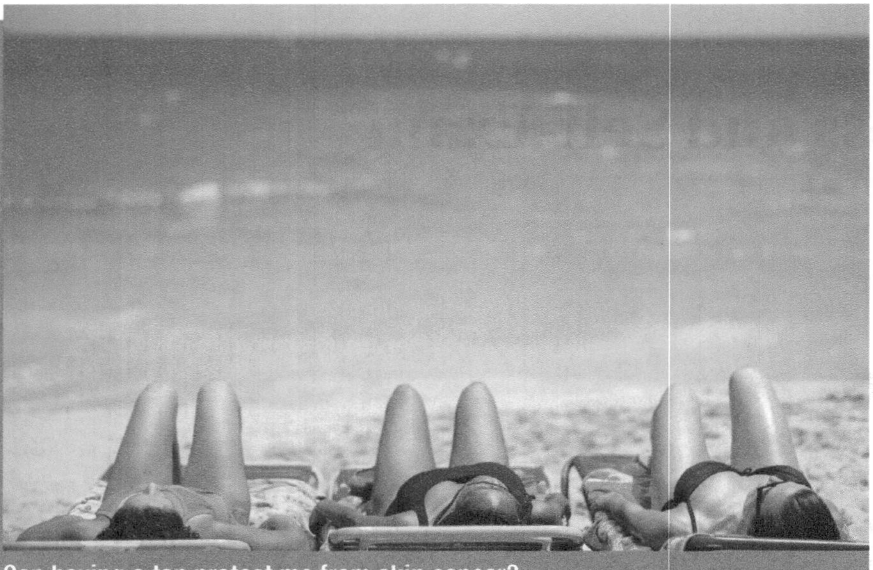

Can having a tan protect me from skin cancer?

It might seem logical that a person's tanned skin would offer protection from the sun's damaging UV rays, but the idea that tanning is healthy and protective has at least three inherent fallacies. First, tanned skin is not healthy but is, by nature, injured skin that has sustained UV-induced damage. Second, a tan isn't protective. According to the American Cancer Society, tanned skin can provide only about the equivalent of sun protection factor (SPF) 4 sunscreen—much too weak to be considered protective. Third, a "base tan" can actually put you at increased risk of sun damage by conferring a false sense of security, leading you to stay out in the sun longer—often without sunscreen.

attention. Surgery may be necessary to remove them, but they are seldom life threatening.

In striking contrast is melanoma, an invasive killer that may appear as a skin lesion whose size, shape, or color changes and that spreads to regional organs and throughout the body. Malignant melanomas account for over 75 percent of all skin cancer deaths. Figure 7 shows melanoma compared to basal cell and squamous cell carcinomas. A simple *ABCD* rule outlines the warning signs of melanoma:

- **Asymmetry.** One half of the mole or lesion does not match the other half.
- **Border irregularity.** The edges are uneven, notched, or scalloped.
- **Color.** Pigmentation is not uniform. Melanomas may vary in color from tan to deeper brown, reddish black, black, or deep bluish black.
- **Diameter.** Greater than 6 millimeters (about the size of a pea).

Treatment of skin cancer depends on its seriousness. Surgery is performed in 90 percent of all cases. Radiation therapy, *electrodesiccation* (tissue destruction by heat), and *cryosurgery* (tissue destruction by freezing) are also common forms of treatment. For melanoma, treatment may involve surgical removal of the regional lymph nodes, radiation, or chemotherapy.

Risk Factors and Prevention Anyone who overexposes himself or herself to ultraviolet radiation without adequate protection is at risk for skin cancer. The risk is greatest for people who fit the following categories:

- Have fair skin; blonde, red, or light brown hair; blue, green, or gray eyes
- Always burn before tanning or burn easily and peel readily
- Don't tan easily but spend lots of time outdoors
- Use no or low–sun protection factor (SPF) sunscreens or old, expired suntan lotions
- Have previously been treated for skin cancer or have a family history of skin cancer
- Have experienced severe sunburns during childhood.

James Stevenson/SPL/Photo Researchers

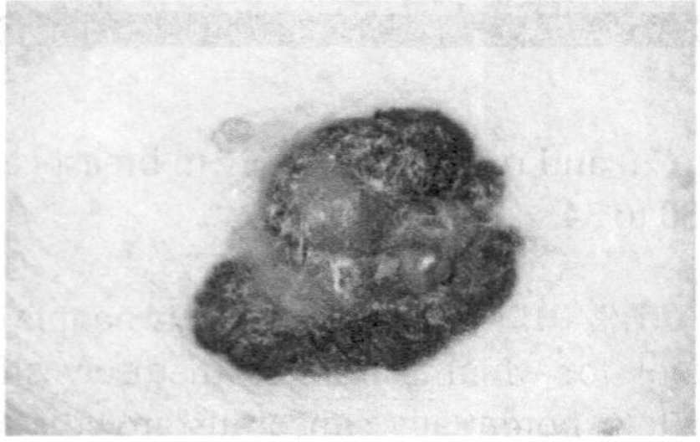

(a) Malignant melanoma

Dr. P. Marazzi/SPL/Photo Researchers

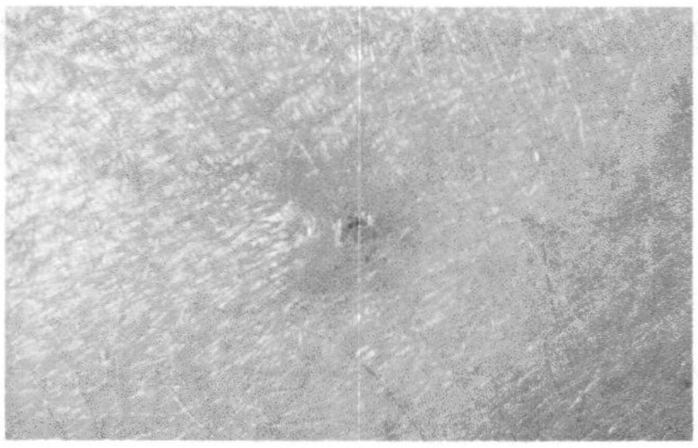

(b) Basal cell carcinoma

Dr. P. Marazzi/SPL/Photo Researchers

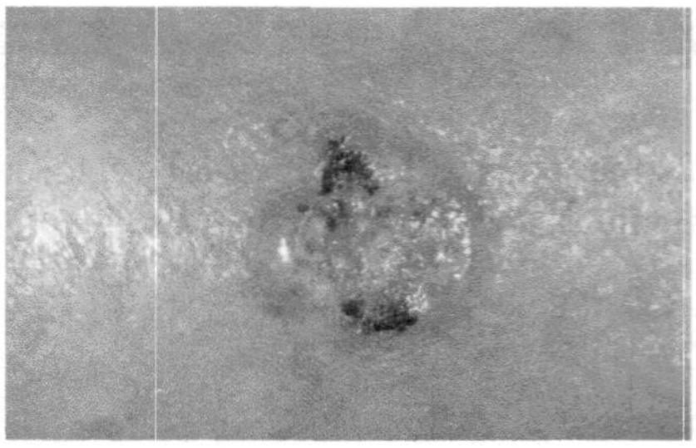

(c) Squamous cell carcinoma

FIGURE 7 **Types of Skin Cancers**

Preventing skin cancer includes keeping a careful watch for any new pigmented growths and for changes to any moles. The ABCD warning signs of melanoma (a) include *asymmetrical* shapes, irregular *borders, color* variation, and an increase in *diameter.* Basal cell carcinoma (b) and squamous cell carcinoma (c) should be brought to your physician's attention but are not as deadly as melanoma.

Preventing skin cancer is a matter of limiting exposure to harmful UV rays found in sunlight. What happens when you expose yourself to sunlight? Biologically, the skin responds to photodamage by increasing its thickness and the number of pigment cells (melanocytes), which produce the "tan" look. The skin's cells that ward off infection are also prone to photodamage, lowering the normal immune protection of our skin and priming it for cancer. Photodamage also causes wrinkling by impairing the elastic substances (collagens) that keep skin soft and pliable. See the **Skills for Behavior Change** box at right for tips on staying safe in the sun.

Although sun exposure risks have been widely reported, over 60 percent of Americans 25 years old and younger report that they are "working on a tan" at some point during the year. Despite the red flag, why do people continue to tan? Recent research suggests a connection between high levels of ultraviolet light and endorphins. Those who tan in the sun or artificially may experience a short "high" for this reason, and tanning can become a type of addiction. For information on the safety of tanning booths and salons, see the **Consumer Health** box on the next page.

Skills for Behavior Change

Safe Sunning

* Avoid the sun or seek shade from 10:00 AM to 2:00 PM, when the sun's rays are strongest. Even on a cloudy day, up to 80 percent of the sun's rays can get through.
* Apply an SPF 15 or higher sunscreen evenly to all uncovered skin before going outside. Look for a "broad-spectrum" sunscreen that protects against both UVA and UVB radiation. Check the label for the correct amount of time you should allow between applying the product and going outdoors. If the label does not specify, apply it 30 minutes before going outside.
* Check the expiration date on your sunscreen. Sunscreens lose effectiveness over time, just like most other products.
* Remember to apply sunscreen to your eyelids, lips, nose, ears, neck, hands, and feet. If you don't have much hair, apply sunscreen to the top of your head, too.
* Reapply sunscreen often. The label will tell you how often you need to do this. If it isn't waterproof, reapply it after swimming, or if you are sweating a lot.
* Wear loose-fitting, light-colored clothing. You can now purchase clothing that has SPF protection in most sporting goods stores. Wear a wide-brimmed, light-colored hat to protect your head and face.
* Use sunglasses with 99 to 100 percent UV protection to protect your eyes. Look for polarization in your shades.
* Check your skin regularly for signs of cancer. Remember to look at the backs of your legs, the undersides of your arms, and between your toes. Check parts that are hard to see—your back, neck, scalp, genitals, and buttocks—with a hand mirror. Look for changes in the size, shape, color, or feel of birthmarks, moles, and spots. If you find any changes or find sores that are not healing, see your doctor.

Source: U.S. Food and Drug Administration, "Sun Safety: Save Your Skin!" Updated July 2009, www.fda.gov/ForConsumers/ConsumerUpdates/ucm049090.htm.

Prostate Cancer

Cancer of the prostate is the most frequently diagnosed cancer in American males today, excluding skin cancer, and is the second leading cause of cancer deaths in men after lung cancer. In 2009, about 192,280 new cases of prostate cancer were diagnosed in the United States. About 1 in 3 men will be diagnosed with prostate cancer during his lifetime, but only 1 in 33 will die of it.[53]

Detection, Symptoms, and Treatment The prostate is a muscular, walnut-sized gland that surrounds part of a man's urethra, the tube that transports urine and sperm out of the body. As part of the male reproductive system, its primary function is to produce seminal fluid. Most symptoms of prostate cancer mimic signs of infection or an enlarged prostate. These may include weak or interrupted urine flow; difficulty starting or stopping urination; feeling the urge to urinate frequently; pain upon urination; blood in the urine; or pain in the low back, pelvis, or thighs. Many men have no symptoms in the early stages.

Men over the age of 40 should have an annual digital rectal prostate examination. The American Cancer Society recommends that men age 50 and over have an annual **prostate-specific antigen (PSA)** test.

Fortunately, 90 percent of all prostate cancers are detected while they are still in the local or regional stages and tend to progress slowly. Over the past 20 years, the 5-year survival rate for all stages combined has increased from 67 percent to almost 99 percent, and the 15-year survival rate is over 76 percent.

Risk Factors and Prevention Chances of developing prostate cancer increase dramatically with age. More than 70 percent of prostate cancers are diagnosed in men over the age of 65. Usually the disease has progressed to the point of displaying symptoms, or, more likely, they are seeing a doctor for other problems and get a screening test or PSA test.

Race is also a risk factor in prostate cancer: African American men are 61 percent more likely to develop prostate cancer than white men and are much more likely to be diagnosed at an advanced stage. Prostate cancer is less common among Asian men and occurs at about the same rates among Hispanic men as it does among white men.

Having a father or brother with prostate cancer more than doubles a man's risk of getting prostate cancer himself (interestingly, the

prostate-specific antigen (PSA) An antigen found in prostate cancer patients.

CONSUMER HEALTH

ARTIFICIAL TANS: SACRIFICING HEALTH FOR BEAUTY?

Tanning is a multibillion-dollar industry that draws more than 28 million Americans into over 25,000 salons each year. Being tan is equated with being healthy, chic, and attractive, leading increasing numbers of men and women, particularly adolescent girls, to seek quick tans in packaged visits to tanning beds.

Most tanning salon patrons incorrectly believe that tanning booths are safer than sitting in the sun. However, the truth is that there is no such thing as a safe tan from *any* source! A tan is visible evidence of skin damage. Every time you tan, whether in the sun or in a salon, you are exposing your skin to harmful UV light rays. Such exposure eventually thins the skin, making it less able to heal, as well as contributing to premature aging. The injury accumulated through years of tanning increases your risk for disfiguring forms of skin cancer, eye problems, and possible death from melanoma. Consider the following:

- Exposure to tanning beds before age 35 increases melanoma risk by 75 percent.
- People who use tanning beds are 2.5 times more likely to develop squamous cell carcinoma and 1.5 times more likely to develop basal cell carcinoma.
- New high-pressure sunlamps used in some salons emit doses of UV radiation that can be as much as 15 times that of the sun.
- Up to 90 percent of visible skin changes commonly blamed on aging are caused by the sun.

Because of the many salons that are springing up across the country, the artificial tanning industry is difficult to monitor and regulate. Although a growing number of states require UV protective eyewear or have machine operators remain present during a client's session, tanning facilities sometimes fail to enforce regulations.

Dermatologists cite additional factors that make tanning in a salon as bad—or even worse—than sitting in the sun:

- Some tanning facilities do not calibrate the ultraviolet output of their tanning bulbs or ensure sufficient rotation of newer and older bulbs, which can lead to more or less exposure than you paid for.
- Tanning facility patrons often try for a total body tan. The buttocks and genitalia are particularly sensitive to UV radiation and are prone to developing skin cancer.
- Shared tanning booths and beds pose significant hygiene risks. Anytime you come in contact with body secretions from others, you run the risk of an infectious disease. Don't assume that those little colored water sprayers used to "clean" the inside of the beds are sufficient to kill organisms. The busier the facility, the more likely you are to come into contact with germs that could make you ill.

Mikhail Pogosov/Shutterstock

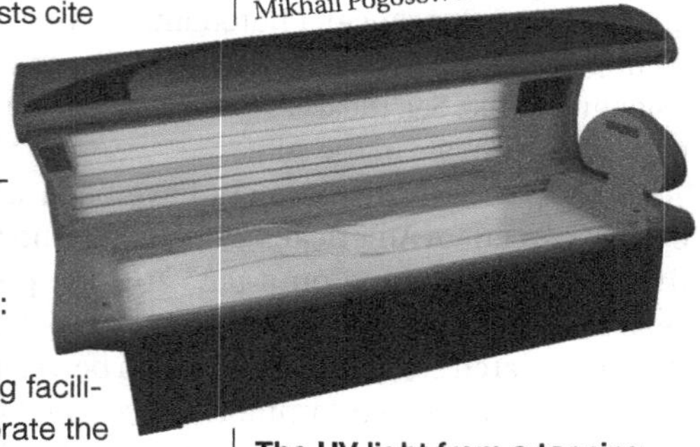

The UV light from a tanning bed is just as harmful and damaging to your skin as that from the sun.

Sources: S. Danoff-Berg and C. E. Mosher, "Prediction of Tanning Salon Use: Behavioral Alternatives for Enhancing Appearance, Relaxing and Socializing," *Journal of Health Psychology* 11, no. 3 (2006): 511–18; Skin Cancer Foundation, "2008 Skin Cancer Facts," 2008, www.skincancer.org/Skin-Cancer/2008-Skin-Cancer-Facts.html.

risk is higher for men with an affected brother than it is for those with an affected father). The genes that predispose men to prostate cancer have not been clearly identified; thus, genetic tests like those for breast cancer in women are not yet available.

Eating more fruits and vegetables, particularly those containing lycopene, a pigment found in tomatoes and other red fruits, may lower the risk of prostate cancer. Some studies suggest that taking 50 mg (400 international units, or IU) of vitamin E and adequate amounts of selenium in your diet may reduce risk, whereas consuming high levels of vitamin A may increase risk.

Ovarian Cancer

Ovarian cancer is the fifth leading cause of cancer deaths for women, with about 21,550 being diagnosed with it in 2009 and 14,600 dying of it.[54] Ovarian cancer causes more deaths than any other cancer of the reproductive system because its insidious, often silent, course means women tend not to discover it until the cancer is at an advanced stage. Overall, 1-year survival rates are 76 percent, and 5-year suvival rates are 45 percent.

The most common symptom of ovarian cancer is enlargement of the abdomen. Women over 40 may experience persistent digestive disturbances, as well. Other symptoms include fatigue, pain during intercourse, unexplained weight loss, unexplained changes in bowel or bladder habits, and incontinence. However, many women have no early symptoms at all.

Primary relatives (mother, daughter, sister) of a woman who has had ovarian cancer are at increased risk. A family or personal history of breast or colon cancer is also associated with increased risk. Women who have never been pregnant are more likely to develop ovarian cancer than those who have had a child. The use of fertility drugs may also increase a woman's risk.

Research shows that using birth control pills, adhering to a low-fat diet, having multiple children, and breast-feeding can all reduce risk of ovarian cancer. General prevention strategies such as focusing on a healthy diet, exercise, sleep, stress management, and weight control are good ideas to lower your risk for this and any of the diseases discussed in this chapter. To protect yourself, getting thorough annual pelvic examinations is important. Women over the age of 40 should have a cancer-related checkup every year. For those with risk factors or unexplained symptoms, uterine ultrasound or a blood test for the tumor marker CA 125 are often recommended.

Cervical and Endometrial (Uterine) Cancer

Most uterine cancers develop in the body of the uterus, usually in the endometrium (lining). The rest develop in the cervix, located at the base of the uterus. In 2009, an estimated 11,270 new cases of cervical cancer and 42,160 cases of endometrial cancer were diagnosed in the United States.[55] The overall incidence of cervical and uterine cancer has been declining steadily over the past decade. This decline may be due to more regular screenings of younger women using the **Pap test,** a procedure in which cells taken from the cervical region are examined for abnormal cellular activity. Although Pap tests are very effective for detecting early-stage cervical cancer, they are less effective for detecting cancers of the uterine lining. Early warning signs of uterine cancer include bleeding outside the normal menstrual period or after menopause or persistent unusual vaginal discharge. These symptoms should be checked by a physician immediately.

Risk factors for cervical cancer include early age at first intercourse, multiple sex partners, cigarette smoking, and certain sexually transmitted infections, including HPV (the cause of genital warts) and herpes. For endometrial cancer, age is a risk factor; however, estrogen and obesity are also strong risk factors. In addition, risks are increased by treatment with tamoxifen for breast cancer, metabolic syndrome, late menopause, never having children, a history of polyps in the uterus or ovaries, a history of other cancers, and race (white women are at higher risk).[56]

Testicular Cancer

Testicular cancer is one of the most common types of solid tumors found in young adult men, affecting nearly 8,400 young men in 2009. Those between the ages of 15 and 35 are at greatest risk. There has been a steady increase in testicular cancer frequency over the past several years in this age group.[57] However, with a 96 percent 5-year survival rate, it is one of the most curable forms of cancer. Although the cause of testicular cancer is unknown, several risk factors have been identified. Men with undescended testicles appear to be at greatest risk, and some studies indicate a genetic influence.

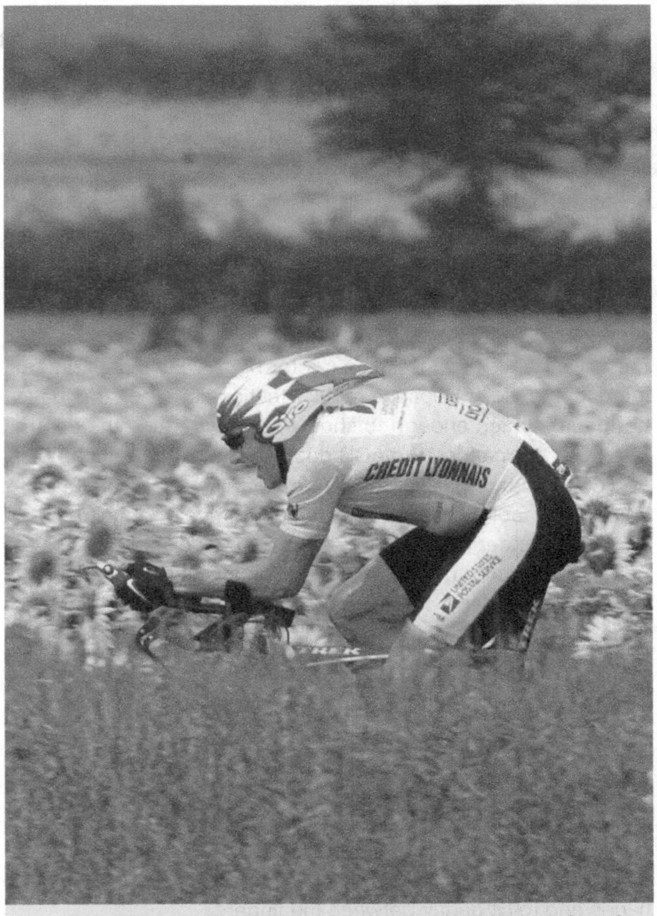

Joel Saget/AFP Photo/Corbis

One of the most remarkable testicular cancer stories is the survival of cyclist Lance Armstrong. After recovering from an invasive form of testicular cancer that spread to several parts of his body, including his brain, Armstrong went on to win the Tour de France seven consecutive times and to create a foundation dedicated to cancer education, research, and advocacy.

In general, testicular tumors first appear as an enlargement of the testis or thickening in testicular tissue. Because this enlargement is often painless, it is important that young men practice regular testicular self-examination (see the **Gender & Health** box on the next page).

Facing Cancer

Based on current rates, about 83 million people in the United States will eventually develop cancer. Despite these gloomy predictions, recent advancements in the diagnosis and treatment of many forms of cancer have reduced some of the fear and mystery that once surrounded this disease.

Detecting Cancer

The earlier cancer is diagnosed, the better the prospect that there is for survival. Make a realistic assessment of your own risk factors; avoid those behaviors that put you at risk; and increase healthy behaviors, such as improving your diet and exercise levels,

Pap test A procedure in which cells taken from the cervical region are examined for abnormal activity.

Gender&Health

Testicular Self-Exam

Most testicular cancers can be found at an early stage. The American Cancer Society (ACS) advises men to be aware of testicular cancer and to see a doctor right away if they find a lump in a testicle. Because regular testicular self-exams have not been studied enough to show that they reduce the death rate from this cancer, the ACS does not have a recommendation on regular testicular self-exams for all men. If you have certain risk factors that increase your chance of developing testicular cancer (e.g., an undescended testicle, previous germ cell tumor in one testicle, or a family history), you should seriously consider monthly self-exams and talk about it with your doctor.

HOW TO EXAMINE YOUR TESTICLES

The best time for you to examine your testicles is during or after a shower, when the skin of the scrotum is relaxed.

* Hold the penis out of the way and examine each testicle separately.
* Hold the testicle between your thumbs and fingers with both hands and roll it gently between the fingers.

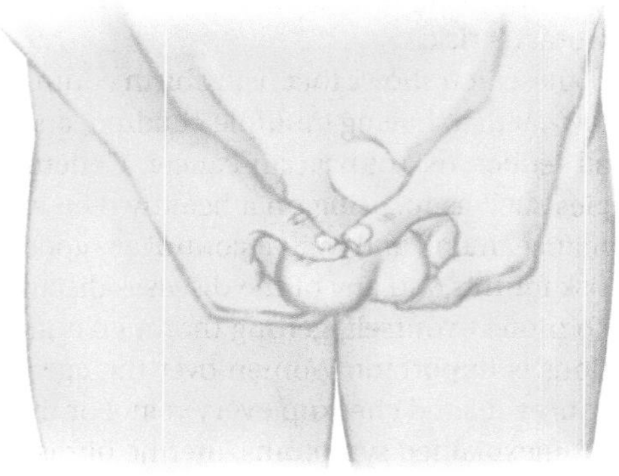

* Look and feel for any hard lumps or nodules (smooth, rounded masses) or any change in the size, shape, or consistency of the testes.

You should be aware that each normal testis has an epididymis, which can feel like a small bump on the upper or middle outer side of the testis. Normal testicles also contain blood vessels, supporting tissues, and tubes that conduct sperm. Some men may confuse these with cancer at first. If you have any concerns, ask your doctor. Note that the ACS recommends a testicular exam as part of a routine cancer-related checkup.

Source: American Cancer Society, "Can Testicular Cancer Be Found Early?," Revised August 3, 2009, www.cancer.org/docroot/CRI/content/CRI_2_4_3X_Can_Testicular_Cancer_Be_Found_Early_41.asp?sitearea=. Reprinted by the permission of the American Cancer Society, Inc. from www.cancer.org.

reducing stress, and getting regular checkups. Even if you have significant risks, there are factors you can control. Do you have a family history of cancer? If so, what types? Make sure you know which symptoms to watch for, and follow the recommendations for self-exams and medical checkups outlined in Table 4 at right. Avoid known carcinogens—such as tobacco—and other environmental hazards, and eat a nutritious diet.

Several high-tech tools to detect cancer have been developed. In **magnetic resonance imaging (MRI),** a huge electromagnet detects hidden tumors by mapping the vibrations of the various atoms in the body on a computer screen. The **computed tomography scan (CT scan)** uses X rays to examine parts of the body. In both of these painless, noninvasive procedures, cross-sectioned pictures can reveal a tumor's shape and location more accurately than can conventional X-ray images.

magnetic resonance imaging (MRI) A device that uses magnetic fields, radio waves, and computers to generate an image of internal tissues of the body for diagnostic purposes without the use of radiation.
computed tomography scan (CT scan) A scan by a machine that uses radiation to view internal organs not normally visible on X-ray images.
radiotherapy Use of radiation to kill cancerous cells.
chemotherapy Use of drugs to kill cancerous cells.

Cancer Treatments

Cancer treatments vary according to the type of cancer and the stage in which it's detected. Surgery, in which the tumor and surrounding tissue are removed, is one common treatment. **Radiotherapy** (the use of radiation) or **chemotherapy** (the use of drugs) to kill cancerous cells are also used. Radiation works by destroying malignant cells or stopping cell growth. It is most effective in treating localized cancer masses. When cancer has spread throughout the body, it is necessary to use some form of chemotherapy.

Whether used alone or in combination, radiotherapy and chemotherapy have side effects, including nausea, nutritional deficiencies, hair loss, and general fatigue. In the process of killing malignant cells, some healthy cells are also destroyed, and long-term damage to the cardiovascular system and other body systems can be significant.

Although surgery, chemotherapy, and radiation therapy remain the most commonly used treatments for all types of cancer and successfully treat about 50 percent of all cancers, several newer techniques either are in clinical trials or have become available in selected cancer centers throughout the country. Promising areas of research include *immunotherapy,* which enhances the body's own disease-fighting mechanisms, *cancer-fighting vaccines* to combat abnormal cells, *gene therapy* to increase the patient's immune response, and treatment with various substances that block cancer-causing events along the *cancer pathway.* Another promising avenue of potential treatment is *stem cell research,* although controversy around the use of stem cells continues to slow research.

TABLE 4

Screening Guidelines for the Early Detection of Cancer in Average-Risk Asymptomatic People

Cancer Site	Population	Test or Procedure	Frequency
Breast	Women, aged 20+	Breast self-examination (BSE)	Beginning in their early 20s, women should be told about the benefits and limitations of BSE. The importance of prompt reporting of any new breast symptoms to a health professional should be emphasized. Women who choose to do BSE should receive instruction and have their technique reviewed on the occasion of a periodic health examination. It is acceptable for women to choose not to do BSE or to do BSE irregularly.
		Clinical breast examination (CBE)	For women in their 20s and 30s, it is recommended that CBE be part of a periodic health examination, preferably at least every 3 years. Asymptomatic women aged 40 and over should continue to receive a CBE as part of a periodic health examination, preferably annually.
		Mammography	Annual, starting at age 40*
Colorectal†	Men and women, aged 50+	Fecal occult blood test (FOBT)‡ with at least 50% test sensitivity for cancer, or fecal immunochemical test (FIT) with at least 50% test sensitivity for cancer, *or*	Annual, starting at age 50
		Stool DNA test	Interval uncertain, starting at age 50
		Flexible sigmoidoscopy, *or*	Every 5 years, starting at age 50
		FOBT‡ and flexible sigmoidoscopy,§ *or*	Annual FOBT (or FIT) and flexible sigmoidoscopy every 5 years, starting at age 50
		Double-contrast barium enema (DCBE), *or*	Every 5 years, starting at age 50
		Colonoscopy	Every 10 years, starting at age 50
		Computerized tomography (CT) colonography	Every 5 years, starting at age 50
Prostate	Men, aged 50+	Digital rectal examination (DRE) and prostate-specific antigen (PSA) test	Health care providers should discuss the potential benefits and limitations of prostate cancer early detection testing with men and offer the PSA blood test and the DRE annually, beginning at age 50, to men who are at average risk of prostate cancer, and who have a life expectancy of at least 10 years.¶
Cervix	Women, aged 18+	Pap test	Cervical cancer screening should begin approximately 3 years after a woman begins having vaginal intercourse, but no later than 21 years of age. Screening should be done every year with conventional Pap tests or every 2 years using liquid-based Pap tests. At or after age 30, women who have had three normal test results in a row may get screened every 2 to 3 years with cervical cytology (either conventional or liquid-based Pap test) alone, or every 3 years with a human papillomavirus (HPV) DNA test plus cervical cytology. Women 70 years of age and older who have had three or more normal Pap tests and no abnormal Pap tests in the past 10 years and women who have had a total hysterectomy may choose to stop cervical cancer screening.
Endometrial	Women, at menopause	At the time of menopause, women at average risk should be informed about risks and symptoms of endometrial cancer and strongly encouraged to report any unexpected bleeding or spotting to their physicians.	
Cancer-Related Checkup	Men and women, aged 20+	On the occasion of a periodic health examination, the cancer-related checkup should include examination for cancers of the thyroid, testicles, ovaries, lymph nodes, oral cavity, and skin, as well as health counseling about tobacco, sun exposure, diet and nutrition, risk factors, sexual practices, and environmental and occupational exposures.	

*Beginning at age 40, annual CBE should be performed prior to mammography.

†Individuals with a personal or family history of colorectal cancer or adenomas, inflammatory bowel disease, or high-risk genetic syndromes should continue to follow the most recent recommendations for individuals at increased or high risk.

‡FOBT as it is sometimes done in physicians' offices, with the single stool sample collected on a fingertip during a DRE, is not an adequate substitute for the recommended at-home procedure of collecting two samples from three consecutive specimens. Toilet bowl FOBT tests also are not recommended. In comparison with guaiac-based tests for the detection of occult blood, immunochemical tests are more patient friendly, and are likely to be equal or better in sensitivity and specificity. There is no justification for repeating FOBT in response to an initial positive finding.

§Flexible sigmoidoscopy, together with FOBT, is preferred compared to FOBT or flexible sigmoidoscopy alone.

¶Information should be provided to men about the benefits and limitations of testing so that an informed decision about testing can be made with the clinician's assistance.

Source: American Cancer Society, *Cancer Facts & Figures 2009* (Atlanta: American Cancer Society, 2009), www.cancer.org. Used with permission. © 2009, American Cancer Society, Inc.

Assess yourself

CVD and Cancer: What's Your Personal Risk?

PEARSON myhealthlab

Fill out this assessment online at www.pearsonhighered.com/myhealthlab or www.pearsonhighered.com/donatelle.

1 Evaluating Your CVD Risk

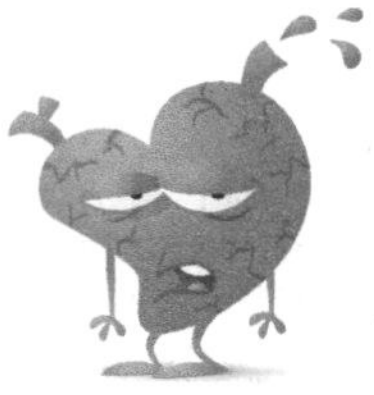

Mark Stay/iStockphoto

Complete each of the following questions and total your points in each section.

A: Your Family Risk for CVD

	Yes (1 point)	No (0 points)	Don't Know
1. Do any of your primary relatives (parents, grandparents, siblings) have a history of heart disease or stroke?	○	○	○
2. Do any of your primary relatives have diabetes?	○	○	○
3. Do any of your primary relatives have high blood pressure?	○	○	○
4. Do any of your primary relatives have a history of high cholesterol?	○	○	○
5. Would you say that your family consumed a high-fat diet (lots of red meat, whole dairy, butter/margarine) during your time spent at home?	○	○	○

Total points: ________

B: Your Lifestyle Risk for CVD

	Yes (1 point)	No (0 points)	Don't Know
1. Is your total cholesterol level higher than it should be?	○	○	○
2. Do you have high blood pressure?	○	○	○
3. Have you been diagnosed as pre-diabetic or diabetic?	○	○	○
4. Would you describe your life as being highly stressful?	○	○	○
5. Do you smoke?	○	○	○

Total points: ________

C: Your Additional Risks for CVD

1. How would you best describe your current weight?
   a. Lower than what it should be for my height and weight (0 points)
   b. About what it should be for my height and weight (0 points)
   c. Higher than it should be for my height and weight (1 point)

2. How would you describe the level of exercise that you get each day?
   a. Less than what I should be exercising each day (1 point)
   b. About what I should be exercising each day (0 points)
   c. More than what I should be exercising each day (0 points)

3. How would you describe your dietary behaviors?
   a. Eating only the recommended number of calories each day (0 points)
   b. Eating less than the recommended number of calories each day (0 points)
   c. Eating more than the recommended number of calories each day (1 point)

4. Which of the following best describes your typical dietary behavior?
   a. I eat from the major food groups, especially trying to get the recommended fruits and vegetables. (0 points)
   b. I eat too much red meat and consume too much saturated and *trans* fats from meat, dairy products, and processed foods each day. (1 point)
   c. Whenever possible, I try to substitute olive oil or canola oil for other forms of dietary fat. (0 points)

Max Delson Martins Santos/iStockphoto

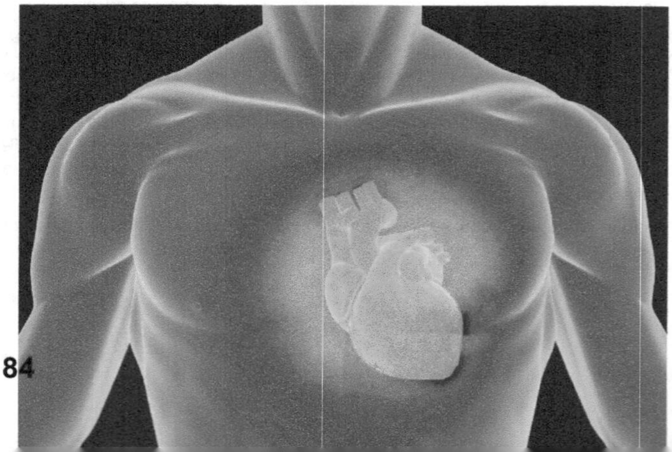

5. Which of the following (if any) describes you?
   a. I watch my sodium intake and try to reduce stress in my life. (0 points)
   b. I have a history of chlamydia infection. (1 point)
   c. I try to eat 5 to 10 mg of soluble fiber each day and try to substitute a soy product for an animal product in my diet at least once each week. (0 points)

Total points: ________

Scoring Part 1

If you scored between 1 and 5 in any section, consider your risk. The higher the number is, the greater your risk will be. If you answered Don't Know for any question, talk to your parents or other family members as soon as possible to find out if you have any unknown risks.

YOUR PLAN FOR CHANGE

The Assessyourself activity evaluated your risk of heart disease. Based on your results and the advice of your physician, you may need to take steps to reduce risk of CVD.

Today, you can:

◯ Get up and move! Take a walk in the evening, use the stairs instead of the escalator, or ride your bike to class. Start thinking of ways you can incorporate more physical activity into your daily routine.

◯ Begin improving your dietary habits by eating a healthier dinner. Replace the meat and processed foods you might normally eat with a serving of fresh fruit or soy-based protein, and green leafy vegetables. Think about the amounts of saturated and *trans* fats you consume—which foods contain them, and how can you reduce consumption of these items?

Within the next 2 weeks, you can:

◯ Begin a regular exercise program, even if you start slowly. Set small goals and try to meet them.

◯ Practice a new stress management technique. For example, learn how to meditate.

◯ Get enough rest. Make sure you get at least 8 hours of sleep per night.

By the end of the semester, you can:

◯ Find out your hereditary risk for CVD. Call your parents and find out if your grandparents or aunts or uncles developed CVD. Ask if they know their latest cholesterol LDL/HDL levels. Do you have a family history of diabetes?

◯ Have your own cholesterol and blood pressure levels checked. Once you know your levels, you'll have a better sense of what risk factors to address. If your levels are high, talk to your doctor about how to reduce them.

2 Evaluating Your Cancer Risk

Read each question and circle the number corresponding to each Yes or No. Individual scores for specific questions should not be interpreted as a precise measure of relative risk, but the totals in each section give a general indication.

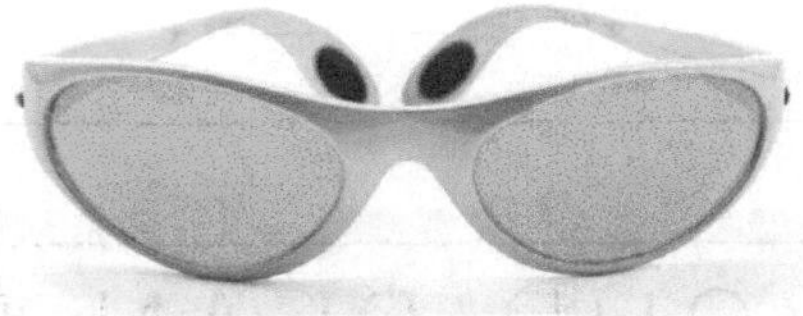

Wojciech Krusinski/iStockphoto

A: Breast Cancer

	Yes	No
1. Do you check your breasts at least monthly using BSE procedures?	1	2
2. Do you look at your breasts in the mirror regularly, checking for any irregular indentations/lumps, discharge from the nipples, or other noticeable changes?	1	2
3. Has your mother, sister, or daughter been diagnosed with breast cancer?	2	1
4. Have you ever been pregnant?	1	2
5. Have you had a history of lumps or cysts in your breasts or underarm?	2	1

Total points: ________

B: Skin Cancer

	Yes	No
1. Do you spend a lot of time outdoors, either at work or at play?	2	1
2. Do you use sunscreens with an SPF rating of 15 or more when you are in the sun?	1	2
3. Do you use tanning beds or sun booths regularly to maintain a tan?	2	1
4. Do you examine your skin once a month, checking any moles or other irregularities, particularly in hard-to-see areas such as your back, genitals, neck, and under your hair?	1	2
5. Do you purchase and wear sunglasses that adequately filter out harmful sun rays?	1	2

Total points: ________

C: Cancers of the Reproductive System

Men

		Yes	No
1.	Do you examine your penis regularly for unusual bumps or growths?	1	2
2.	Do you perform regular testicular self-examinations?	1	2
3.	Do you have a family history of prostate or testicular cancer?	2	1
4.	Do you practice safe sex and wear condoms during every sexual encounter?	1	2
5.	Do you avoid exposure to harmful environmental hazards such as mercury, coal tars, benzene, chromate, and vinyl chloride?	1	2

Total points: ________

Women

		Yes	No
1.	Do you have regularly scheduled Pap tests?	1	2
2.	Have you been infected with HPV, Epstein-Barr virus, or other viruses believed to increase cancer risk?	2	1
3.	Has your mother, sister, or daughter been diagnosed with breast, cervical, endometrial, or ovarian cancer (particularly at a young age)?	2	1
4.	Do you practice safer sex and use condoms with every sexual encounter?	1	2
5.	Are you obese, taking estrogen, or consuming a diet that is very high in saturated fats?	2	1

Total points: ________

D: Cancers in General

		Yes	No
1.	Do you smoke cigarettes on most days of the week?	2	1
2.	Do you consume a diet that is rich in fruits and vegetables?	1	2
3.	Are you obese, or do you lead a primarily sedentary lifestyle?	2	1
4.	Do you live in an area with high air pollution levels or work in a job where you are exposed to several chemicals on a regular basis?	2	1
5.	Are you careful about the amount of animal fat in your diet, substituting olive oil or canola oil for animal fat whenever possible?	1	2
6.	Do you limit your overall consumption of alcohol?	1	2
7.	Do you eat foods rich in lycopenes (such as tomatoes) and antioxidants?	1	2
8.	Are you "body aware" and alert for changes in your body?	1	2
9.	Do you have a family history of ulcers or of colorectal, stomach, or other digestive system cancers?	2	1
10.	Do you avoid unnecessary exposure to radiation, cell phone emissions, and microwave emissions?	1	2

Total points: ________

Scoring Part 2

Look carefully at each question for which you received a 2. Are there any areas in which you received mostly 2s? Did you receive total points of 6 or higher in A through C? Did you receive total points of 11 or higher in D? If so, you have at least one identifiable risk. The higher the score is, the more risks you may have.

YOUR PLAN FOR CHANGE

The Assess yourself activity identified certain factors and behaviors that can contribute to increased cancer risks. If you engage in potentially risky behaviors, consider steps you can take to change these risks and improve your future health.

Today, you can:

- ◯ Perform a breast or testicular self-exam and commit to doing one every month.
- ◯ Take advantage of the salad bar in your dining hall for lunch or dinner, and load up on greens, or request veggies such as steamed broccoli or sautéed spinach.

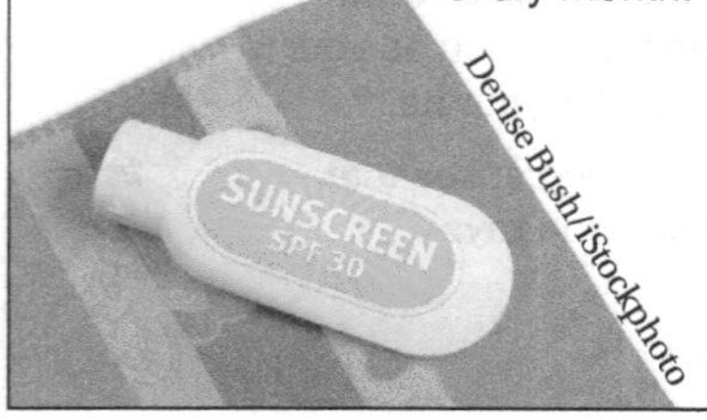

Denise Bush/iStockphoto

Within the next 2 weeks, you can:

- ◯ Buy a bottle of sunscreen (with SPF 15 or higher) and begin applying it as part of your daily routine. (Be sure to check the expiration date, particularly on sale items!)
- ◯ Find out your family health history. Talk to your parents, grandparents, or an aunt or uncle to find out if family members have developed cancer. This will help you assess your own genetic risk.

By the end of the semester, you can:

- ◯ Work toward achieving a healthy weight. If you aren't already engaged in a regular exercise program, begin one now. Maintaining a healthy body weight and exercising regularly will lower your risk for cancer.
- ◯ Stop smoking, avoid secondhand smoke, and limit your alcohol intake.

Summary

* The cardiovascular system consists of the heart and a network of vessels that supplies the body with nutrients and oxygen. Cardiovascular diseases include atherosclerosis, coronary heart disease, angina pectoris, arrhythmias, congestive heart failure, and stroke.
* *Cardiometabolic risks* refer to combined factors that increase a person's chances of CVD and diabetes. *Metabolic syndrome* is a term for when a person possesses three or more cardiometabolic risk factors.
* Many risk factors for CVD can be controlled, such as cigarette smoking, high blood cholesterol and triglyceride levels, hypertension, lack of exercise, obesity, diabetes, and emotional stress. Some risk factors, such as age, gender, and heredity, cannot be controlled. Other factors being studied include inflammation and homocysteine levels.
* New methods developed for treating heart blockages include coronary bypass surgery and angioplasty. Drugs can reduce high blood pressure and treat other symptoms.
* Cancer is a group of diseases characterized by uncontrolled growth and spread of abnormal cells. These cells may create tumors. Malignant (cancerous) tumors can spread to other parts of the body through metastasis.
* Lifestyle factors for cancer risk include smoking and obesity. Biological factors include inherited genes and gender. Components of the environment that may act as carcinogens include asbestos, radiation, preservatives, and pesticides. Infectious diseases that may lead to cancer include hepatitis and human papillomavirus.
* Common cancers include lung, breast, colon and rectal, skin, prostate, ovarian, uterine, and testicular cancers.
* Early diagnosis improves cancer survival rate. Self-exams aid early diagnosis. New types of cancer treatments include combinations of radiotherapy, chemotherapy, and immunotherapy.

Pop Quiz

1. The function of the aorta is to
   a. return the blood from the lungs.
   b. pump the blood to the arteries in the rest of the body.
   c. pump blood to the lungs.
   d. return blood back to the heart.

2. Severe chest pain due to reduced oxygen flow to the heart is called
   a. angina pectoris.
   b. arrhythmias.
   c. myocardial infarction.
   d. congestive heart failure.

3. Atherosclerosis is referred to as
   a. hardening of the arteries.
   b. heart attack.
   c. high blood pressure.
   d. plaque.

4. A stroke results
   a. when a heart stops beating.
   b. when cardiopulmonary resuscitation has failed to revive the stopped heart.
   c. when blood to the brain has been blocked off.
   d. when the blood pressure rises too high.

5. Which of the following are major causes of cancer?
   a. Sex and socioeconomic status
   b. Environment and genetics
   c. Geographic locations
   d. High-carbohydrate foods

6. The "bad" type of cholesterol found in the bloodstream is known as
   a. high-density lipoprotein.
   b. low-density lipoprotein.
   c. total cholesterol.
   d. triglyceride.

7. The greatest number of cancer deaths for both sexes is caused by
   a. colorectal cancer.
   b. leukemia.
   c. lung cancer.
   d. skin cancer.

8. The more serious, life-threatening type of skin cancer is
   a. basal cell carcinoma.
   b. squamous cell carcinoma.
   c. malignant melanoma.
   d. non-Hodgkin lymphoma.

9. Suspected cancer-causing genes are
   a. epigenes.
   b. oncogenes.
   c. primogenes.
   d. metastogenes.

10. The fecal occult blood test is the most basic screening test used for
    a. lung cancer.
    b. prostate cancer.
    c. cervical cancer.
    d. colorectal cancer.

Answers to Chapter Review Questions
1. b; 2. a; 3. a; 4. c; 5. b;
6. b; 7. c; 8. c; 9. b; 10. d

Think about It!

1. List the different types of CVD. Compare and contrast their symptoms, risk factors, prevention, and treatment.
2. Discuss the role that exercise, stress management, dietary changes, medical checkups, and other factors can play in reducing risk for CVD. What role may chronic infections play in CVD risk?
3. Describe some of the diagnostic and treatment alternatives for CVD. If you had a heart attack today, which treatment would you prefer?
4. List the likely causes of cancer. Do any of them put you personally at greater risk? What can you do to reduce your risk? What risk factors do you share with family members? With friends?

5. What are the symptoms of lung, breast, prostate, and testicular cancer? What can you do to reduce your risk of developing these cancers or increase your chances of surviving them?
6. Why are breast and testicular self-exams important for women and men?

Accessing Your Health on the Internet

The following websites explore further topics and issues related to personal health. For links to the websites below, visit the Companion Website for *Health: The Basics,* Green Edition at www.pearsonhighered.com/donatelle.

1. *American Heart Association.* Home page for the leading private organization dedicated to heart health. This site provides information, statistics, and resources regarding cardiovascular care. www.americanheart.org
2. *National Heart, Lung, and Blood Institute.* A valuable resource for information on all aspects of cardiovascular health and wellness. www.nhlbi.nih.gov
3. *American Cancer Society.* Resources from the leading private organization dedicated to cancer prevention. This site provides information, statistics, and resources regarding cancer. www.cancer.org
4. *National Cancer Institute.* Check here for valuable information on clinical trials and the Physician Data Query (PDQ), a comprehensive database of cancer treatment information. www.cancer.gov
5. *Oncolink.* Sponsored by the Abramson Cancer Center of the University of Pennsylvania, this site offers information on cancer support services, cancer causes, screening, and prevention. www.oncolink.com

References

1. Centers for Disease Control and Prevention, "Chronic Disease Overview," Modified October 7, 2009, www.cdc.gov/nccdphp/overview.htm.
2. R. DeVol and A. Bedroussian, *An Unhealthy America: The Economic Burden of Chronic Disease, Charting a New Course to Save Lives and Increase Productivity and Economic Growth* (Santa Monica, CA: Milken Institute, 2007).
3. American Heart Association, *Heart Disease and Stroke Statistics—2009 Update At-A-Glance* (Dallas: American Heart Association, 2009).
4. American Heart Association, *Heart Disease and Stroke Statistics—2009 Update At-A-Glance,* 2009; Centers for Disease Control and Prevention, "Chronic Disease Overview," Updated November 20, 2008, www.cdc.gov/nccdphp/overview.htm.
5. D. Lloyd-Jones et al., "Heart Disease and Stroke Statistics—2009 Update: A Report from the AHA Statistics Committee and the Stroke Statistics Subcommittee." *Circulation* 199, no. 3 (2009): 480–86
6. American Heart Association, *Heart Disease and Stroke Statistics—2009 Update At-A-Glance,* 2009.
7. Ibid.
8. Ibid.
9. Ibid.
10. Ibid.
11. Ibid.
12. Ibid.
13. J. Despres et al., "Abdominal Obesity and Metabolic Syndrome: Contribution to Global Cardiometabolic Risk," *Arteriosclerosis, Thrombosis, and Vascular Biology* 28, no. 6 (2008): 1039–42; S. Haffner, "Epidemiology of Cardiometabolic Diseases," *Mechanisms and Syndromes of Cardiometabolic Disease: Emerging Science in Atherosclerosis Hypertension and Diabetes,* 2009, Medscape CME, http://cme.medscape.com; American Heart Association, *Heart Disease and Stroke Statistics—2009 Update At-A-Glance,* 2009; J. Rosenzwigg, et al., "Primary Prevention of Cardiovascular Disease and Type 2 Diabetes in Patients at Metabolic Risk: An Endocrine Society Clinical Practice Guideline," *Journal of Clinical Endocrinology and Metabolism* 93, no. 10 (2008): 3671–89.
14. S. Haffner, "Epidemiology of Cardiometabolic Diseases," 2009; J. Despres et al., "Abdominal Obesity and Metabolic Syndrome, 2008; A. Gami et al., "Metabolic Syndrome and Risk of Incident Cardiovascular Events and Death: A Systematic Review and Meta-Analysis of Longitudinal Studies," *Journal of the American College of Cardiology* 49, no. 4 (2007): 403–14.
15. U. R. Ximena et al., "High Blood Pressure in Schoolchildren: Prevalence and Risk Factors," *BMC Pediatrics* 6 (2006): 32; R. Din-Dzietham et al., "High Blood Pressure Trends in Children and Adolescents in National Surveys, 1963–2002," *Circulation* 116 (2007): 1488–91; L. Yong, M. Bielo, and F. Shamsa, "Kid's Elevated Blood Pressure Prevalence Linked to Rise in Obesity," *American Heart Association Rapid Access Journal Report,* 2007, www.americanheart.org/presenter.jhtml?identifier=3050261; T. Huang et al., "Metabolic Syndrome and Related Disorders in College Students: Prevalence and Gender Differences," *Metabolic Syndrome and Related Disorders* 5, no. 4 (2007): 365–72.
16. National Center for Health Statistics, *Health, United States, 2008 with Chartbook on Trends in the Health of Americans* (Hyattsville, MD: National Center for Health Statistics, 2009).
17. American Heart Association, *Heart Disease and Stroke Statistics—2009 Update At-A-Glance,* 2009.
18. B. Howard et al., "Low Fat Diet and Risk of Cardiovascular Disease," *JAMA* 295, no. 6 (2006): 655–66; American Heart Association, *Heart Disease and Stroke Statistics—2009 Update At-A-Glance,* 2009.
19. C. A. Garza et al., "The Association between Lipoprotein-Associated Phospholipase A_2 and Cardiovascular Disease: A Systematic Review," *Mayo Clinic Proceedings* 82, no. 2 (2007):159–65.
20. P. J. Barter et al., "Apo B versus Cholesterol in Estimating Cardiovascular Risk and in Guiding Therapy: Report of the Thirty-Person/Ten-Country Panel," *Journal of Internal Medicine* 259, no. 3 (2006): 247–58; E. Ingelsson et al., "Clinical Utility of Different Lipid Measures for Prediction of Coronary Heart Disease in Men and Women," *JAMA* 298, no. 7 (2007): 776–85; M. McQueen et al., "Lipids, Lipoproteins and Apolipoproteins as Risk Markers of Myocardial Infarction in 52 Countries (The INTERHEART Study): A Case-Control Study," *Lancet* 372, no. 9634 (2008): 244–33.
21. American Heart Association, *Heart Disease and Stroke Statistics—2009 Update At-A-Glance,* 2009.
22. C. H. Saely, P. Rein, and H. Drexel, "The Metabolic Syndrome and Risk of Cardiovascular Disease and Diabetes: Experiences with the New Diagnostic Criteria from the International Diabetes Federation," *Hormone and Metabolic Research* 39 (2007): 642–50; K. Galassi, K. Reynolds, and J. He, "Metabolic Syndrome and Risk of

Cardiovascular Disease: A Meta-Analysis," *American Journal of Medicine* 119, no. 10 (2007): 812–19.
23. American Heart Association, *Heart Disease and Stroke Statistics—2009 Update At-A-Glance*, 2009.
24. Ibid.
25. M. Esler et al., "Chronic Mental Stress Is a Cause of Essential Hypertension: Presence of Biological Markers of Stress," *Clinical and Experimental Pharmacology and Physiology* 35, no. 4 (2008): 498–502; A. Flaa, I. Eide, S. Kjeldsen, and M. Rostrup, "Sympathoadrenal Stress Reactivity Is a Predictor of Future Blood Pressure. An 18 Year Follow-Up Study," *Hypertension* 52 (2008): 336–41; T. Chadola et al., "Work Stress and Coronary Heart Disease: What Are the Mechanisms," *European Heart Journal* 29, no. 5 (2008): 640–48; J. Yarnell, "Stress at Work—an Independent Risk Factor for Coronary Heart Disease?" *European Heart Journal* 29, no. 5 (2008): 579–81; P. Surtees et al., "Psychological Distress, Major Depressive Disorder, and Risk of Stroke," *Neurology* 70 (2008): 788–94; J. Dimsdale, "Psychological Stress and Cardiovascular Disease," *Journal of the American College of Cardiology* 51 (2008): 1237–46.
26. J. Murabito et al., "Sibling Cardiovascular Disease as a Risk Factor for Cardiovascular Disease in Middle-Aged Adults," *JAMA* 294, no. 24 (2005): 3117–23.
27. J. Ordovas, "Genetic Interactions with Diet Influence the Risk of CVD. Supplement: Living Well to 100: Nutrition, Genetics, Inflammation," *American Journal of Clinical Nutrition* 83, no. 2 (2006): 443S–446S; J. Lovegrove and R. Gitau, "Nutrigenetics and CVD: What Does the Future Hold?" *Proceedings of the Nutrition Society* 67, no. 2 (2008): 206–13.
28. O. Ben-Yehuda, "High-Sensitivity C-Reactive Protein in Every Chart?: The Use of Biomarkers in Individual Patients," *Journal of the American College of Cardiology* 49, no. 21 (2007): 2139–41; D. D. Sin and S. F. P. Man, "Biomarkers in COPD: Are We There Yet?" *Chest* 133, no. 6 (2008): 1296–98; B. Zethelius et al., "Use of Multiple Biomarkers to Improve the Prediction of Death from Cardiovascular Causes," *New England Journal of Medicine* 358, no. 20 (2008): 2107–16; L. Mosca et al., "Narrative Review: Assessment of C-Reactive Protein in Risk Prediction for Cardiovascular Disease," *Annals of Internal Medicine* 145 (2006): 35–42.
29. F. Sofi et al., "Homocysteine-Lowering Therapy and Risk for Venous Thromboembolism: A Randomized Trial," *Annals of Internal Medicine* 146 (2007): 761–67.
30. American Heart Association, "Homocysteine, Folic Acid, and Cardiovascular Disease," 2009, www.americanheart.org/presenter.jhtml?identifier=4677; R. Clarke et al., "Effects of B-Vitamins on Plasma Homocysteine Concentrations and on Risk of Cardiovascular Disease and Dementia," *Current Opinion in Clinical Nutrition and Metabolic Care* 10, no. 1 (2007): 32–39.
31. C. Campbell, S. Smyth, G. Montalescot, and S. Steinhubl, "Aspirin Dose for the Prevention of Cardiovascular Disease: A Systematic Review," *JAMA* 297, no. 18 (2007): 2018–24.
32. American Cancer Society, *Cancer Facts & Figures 2009* (Atlanta: American Cancer Society, 2009).
33. Ibid.
34. Ibid.
35. Ibid.
36. Ibid.
37. Ibid.
38. Centers for Disease Control and Prevention, "Tobacco Use: Targeting The Nation's Leading Killer—at a Glance 2009," 2009, www.cdc.gov/NCCDPHP/publications/aag/osh.htm; World Health Organization, *WHO Report on Global Tobacco Epidemic, 2008: The MPOWER Package* (Geneva, Switzerland: World Health Organization, 2008).
39. K. Flegal et al., "Cause-Specific Excess Deaths Associated with Underweight, Overweight, and Obesity," *Gynecology Obstetrical & Gynecological Survey* 63, no. 3 (2008): 157–59; A. Rehehan, "Body Mass Index and Incidence of Cancer: A Systematic Review and Meta-Analysis of Prospective Observational Studies," *Lancet* 371, no. 9612 (2008): 568–78; G. Reeves et al., "Cancer Incidence and Mortality in Relation to BMI in the Million Women Study: Cohort Study," *BMJ (British Medical Journal)* 1, no. 335 (2007):1134–42; S. Larsson and A. Wolk, "Obesity and Colon and Rectal Cancer Risk: A Meta-Analysis of Prospective Studies," *American Journal of Clinical Nutrition* 86, no. 3 (2008): 556–65.
40. K. Rapp et al., "Obesity and Incidence of Cancer: A Large Cohort Study of over 145,000 Adults in Austria," *British Journal of Cancer* 93 (2005): 1062–67; S. Feedland, "Obesity and Prostate Cancer: A Growing Problem," *Clinical Cancer Research* 11, no. 19 (2005): 6763–66; R. MacInnis et al., "Body Size and Composition and Colon Cancer Risk in Women," *International Cancer Journal* 118 no. 6 (2005): 1496–500; C. Samanic et al., "Relation of Body Mass Index to Cancer Risk in 362,552 Swedish Men," *Cancer Causes and Control* 17, no. 7 (2005): 10552–600; M. McCullough et al., "Risk Factors for Fatal Breast Cancer in African American Women and White Women in a Large U.S. Prospective Cohort," *American Journal of Epidemiology* 162, no. 8 (2005): 734–42; P. Soliman et al., "Risk Factors for Young Premenopausal Women with Endometrial Cancer," *Obstetrics and Gynecology* 105 (2005): 575–80.
41. E. Reiche, H. Morimoto, and S. Nunes, "Stress and Depression-Induced Immune Dysfunction—Implications for the Development and Progress of Cancer," *International Review of Psychiatry* 17, no. 6 (2005): 515–27; K. Ross, "Mapping Pathways from Stress to Cancer Progression," *Journal of the National Cancer Institute* 100, no. 13 (2008): 914–17; B. Eliyahui, "Stress and Fear Can Affect Cancer's Recurrence," *Science Daily* (February 29, 2008), www.sciencedaily.com/releases/2008/02/080227142656.htm.
42. American Cancer Society, *Cancer Facts & Figures*, 2009.
43. S. Joachim et al., "Cellular Telephone Use and Cancer Risk: Update of a Nationwide Danish Cohort," *Journal of the National Cancer Institute* 98, no. 23 (2006): 1707–13.
44. American Cancer Society, "New Report Estimates 12 Million Cancer Cases Worldwide in 2007," *Science Daily* (December 18, 2008), www.sciencedaily.com/releases/2007/12/071217092929.htm.
45. American Cancer Society, *Cancer Facts & Figures*, 2009.
46. Ibid.
47. H. A. Wakelee et al., "Lung Cancer Incidence in Never Smokers," *Journal of Clinical Oncology* 25, no. 5 (2007): 472–78.
48. American Cancer Society, *Cancer Facts and Figures*, 2009.
49. Ibid.
50. C. M. Dallal et al., "Long-Term Recreational Physical Activity and Risk of Invasive and In Situ Breast Cancer," *Archives of Internal Medicine* 167, no. 4 (2007): 408–15.
51. American Cancer Society, *Cancer Facts & Figures*, 2009.
52. Ibid.
53. Ibid.
54. Ibid.
55. Ibid.
56. National Cancer Institute, "Endometrial Cancer," Accessed August 2009, www.cancer.gov/cancertopics/types/endometrial.
57. National Cancer Institute, "Testicular Cancer," Accessed August 2009, www.cancer.gov/cancertopics/types/testicular.

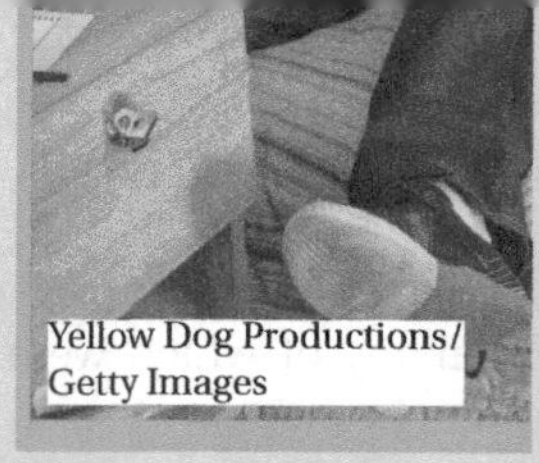

Yellow Dog Productions/ Getty Images

Why are vaccinations important?

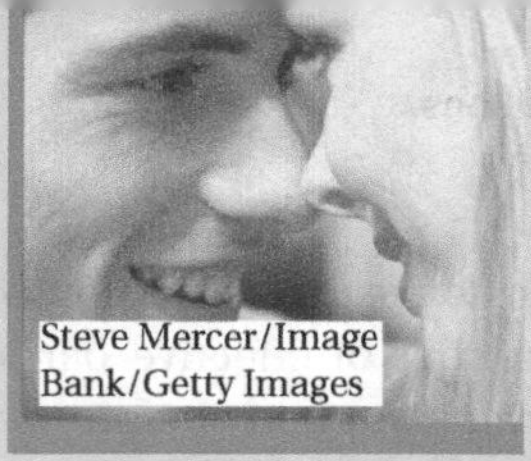

Steve Mercer/Image Bank/Getty Images

How can I tell if someone I'm dating has an STI?

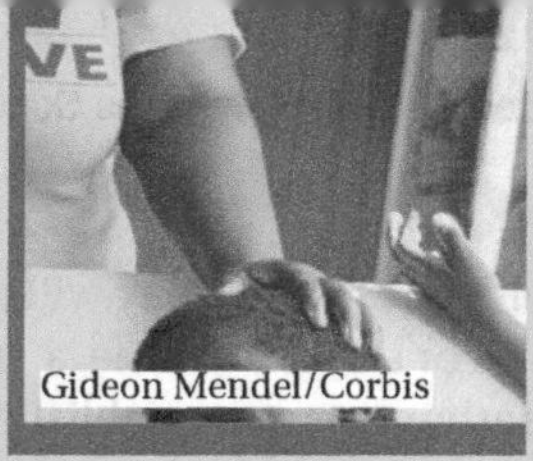

Gideon Mendel/Corbis

Is HIV/AIDS still an epidemic?

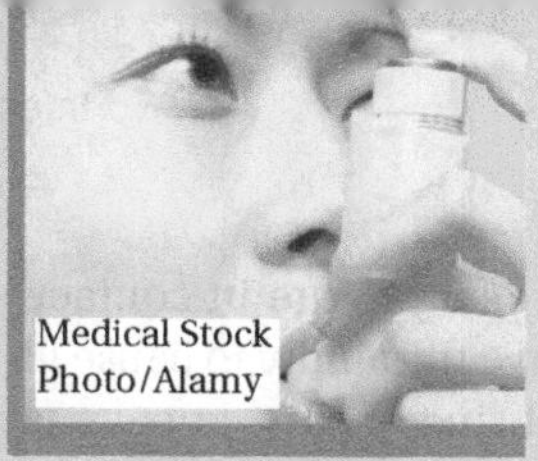

Medical Stock Photo/Alamy

What causes asthma?

Infectious and Noninfectious Conditions

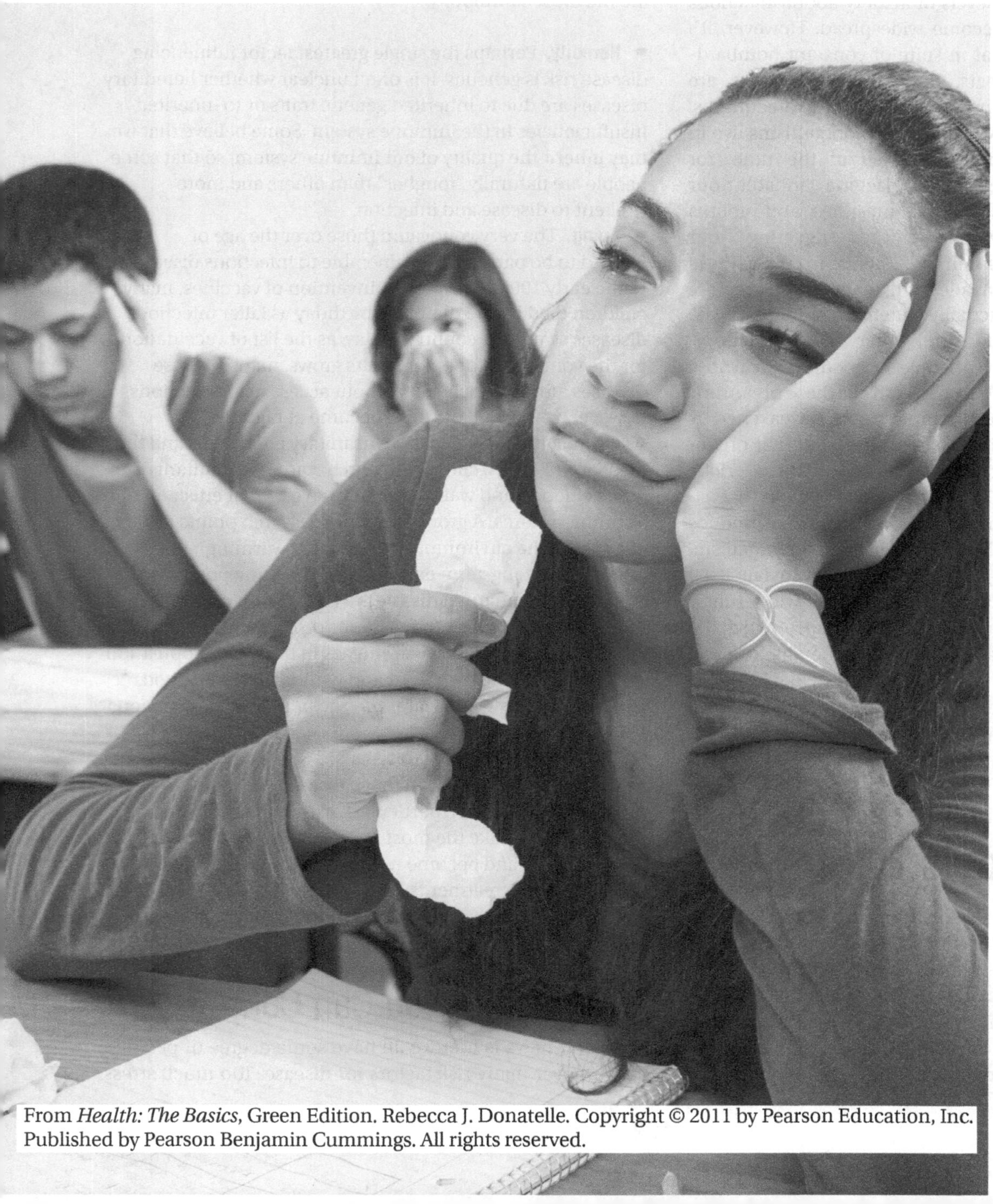

Somos/Veer/Getty Images

Objectives

* Explain how your immune system works to protect you and what you can do to boost its effectiveness.
* Describe the most common pathogens infecting humans today and the typical diseases each causes.
* Discuss the various sexually transmitted infections, their means of transmission, and actions that can be taken to prevent their spread.
* Discuss human immunodeficiency virus (HIV) and acquired immunodeficiency syndrome (AIDS), trends in infection and treatment, and the impact of the disease on special populations.
* Discuss common noninfectious conditions, including asthma and low back pain.

Every moment of every day, you are in contact with microscopic organisms that have the ability to cause illness or even death. These disease-causing agents, known as **pathogens,** are found in air and food and on nearly every object and person with whom you come in contact. New varieties of pathogens arise all the time, and scientific evidence indicates that many have existed for as long as there has been life on the planet. Throughout history, infectious diseases have at times wiped out whole groups of people through **epidemics** such as the Black Death, or bubonic plague, which killed up to one-third of the population of Europe in the 1300s. A **pandemic,** or global epidemic, of influenza killed an estimated 30 to 50 million people in 1918, whereas strains of tuberculosis and cholera continue to cause premature death throughout the world.

At times, fear and high levels of anxiety about infectious diseases such as the flu become widespread. However, it's important to remember that in spite of constant bombardment by pathogenic threats, our immune systems are remarkably resilient and amazingly adept at protecting us. Millions of microorganisms live in our bodies all of the time; for example, bacteria inhabit our stomachs, intestines, and mouths without ever triggering our immune systems to fight these invaders. In many cases they are actually beneficial, aiding in digestion and other bodily functions. For people in good health whose immune systems are functioning effectively, these organisms are harmless; however, if the immune system is weakened by other pathogens or chronic diseases, these internal organisms can grow rapidly, overcome the host, and cause serious illness.

pathogen A disease-causing agent.
epidemic Disease outbreak that affects many people in a community or region at the same time.
pandemic Global epidemic of a disease.
virulent Strong enough to overcome host resistance and cause disease.
immunocompromised Having an immune system that is impaired.

When pathogens gain entry to the body, they may produce varying degrees of illness. The more **virulent** the organism, the greater the chance that it can gain entry and sustain itself in the host, and the more likely it is that illness will result. If your immune system is weak, or **immunocompromised,** the greater the chances are that pathogens will be able to overcome your arsenal of immune defenses and make you sick. Keeping your immune system healthy will greatly reduce your chances of developing an infectious disease.

The Process of Infection and Your Body's Defenses

For a disease to occur in a person, or *host,* the host must be *susceptible,* which means that the immune system must be immunocompromised; an *agent* capable of *transmitting* a disease must be present; and the *environment* must be *hospitable* to the pathogen in terms of temperature, light, moisture, and other requirements. Although all pathogens pose a threat if they take hold in your body, the chances that they will do so are actually quite small. First, they must overcome a number of effective barriers, many of which were established in your body before you were born. Figure 1 summarizes some of the body's defenses that help protect you against invasion and decrease your susceptibility to disease. Many of these defenses can be improved, meaning that there are actions you can take to make your body's defenses more effective.

Risk Factors You Typically Cannot Control

Unfortunately, some of the factors that make you susceptible to a certain disease are beyond your control. The following are the most common:

- **Heredity.** Perhaps the single greatest factor influencing disease risk is genetics. It is often unclear whether hereditary diseases are due to inherited genetic traits or to inherited insufficiencies in the immune system. Some believe that we may inherit the quality of our immune system, so that some people are naturally "tougher" than others and more resilient to disease and infection.
- **Aging.** The very young and those over the age of 65 tend to be particularly vulnerable to infectious diseases. In the early 1900s, prior to the invention of vaccines, many children died before their fifth birthday as killer infectious diseases swept the country. Today, as the list of vaccinations for the young and for older adults grows, many of these diseases are kept in check. Without access to vaccinations, however, young and old alike become at high risk.
- **Environmental conditions.** Unsanitary conditions and the presence of drugs, chemicals, and hazardous pollutants and wastes in food and water probably have a great effect on our immune systems. A growing body of research points to changes in the environment (like global warming), the potential for long-term exposure to a "melting pot" of toxic chemicals, and natural disasters as significant contributors to increasing numbers of infectious diseases. Add to that the large numbers of displaced refugees in the world population and persons living in squalor and without access to food, clean water, or medical care, and the potential for infectious disease skyrockets.
- **Organism virulence and resistance.** Some organisms, such as the foodborne organism that causes *botulism* (a severe foodborne illness), are particularly virulent, and even tiny amounts may make the most hardy of us ill. Other organisms have mutated and become resistant to the body's defenses and to medical treatments. Multidrug-resistant strains of tuberculosis, *Staphylococcus,* and other organisms are emerging in many parts of the world.

Risk Factors You Can Control

The good news is that we all have some degree of personal control over many risk factors for disease. Too much stress,

TEARS
Wash away irritating substances and microbes
Lysozyme kills many bacteria

STOMACH
Acid kills organisms

BLADDER
Urine washes microbes from urethra

IMMUNE SYSTEM
B cells produce antibodies in response to specific antigens (humoral immunity)
T cells attack and destroy foreign cells or cells that have been infected by foreign antigens (cell-mediated immunity)
Memory cells remain to mobilize quick response to future invasion by the same pathogen

SALIVA
Washes microbes from the teeth and mucous membranes of the mouth

SKIN
Provides a physical barrier to the entrance of microbes
Acidic pH discourages the growth of organisms
Sweat and oil gland secretions kill many bacteria

RESPIRATORY TRACT
Mucus traps organisms
Cilia sweep away trapped organisms

LARGE INTESTINE
Normal bacterial inhabitants keep invaders in check

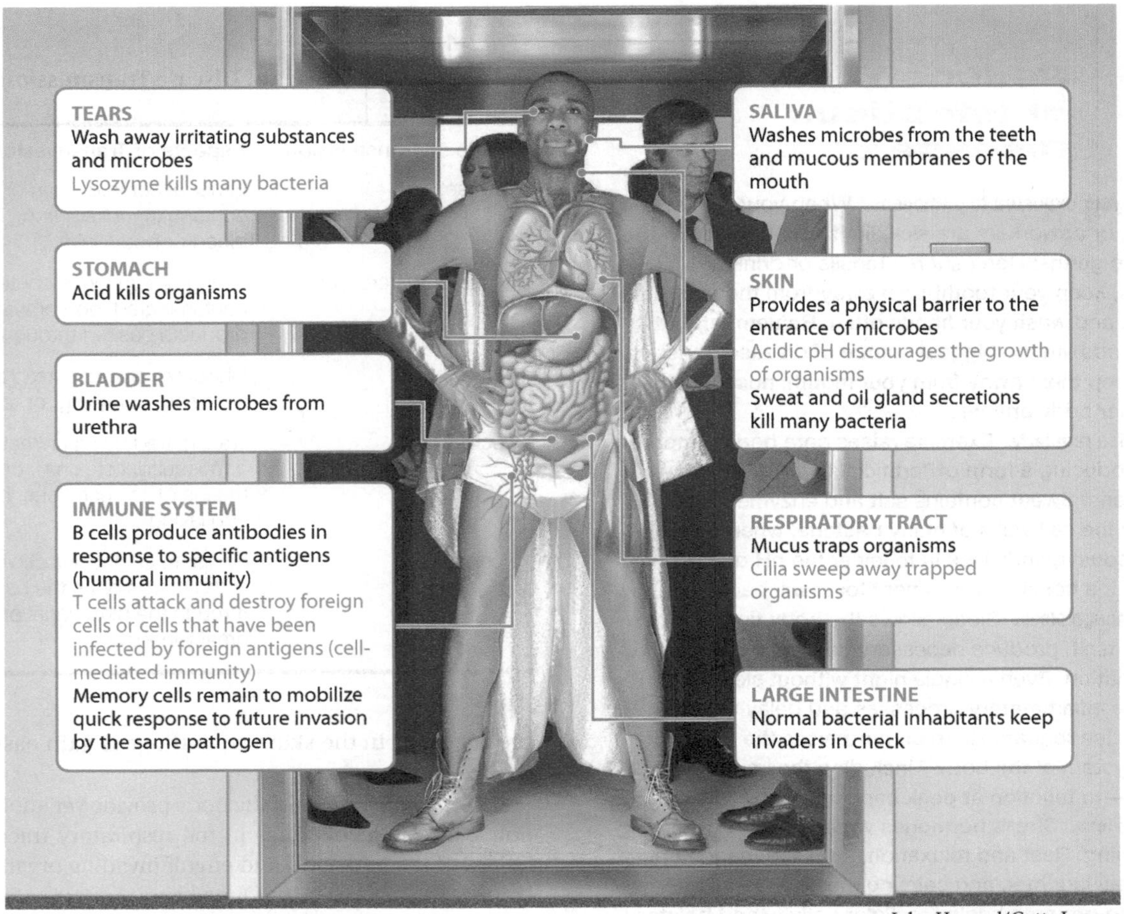

John Howard/Getty Images

FIGURE 1 The Body's Defenses against Disease-Causing Pathogens
In addition to the defenses listed, many of the body's secretions and fluids, such as earwax, mucus, and blood, contain enzymes and other proteins that can kill some invading pathogens or prevent or slow their reproduction.

inadequate nutrition, a low fitness level, lack of sleep, misuse or abuse of legal and illegal drugs and alcohol, poor personal hygiene, high-risk behaviors, exposure to products and services that increase your risk, and other variables significantly increase the risk for many diseases. Fortunately, there are things you can do to eliminate, reduce, or change your susceptibility to various pathogens. The Skills for Behavior Change lists some actions you can take and lifestyle changes you can adopt to keep your body's defenses in top form for warding off infections. There are also changes you can make in your community to clean up toxins, set policies on contaminant levels, and reduce the likelihood of being exposed to pathogens or things that could harm the immune system.

what do you think?

Do you have any risks for infectious disease that may be hereditary? Do you have any that are the result of your lifestyle? ● What actions can you take to reduce your risks? ● Are your risks greater today than before you entered college? Why or why not?

Routes of Transmission

Pathogens enter the body in several ways. They may be transmitted by *direct contact* between infected persons, such as during sexual relations, kissing, or touching, or by *indirect contact*, such as by touching an object the infected person has had contact with. Table 1 on the next page lists common routes of transmission. You may also **autoinoculate** yourself, or transmit a pathogen from one part of your body to another. For example, you may touch a sore on your lip that is teeming with viral herpes and then transmit the virus to your eye when you scratch your itchy eyelid.

Your best friend may be the source of *animalborne pathogens*. Dogs, cats, livestock, and wild animals can spread numerous diseases through their bites or feces or by carrying infected insects into living areas and transmitting diseases either directly or indirectly. Although *interspecies transmission* of diseases (diseases passed from humans to animals and vice versa) is rare, it does occur.

autoinoculate Transmit a pathogen from one part of your own body to another part.

Skills for Behavior Change

Reduce Your Risk of Infectious Disease

* **Limit your exposure to pathogens.** When your family, friends, or coworkers are sick, limit your contact with possible germs: Don't share utensils or drinking glasses, keep your toothbrush away from those of other people, and wash your hands often. Remember that your hands are the biggest source of disease transmission. Keep them away from your mouth, nose, eyes, and other body orifices.
* **Exercise regularly.** Exercise raises core body temperature, producing a form of "artificial fever" that kills pathogens. Sweat contains salt and enzymes that destroy the cell walls of many bacteria, whereas the oil (sebaceous) glands kick in to lower the pH of the skin, making it a hostile environment for many bacteria.
* **Get enough sleep.** Sleep allows the body time to refresh itself, produce necessary cells, and reduce inflammation. Even a single night without sleep can increase inflammatory processes and delay wound healing. Inadequate sleep compromises the ability of every system of the body—including the immune system—to function at peak capacity.
* **Stress less.** Stress hormones wreak havoc on immune functioning. Rest and relaxation, stress management practices, laughter, and calming music have all been shown to promote healthy cellular activity and bolster immune functioning.
* **Optimize eating.** Enjoy a healthy diet, including adequate amounts of water, protein, and complex carbohydrates. Eat more omega-3 fatty acids to reduce inflammation, and restrict saturated fats, replacing them with good fats such as olive oil. Antioxidants are believed to be important in immune functioning, so make sure you get your daily fruits and vegetables.

TABLE 1 **Routes of Disease Transmission**

Mode of Transmission	Aspects of Transmission
Contact	Either *direct* (e.g., skin or sexual contact) or *indirect* (e.g., infected blood or body fluid)
Food- or waterborne	Eating or coming in contact with contaminated food or water or products passed through them
Airborne	Inhalation; droplet spread as through sneezing, coughing, or talking
Vectorborne	Transmitted by an animal, such as a mosquito, tick, snail, or bird, by means of its secretions, biting, or egg laying
Perinatal	Similar to contact infection; happens in the uterus or as the baby passes through the birth canal or through breast-feeding

Physical and Chemical Defenses: Your Body Responds

Our single most critical early defense system is the skin. Layered to provide an intricate web of barriers, the skin allows few pathogens to enter. Enzymes in body secretions such as sweat provide additional protection, destroying microorganisms on skin surfaces by producing inhospitable pH levels. In either case, microorganisms that flourish at a selected pH will be weakened or destroyed as these changes occur. Only when cracks or breaks occur in the skin can pathogens gain easy access to the body.

antigen Substance capable of triggering an immune response.
antibodies Substances produced by the body that are individually matched to specific antigens.
humoral immunity Aspect of immunity that is mediated by the secretion of antibodies that target cells for destruction.
toxins Poisonous substances produced by certain microorganisms that cause various diseases.

The internal linings of the body provide yet another protection. Mucous membranes in the respiratory tract and other linings of the body trap and engulf invading organisms. *Cilia,* hairlike projections in the lungs and respiratory tract, sweep invaders toward body openings, where they are expelled. Tears, nasal secretions, earwax, and other secretions found at body entrances contain enzymes designed to destroy or neutralize pathogens. Finally, any organism that manages to breach these initial lines of defense faces a formidable specialized network of defenses thrown up by the immune system.

The Immune System: Your Body Fights Back

Immunity is a condition of being able to resist a particular disease by counteracting the substance that produces the disease. Any substance capable of triggering an immune response is called an **antigen.** An antigen can be a virus, a bacterium, a fungus, a parasite, a toxin, or a tissue or cell from another organism. When invaded by an antigen, the body responds by forming substances called **antibodies** that are matched to that specific antigen, much as a key is matched to a lock.

Once an antigen breaches the body's initial defenses, the body begins a process of antigen analysis. It considers the size and shape of the invader, verifies that the antigen is not part of the body itself, and then produces a specific antibody to destroy or weaken the antigen. This process, which is much more complex than described here, is part of a system called *humoral immune responses.* **Humoral immunity** is the body's major defense against many bacteria and the poisonous substances, called **toxins,** that they produce.

Cell-mediated immunity is characterized by the formation of a population of **lymphocytes** (specialized white blood cells) that can attack and destroy the foreign invader. These lymphocytes constitute the body's main defense against viruses, fungi, parasites, and some bacteria, and they are found in the blood, lymph nodes, bone marrow, and certain glands. Other key players in this immune response are **macrophages** (a type of phagocytic, or cell-eating, white blood cell).

Two forms of lymphocytes in particular, the *B lymphocytes* (B cells) and *T lymphocytes* (T cells), are involved in the immune response. T cells assist the immune system in several ways. *Helper T cells* are essential for activating B cells to produce antibodies. They also activate other T cells, and macrophages. Another form of T cell, known as the *killer T cell* directly attacks infected or malignant cells. Killer T cells enable the body to rid itself of cells that have been infected by viruses or transformed by cancer; they are also responsible for rejecting tissue and organ grafts. *Suppressor T cells* turn off or suppress the activity of B cells, killer T cells, and macrophages. After a successful attack on a pathogen, some of the attacker T and B cells are preserved as *memory T* and *B cells,* enabling the body to recognize and respond quickly to subsequent attacks by the same kind of organism at a later time.

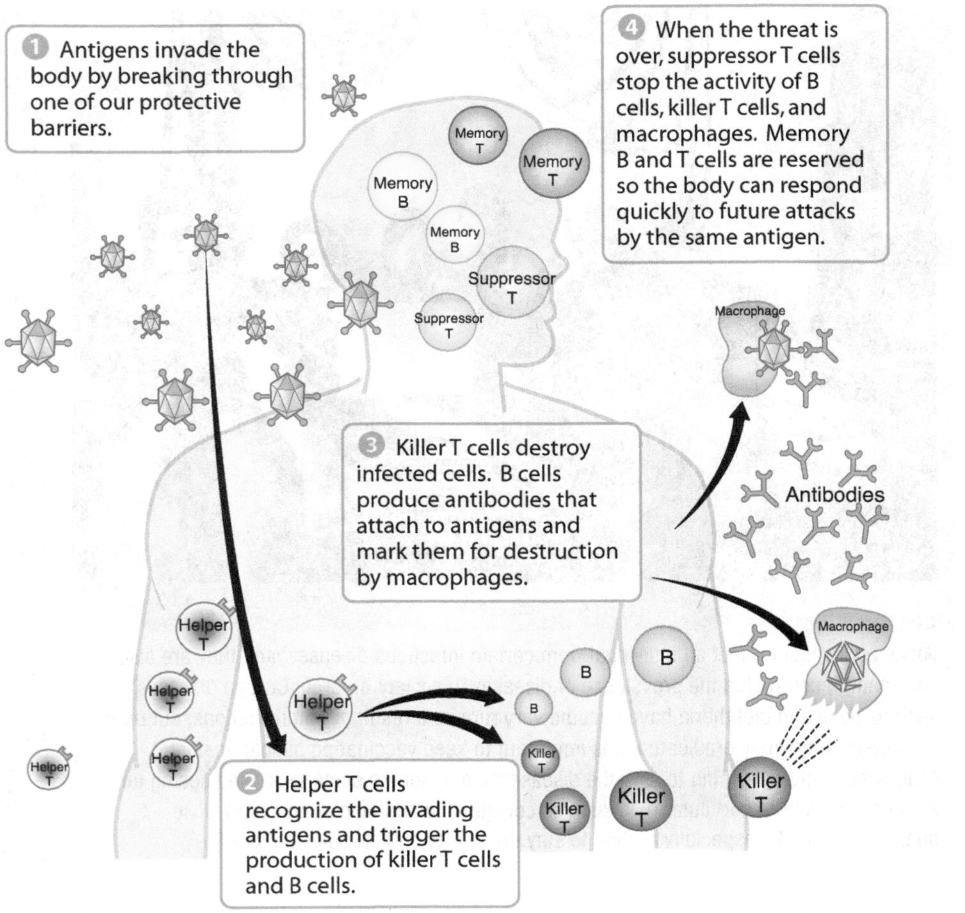
1 Antigens invade the body by breaking through one of our protective barriers.
2 Helper T cells recognize the invading antigens and trigger the production of killer T cells and B cells.
3 Killer T cells destroy infected cells. B cells produce antibodies that attach to antigens and mark them for destruction by macrophages.
4 When the threat is over, suppressor T cells stop the activity of B cells, killer T cells, and macrophages. Memory B and T cells are reserved so the body can respond quickly to future attacks by the same antigen.
Memory T
Memory T
Memory B
Memory B
Suppressor T
Suppressor T
Macrophage
Antibodies
Macrophage
Helper T
Helper T
Helper T
Helper T
Helper T
B
B
B
Killer T
Killer T
Killer T
Killer T

FIGURE 2 **The Immune Response**

Once people have survived certain infectious diseases, they become immune to those diseases, meaning that in all probability they will not develop them again. Upon subsequent attack by the same disease-causing microorganisms, their memory T and B cells are quickly activated to come to their defense. Figure 2 provides a summary of the cell-mediated immune response.

Autoimmune Diseases Although white blood cells and the antigen–antibody response generally work in our favor, the body sometimes makes a mistake and targets its own tissue as the enemy, builds up antibodies against that tissue, and attempts to destroy it. This is known as **autoimmune disease** (*auto* means "self"). Common autoimmune disorders include rheumatoid arthritis, systemic lupus erythematosus (SLE), type 1 diabetes, and multiple sclerosis.

Inflammatory Response, Pain, and Fever If an infection is localized, pus formation, redness, swelling, and irritation often occur. These symptoms are components of the body's inflammatory response, and they indicate that the invading organisms are being fought systematically. The four cardinal signs of inflammation are redness, swelling, pain, and heat.

Pain is often one of the earliest signs that an injury or infection has occurred and it can cause the person to avoid activity that may aggravate the injury or site of infection, thereby protecting against further damage. Although pain doesn't feel good, it plays a valuable role in the body's response to injury or invasion. Pathogens can kill or injure tissue at the site of infection, causing swelling that puts pressure on nerve endings in the area, causing pain to occur.

In addition to inflammation, another frequent indicator of infection is the development of a *fever,* or a rise in body temperature above the average norm of 98.6°F. Fever is frequently caused by toxins secreted by pathogens that interfere with the control of body temperature. Although extremely elevated temperatures are harmful to the body, a mild fever is protective: Raising body temperature by one or two degrees provides an environment that destroys some disease-causing organisms. A fever also stimulates the body to produce more white blood cells,

cell-mediated immunity Aspect of immunity that is mediated by specialized white blood cells that attack pathogens and antigens directly.
lymphocyte A type of white blood cell involved in the immune response.
macrophage A type of white blood cell that ingests foreign material.
autoimmune disease Disorders in which the body's tissues are attacked by its own immune system.

Yellow Dog Productions/Getty Images

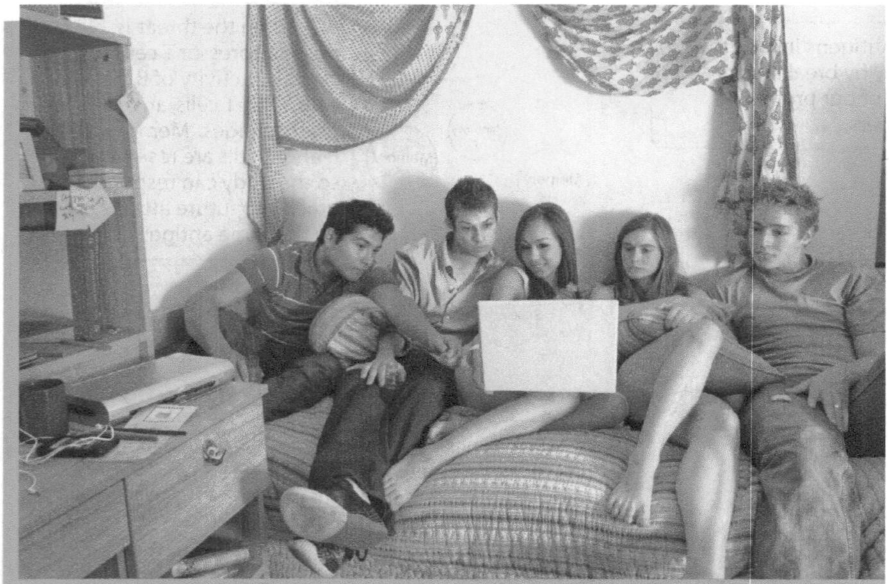

Why are vaccinations important?

Vaccinations can protect an individual from certain infectious diseases, and they are also important in controlling the prevalence of diseases in society at large. Certain diseases such as polio and diphtheria have become very rare as a result of immunizations, but until a disease is completely eradicated, it is important to keep vaccinating people against it. Otherwise, there is nothing to stop the disease from making a comeback and causing an epidemic. People at particular risk, such as college students who often live in close quarters, should be especially certain to stay up to date on their vaccinations.

which destroy more invaders. Of course, as fevers increase beyond 101 or 102 degrees Fahrenheit, risks to the patient outweigh any benefits. In these cases, medical treatment should be obtained. Misuse of aspirin in the early stage of (low) fever may inadvertently sabotage the immune system's defenses by keeping temperature ideal for pathogen growth.

Vaccines: Bolstering Your Immunity

Recall that once people have been exposed to a specific pathogen, subsequent attacks will activate their memory T and B cells, thus giving them immunity. This is the principle on which **vaccination** is based.

vaccination Inoculation with killed or weakened pathogens or similar, less dangerous antigens to prevent or lessen the effects of some disease.
allergy Hypersensitive reaction to a specific antigen in which the body produces antibodies to a normally harmless substance in the environment.
allergen An antigen that induces a hypersensitive immune response.
histamine Chemical substance that dilates blood vessels, increases mucous secretions, and produces other symptoms of allergies.

A vaccine consists of killed or weakened versions of a disease-causing microorganism or an antigen that is similar to but less dangerous than the disease antigen. It is administered to stimulate the person's immune system to produce antibodies against future attacks—without actually causing the disease (or by causing a very minor case of it). Vaccines typically are given orally or by injection, and this form of immunity is termed *artificially acquired active immunity*, in contrast to *naturally acquired active immunity* (which is obtained by exposure to antigens in the normal course of daily life) or *naturally acquired passive immunity* (as occurs when a mother passes immunity to her fetus via their shared blood supply or to an infant via breast milk).

Depending on the organism's virulence, vaccines containing live, attenuated (weakened), or dead organisms are given for specific diseases. Regardless of the type of vaccine, specific schedules have been established for optimal vaccine performance in protecting against typical diseases that affect children and adults. Figure 3 shows the recommended schedule for adult vaccinations. Childhood vaccine schedules are available at the Centers for Disease Control and Prevention (CDC) website. Concerns about potential dangers related to vaccines have caused some parents to refuse to vaccinate their children, a potentially dangerous choice that could lead to reemergence of previously eradicated diseases.

Because of their close living quarters and frequent interaction with people from many different places and backgrounds, college students face higher than average risks of infections from diseases that are largely preventable. Recent increases in some childhood diseases among the general public have prompted campuses across the country to require immunizations against diseases that should no longer plague U.S. citizens, particularly measles, German measles (rubella), and tetanus/diphtheria.

Allergies: The Immune System Overreacts

An **allergy** occurs as part of the body's attempt to defend itself against a specific *antigen* or **allergen** by producing specific *antibodies*. Under normal conditions, the production of antibodies is a positive element in the body's defense system. However, for unknown reasons, in some people the body overreacts by developing an overly protective mechanism against relatively harmless substances. The resulting *hypersensitivity reaction* is fairly common, as anyone who has awakened with a runny nose or itchy eyes will testify. Most commonly, these hypersensitivity, or allergic, reactions occur as a response to environmental antigens such as molds, animal dander (hair and dead skin), pollen, ragweed, or dust. Some people are also allergic to certain foods. Once excessive antibodies to allergens are produced, they trigger the release of **histamine,** a chemical that dilates blood vessels, increases mucous secretions, causes tissues to swell, and produces rashes, difficulty breathing, and

Vaccine	Age group				
	19–26 years	27–49 years	50–59 years	60–64 years	≥ 65 years
Tetanus, diphtheria, pertussis (Td/Tdap)*	Substitute 1-time dose of Tdap for Td booster; then boost with Td every 10 years				Td booster every 10 years
Human papillomavirus (HPV)*	3 doses (females)				
Varicella*	2 doses				
Zoster				1 dose	
Measles, mumps, rubella (MMR)*	1 or 2 doses		1 dose		
Influenza*	1 dose annually				
Pneumococcal (polysaccharide)	1 or 2 doses				1 dose
Hepatitis A*	2 doses				
Hepatitis B*	3 doses				
Meningococcal*	1 or more doses				

*Covered by the Vaccine Injury Compensation Program

For all persons in this category who meet the age requirements and who lack evidence of immunity (e.g., lack documentation of vaccination or have no evidence of prior infection)

Recommended if some other risk factor is present (e.g., on the basis of medical, occupational, lifestyle, or other indications)

No recommendation

FIGURE 3 **Recommended Adult Immunization Schedule, by Vaccine and Age Group, 2009**

Note that there are important explanations and additions to these recommendations that should be consulted by checking the latest schedule at www.cdc.gov/vaccines/recs/schedules/adult-schedule.htm.

Source: Centers for Disease Control and Prevention, "Recommended Adult Immunization Schedule—United States, 2009," *MMWR Weekly* 57, no. 53 (2009): 1–4.

other allergy symptoms. Many people have found that **immunotherapy** treatment, or "allergy shots," somewhat reduce the severity of their symptoms. In most cases, once the offending antigen has disappeared, allergy-prone people suffer few symptoms.

Hay Fever **Hay fever,** or *pollen allergy,* occurs throughout the world and is one of the most common chronic diseases in the United States, affecting over 25 million Americans each year (about 8% of all adults and 10% of children).[1] It is usually considered a seasonal disease, because it is most prevalent when ragweed and flowers are blooming. Symptoms include sneezing and itchy, watery eyes and nose, and they make countless people miserable for weeks at a time every year. As with other allergies, hay fever results from a hypersensitive immune system and an inherited tendency to have this hypersensitivity.

Avoiding the environmental triggers is the best way to prevent hay fever. If you can't prevent it, shots or antihistamines often provide relief. Decongestants can reduce symptoms, as can air-conditioning and air purifiers. Rinsing out your nose can also bring relief. Over-the-counter nose sprays are usually of limited value, and their prolonged use may actually cause symptoms or make them worse. Inhaled steroids are often effective and may be prescribed, as are specific desensitizing injections.[2]

Types of Pathogens and Diseases They Cause

We can categorize pathogenic microorganisms into six major types: bacteria, viruses, fungi, protozoans, parasitic worms, and prions. Each pathogen has a particular route of transmission and characteristic elements that make it unique. In the following pages, we discuss each of these categories and give an overview of some diseases they cause that have a significant impact on public health. Figure 4 shows examples of several of these pathogens.

Bacteria

Bacteria (singular: *bacterium*) are simple, single-celled microscopic organisms. There are three major types of bacteria, as classified by their shape: cocci, bacilli, and spirilla. Although there are several thousand known species of bacteria (and many thousands more that are unknown), just over 100 cause diseases in humans. In

immunotherapy Treatment strategies based on the concept of regulating the immune system, as by administering antibodies or desensitization shots of allergens.

hay fever A chronic allergy-related respiratory disorder that is most prevalent when ragweed and flowers bloom.

bacteria (singular: *bacterium*) Simple, single-celled microscopic organisms. About 100 known species of bacteria cause disease in humans.

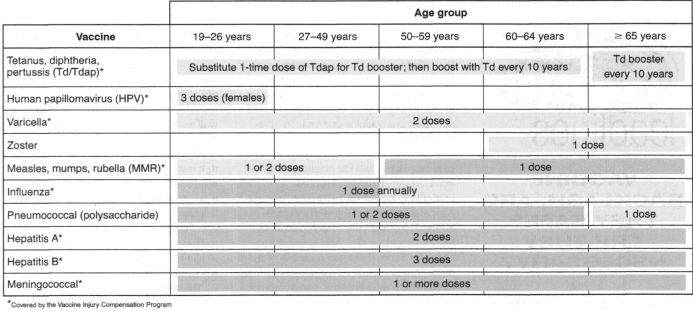

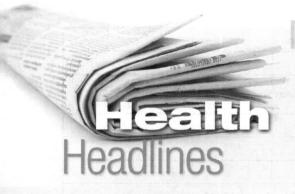

Health Headlines

VACCINE BACKLASH: ARE THEY SAFE? ARE THEY NECESSARY?

Immunizations against widespread infectious diseases are one of the greatest public health success stories of all time—so successful, in fact, that most people have never seen or heard of anyone having the diseases that once wiped out entire populations. As fear of getting these diseases waned, as numbers of vaccines recommended increased, as medical costs increased, and as distrust of all things related to government increased, many people have questioned the ethics, safety, and necessity of these shots. Misinformation and fearmongering about potential hazards of vaccines have prompted more and more people to forgo their shots. How serious a problem is this? In some communities, such as Ashland, Oregon, parents of up to 25 percent of kindergartners opted their children out of at a least one vaccine last year. In other U.S. school districts and counties, these rates are even higher, and a general trend of exemptions from vaccinations is growing. Undervaccination rates are particularly high in non-Hispanic, college-educated white families with incomes above $75,000 a year. Religious tenets, fear of vaccine safety, and worry about vaccine overload are among some of the more common reasons for parents' refusal to vaccinate their children. Others object to mandatory vaccinations because they consider them to be a government intrusion into their individual rights.

The vaccine concerns receiving the most attention include fear that the measles, mumps, rubella (MMR) vaccine can lead to autism; fear that the hepatitis B vaccine is related to multiple sclerosis (MS); and fear that the tetanus, diphtheria, pertussis (Td/Tdap vaccine) can cause sudden infant death syndrome (SIDS). Are these concerns valid? While research is ongoing, there is no clear evidence that the MMR vaccine causes autism, that hepatitis B shots are the culprit behind MS, or that the Tdap vaccine leads to SIDS. Virtually all medical and public health organizations support vaccinations, pointing to stringent safety controls in the manufacturing and testing of vaccines, as well as ongoing safety monitoring, the long history of vaccines in wiping out killer diseases across the globe, and the fact that risks from the diseases the themselves are almost always much greater than any risks associated with a vaccine. If large numbers of people were to avoid vaccinations, old killers would be likely to reemerge, and those people who were already sick or weak from other conditions would be extremely vulnerable.

The reasons for vaccination far outweigh any arguments against. That said, it's important to note that, despite extensive testing, no vaccine is completely safe and effective and that there are often risks from temporary, minor side effects from any given vaccine. Local rashes and reactions at injection sites, low-grade fever, discomfort, and even allergic reactions can occur. Major risks from getting vaccinations are extremely rare and studies supporting the "antivaccine" rhetoric are unsubstantiated. The official positions of the international community, the U.S. government, and research groups are in support of vaccine efficacy.

many cases, it is not the bacteria themselves that cause disease but rather the toxins that they produce.

antibiotics Medicines used to kill microorganisms, such as bacteria.
antibiotic resistance The ability of bacteria or other microbes to withstand the effects of an antibiotic.
staphylococci A group of round bacteria, usually found in clusters, that cause a variety of diseases in humans and other animals.
colonization The process of bacteria or some other infectious organisms establishing themselves on a host without causing infection.
infection The state of pathogens being established in or on a host and causing disease.
methicillin-resistant staphylococcus aureus (MRSA) Highly resistant form of staph infection that is growing in international prevalence.

Diseases caused by bacteria are often easily treatable with **antibiotics;** penicillin is one of the oldest and historically most well-known antibiotics. However, today's arsenal of antibiotics is becoming less effective, as antibiotic-resistant strains of bacteria become more common. Such "superbugs" can result when successive generations of bacteria mutate to develop **antibiotic resistance,** meaning they are able to withstand the effects of specific drugs. The following are the most common bacterial infections, some of which pose new threats through especially virulent, resistant strains.

Staphylococcal Infections **Staphylococci** are normally present on the skin or in the nostrils of 20 to 30 percent of us at any given time. Usually they cause no problems for otherwise healthy persons. The presence of bacteria on or in a person without infection is called **colonization.** A person can be colonized and spread the infection to others, yet not ever develop the disease. In contrast, when the pathogen is present and there is a cut or break in the *epidermis,* or outer layer of the skin, staphylococci may enter the system and cause an **infection.** If you have ever suffered from acne, boils, styes (infections of the eyelids), or infected wounds, you have probably had a "staph" infection.

Although most of these infections are readily defeated by your immune system, resistant forms of staph bacteria are on the rise. These infections pose serious risks and must be treated with specific antibiotics, of which fewer and fewer remain effective. One of these resistant forms of staph, **methicillin-resistant staphylococcus aureus (MRSA),** has come under intense international scrutiny as numerous cases have arisen around the world, especially in the United States.[3] One form,

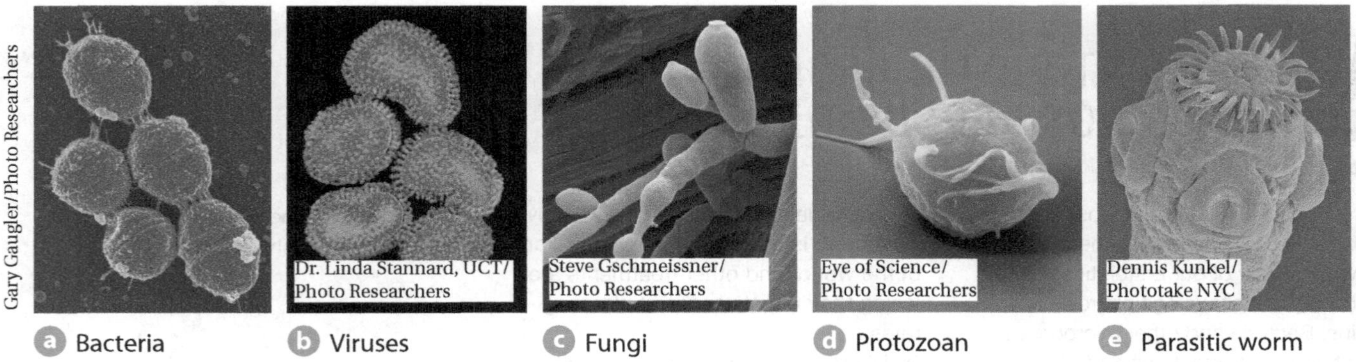

FIGURE 4 **Example of 5 Major Types of Pathogens**

(a) Color-enhanced scanning electron micrograph (SEM) of *Streptococcus* bacteria, magnified 40,000×. (b) Colored transmission electron micrograph (TEM) of influenza (flu) viruses, magnified 32,000×. (c) Color SEM of *Candida albicans,* a yeast fungus, magnified 50,000×. (d) Color TEM of *Trichomonas vaginalis*, a protozoan, magnified 9,000×. (e) Color-enhanced SEM of the adult head (scolex) of a mammalian intestinal tapeworm, magnified 20×.

healthcare associated (HA-MRSA), makes up the vast majority of cases and is particularly worrisome in hospitals, nursing homes, and other settings where invasive treatments, persons with weakened immune systems, and other infections are common. A second form, *community acquired (CA-MRSA),* is on the rise in otherwise healthy people who are exposed to the pathogen and can't fight it effectively on their own.

Symptoms of MRSA often start with a rash or pimplelike skin irritation. Within hours, these early symptoms may progress to redness, inflammation, pain, and deeper wounds. If untreated, the MRSA may invade the blood, bones, joints, surgical wounds, heart valves, and lungs and can be fatal. There are only a few antibiotics, such as vancomycin, that are effective—yet even vancomycin is showing signs of weakness against tougher strains of MRSA. For more information on antibiotic-resistant pathogens, including preventive measures, see the **Health Today** box on the following pages.

Streptococcal Infections At least five types of the **streptococcus** microorganism are known to cause bacterial infections. Group A streptococci (GAS) cause the most common diseases, such as streptococcal pharyngitis ("strep throat") and scarlet fever, which is often preceded by a sore throat.[4] One particularly virulent group of GAS can lead to a disease known as *necrotizing faciitis* (often referred to as "flesh-eating strep"), a rare, but serious, disease that leads to death in about 30 percent of all cases, even with vigorous antibiotic treatment.[5] Group B streptococci can cause illness in newborn babies, pregnant women, older adults, and adults with other illnesses such as diabetes or liver disease.

Meningitis **Meningitis** is an infection and inflammation of the *meninges,* the membranes that surround the brain and spinal cord. Some forms of bacterial meningitis are contagious and can be spread through contact with saliva, nasal discharge, feces, or respiratory and throat secretions. *Pneumococcal meningitis,* the most common form of meningitis, is the most dangerous form of bacterial meningitis. Approximately 6,000 cases of pneumococcal meningitis are reported in the United States each year. *Meningococcal meningitis,* a virulent form of meningitis, has risen dramatically on college campuses in recent years.[6] College students living in dormitories have a higher risk of contracting this disease than those who live off campus.

The signs of meningitis are sudden fever, severe headache, and a stiff neck, particularly causing difficulty touching your chin to your chest. Persons who are suspected of having meningitis should receive immediate, aggressive medical treatment. Vaccines are available for some types of meningitis.

Pneumonia In the early twentieth century, **pneumonia** was a leading cause of death in the United States. This lung disease is characterized by chronic cough, chest pain, chills, high fever, fluid accumulation, and eventual respiratory failure. One of the most common forms of pneumonia is caused by bacterial infection and responds readily to antibiotic treatment in the early stages. Other forms are caused by viruses, chemicals, or other substances in the lungs and are more difficult to treat. Although medical advances have reduced the overall incidence of pneumonia, it continues to be a major threat in the United States and throughout the world. Vulnerable populations include the poor, older adults, and people already suffering from other illnesses.

streptococcus A round bacterium, usually found in chain formation.
meningitis An infection of the meninges, the membranes that surround the brain and spinal cord.
pneumonia Disease of the lungs characterized by chronic cough, chest pain, chills, high fever, and fluid accumulation; may be caused by bacteria, viruses, chemicals, or other substances.
tuberculosis (TB) A disease caused by bacterial infiltration of the respiratory system.

Tuberculosis A major killer in the United States in the early twentieth century, **tuberculosis (TB)** was largely controlled in America by 1950 as a result of improved sanitation, isolation of infected persons, and treatment with drugs such as *rifampin* or *isoniazid.* Though many health professionals assumed that TB had been conquered, that

HEALTH Today

ANTIBIOTIC RESISTANCE: BUGS VERSUS DRUGS

Antibiotics typically wipe out bacteria that are susceptible to them. However, many of our antibiotics are becoming ineffective against resistant strains. Bacteria and other microorganisms that cause infections and diseases are remarkably resilient and continue developing ways to survive drugs that should kill or weaken them. This means that some of the bacteria and microorganisms are becoming "superbugs" that cannot be stopped with medications. Drug resistance is exacerbated by several factors, including over-prescription, underuse, and misuse (poor patient compliance). Consider these examples:

* Strains of *Staphylococcus aureus* resistant to most antibiotics, such as methicillin-resistant staphylococcus aureus (MRSA), are endemic in many hospitals today. In some cities, 31 percent of staph infections are resistant to antibiotics, and in nursing homes as many as 71 percent of staph infections defy traditional antibiotic regimens.
* The species *Streptococcus pneumoniae* causes thousands of cases of meningitis and pneumonia and 7 million cases of ear infections in the United States each year. Currently, about 30 percent of these cases are resistant to penicillin, the primary drug for treatment. Many penicillin-resistant strains are also resistant to other antibiotics.
* An estimated 500 million people worldwide are infected with parasites that cause malaria, and an estimated 700,000 to 2.7 million people die each year from that disease. Resistance to chloroquine, once a widely used and highly effective treatment, is now found in most regions of the world, and other treatments are losing their effectiveness at alarming rates.
* Diarrheal diseases cause almost 3 million deaths per year—mostly in developing countries where resistant forms of *Campylobacter, Shigella, Escherichia coli, Vibrio cholerae,* and *Salmonella* food poisoning have emerged. In some areas, as much as 50 percent of the *Campylobacter* cases are resistant to Cipro, the most effective treatment. A potentially deadly "superbug" called *Salmonella enterica typhimurium* is resistant to most antibiotics and has appeared in Europe, Canada, and the United States.

WHY IS THIS HAPPENING?

In the battle between drugs and bugs, the bugs are clearly scoring some big wins. Why is antibiotic resistance on the rise? Reasons include the following:

1. **Improper use of antibiotics and growth of superbugs.** When used improperly, antibiotics kill only the weak bacteria and leave the strongest versions to thrive and replicate. Because bacteria can swap genes with one another under the right conditions, hardy drug-resistant germs can share their resistance mechanisms with other germs. They adapt, change, and mutate, and eventually an entire colony of resistant bugs grows and passes on its resistance traits to new generations of bacteria. Over time, most pathogens evolve. Human negligence just speeds the healthy ones on their journey.

   For example, patients may begin an antibiotic regimen, start to feel better, and stop taking the drug. The surviving bacteria then build immunity to the drugs used to treat them. Also, doctors have overused antibiotics; the Centers for Disease Control and Prevention (CDC) estimates that one-third of the 150 million prescriptions written each year are unnecessary, resulting in bacterial strains that are tougher than the drugs used to fight them.

To prevent the spread of infectious disease, wash your hands!

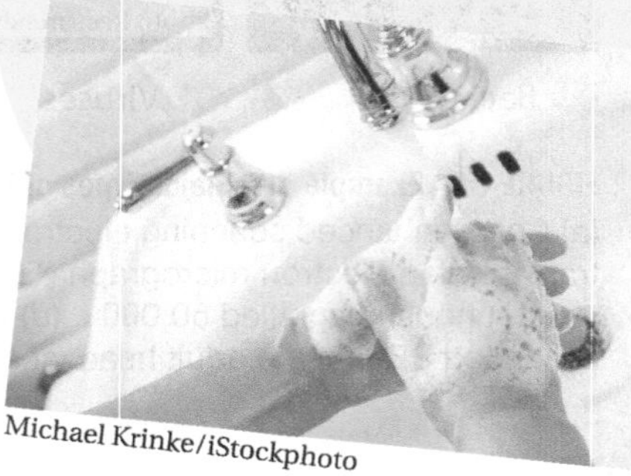

Michael Krinke/iStockphoto

2. **Overuse of antibiotics in food production.** About 70 percent of antibiotic production today is used to treat sick animals and encourage growth in livestock and poultry. Farmed fish may be given antibiotics to fight off disease in controlled water areas. Although research is only in its infancy, many believe that ingesting meats, animal products, and fish that are rich in antibiotics may contribute to antibiotic resistance in humans. In addition, water runoff from feedlots and sewage

appears not to be the case. During the past 20 years, several factors have led to an epidemic rise in the disease: deteriorating social conditions, including overcrowding and poor sanitation; failure to isolate active cases of TB; a weakening of public health infrastructure, which has led to less funding for screening; and migration of TB to the United States through immigration and international travel. In 2007, the most recent year for which data are available, there were 13,299 active cases of TB in the United States, compared to 85,000 in 1950.[7]

How serious is the TB threat today? The World Health Organization (WHO) reports that almost 2 billion people (a third of the world's entire population) have been exposed to TB, with 9.3 million becoming ill and 2 million dying each year. Some 80 percent of tuberculosis-related deaths occur in developing countries, where it accounts for 26 percent of preventable deaths.[8] TB is the number one infectious killer of women of reproductive age worldwide, as well as the leading cause of death among HIV-positive patients.

can contaminate the water in our rivers and streams with antibiotics.

3. Misuse and overuse of antibacterial soaps and other cleaning products. Preying on the public's fear of germs and disease, the cleaning industry adds antibacterial ingredients to many of their dish soaps, hand cleaners, shower scrubs, surface scrubs, and most household products. Just how much these products contribute to overall resistance is difficult to assess; as with antibiotics, the germs these products do not kill may become stronger than before.

WHO IS AT RISK?

In general, anyone who comes in contact with superbugs such as MRSA can become infected. However, certain groups are at particular risk for these new strains of antibiotic-resistant bugs. Among these are

- Health care workers
- People with weakened immune systems
- Surgical patients and anyone in a hospital with incisions and tissue exposure or persons staying in a health care facility for an extended period of time
- Young children and the elderly
- Diabetics
- People participating in contact sports
- Prisoners or anyone living in confined space with other people

HOW CAN YOU AVOID SUPERBUGS?

Prevention of MRSA and other drug-resistant pathogens involves common infection-control measures in your everyday activities. If someone you know has MRSA or another drug-resistant pathogen, extra precautions may be necessary:

- **Wash your hands often.** Use regular soap and water, wash for at least 10 to 30 seconds, and be sure to scrub the back of the hands and under the fingernails. If you are caring for a patient at home, wash your hands before leaving the house.
- **Keep personal items personal.** Don't share lip balm, makeup, razors, or other personal hygiene implements.
- **Keep wounds clean, sterile, and covered.** Use disposable latex gloves when treating wounds or bandaging. Wash your hands after taking gloves off.
- **Keep surfaces and linens clean.** Any surface that is in frequent contact with an infected person should be washed often with hot, soapy water. Use towels only once and change linens regularly.
- **Take precautions in public athletic facilities.** At the gym, wipe down surfaces you touch with antibiotic washes. Launder your clothes after touching weight machines and other surfaces. Wash hands after touching your dirty clothes. If you are involved in intramural or competitive athletics, shower with hot, soapy water after all contact with individuals, mats, and equipment.
- **Inform others.** If you suspect infection, tell your close friends and health care providers. They can all take precautions to prevent the spread of disease.

WHAT CAN YOU DO ABOUT ANTIBIOTIC RESISTANCE?

To help prevent antibiotic resistance, use antimicrobial drugs only for bacterial, not viral, infections. Take medications as prescribed and finish the full course. Consult with your health care provider if you feel it is necessary to stop your medication. It is also important that you do not keep medication for the next time you are sick. This can lead to an improper dosage, potentially contributing to future antibiotic resistance.

Prescription medications are not the only potential contributors to antibiotic resistance. Next time you go to the grocery store, take note of the multitude of cleaning products that are designed to kill just about any bacterium you face. Some experts say that these antibacterial products do more harm than good. Research suggests that antibacterial agents contained in soaps actually may kill normal bacteria, thus creating an environment for resistant, mutated bacteria that are impervious to antibacterial cleaners and antibiotics.

Sources: Centers for Disease Control and Prevention, National Center for Preparedness, Detection, and Control of Infectious Diseases/Division of Healthcare Quality Promotion, "Antibiotic/Antimicrobial Resistance: Diseases Connected to Antibiotic Resistance," Updated July 2008, www.cdc.gov/drugresistance/diseases.htm; Centers for Disease Control and Prevention, National Center for Immunization and Respiratory Diseases, Division of Bacterial Diseases, "Antibiotic Resistance Questions & Answers," Updated June 2009, www.cdc.gov/getsmart/antibiotic-use/anitbiotic-resistance-faqs.html.

Tuberculosis is caused by bacterial infiltration of the respiratory system that results in a chronic inflammatory reaction in the lungs. Airborne transmission via the respiratory tract is the primary and most efficient mode of transmitting TB. Symptoms include persistent coughing, weight loss, fever, and spitting up blood. Infected people can be contagious without actually showing any symptoms themselves and can transmit the disease while talking, coughing, sneezing, or singing.

Fortunately, TB is fairly difficult to catch, and prolonged exposure, rather than single exposure, is the typical mode of infection. Those at highest risk for TB include the poor, especially children, and the chronically ill. People residing in crowded prisons and homeless shelters with poor ventilation who continuously inhale the same contaminated air are at higher risk. Persons with compromised immune systems are also at high risk, as are those recovering from surgery, cancer therapy, and other situations where comorbidity exists. Treatments are effective for most nonresistant cases and usually include rest, careful infection-control procedures, and anti-TB drug regimens.

As with many bacterial diseases, resistant forms of TB are increasing in the global population. **Multidrug resistant TB (MDR-TB)** is a form of TB that is currently resistant to at least two of the best anti-TB drugs in use today. An even more dangerous form, **extensively drug resistant TB (XDR-TB),** is resistant to nearly all first- and second-line drug defenses against it and is extremely difficult to treat. Fatalities from XDR are increasing globally.

Tickborne Bacterial Diseases In the past few decades, certain tickborne diseases have become major health threats in the United States. Those that are most noteworthy include two bacterially caused diseases, **Lyme disease** and *ehrlichiosis,* each of which spike in the summer months in many states and which can cause significant disability and threats to humans and animals.

Once believed to be closely related to viruses, **rickettsia** are now considered a small form of bacteria. They produce toxins and multiply within small blood vessels, causing vascular blockage and tissue death. Rickettsia require an insect vector (carrier) for transmission to humans. Two common forms of human rickettsial disease are *Rocky Mountain spotted fever* (RMSF), carried by a tick; and *typhus,* carried by a louse, flea, or tick. These diseases produce similar symptoms, including high fever, weakness, rash, and coma, and both can be life threatening.

multidrug resistant TB (MDR-TB) Form of TB that is resistant to at least two of the best antibiotics available.
extensively drug resistant TB (XDR-TB) Form of TB that is resistant to nearly all existing antibiotics.
Lyme disease A bacterial disease transmitted to humans by the bite of an infected tick.
rickettsia A small form of bacteria that lives inside other living cells.
viruses Microbes consisting of DNA or RNA that invade a host cell and use the cell's resources to reproduce themselves.
incubation period The time between exposure to a disease and the appearance of symptoms.
endemic Describing a disease that is always present to some degree.
influenza A common viral disease of the respiratory tract.

For all insectborne diseases, the best protection is to stay indoors at dusk and early morning to avoid hours when insects are especially active. If you must go out, wear protective clothing or use bug sprays containing natural oils, pyrethrins, or DEET (diethyl tolumide), all products regarded as generally safe.

Viruses

Viruses are the smallest known pathogens, approximately 1/500th the size of bacteria. Essentially, a virus consists of a protein structure that contains either *ribonucleic acid (RNA)* or *deoxyribonucleic acid (DNA).* Viruses are incapable of carrying out any life processes on their own. To reproduce, they must invade and inject their own DNA and RNA into the host cell, take it over, and force it to make copies of themselves. The new viruses then erupt out of the host cell and seek other cells to infect.

Viral diseases can be difficult to treat because many viruses can withstand heat, formaldehyde, and large doses of radiation with little effect on their structure. Some viruses have **incubation periods** (the length of time required to develop fully and cause symptoms in their hosts) that last for years, which delays diagnosis. Drug treatment for viral infections is also limited. Drugs powerful enough to kill viruses generally kill the host cells too, although some medications block stages in viral reproduction without damaging host cells.

The Common Cold Colds are responsible for more days lost from work and more uncomfortable days spent at work than any other ailment. Caused by any number of viruses (some experts claim there may be over 200 different viruses responsible), colds are **endemic** (always present to some degree) throughout the world. Current research indicates that otherwise healthy people carry cold viruses in their noses and throats most of the time. These viruses are held in check until the host's resistance is lowered. In the true sense of the word, it is possible to "catch" a cold—from the airborne droplets of another person's sneeze or from skin-to-skin or mucous membrane contact—although the hands are the greatest avenue for transmitting colds and other viruses. Contrary to common thinking, you won't "catch" a cold from getting a chill, but the chill may lower your immune system's resistance to the cold virus or other pathogens.

Influenza In otherwise healthy people, **influenza,** or flu, is usually not life threatening. However, for certain vulnerable populations, such as individuals with respiratory problems or heart disease, older adults (over age 65), or young children (under age 5), the flu can be very serious. Five to 20 percent of Americans get the flu each year, and of these, 200,000 will need hospitalization.[9] Once a person gets the flu, treatment is *palliative,* meaning that it is focused on relief of symptoms, rather than cure.

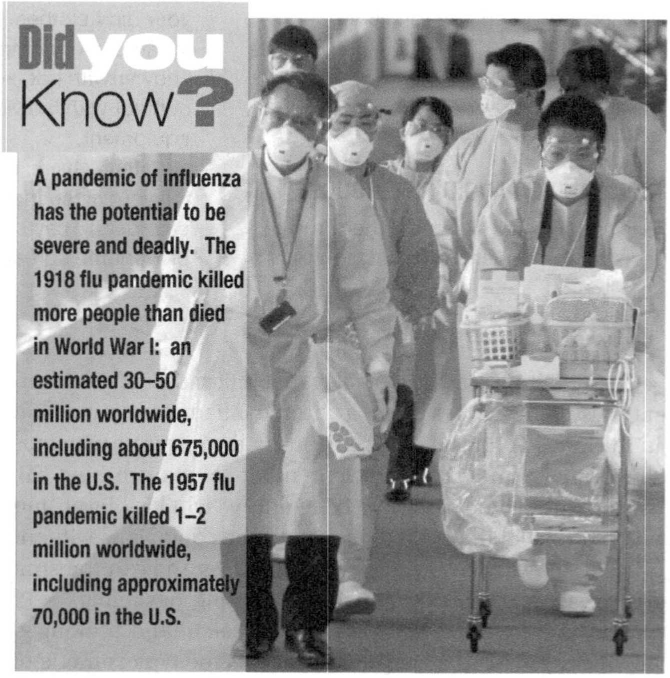

Did you Know?

A pandemic of influenza has the potential to be severe and deadly. The 1918 flu pandemic killed more people than died in World War I: an estimated 30–50 million worldwide, including about 675,000 in the U.S. The 1957 flu pandemic killed 1–2 million worldwide, including approximately 70,000 in the U.S.

Dai Kurokawa/epa/Corbis

Skills for Behavior Change

What You Can Do to Avoid H1N1 and Other Forms of the Flu

Whether it's the H1N1 flu virus or other strains, there are steps you can take to reduce your risk of contracting the flu, including:

- **Stay informed. Use the Centers for Disease Control and Prevention (CDC) and your state's health division's websites to keep up with the latest information about vaccinations, flu transmission, and ways to protect yourself.**
- **Take everyday actions to stay healthy. Influenza is thought to spread mainly person to person through coughing or sneezing.**
- **Cover your nose and mouth with a tissue when you cough or sneeze, or sneeze into your sleeve. Throw the tissue in the trash after you use it.**
- **Wash your hands often with soap and water, especially after you cough or sneeze. Alcohol-based hand cleaners are also effective.**
- **Avoid touching your eyes, nose, or mouth.**
- **Stay home if you get sick, and limit contact with others to keep from infecting them.**
- **Follow public health advice regarding school closures, avoiding crowds, and other social distancing measures.**

Source: Centers for Disease Control and Prevention, "2009 H1N1 Flu (Swine Flu)," Updated November 2009, www.cdc.gov/h1n1flu.

To date, three major varieties of flu virus have been discovered, with many different strains existing within each variety. The A form of the virus is generally the most virulent, followed by the B and C varieties. If you contract one form of influenza you may develop immunity to it, but you will not necessarily be immune to other forms of the disease.

36,000 **Americans die of the flu each year.**

Some vaccines have proven effective against certain strains of flu virus, but they are totally ineffective against others. In spite of minor risks, people over age 65, pregnant women, people with heart or lung disease, and people with certain other illnesses should be vaccinated. Flu shots take 2 to 3 weeks to become effective, so people at risk should get these shots in the fall before the flu season begins.

New strains of influenza are appearing all the time. In 2009, one flu in particular, **H1N1,** the so-called swine flu, captured world attention and rose to pandemic levels. For more about how to avoid H1N1 and other forms of the flu, see the **Skills for Behavior Change** box at left.

Hepatitis One of the most highly publicized viral diseases is **hepatitis,** a virally caused inflammation of the liver. Hepatitis symptoms include fever, headache, nausea, loss of appetite, skin rashes, pain in the upper right abdomen, dark yellow (with brownish tinge) urine, and jaundice. Internationally, viral hepatitis is a major contributor to liver disease and accounts for high morbidity and mortality. Currently, there are seven known forms, with hepatitis A, B, and C having the highest rates of incidence.

Hepatitis A (HAV) is contracted from eating food or drinking water contaminated with human feces. Since vaccinations became available, HAV rates have declined by nearly 90 percent in the United States. However, over 25,000 people per year are still infected.[10] Handlers of infected food, children at day care centers, those who have sexual contact with HAV-positive individuals, or those who travel to international regions where HAV is endemic are at higher risk. In addition, those who ingest seafood from contaminated water, and people who use contaminated needles are also at risk. Fortunately, individuals infected with hepatitis A do not become chronic carriers, and vaccines for the disease are available. Many who contract HAV are asymptomatic.

Hepatitis B (HBV) is spread primarily through body fluids being shared through unprotected sex. However, it is also contracted via sharing needles when injecting drugs; through needlesticks on the job; or, in the case of a newborn baby, from an infected mother. Hepatitis B can lead to chronic liver disease or liver cancer.

H1N1 or "swine flu" A strain of potentially virulent influenza identified in 2009.

hepatitis A viral disease in which the liver becomes inflamed, producing symptoms such as fever, headache, and possibly jaundice.

In spite of vaccine availability since 1982, there are over 43,000 new cases of HBV in the United States each year. Vaccines for HAV and HBV are now available on most college campuses and large numbers of students have been vaccinated. As such, HBV is now one of the only vaccine-preventable forms of sexually transmitted infections. Globally, HBV infections are on the decline, but they continue to be a major health problem, with over 350 million chronic carriers and over 1 million deaths each year. Three-quarters of the world's population live in areas where there are high rates of infection.[11]

Hepatitis C (HCV) infections are on an epidemic rise in many regions of the world as resistant forms of the virus are emerging. Some cases can be traced to blood transfusions or organ transplants. Currently, an estimated 17,000 new cases of HCV are diagnosed in the United States each year, with over 3.2 million people chronically infected.[12] Over 85 percent of those infected develop chronic infections; if the infection is left untreated, the person may develop cirrhosis of the liver, liver cancer, or liver failure. Liver failure resulting from chronic hepatitis C is the leading reason for liver transplants in the United States. Currently, there is no vaccine for HCV, although efforts to develop one have been under way for the past decade.

Other Pathogens

Although bacteria and viruses account for many of the common diseases in both adults and children, they don't account for all of them. Other very small or microscopic organisms can also infect and cause disease symptoms in a host. Among these are fungi, protozoans, parasitic worms, and prions.

Fungi Our environment is inhabited by thousands of species of **fungi,** multicellular or unicellular organisms that obtain their food by infiltrating the bodies of other organisms, both living and dead. Many fungi are useful to humans, such as edible mushrooms, penicillin, and the yeast used in making bread, but some species of fungi can produce infections. *Candidiasis* (a vaginal yeast infection), athlete's foot, ringworm, and jock itch are examples of fungal diseases. With most fungal diseases, keeping the affected area clean and dry plus treating it with appropriate medications will generally bring prompt relief.

Protozoans **Protozoans** are microscopic single-celled organisms that are generally associated with tropical diseases such as African sleeping sickness and malaria. Although these pathogens are prevalent in nonindustrialized countries, they are largely controlled in the United States. The most common protozoan disease in the United States is *trichomoniasis,* which we will discuss later in this chapter's section on sexually transmitted infections. A common waterborne protozoan disease in many regions of the country is *giardiasis.*

Parasitic Worms **Parasitic worms** are the largest of the pathogens. Ranging in size from the small pinworms typically found in children to the relatively large tapeworms that can be found in all warm-blooded animals, most parasitic worms are more a nuisance than a threat. Of special note today are the worm infestations associated with eating raw fish (as in sashimi). Cooking fish and other foods to temperatures sufficient to kill the worms and their eggs can prevent this.

Prions A **prion** is a self-replicating, protein-based agent that can infect humans and other animals. One such prion is believed to be the underlying cause of spongiform diseases such as *bovine spongiform encephalopathy* (BSE, or "mad cow disease"). Evidence indicates that there is a relationship between outbreaks of BSE in Europe and a disease in humans called *variant Creutzfeldt-Jakob disease* (vCJD).[13] Both disorders are invariably fatal brain diseases with unusually long incubation periods measured in years, and both are caused by prions. To date, there have been no known human infections from U.S. beef; however, infected cattle have been found.

fungi A group of multicellular and unicellular organisms that obtain their food by infiltrating the bodies of other organisms, both living and dead; several microscopic varieties are pathogenic.
protozoans Microscopic single-celled organisms that can be pathogenic.
parasitic worms The largest of the pathogens, most of which are more a nuisance than a threat.
prion A recently identified self-replicating, protein-based pathogen.

Emerging and Resurgent Diseases

Although our immune systems are remarkably adept at responding to challenges, microbes and other pathogens appear to be gaining ground. Old scourges are back, and new ones are emerging. Within the past decades, rates for infectious diseases have rapidly increased, particularly for reemerging diseases such as tuberculosis. This trend can be attributed to a combination of overpopulation, inadequate health care systems, increasing poverty, extreme environmental degradation, and drug resistance. As international travel increases (over 1 million people per day cross international boundaries), with germs transported from remote regions to huge urban centers within hours, the likelihood of infection by pathogens previously unknown on U.S. soil increases.

West Nile Virus Until 1999, few Americans had heard of *West Nile virus (WNV),* which is spread by the bite of an infected mosquito. Today, only Alaska and Hawaii remain free of the disease. Several thousand active cases of WNV surface in the United States every year. The elderly and those with impaired immune systems bear the brunt of the disease burden.[14]

Most people who become infected with West Nile virus will have mild symptoms or none at all. Rarely, WNV infection can result in severe and sometimes fatal illness. Symptoms include fever, headache, and body aches, often with skin rash and swollen lymph glands, and a form of encephalitis (inflammation of the brain). There is no vaccine or specific treatment for WNV, but avoiding mosquito bites is the best way to prevent it: using Environmental Protection Agency (EPA)-registered insect repellents such as those with DEET or eucalyptus; wearing long-sleeved clothing and long pants when outdoors; staying indoors during dawn, dusk, and other peak mosquito feeding times; and removing any standing water sources around the home.

Avian (Bird) Flu *Avian influenza* is an infectious disease of birds. There has been considerable media flurry in the past few years over a strain of avian (bird) flu, H5N1, that is highly pathogenic and is capable of crossing the species barrier and causing severe illness in humans. This virulent flu strain began to emerge in bird populations throughout Asia, including domestic birds such as chickens and ducks, as early as 1997. By 2007, H5N1 bird flu had spread to birds in parts of western Europe, eastern Europe, Russia, and northern Africa. Although the virus has yet to mutate into a form highly infectious to humans, outbreaks have occurred in rural areas of the world (where people often live in close proximity to poultry and other animals). As of September 2009, bird flu had caused 262 human deaths worldwide.[15]

Escherichia coli O157:H7 *Escherichia coli* O157:H7 is one of over 170 types of *E. coli* bacteria that can infect humans. Most *E. coli* organisms are harmless and live in the intestines of healthy animals and humans; *E. coli* O157:H7, however, produces a lethal toxin and can cause severe illness or death.

E. coli O157:H7 can live in the intestines of healthy cattle and then contaminate food products at slaughterhouses. Eating ground beef that is rare or undercooked, drinking unpasteurized milk or juice, or swimming in sewage-contaminated water or public pools can cause infection through ingestion of feces that contain *E. coli*.

Although *E. coli* organisms continue to pose threats to public health, strengthened regulations on the cooking of meat and regulation of chlorine levels in pools have helped. However, the 2006 *E. coli* outbreak linked to contaminated spinach and other outbreaks in recent years have caused the U.S. Department of Agriculture (USDA) and others in the agriculture industry to consider new safety measures.

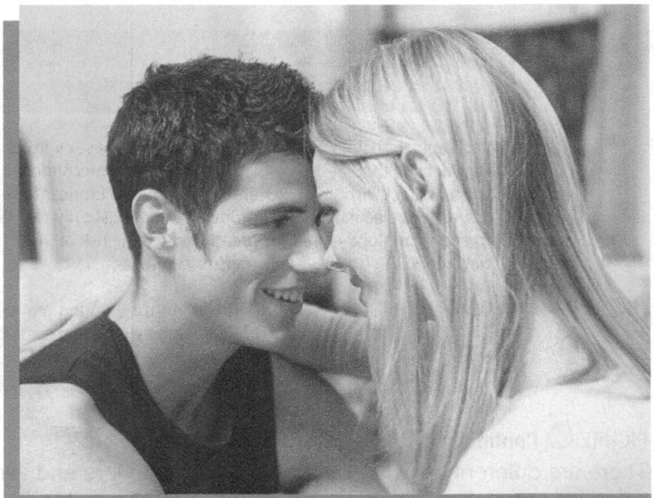

Steve Mercer/Image Bank/Getty Images

How can I tell if someone I'm dating has an STI?

You can't tell if someone has an STI just by looking at them; it isn't something broadcast on a person's face, and many people with STIs are unaware of the infection because it is asymptomatic. The only way to know for sure is to go to a clinic and get tested. In addition, partners need to be open and honest with each other about their sexual histories, and practice safer sex.

Sexually Transmitted Infections

Sexually transmitted infections (STIs) have been with us since our earliest recorded days on Earth. Today, there are more than 20 known types of STIs. Once referred to as *venereal diseases* and then *sexually transmitted diseases,* the current terminology is more reflective of the number and types of these communicable diseases, and also of the fact that they are caused by infecting pathogens. More virulent strains and antibiotic-resistant forms spell trouble in the days ahead.

65 million people are currently living with an incurable STI.

Sexually transmitted infections affect men and women of all backgrounds and socioeconomic levels. However, they disproportionately affect women, minorities, and infants. In addition, STIs are most prevalent in teens and young adults.[16] In the United States alone, an estimated 19 million new cases of STIs are reported each year.[17]

Early symptoms of an STI are often mild and unrecognizable. Left untreated, some of these infections can have grave consequences, such as sterility, blindness, central nervous system destruction, disfigurement, and even death. Infants born to mothers carrying the organisms for these infections are at risk for a variety of health problems.

As with many communicable diseases, much of the pain, suffering, and anguish associated with STIs can be eliminated through education, responsible action, simple preventive strategies, and prompt treatment. Although STIs can happen to anyone, you can avoid them if you take appropriate precautions when you decide to engage in a sexual relationship.

What's Your Risk?

Several reasons have been proposed to explain the present high rates of STIs. The first relates to the moral and social stigma associated with these infections. Shame and embarrassment often keep infected people from seeking treatment. Unfortunately, they usually continue to be sexually active, thereby infecting unsuspecting partners. People who are uncomfortable discussing sexual issues may also be less likely to use and ask their partners to use condoms to protect against STIs and pregnancy.

Another reason proposed for the STI epidemic is our culture's casual attitude about sex. Bombarded by media hype that glamorizes easy sex, many people take sexual partners without considering the consequences. Generally, the more sexual partners a person has, the greater the risk for contracting an STI.

Ignorance—about the infections, their symptoms, and the fact that someone can be asymptomatic but still infected—is also a factor. A person who is infected but asymptomatic can unknowingly spread an STI to an unsuspecting partner, who may, in turn, ignore or misinterpret any symptoms. By the time either partner seeks medical help, he or she may have infected several others. In addition, many people mistakenly believe that certain sexual practices—oral sex, for example—carry no risk for STIs. In fact, oral sex practices among young adults may be

sexually transmitted infections (STIs) Infectious diseases caused by pathogens transmitted through some form of intimate, usually sexual, contact.

High-risk behaviors	Moderate-risk behaviors	Low-risk behaviors	No-risk behaviors
Unprotected vaginal, anal, and oral sex—any activity that involves direct contact with bodily fluids, such as ejaculate, vaginal secretions, or blood—are high-risk behaviors.	Vaginal, anal, or oral sex with a latex or polyurethane condom and a water-based lubricant used properly and consistently can greatly reduce the risk of STI transmission. Dental dams used during oral sex can also greatly reduce the risk of STI transmission.	Mutual masturbation, if there are no cuts on the hand, penis or vagina, is very low risk. Rubbing, kissing, and massaging carry low risk, but herpes can be spread by skin-to-skin contact from an infected partner.	Abstinence, phone sex, talking, and fantasy are all no-risk behaviors.

FIGURE 5 **Continuum of Risk for Various Sexual Behaviors**
There are different levels of risk for various behaviors and various sexually transmitted infections (STIs); however, no matter what, any sexual activity involving direct contact with blood, semen, or vaginal secretions is high risk.

responsible for increases in herpes and other STIs. Figure 5 shows the continuum of risk for various sexual behaviors, and the **Skills for Behavior Change** box on the next page offers tips for ways to practice safer sex.

Routes of Transmission

Sexually transmitted infections are generally spread through some form of intimate sexual contact. Sexual intercourse, oral–genital contact, hand–genital contact, and anal intercourse are the most common modes of transmission. Less likely, but still possible, modes of transmission include mouth-to-mouth contact, or contact with fluids from body sores that may be spread by the hands. Although each STI is a different infection caused by a different pathogen, all STI pathogens prefer dark, moist places, especially the mucous membranes lining the reproductive organs. Most of them are susceptible to light, excess heat, cold, and dryness, and many die quickly on exposure to air. Like other communicable infections, STIs have both pathogen-specific incubation periods and periods of time during which transmission is most likely, called *periods of communicability.*

Chlamydia

Chlamydia, an infection caused by the bacterium *Chlamydia trachomatis* that often presents no symptoms, is the most commonly reported STI in the United States. Chlamydia infects about 2.2 million Americans annually, the majority of them women.[18] Public health officials believe that the actual number of cases is probably higher, because these figures represent only those cases reported.

chlamydia Bacterially caused STI of the urogenital tract.
gonorrhea Bacterial infection that is the second most common STI in the United States; if untreated, may cause sterility.

Signs and Symptoms In men, early symptoms may include painful and difficult urination; frequent urination; and a watery, puslike discharge from the penis. Symptoms in women may include a yellowish discharge, spotting between periods, and occasional spotting after intercourse. However, many chlamydia victims display no symptoms and therefore do not seek help until the disease has done secondary damage. Women are especially likely to be asymptomatic; over 70 percent do not realize they have the disease until secondary damage occurs.

Complications The secondary damage resulting from chlamydia is serious in both men and women. Men can suffer injury to the prostate gland, seminal vesicles, and bulbourethral glands, and they can suffer from arthritis-like symptoms and inflammatory damage to the blood vessels and heart. Men can also experience epididymitis, inflammation of the area near the testicles. In women, chlamydia-related inflammation can injure the cervix or fallopian tubes, causing sterility, and it can damage the inner pelvic structure, leading to pelvic inflammatory disease (PID) (see the **Gender & Health** box). If an infected woman becomes pregnant, she has a high risk for miscarriage and stillbirth. Chlamydia may also be responsible for one type of *conjunctivitis,* an eye infection that affects not only adults but also infants, who can contract the disease from an infected mother during delivery. Untreated conjunctivitis can cause blindness.[19]

Diagnosis and Treatment Diagnosis of chlamydia is determined through a laboratory test. A sample of urine or fluid from the vagina or penis is collected to identify the presence of the bacteria. Unfortunately, chlamydia tests are not a routine part of many health clinics' testing procedures. Usually a person must specifically request it. If detected early, chlamydia is easily treatable with antibiotics such as tetracycline, doxycycline, or erythromycin.

Gonorrhea

Gonorrhea is one of the most common STIs in the United States, surpassed only by chlamydia in number of cases. The CDC estimates that there are over 700,000 cases per year, plus

Skills for Behavior Change

Safe Is Sexy

Practicing the following behaviors will help you reduce your risk of contracting a sexually transmitted infection (STI):

- **Avoid casual sexual partners. All sexually active adults who are not in a lifelong monogamous relationship should practice safer sex.**
- **Use latex condoms consistently and correctly. Remember that condoms do not provide 100 percent protection against all STIs.**
- **Postpone sexual involvement with someone until you are assured that your partner is not infected by discussing past sexual history and getting testing.**
- **Avoid injury to body tissue during sexual activity. Some pathogens can enter the bloodstream through microscopic tears in anal or vaginal tissues.**
- **Avoid unprotected oral, anal, or vaginal sexual activity in which semen, blood, or vaginal secretions could penetrate mucous membranes or enter through breaks in the skin.**
- **Always use a condom or a dental dam (a sensitive latex sheet, about the size of a tissue, that can be placed over the female genitals to form a protective layer) during oral sex.**
- **Avoid using drugs and alcohol, which can dull your senses and affect your ability to take responsible precautions with potential sex partners.**
- **Wash your hands before and after sexual encounters. Urinate after sexual relations and, if possible, wash your genitals.**
- **Although total abstinence is the only absolute means of preventing the transmission of STIs, abstinence can be a difficult choice to make. If you have any doubt about the potential risks of having sex, consider other means of intimacy (at least until you can assure your safety)—massage, dry kissing, hugging, holding and touching, and masturbation (alone or with a partner).**
- **If you are worried about your own HIV or STI status, have yourself tested. Don't risk infecting others.**

Source: The American College of Obstetricians and Gynecologists, *How to Prevent Sexually Transmitted Diseases* (Atlanta: The American College of Obstetricians and Gynecologists, 2008).

numbers that go unreported.[20] Caused by the bacterial pathogen *Neisseria gonorrhoeae,* gonorrhea primarily infects the linings of the urethra, genital tract, pharynx, and rectum. It may spread to the eyes or other body regions by the hands or through body fluids, typically during vaginal, oral, or anal sex. Most cases occur in individuals between the ages of 20 and 24.[21]

Signs and Symptoms In men, a typical symptom is a white, milky discharge from the penis accompanied by painful, burning urination 2 to 9 days after contact (Figure 6). Epididymitis can also occur as a symptom of infection. However, about 20 percent of all men with gonorrhea are asymptomatic.

In women, the situation is just the opposite: only 20 percent experience any discharge, and few develop a burning sensation on urinating until much later in the course of the infection (if ever). The organism can remain in the woman's vagina, cervix, uterus, or fallopian tubes for long periods with no apparent symptoms other than an occasional slight fever. Thus a woman can be unaware that she has been infected and that she is infecting her sexual partners.

Complications In a man, untreated gonorrhea may spread to the prostate, testicles, urinary tract, kidney, and bladder. Blockage of the vasa deferentia due to scar tissue may cause sterility. In some cases, the penis develops a painful curvature during erection. If the infection goes undetected in a woman, it can spread to the fallopian tubes and ovaries, causing sterility or, at the very least, severe inflammation and PID. The bacteria can also spread up the reproductive tract or, more rarely, through the blood and infect the joints, heart valves, or brain. If an infected woman becomes pregnant, the infection can be transmitted to her baby during delivery, potentially causing blindness, joint infection, or a life-threatening blood infection.

Diagnosis and Treatment Diagnosis of gonorrhea is similar to that of chlamydia, requiring a sample of either urine or fluid from the vagina or penis to detect the presence of the bacteria. If detected early, gonorrhea is treatable with antibiotics, but the *Neisseria gonorrhoeae* bacterium has

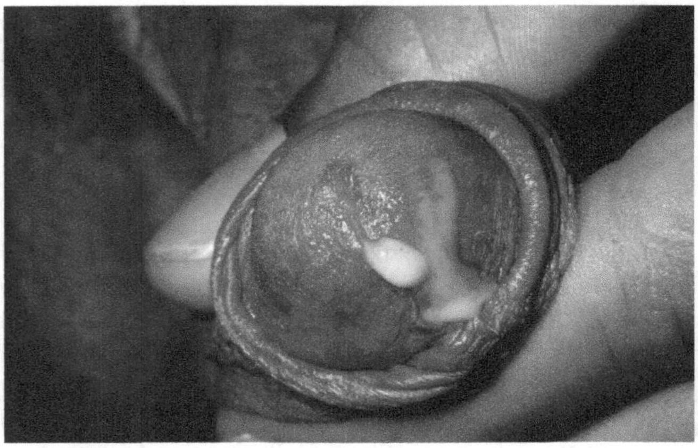

Centers for Disease Control and Prevention

FIGURE 6 **Gonorrhea**
One common symptom of gonorrhea in men is a milky discharge from the penis, accompanied by burning sensations during urination. Whereas these symptoms will cause most men to seek diagnosis and treatment, women with gonorrhea are often asymptomatic, so they may not be aware they are infected.

Gender&Health

Complications of STIs in Women: PID and UTIs

Women disproportionately experience the long-term consequences of STIs. If not treated, up to 40 percent of women who are infected with *Neisseria gonorrhoeae* or *Chlamydia trachomatis* may develop pelvic inflammatory disease (PID). Pelvic inflammatory disease is a catchall term for a number of infections of the uterus, fallopian tubes, and ovaries that are complications resulting from an untreated STI.

Symptoms of PID vary but generally include lower abdominal pain, fever, unusual vaginal discharge, painful intercourse, painful urination, and irregular menstrual bleeding. The vague symptoms associated with chlamydial and gonococcal PID cause 85 percent of women to delay seeking medical care, thereby increasing the risk of permanent damage and scarring that can lead to infertility and ectopic pregnancy. Among women with PID, ectopic pregnancy (in which an embryo begins to develop outside of the uterus, usually in a fallopian tube) occurs in 9 percent, and chronic pelvic pain in 18 percent.

Women are also at greater risk than men for developing a general urinary tract infection (UTI). Urinary tract infections can be caused by various factors, including untreated STIs. Women are more disproportionately affected by UTIs because a woman's urethra is much shorter than a man's, making it easier for bacteria to enter the bladder. In addition, a woman's urethra is closer to her anus than is a man's, allowing bacteria to spread into her urethra and cause an infection.

Symptoms of a UTI include burning sensation during urination and lower abdominal pain. A UTI can be diagnosed through a urine test and treated by antibiotics. If left untreated, UTIs can cause kidney damage.

These serious complications that can result from untreated STIs in women further illustrate the need for early diagnosis and treatment. Regular screening is particularly important, because women are often asymptomatic, increasing their risk of complications such as PID and UTIs. Therefore, it is recommended that all sexually active women should be screened regularly. Data from a randomized trial of chlamydia screening in a managed care setting suggested that screening programs can reduce the incidence of PID by as much as 60 percent.

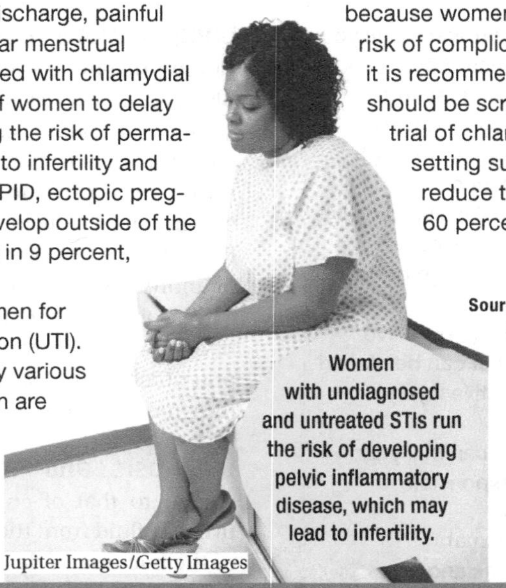

Jupiter Images/Getty Images

Women with undiagnosed and untreated STIs run the risk of developing pelvic inflammatory disease, which may lead to infertility.

Sources: MedlinePlus, "Pelvic Inflammatory Disease (PID)," Updated September 2009, www.nlm.nih.gov/medlineplus/ency/article/000888.htm; Mayo Clinic Staff, "Urinary Tract Infection: Risk Factors," June 2008, Available online: www.mayoclinic.com/health/urinary-tract-infection/DS00286/DSECTION=risk-factors; Centers for Disease Control and Prevention, Division of STD Prevention, National Center for HIV/AIDS, Viral Hepatitis, STD, and TB Prevention, "STDs in Women and Infants," Updated January 2009, www.cdc.gov/std/stats07/womenandinf.htm.

begun to develop resistance to some antibiotics. It is also important to recognize that chlamydia and gonorrhea often occur at the same time, but different antibiotics are needed to treat each infection separately.[22]

Syphilis

Syphilis is caused by a bacterium, the spirochete called *Treponema pallidum*. The incidence of syphilis is highest in women aged 20 to 24 and men aged 35 to 39. The incidence of syphilis in newborns has continued to increase in the United States.[23] Because it is extremely delicate and dies readily upon exposure to air, dryness, or cold, the organism is generally transferred only through direct sexual contact or from mother to fetus.

syphilis One of the most widespread STIs; characterized by distinct phases and potentially serious consequences.
chancre Sore often found on the site of primary syphilis infection.

Signs and Symptoms Syphilis is known as the "great imitator," because its symptoms resemble those of several other infections. It should be noted, however, that some people experience no symptoms at all. Syphilis can occur in four distinct stages:[24]

- **Primary syphilis.** The first stage of syphilis, particularly for men, is often characterized by the development of a **chancre** (pronounced "shank-er"), a sore located most frequently at the site of initial infection that usually appears 3 to 4 weeks after initial infection (Figure 7). In men, the site of the chancre tends to be the penis or scrotum; in women, the site of infection is often internal, on the vaginal wall or high on the cervix where the chancre is not readily apparent and the likelihood of detection is not great. Whether or not it is detected, the chancre is oozing with bacteria, ready to infect an unsuspecting partner. In both men and women, the chancre will completely disappear in 3 to 6 weeks.
- **Secondary syphilis.** If the infection is left untreated, a month to a year after the chancre disappears, secondary symptoms may appear, including a rash or white patches on the skin or on the mucous membranes of the mouth, throat, or genitals. Hair loss may occur, lymph nodes may enlarge,

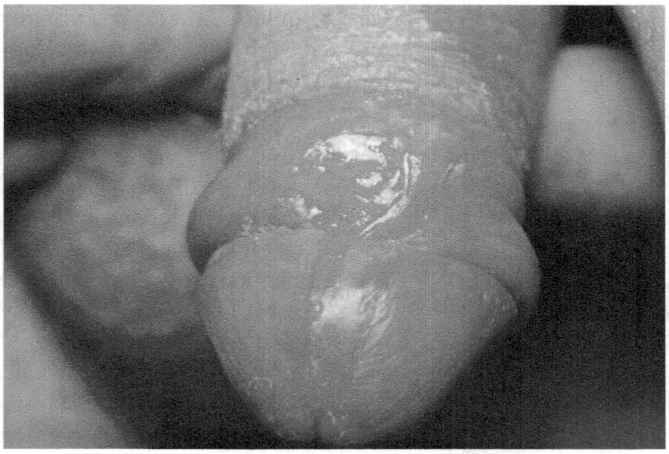

SPL/Photo Researchers

FIGURE 7 **Syphilis**
A chancre on the site of the initial infection is a symptom of primary syphilis.

and the victim may develop a slight fever or headache. In rare cases, sores develop around the mouth or genitals. As during the active chancre phase, these sores contain infectious bacteria, and contact with them can spread the infection.

- **Latent syphilis.** After the secondary stage, if the infection is left untreated, the syphilis spirochetes begin to invade body organs, causing lesions called *gummas*. The infection now is rarely transmitted to others, except during pregnancy, when it can be passed to the fetus.
- **Tertiary/late syphilis.** Years after syphilis has entered the body, its effects become all too evident if still untreated. Late-stage syphilis indications include heart and central nervous system damage, blindness, deafness, paralysis, premature senility, and, ultimately, dementia.

Complications Pregnant women with syphilis can experience complications including premature births, miscarriages, and stillbirths. An infected pregnant woman may transmit the syphilis to her unborn child. The infant will then be born with *congenital syphilis*, which can cause death; severe birth defects such as blindness, deafness, or disfigurement; developmental delays; seizures; and other health problems. Because in most cases the fetus does not become infected until after the first trimester, treatment of the mother during this time will usually prevent infection of the fetus.

Diagnosis and Treatment There are two methods that can be used to diagnose syphilis. In the primary stage, a sample from the chancre is collected to identify the bacteria. Another method of diagnosing syphilis is through a blood test. Syphilis can easily be treated with antibiotics, usually penicillin, for all stages except the late stage.

Herpes

Herpes is a general term for a family of infections characterized by sores or eruptions on the skin and caused by herpes simplex virus. The herpes family of diseases is not transmitted exclusively by sexual contact. Kissing or sharing eating utensils can also exchange saliva and transmit the infection. Herpes infections range from mildly uncomfortable to extremely serious. **Genital herpes** affects over 45 million Americans aged 12 and older.[25]

There are two types of herpes simplex virus. Only about one in six Americans currently has HSV-2; however, nearly 58 percent have HSV-1, usually appearing as cold sores on their mouths. Both herpes simplex types 1 and 2 can infect any area of the body, producing lesions (sores) in and around the vaginal area; on the penis; and around the anal opening, buttocks, thighs, or mouth (see Figure 8 on the next page). Whether you contract HSV-1 or HSV-2 on your genitals, the net results may be just as painful, just as long term, and just as infectious for future partners. Herpes simplex virus remains in certain nerve cells for life and can flare up when the body's ability to maintain itself is weakened.

Signs and Symptoms The precursor phase of a herpes infection is characterized by a burning sensation and redness at the site of infection. During this time, prescription medicines such as acyclovir and over-the-counter medications such as Abreva will often keep the disease from spreading. However, this phase of the disease is quickly followed by the second phase, in which a blister filled with a clear fluid containing the virus forms. If you pick at this blister or otherwise touch the site and spread this fluid with fingers, lipstick, lip balm, or other products, you can autoinoculate other body parts. Particularly dangerous is the possibility of spreading the infection to your eyes, for a herpes lesion on the eye can cause blindness.

Over a period of days, the unsightly blister will crust over, dry up, and disappear, and the virus will travel to the base of an affected nerve supplying the area and become dormant. Only when the victim becomes overly stressed, when diet and sleep are inadequate, when the immune system is overworked, or when excessive exposure to sunlight or other stressors occurs will the virus become reactivated (at the same site every time) and begin the blistering cycle all over again. Each time a sore develops, it casts off (sheds) viruses that can be highly infectious. However, it is important to note that a herpes site can shed the virus even when no overt sore is present, particularly during the interval between the earliest symptoms and blistering. People may get genital herpes by having sexual contact with others who don't know they are infected or who are having outbreaks of herpes without any sores. A person with genital herpes can also infect a sexual partner during oral sex. The virus is spread only rarely, if at all, by touching objects such as a toilet seat or hot tub seat.

genital herpes STI caused by the herpes simplex virus.

Complications Genital herpes is especially serious in pregnant women because the baby can be infected as it passes through the vagina during birth. Many physicians

National Archives and Records Administration

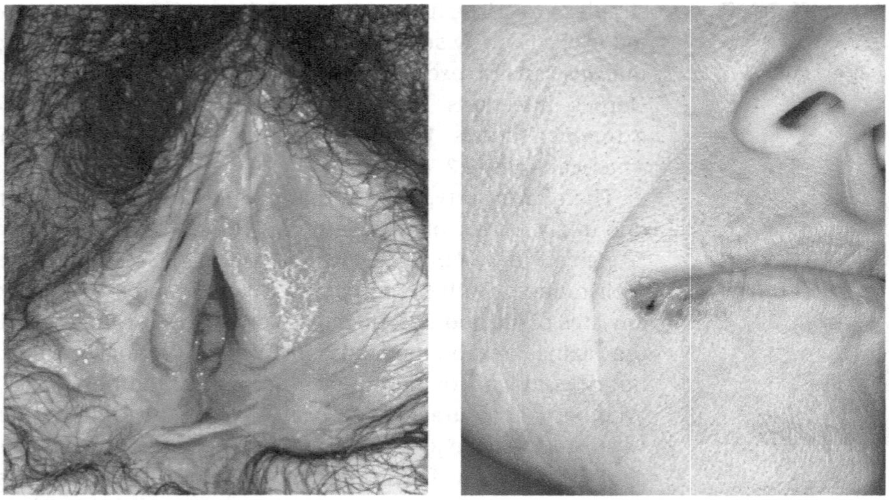

ISM/Phototake NYC

a Genital herpes is a highly contagious and incurable STI. It is characterized by recurring cycles of painful blisters on the genitalia.

b Oral herpes is also extremely contagious and can cause recurrent painful cold sores or fever blisters around the mouth.

FIGURE 8 **Herpes**
Herpes can be caused by herpes simplex virus types 1 or 2.

recommend cesarean deliveries for infected women. Additionally, women with a history of genital herpes appear to have a greater risk of developing cervical cancer.

Diagnosis and Treatment Diagnosis of herpes can be determined by collecting a sample from the suspected sore or by performing a blood test to identify an HSV-1 or HSV-2 infection. Although there is no cure for herpes at present, certain drugs can be used to treat symptoms. Unfortunately, they seem to work only if the infection is confirmed during the first few hours after contact. The effectiveness of other treatments, such as L-lysine, is largely unsubstantiated. Over-the-counter medications may reduce the length of time you have sores/symptoms. Other drugs, such as famciclovir (FAMVIR), may reduce viral shedding between outbreaks. This means that if you have outbreaks, you may reduce risks to your sexual partners.[26]

Human Papillomavirus and Genital Warts

Genital warts (also known as *venereal warts* or *condylomas*) are caused by a group of viruses known as **human papillomavirus (HPV).** There are over 100 different types of HPV; more than 30 types are sexually transmitted and are classified as either low risk or high risk. A person becomes infected when certain types of HPV penetrate the skin and mucous membranes of the genitals or anus. This is among the most common forms of STI, with 20 million Americans currently infected with genital HPV and approximately 6.2 million new cases each year.[27]

genital warts Warts that appear in the genital area or the anus; caused by the human papillomavirus (HPV).
human papillomavirus (HPV) A group of viruses, many of which are transmitted sexually; some types of HPV can cause genital warts or cervical cancer.

Signs and Symptoms Genital HPV appears to be relatively easy to catch. The typical incubation period is 6 to 8 weeks after contact. People infected with low-risk types of HPV may develop genital warts, a series of bumps or growths on the genitals, ranging in size from small pinheads to large cauliflower-like growths (Figure 9).

Complications Infection with high-risk types of HPV poses a significant risk for cervical cancer in women. It may lead to *dysplasia,* or changes in cells that may lead to a precancerous condition. Exactly how high-risk HPV infection leads to cervical cancer is uncertain. It is known that within 5 years after infection, 30 percent of all HPV cases will progress to the precancerous stage. Of those cases that become precancerous and are left untreated, 70 percent will eventually result in actual cancer. In addition, HPV may pose a threat to a fetus that is exposed to the virus during birth. Cesarean deliveries may be considered in serious cases. New research has also implicated HPV as a possible risk factor for coronary artery disease. It is hypothesized that HPV causes an inflammatory response in the artery walls, which leads to cholesterol and plaque buildup.

Diagnosis and Treatment Diagnosis of genital warts from low-risk types of HPV is determined through a visual examination by a health care provider. High-risk types can be diagnosed in women through microscopic analysis of cells from a Pap smear or by collecting a sample from the cervix to test for HPV DNA. There is currently no HPV DNA test for men.

Treatment is only available for the low-risk forms of HPV that cause genital warts. The warts can be treated with topical medication or can be frozen with liquid nitrogen and then removed. Large warts may require surgical removal.

HPV Vaccination In 2006, the Food and Drug Administration (FDA) approved a vaccine that protects against four types of HPV. Two of these are low-risk types, 6 and 11, that cause 40 percent of cases of genital warts, and the other two are high-risk types, 16 and 18, that lead to 70 percent of cervical cancer cases. The vaccine is meant primarily for girls and women aged 9 to 26 and is administered as a series of three shots over a 6-month period. See the **Health Headlines** box for more information about this vaccine.

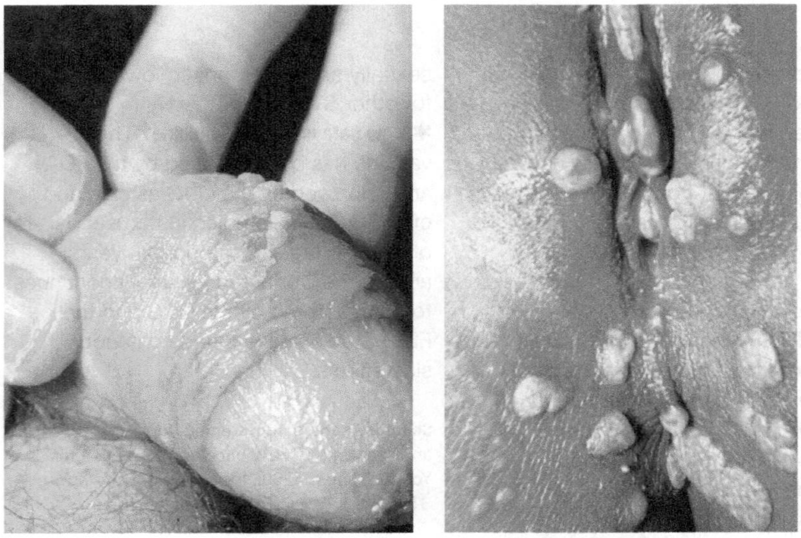

Dr. P. Marazzi/Science Photo Library/Photo Researchers

Centers for Disease Control and Prevention (CDC)

FIGURE 9 **Genital Warts**
Genital warts are caused by certain types of human papillomavirus (HPV).

Candidiasis (Moniliasis)

Most STIs are caused by pathogens that come from outside the body; however, the yeastlike fungus *Candida albicans* is a normal inhabitant of the vaginal tract in most women. (See Figure 4c for a micrograph of this fungus.) Only when the normal chemical balance of the vagina is disturbed will these organisms multiply and cause the fungal disease **candidiasis,** also sometimes called *moniliasis* or a *yeast infection.*

Signs and Symptoms Symptoms of candidiasis include severe itching and burning of the vagina and vulva, and a white, cheesy vaginal discharge.[28] When this microbe infects the mouth, whitish patches form, and the condition is referred to as *thrush.* Thrush infection can also occur in men and is easily transmitted between sexual partners. Symptoms of candidiasis can be aggravated by contact with soaps, douches, perfumed toilet paper, chlorinated water, and spermicides.

Diagnosis and Treatment Diagnosis of candidiasis is usually made by collecting a vaginal sample and analyzing it to identify the pathogen. Antifungal drugs applied on the surface or by suppository usually cure candidiasis in just a few days.

Trichomoniasis

Unlike many STIs, **trichomoniasis** is caused by a protozoan, *Trichomonas vaginalis.* (See Figure 4d for a micrograph of this organism.) Although as many as half of the men and women in the United States may carry this organism, most remain free of symptoms until their bodily defenses are weakened.

Signs and Symptoms Symptoms among women include a foamy, yellowish, unpleasant-smelling discharge accompanied by a burning sensation, itching, and painful urination. Most men with trichomoniasis do not have any symptoms, though some men experience irritation inside the penis, mild discharge, and a slight burning after urinating.[29] Although usually transmitted by sexual contact, the "trich" organism can also be spread by toilet seats, wet towels, or other items that have discharged fluids on them.

Diagnosis and Treatment Diagnosis of trichomoniasis is determined by collecting fluid samples from the penis or vagina to test for the presence of the protozoan. Treatment includes oral metronidazole, usually given to both sexual partners to avoid the possible "ping-pong" effect of repeated cross-infection typical of STIs.

Pubic Lice

Pubic lice, often called "crabs," are small parasitic insects that are usually transmitted during sexual contact (Figure 10). More annoying than dangerous, they move easily from partner to partner during sex. They have an affinity for pubic hair and attach themselves to the base of these hairs, where they deposit their eggs (nits). One to 2 weeks later, these nits develop into adults that lay eggs and migrate to other body parts, thus perpetuating the cycle.

candidiasis Yeastlike fungal infection often transmitted sexually; also called *moniliasis* or *yeast infection.*
trichomoniasis Protozoan STI characterized by foamy, yellowish discharge and unpleasant odor.
pubic lice Parasitic insects that can inhabit various body areas, especially the genitals.

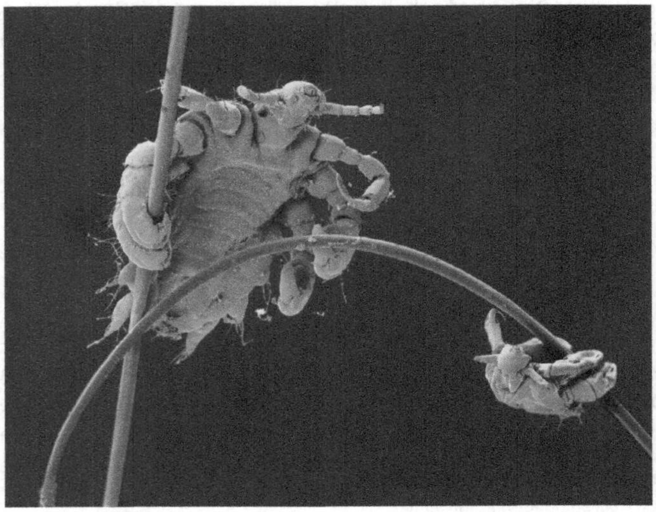

Eye of Science/Photo Researchers

FIGURE 10 **Pubic Lice**
Pubic lice, also known as "crabs," are small, parasitic insects that attach themselves to pubic hair.

Health Headlines

Q & A ON THE HPV VACCINE

Most sexually active people will contract some form of human papillomarvirus (HPV) at some time in their lives, though they may never even know it. There are about 40 types of sexually transmitted HPV, most of which cause no symptoms and go away on their own. But some high-risk types can cause cervical cancer in women and other less common genital cancers—like cancers of the anus, vagina, and vulva (area around the opening of the vagina). Every year in the United States, about 12,000 women are diagnosed with cervical cancer, and almost 4,000 die from this disease. The new HPV vaccine can help prevent women from becoming infected with HPV and subsequently developing cervical cancer.

✱ **Who should get the HPV vaccine?** The HPV vaccine is recommended for 11- and 12-year-old girls and can also be given to girls 9 or 10 years of age. It is also recommended for girls and women aged 13 through 26 who have not yet been vaccinated or completed the vaccine series. Ideally, females should get the vaccine before they become sexually active. Females who are sexually active may get less benefit from it, because they may have already gotten an HPV type targeted by the vaccine. However they would still get protection from those types they have not yet contracted.

✱ **Why is the HPV vaccine only recommended for girls and women through the age of 26?** The vaccine has been widely tested in girls and women aged 9 through 26 years. New research is being done on the vaccine's safety and efficacy in women older than 26. The FDA will consider licensing the vaccine for these women when there is enough research to show that it is safe and effective for them.

✱ **What about vaccinating boys and men?** Studies are now being done to find out if the vaccine works to prevent HPV infection and disease in males. It is possible that vaccinating men will have health benefits for them by preventing genital warts and rare cancers, such as penile and anal cancer.

✱ **What does the vaccine *not* protect against?** The vaccine does not protect against all types of HPV—so it will not prevent all cases of cervical cancer. About 30 percent of cervical cancers will not be prevented by the vaccine, so it will be important for women to continue getting screened for cervical cancer (through regular Pap tests). Also, the vaccine does not prevent other sexually transmitted infections (STIs), so it is still important for sexually active persons to lower their risk for other STIs.

✱ **How safe is the HPV vaccine?** This vaccine has been licensed by the FDA and approved by the CDC as safe and effective. It was studied in thousands of females (aged 9 through 26 years) around the world and its safety continues to be monitored by the CDC and the FDA. Studies have found no serious side effects.

Source: Adapted from Centers for Disease Control and Prevention, "HPV Vaccine Information for Young Women," 2008, www.cdc.gov/std/hpv/STDFact-HPV-vaccine-young-women.htm.

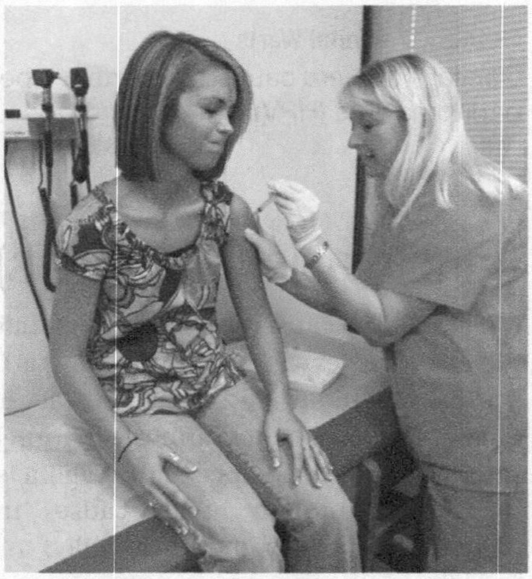

John Amis/Associated Press

The HPV vaccine is recommended for girls and women aged 9 to 26 as a preventive against cervical cancer. Many state health departments and college campuses offer free or low-cost vaccines for those whose insurance does not cover the cost.

Signs and Symptoms Symptoms of pubic lice infestation include itchiness in the area covered by pubic hair, bluish-gray skin color in the pubic region, and sores in the genital area.

Diagnosis and Treatment Diagnosis of pubic lice involves an examination by a health care provider to identify the eggs in the genital area. Treatment includes washing clothing, furniture, and linens that may harbor the eggs. It usually takes 2 to 3 weeks to kill all larval forms. Although sexual contact is the most common mode of transmission, you can "catch" pubic lice from lying on sheets or sitting on a toilet seat that an infected person has used.

acquired immunodeficiency syndrome (AIDS) A disease caused by a retrovirus, the human immunodeficiency virus (HIV), that attacks the immune system, reducing the number of helper T cells and leaving the victim vulnerable to infections, malignancies, and neurological disorders.

human immunodeficiency virus (HIV) The virus that causes AIDS.

HIV/AIDS

Acquired immunodeficiency syndrome (AIDS) is a significant global health threat. Since 1981, when AIDS was first recognized, approximately 65 million people in the world have become infected with **human immunodeficiency virus (HIV)**, the virus that causes AIDS. At the end of 2008, there were approximately 33.4 million people worldwide living with HIV.[30]

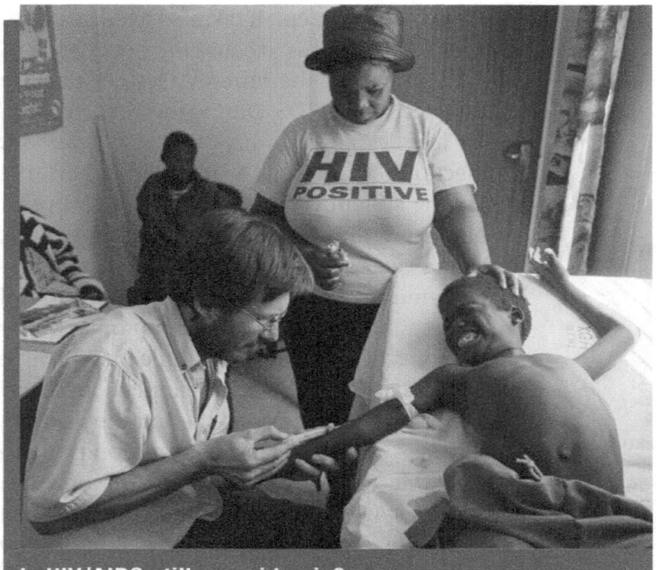

Is HIV/AIDS still an epidemic?

Yes! With swine flu and other emerging diseases dominating the news, it may seem like HIV/AIDS is no longer a problem; however, nothing could be further from the truth. In North America, 1.4 million people are living with HIV, and HIV and AIDS are still at epidemic levels all over the world, especially in developing nations. Sub-Saharan Africa has been hit hardest: 22.4 million people in the region are living with the disease. Another 3.8 million in south/southest Asia are infected and 2 million in Latin America. The epidemic is spreading most rapidly in eastern Europe and central Asia, where 1.5 million people currently have HIV.

95% of people with HIV worldwide live in developing nations.

In the United States, there have been approximately 1.1 million people infected with HIV and at least 583,000 have died.[31] In their most recent incidence reports, the CDC estimated that in 2006, there were approximately 56,300 new HIV/AIDS cases diagnosed in the United States.[32]

Initially, people with HIV were diagnosed as having AIDS only when they developed blood infections, the cancer known as Kaposi's sarcoma, or any of 21 other indicator diseases, most of which were common in male AIDS patients. The CDC has expanded the indicator list to include pulmonary tuberculosis, recurrent pneumonia, and invasive cervical cancer. Perhaps the most significant indicator today is a drop in the level of the body's master immune cells, CD4 cells (also called helper T cells), to one-fifth the level in a healthy person.

AIDS cases have been reported state by state throughout the United States since the early 1980s. Today, the CDC recommends that all states report HIV infections as well as AIDS. Because of medical advances in treatment and increasing numbers of HIV-infected persons who do not progress to AIDS, it is believed that AIDS incidence statistics may not provide a true picture of the epidemic, the long-term costs of treating HIV-infected individuals, and other key information.

How HIV Is Transmitted

HIV typically enters one person's body when another person's infected body fluids (e.g., semen, vaginal secretions, blood) gain entry through a breach in body defenses. Mucous membranes of the genital organs and the anus provide the easiest route of entry. If there is a break in the mucous membranes (as can occur during sexual intercourse, particularly anal intercourse), the virus enters and begins to multiply. After initial infection, HIV multiplies rapidly, invading the bloodstream and cerebrospinal fluid. It progressively destroys helper T cells (recall that these cells call the rest of the immune response to action), weakening the body's resistance to disease.

Despite some myths, HIV is not highly contagious. Studies of people living in households with an AIDS patient have turned up no documented cases of HIV infection resulting from casual contact.[33] Other investigations provide overwhelming evidence that insect bites do not transmit HIV.

Engaging in High-Risk Behaviors AIDS is not a disease of gay people or minority groups. Although during the early days of the epidemic it appeared that HIV infected only homosexuals, it quickly became apparent that the disease was not confined to groups of people, but rather was related to high-risk behaviors such as unprotected sexual intercourse and sharing needles (see the **Gender & Health** box). People who engage in high-risk behaviors increase their risk for the disease; people who do not engage in these behaviors have minimal risk. Figure 11 shows the breakdown of sources of HIV infection among U.S. men and women. The majority of HIV infections arise from the following high-risk behaviors:

- **Exchange of body fluids.** The greatest risk factor is the exchange of HIV-infected body fluids during vaginal or anal intercourse. Substantial research indicates that blood, semen, and vaginal secretions are the major fluids of concern. In rare instances, the virus has been found in saliva, but most health officials state that saliva is a less significant risk than other shared body fluids.
- **Injecting drugs.** A significant percentage of AIDS cases in the United States result from sharing or using HIV-contaminated needles and syringes. Though users of illegal drugs are commonly considered the only members of this category, others may also share needles—for example, people with diabetes who inject insulin or athletes who inject steroids. People who share needles and also engage in sexual activities with members of high-risk groups, such as those who exchange sex for drugs, increase their risks dramatically. Tattooing and piercing can also be risky (see the **Consumer Health** box).

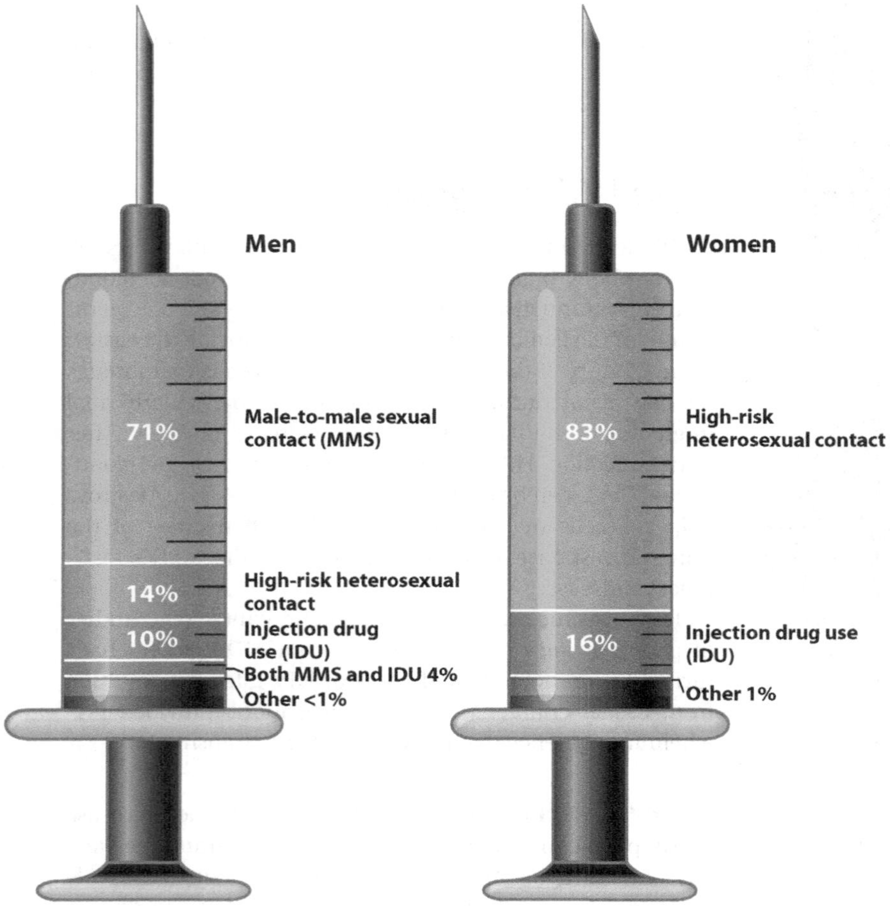

FIGURE 11 **Sources of HIV Infection in Men and Women in the United States**

Source: Data are from AVERT, "United States—Statistics by Transmission Route and Gender," Updated August 2009, www.avert.org/usa-transmission-gender.htm.

Blood Transfusion Prior to 1985 A small group of people have become infected after receiving blood transfusions. In 1985, the Red Cross and other blood donation programs implemented a stringent testing program for all donated blood. Today, because of these massive screening efforts, the risk of receiving HIV-infected blood is almost nonexistent in developed countries, including the United States.

Mother-to-Child (Perinatal) Transmission Mother-to-child transmission occurs when an HIV-positive woman passes the virus to her baby. This can occur during pregnancy, during labor and delivery, or through breast-feeding. Without antiretroviral treatment, approximately 25 percent of HIV-positive pregnant women will transmit the virus to their infant.[34]

Symptoms of HIV/AIDS

A person may go for months or years after infection by HIV before any significant symptoms appear. The incubation time varies greatly from person to person. For adults who receive no medical treatment, it takes an average of 8 to 10 years for the virus to cause the slow, degenerative changes in the immune system that are characteristic of AIDS. During this time, the person may experience *opportunistic infections* (infections that gain a foothold when the immune system is not functioning effectively). Colds, sore throats, fever, tiredness, nausea, night sweats, and other generally non–life-threatening conditions commonly appear and are described as pre-AIDS symptoms. Other symptoms of progressing HIV infection include wasting syndrome, swollen lymph nodes, and neurological problems. As the immune system continues to decline, the body becomes more vulnerable to infection. A diagnosis of AIDS, the final stage of HIV infection, is made when the infected person has either a dangerously low CD4 (helper T) cell count (below 200 cells per cubic milliliter of blood) or has contracted one or more opportunistic infections characteristic of the disease (such as Kaposi's sarcoma or *Pneumocystis carinii* pneumonia).

Testing for HIV Antibodies

Once antibodies have formed in reaction to HIV, a blood test known as the *ELISA* (enzyme-linked immunosorbent assay) may detect their presence. It can take 3 to 6 months after initial infection for sufficient antibodies to develop in the body to show a positive test result. Therefore, individuals with negative test results should be retested within 6 months. If sufficient antibodies are present, the test will be positive. When a person who previously tested *negative* (no HIV antibodies present) has a subsequent test that is *positive*, seroconversion is said to have occurred. In such a situation, the person would typically take another ELISA test, followed by a more precise test known as the *Western blot*, to confirm the presence of HIV antibodies.

It should be noted that these tests are not AIDS tests per se. Rather, they detect antibodies for HIV, indicating the presence of the virus in the person's system. Whether the person will develop AIDS depends to some extent on the strength of the immune system. Although we have made remarkable progress in prolonging the relatively symptom-free period between infection, HIV-positive status, and progression to symptomatic AIDS, it is important to

what do you think?

Do you favor mandatory reporting of HIV and AIDS cases? ● On the one hand, if you knew that your name and vital statistics would be "on file" if you tested positive for HIV, would you be less likely to take the HIV test? ● On the other hand, do people who carry this contagious fatal disease have a responsibility to inform the general public and the health professionals who provide their care?

Gender&Health

Women and HIV/AIDS

Women are four to ten times more likely than men to contract HIV through unprotected heterosexual intercourse with an infected partner, because the vaginal area is more susceptible to microtears. Also, during intercourse, a woman is exposed to more semen than a man is to vaginal fluids. Women who have sexually transmitted infections (STIs) are more likely to be asymptomatic and therefore unaware they have an infection; preexisting STIs increase the risk of HIV transmission.

Women have been underrepresented in clinical trials for HIV treatment and prevention and may be less likely to seek medical treatment because of caregiving burdens, transportation problems, and lack of money. In some countries, women have few rights regarding sexual relationships and the family. Instead, men are in charge of making the majority of decisions, such as whom they will marry and whether the man will have more than one sexual partner. This power imbalance means that it can be especially difficult for women to protect themselves from getting infected with HIV/AIDS. A woman may not be able to negotiate the use of a condom if her husband makes the decisions. Efforts must be initiated to help women take control of their sexual health and participate actively in sexual decisions with their partners.

In addition, millions of women have been indirectly affected by the HIV/AIDS pandemic. Women's childbearing role means that they have to contend with issues such as mother-to-child transmission of HIV. The responsibility of caring for AIDS patients and orphans is also an issue that has a greater effect on women.

As more and more women become infected with HIV/AIDS, global efforts of aid and prevention need to increase. These efforts should include the promotion and protection of women's human rights; an increase in education and awareness among women; and the development of new, preventive technologies such as microbicides, gels, or creams that could be applied vaginally without a partner even knowing it, to prevent HIV infection. Research has been underway for a number of years, but there is still no microbicide that is currently available.

Sources: Centers for Disease Control and Prevention, Divisions of HIV/AIDS Prevention National Center for HIV/AIDS, Viral Hepatitis, STD, and TB Prevention, "HIV/AIDS among Women," Revised August 2008, www.cdc.gov/hiv/topics/women/resources/factsheets/women.htm; AVERT, "Women, HIV and AIDS," Updated August 2009, www.avert.org/women.htm.

note that a cure does not yet exist. The vast majority of infected people eventually develop some form of the disease.

Health officials distinguish between *reported* and *actual* cases of HIV infection because it is believed that many HIV-positive people avoid being tested. One reason is fear of knowing the truth. Another is the fear of recrimination from employers, insurance companies, and medical staff. However, early detection and reporting are important, because immediate treatment for someone in the early stages of HIV disease is critical.

New Hope and Treatments

New drugs have slowed the progression from HIV to AIDS and have prolonged life expectancies for most AIDS patients. Current treatments combine selected drugs, especially protease inhibitors and reverse transcriptase inhibitors. *Protease inhibitors* (e.g., amprenavir, ritonavir, and saquinavir) act to prevent the production of the virus in chronically infected cells that HIV has already invaded. Other drugs, such as AZT, ddI, ddC, d4T, and 3TC, inhibit the HIV enzyme *reverse transcriptase* before the virus has invaded the cell, thereby preventing the virus from infecting new cells. All of the protease drugs seem to work best in combination with other therapies. These combination treatments are still quite experimental, and no combination has proven to be absolute for all people.

Although these drugs provide new hope and longer survival rates for people living with HIV, it is important to maintain caution. We are still a long way from a cure. Apathy and carelessness may abound if too much confidence is placed in these treatments. Newer drugs that held much promise are becoming less effective as HIV develops resistance to them. Costs of taking multiple drugs are prohibitive, and side effects common. Furthermore, the number of people becoming HIV-infected each year has increased in some communities, meaning that we are still a long way from beating this disease.

Preventing HIV Infection

Although scientists have been working on a variety of HIV vaccine trials, none is currently available. The only way to prevent HIV infection is through the choices you make in sexual behaviors and drug use and by taking responsibility for your own health and the health of your loved ones.

Unfortunately, the message has not gotten through to many Americans. They assume that because they are heterosexual, do not inject illegal drugs, and do not have sex with sex workers, they are not at risk. They couldn't be more wrong. Anyone who engages in unprotected sex is at risk, especially if they have sex with a partner who has engaged in other high-risk behaviors. Sex with multiple partners is the greatest threat. You can't determine the presence of HIV by looking at a person; you can't tell by questioning the person, unless he or she has been tested recently, is HIV-negative, and is giving an honest answer. So what should you do?

CONSUMER HEALTH

BODY PIERCING AND TATTOOING: POTENTIAL RISKS

A look around any college campus reveals many examples of "body art," the widespread trend of using body piercing and tattoos as a form of self-expression. Although the practice can be done safely, health professionals cite several health concerns. The most common problems include skin reactions, infections, allergic reactions, and scarring. Of even greater concern is the potential transmission of dangerous pathogens that can occur with any puncture of the skin. The use of unsterile needles—which can cause serious infections and can transmit staph, HIV, hepatitis B and C, tetanus, and a host of other diseases—poses a very real risk.

Stonehill/zefa/Corbis

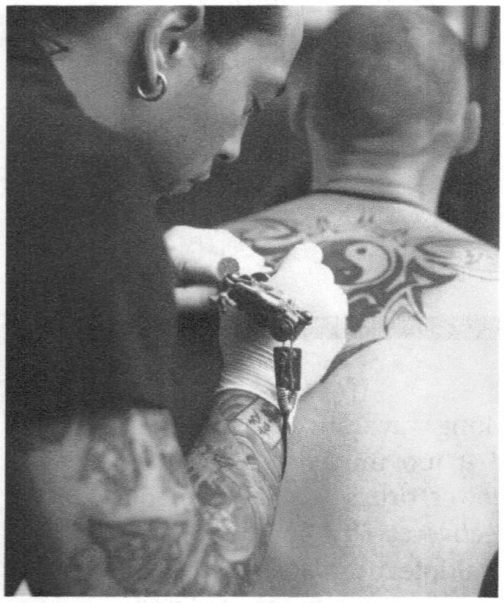

Like any activity that involves bodily fluids, tattooing carries some risk of disease transmission.

Laws and policies regulating body piercing and tattooing vary greatly by state. Standards for safety usually include minimum age of clientele, standards of sanitation, use of aseptic techniques, sterilization of equipment, record keeping, informed risks, instructions for skin care, and recommendations for dealing with adverse reactions. Because of the lack of universal regulatory standards and the potential for transmission of dangerous pathogens, anyone who receives a tattoo, body piercing, or permanent makeup tattoo cannot donate blood for 1 year.

Before deciding on a body artist to do your tattoo or piercing, you may want to watch the artist working on another client to evaluate the person's safety and skill. If you opt for tattooing or body piercing, remember to take the following safety precautions:

* Look for clean, well-lighted work areas, and inquire about sterilization procedures. Ask to see the autoclave used for sterilizing the instruments. Be wary of establishments that are reluctant to show you their autoclave or to discuss their sterilization procedures.
* Packaged, sterilized needles should be used only once and then discarded. A piercing gun should not be used, because it cannot be sterilized properly. Watch that the artist uses new needles and tubes from a sterile package before your procedure begins. Ask to see the sterile confirmation logo on the bag itself.
* Immediately before piercing or tattooing, the body area should be carefully sterilized. The artist should wash his or her hands and put on new latex gloves for each procedure. Make sure the artist changes those gloves if he or she needs to touch anything else, such as the telephone, while working.
* Leftover tattoo ink should be discarded after each procedure. Do not allow the artist to reuse ink that has been used for other customers. Used needles should be disposed of in a "sharps" container, a plastic container with the biohazard symbol clearly marked on it.
* If any signs of pus, swelling, redness, or discoloration persist after a piercing, remove the piercing object, and contact a physician.

Sources: Mayo Clinic Staff, "Tattoos: Risks and Precautions to Know First," February 2008, www.mayoclinic.com/health/tattoos-and-piercings/MC00020; Center for Food Safety and Applied Nutrition, "Tattoos and Permanent Makeup," *Office of Cosmetics Fact Sheet*, Updated June 2008, www.fda.gov/Cosmetics/ProductandIngredientSafety/ProductInformation/ucm108530.htm.

Of course, the simplest answer is abstinence. If you don't exchange body fluids, you won't get the disease. As a second line of defense, if you decide to be intimate, the next best option is to use a condom. However, in spite of all the educational campaigns, surveys consistently indicate that most college students throw caution to the wind if they think they "know" someone—and they have unprotected sex. The **Skills for Behavior Change** box at right presents ways to talk to your sexual partner about protecting yourselves from HIV and other STIs.

Noninfectious Conditions

Typically, when we think of major noninfectious ailments, we think of "killer" diseases such as cancer and heart disease. Clearly, these diseases make up the major portion of life-threatening diseases—accounting for nearly two-thirds of all deaths. Although these diseases capture much media attention, other chronic conditions can also cause pain, suffering, and disability.

Generally, noninfectious diseases are not transmitted by a pathogen or by any form of personal contact. Lifestyle and personal health habits are often implicated as underlying causes. Healthy changes in lifestyle and public health efforts aimed at research, prevention, and control can minimize the effects of these diseases.

Chronic Lung Diseases

Lung disease is the number three killer in the United States, right behind heart disease and cancer, and is responsible for one in six deaths, or nearly 400,000 people per year. Today, more than 35 million Americans are living with chronic lung disease such as asthma and chronic obstructive pulmonary

Skills for Behavior Change

Communicating about Safer Sex

At no time in your life is it more important to communicate openly than when you are considering an intimate relationship. The following will help you communicate with your partner about potential risks:

- **Plan to talk before you find yourself in an awkward situation.**
- **Select the right moment and place for both of you to discuss safer sex; choose a relaxing environment in a neutral location, free of distractions.**
- **Remember that you have a responsibility to your partner to disclose your own health status. You also have a responsibility to yourself to stay healthy.**
- **Be direct, honest, and determined in talking about sex before you become involved. Do not act silly or evasive. Get to the point, ask clear questions, and do not be put off in receiving a response.**
- **Discuss the issues without sounding defensive or accusatory. Be prepared with complete information, and articulate your feelings clearly. Reassure your partner that your reasons for desiring abstinence or safer sex arise from respect and not distrust.**
- **Analyze your own beliefs and values ahead of time. Know where you will draw the line on certain actions, and be very clear with your partner about what you expect. If you believe that using a condom is necessary, make sure you communicate this.**
- **Decide what you will do if your partner does not agree with you. Anticipate potential objections or excuses, and prepare your responses accordingly.**

Sources: Queensland Health, "Talking to Your Partner about Sex. 2009, www.health.qld.gov.au/istaysafe/content/letsTalk/talkingToYourPartner.html.

disease (COPD), otherwise known as emphysema and chronic bronchitis.[35]

Any disease or disorder in which lung function is impaired is considered a lung disease. The lungs can be damaged by a single exposure to a toxic chemical or severe heat, or they can be impaired from years of inhaling the tar and chemicals in tobacco smoke. Occupational or home exposure to asbestos, silica dust, paint fumes and lacquers, pesticides, and a host of other environmental substances can cause lung deterioration. Of course, cancers, infections, and degenerative changes can also wreak havoc with lung function. When the lungs are impaired, a condition known as **dyspnea,** or a choking type of breathlessness can occur, even with mild exertion. As the lungs are oxygen deprived, the heart is forced to work harder and, over time, cardiovascular problems, suffocation, and death can occur.

Chronic Obstructive Pulmonary Diseases

Chronic obstructive pulmonary diseases (COPDs) include chronic bronchitis and emphysema. Since these conditions often occur together, the abbreviation *COPD* is often preferred by health professionals; COPD does not include other obstructive diseases such as asthma. Currently, about 24 million U.S. adults have impaired lung function, with over 12 million believed to have COPD. Eighty to 90 percent of persons with COPD have a history of smoking.[36] Occupational exposure to certain industrial fumes or gases and exposure to dusts and other lung irritants increases risks, whether this exposure comes in one big dose or over months and years.

Bronchitis

Bronchitis refers to an inflammation of the lining of the bronchial tubes. These tubes, the bronchi, connect the windpipe with the lungs. When the bronchi become inflamed or infected, less air is able to flow from the lungs, and heavy mucus begins to form. *Acute bronchitis* is the most common of the bronchial diseases, and symptoms often improve in a week or two.

When the symptoms of bronchitis last for at least 3 months of the year for 2 consecutive years, the condition is considered *chronic bronchitis.* In some cases, this chronic inflammation and irritation goes undiagnosed for years, particularly in smokers who feel it's a normal part of their lives. By the time these individuals receive medical care, the damage to their lungs is severe and may lead to heart and respiratory failure or to a chronic need to carry oxygen to aid in breathing. Nearly 10 million Americans suffer from chronic bronchitis.[37]

Emphysema

Emphysema involves the gradual, irreversible destruction of the **alveoli** (tiny air sacs through which gas exchange occurs) of the lungs. Over 4.1 million Americans suffer from emphysema, with nearly 70 percent of cases occurring in men.[38] As the alveoli are destroyed, the affected person finds it more and more difficult to exhale, struggling to take in a fresh supply of air before the air held in the lungs has been expended. The chest cavity gradually begins to expand, producing a barrel-shaped chest.

Asthma

Asthma is a long-term, chronic inflammatory disorder that blocks air flow into and out of the lungs. Asthma causes tiny airways in the lung to overreact with spasms in response to certain triggers. Symptoms include wheezing, difficulty breathing, shortness of breath,

dyspnea Shortness of breath, usually associated with disease of the heart or lungs.
chronic obstructive pulmonary diseases (COPDs) A collection of chronic lung diseases including emphysema and chronic bronchitis.
bronchitis Inflammation of the lining of the bronchial tubes.
emphysema A respiratory disease in which the alveoli become distended or ruptured and are no longer functional.
alveoli Tiny air sacs of the lungs where gas exchange occurs (oxygen enters the blood and carbon dioxide is removed).
asthma A chronic respiratory disease characterized by attacks of wheezing, shortness of breath, and coughing spasms.

and coughing spasms. Although most asthma attacks are mild and non–life-threatening, severe attacks can trigger bronchospasms (contractions of the bronchial tubes in the lungs) that are so severe that, without rapid treatment, death may occur. Between attacks, most people have few symptoms.

Asthma falls into two distinctly different types. The more common form of asthma, known as *extrinsic* or *allergic asthma*, is typically associated with allergic triggers; it tends to run in families and develop in childhood. Often by adulthood, a person has few episodes, or the disorder completely goes away. *Intrinsic* or *nonallergic asthma* may be triggered by anything except an allergy.

Several factors can increase your risk of developing asthma: living in a large urban area; being exposed to secondhand smoke during childhood; or having respiratory infections in childhood, low birth weight, obesity, gastroesophageal reflux disease, or one or both parents with asthma.[39] Asthma attacks can be triggered by exposure to irritants or allergens such as tobacco smoke, occupational chemicals, pollen, cockroaches, feathers, foods, molds, dust, or pet dander. In some individuals, stress, exercise, certain medications, cold air, and sulfites are also potential triggers. Interestingly, one in five asthmatics can suffer an attack from taking aspirin.[40]

Custom Medical Stock Photo/Alamy

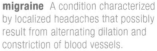

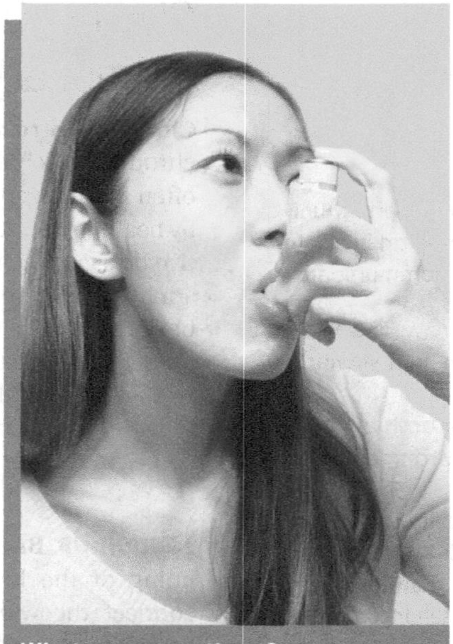

What causes asthma?

Asthma is caused by inflammation of the airways in the lungs, restricting them and leading to wheezing, chest tightness, shortness of breath, and coughing. In most people, asthma is brought on by contact with allergens or irritants in the air; some people also have exercise-induced asthma. People with asthma can generally control their symptoms through the use of inhaled medications, and most asthmatics keep a "rescue" inhaler of bronchodilating medication on hand to use in case of a flare-up.

Approximately 23 million people in the United States currently have asthma, making it one of the most prevalent respiratory diseases.[41] Asthma can occur at any age but is most likely to appear in children between infancy and age 5 and in adults before age 40. In childhood, asthma strikes more boys than girls; in adulthood, it strikes more women than men. The asthma rate is 50 percent higher among African Americans than whites, and four times as many African Americans die of asthma as do whites.[42]

25% of all school absences are due to asthma.

In the past few decades, asthma rates have risen dramatically, increasing by more than 65 percent since the 1980s.[43] Asthma has become the most common chronic disease of childhood, affecting more than 1 child in 20. Among adults, asthma is the fourth leading cause of work absence, resulting in over 10 million lost workdays per year. The annual direct costs of asthma are nearly $20 billion.

Determining whether a specific allergen provokes asthma attacks, taking steps to reduce exposure, and avoiding triggers such as certain types of exercise or stress are important steps in asthma prevention. The **Green Guide** at right offers suggestions for ways to green your home and reduce potential asthma and allergy triggers. In addition to avoiding triggers, finding the most effective medications can help asthmatics control their condition and avoid severe attacks.

migraine A condition characterized by localized headaches that possibly result from alternating dilation and constriction of blood vessels.

Headaches

Almost all of us have experienced at least one major headache. In fact, more than 80 percent of women and 65 percent of men experience headaches on a regular basis.[44] Over 90 percent of all headaches are of three major types: tension headaches, migraines, and cluster headaches.

Tension Headaches

Tension headaches are generally caused by muscle contractions or tension in the neck or head. This tension may be caused by actual strain placed on neck or head muscles due to overuse, to holding static positions for long periods, or to tension triggered by stress. Other possible triggers include red wine, lack of sleep, fasting, and menstruation. Relaxation, hot water treatment, and massage are holistic treatments. Aspirin, ibuprofen, acetaminophen, and naproxen sodium remain the old standby medicinal treatments for pain relief.

Migraine Headaches

Nearly 30 million Americans—three times more women than men—suffer from **migraines,** a type of headache that often has severe, debilitating symptoms. One out of 4 households has a migraine sufferer.[45] If one parent has migraines, his or her children have a 50 percent chance of having them. If both parents have them, there is a 75 percent chance their children will have them. Usually migraine incidence peaks in young adulthood, people aged 20 to 45.

Symptoms vary greatly by individual, and attacks typically last anywhere from 4 to 72 hours, with distinct phases of symptoms. In about 15 percent of cases, migraines are preceded by a sensory warning sign known as an *aura,* such as flashes of light, flickering vision, blind spots, tingling in arms or legs, or sensation of odor or taste. Sometimes nausea, vomiting, and extreme sensitivity to light and sound are present. Symptoms of migraine include excruciating pain behind or around one eye and usually on the same side of the head. In some people, there is sinus pain, neck pain, or an aura without headache.

GREEN GUIDE

Be Eco-Clean and Allergen Free

Exposure to household chemicals, dust, and pet dander may exacerbate asthma, allergies, and other respiratory problems. You can reduce exposure to noxious household chemicals and create a clean, comfortable home by practicing green cleaning. This involves using cleaning supplies and household products that are less toxic to one's home environment and less of a burden on water resources. Because some companies may want you to believe their product is greener than it actually is, read the labels carefully and look for independent certifications such as Green Seal and the EPA's Design for the Environment program.

Making your own cleaners is often less expensive than purchasing them at the store, and it is the best way to ensure a cleaner will not harm your health or the environment. Here are a few practical recipes:

* For a handy glass and surface cleaner, mix one-half cup white vinegar to 4 cups water. Pour the solution into a spray bottle and keep the remainder for a quick and cheap refill.
* Use 2 tablespoons lemon juice to 4 cups water for a surface cleaner.
* Baking soda works as a great deodorizer and cleaner. Use it to remove carpet odors and to scour sinks, toilets, and bathtubs.
* Because chlorine can damage lungs, skin, and eyes, and chlorine production adds toxic chemicals such as carcinogenic dioxins to our environment, use a chlorine bleach alternative. For example, use one-half cup of hydrogen peroxide in your laundry or use oxygen-based bleaches that can be found in most grocery stores.
* An all-purpose cleaner can be made of one-half cup borax (a natural mineral you can find in the laundry aisle) to 1 gallon of hot water.
* For green air fresheners, use essential oils, such as lemon or lavender. Many store-bought air fresheners contain phthalates, often called "fragrance," that are related to respiratory problems and other noninfectious conditions. Place a few drops of essential oils on a piece of tissue paper, in a bowl of warm water, or in a store-bought diffuser.

As you transition to green cleaning, do not just throw old products in the trash, as these can wind up polluting landfills and leaching into water supplies. Instead, take them to a hazardous chemical recycling facility.

The cause of migraines is unknown, but some research suggests they may occur when blood vessels dilate in the membrane that surrounds the brain. Critics of the blood vessel dilation theory question why only blood vessels of the head dilate in these situations. These researchers suggest that migraines originate in the cortex of the brain, where certain pain sensors are stimulated.

Historically, treatments have centered on reversing or preventing blood vessel dilation, with the most common treatment derived from the rye fungus *ergot*. Today, fast-acting ergot compounds are available by nasal spray, vastly increasing the speed of relief. However, ergot drugs have many side effects, not the least of which may be that they are habit forming. Other drugs that are sometimes prescribed include lidocaine, a new group of drugs called triptans, and Imitrex, a drug tailor-made for migraines.

Cluster Headaches

The pain of a cluster headache is often severe and has been described as "killer" or "suicidal." Usually these headaches cause stabbing pain on one side of the head, behind the eye, or in one defined spot. Other typical cluster headache characteristics include nasal discharge and congestion, tearing of the eye on the same side as the pain, a swollen or drooping eyelid and contracted pupil, flushing of the face on the affected side, and excessive sweating. Fortunately, cluster headaches are among the more rare forms of headache, affecting less than 1 percent of people, usually men. Young adults in their twenties tend to be particularly susceptible.[46]

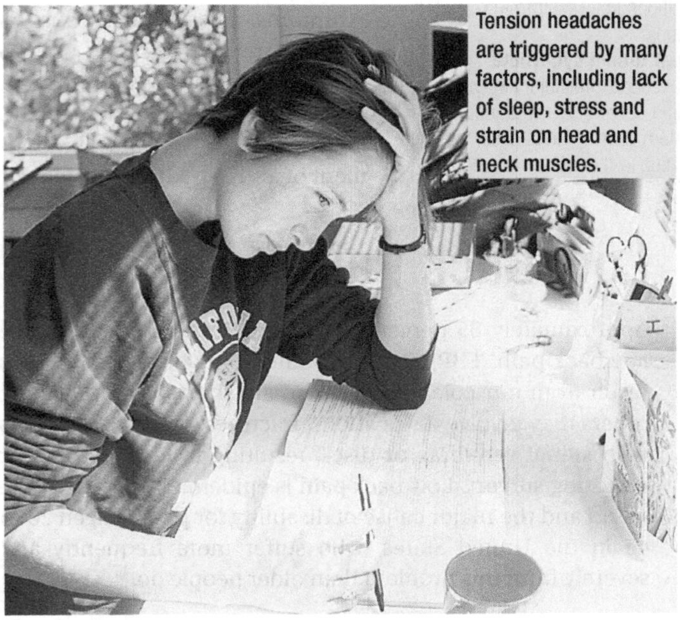

Tension headaches are triggered by many factors, including lack of sleep, stress and strain on head and neck muscles.

Elena Dorfman

Cluster headaches can last for weeks and disappear quickly. However, more commonly they last for 40 to 90 minutes and often occur in the middle of the night, usually during rapid eye movement (REM) sleep. Oxygen therapy, drugs, and even surgery have been used to treat severe cases.

Chronic Fatigue Syndrome

Since the late 1980s, several U.S. clinics have noted a characteristic set of symptoms that include chronic fatigue, headaches, fever, sore throat, enlarged lymph nodes, depression, poor memory, general weakness, and nausea. Researchers initially believed these symptoms were caused by the Epstein-Barr virus, the same one that causes mononucleosis. Since those initial studies, however, researchers have all but ruled out the Epstein-Barr virus. Despite extensive testing, no viral cause has been found.

Today, in the absence of a known pathogen, many researchers believe that the illness, now commonly referred to as **chronic fatigue syndrome (CFS),** may have strong psychosocial roots. Our heightened awareness of health makes some of us scrutinize our bodies so carefully that the slightest deviation becomes amplified. In addition, the growing number of people who suffer from depression seem to be good candidates for chronic fatigue syndrome. Experts worry, however, that too many scientists approach CFS as something that is "in the person's head" and that such an attitude may prevent them from doing the serious research needed to find a cure.

The diagnosis of chronic fatigue syndrome depends on two major criteria and eight or more minor criteria. The major criteria are (1) debilitating fatigue that persists for at least 6 months, and (2) the absence of other illnesses that could cause the symptoms. Minor criteria include headaches, fever, sore throat, painful lymph nodes, weakness, fatigue after exercise, sleep problems, and rapid onset of these symptoms. Because the cause is not apparent, treatment of CFS focuses on improved nutrition, rest, counseling for depression, judicious exercise, and development of a strong support network.

chronic fatigue syndrome (CFS) A condition of unknown cause characterized by extreme fatigue.
repetitive motion disorders (RMDs) A family of painful muscular conditions that result from repeated motions.
carpal tunnel syndrome A common occupational injury in which the median nerve in the wrist becomes irritated, causing numbness, tingling, and pain in the fingers and hands.

Low Back Pain

Approximately 85 percent of all Americans will experience low back pain (LBP) at some point. Some of these episodes result from muscular damage and are short lived and acute; others may involve dislocations, fractures, or other problems with spinal vertebrae or discs, resulting in chronic pain or requiring surgery. Low back pain is epidemic throughout the world and the major cause of disability for people aged 20 to 45 in the United States, who suffer more frequently and severely from this problem than older people do.[47]

Almost 90 percent of all back problems occur in the lumbar spine (lower back). You can avoid many problems by consciously maintaining good posture. Numerous studies have shown that wearing heavy backpacks, particularly among younger, school-aged children, can result in back pain. It is likely that carrying books and computers all day may also be a cause for concern among college students. Although no clear research has pointed this out, common sense suggests you use caution, making sure you purchase a good quality backpack that has straps to off-load some of the weight to your hips, rather than on your shoulders and back. Other things you can do to reduce risks of back pain include the following:

- Purchase a high-quality, supportive mattress, and avoid sleeping on your stomach.
- Avoid high-heeled shoes, which tilt the pelvis forward, and wear shoes with good arch support.
- Control your weight. Extra weight puts increased strain on knees, hips, and your back.
- Warm up and stretch before exercising or lifting heavy objects.
- When lifting something heavy, use your leg muscles and proper form. Do not bend from the waist or take the weight load on your back.
- Buy a chair with good lumbar support for doing your work.
- Move your car seat forward so your knees are elevated slightly.
- Exercise regularly, particularly exercises that strengthen the abdominal muscles and stretch the back muscles.

Repetitive Motion Disorders

It's the end of the term, and you have finished the last of several papers. After hours of nonstop typing, your hands are numb and you feel an intense, burning pain that makes the thought of typing one more word almost unbearable. If this happens, you may be suffering from one of several **repetitive motion disorders (RMDs).** Repetitive motion disorders include carpal tunnel syndrome, bursitis, tendonitis, ganglion cysts, and others.[48] Twisting of the arm or wrist, overexertion, and incorrect posture or position are usually contributors. The areas most likely to be affected are the hands, wrists, elbows, and shoulders, but the neck, back, hips, knees, feet, ankles, and legs can be affected, too. Over time, RMDs can cause permanent damage to nerves, soft tissue, and joints.

One of the most common RMDs is **carpal tunnel syndrome,** a product of spending hours typing at the computer, flipping groceries through computerized scanners, or other jobs requiring repeated hand and wrist movements that can irritate the median nerve in the wrist, causing numbness, tingling, and pain in the fingers and hands. Although carpal tunnel syndrome risk can be reduced by proper placement of the keyboard, mouse, wrist pads, and other techniques, it is often overlooked until significant damage has been done. Better education and ergonomic workplace designs can eliminate many injuries of this nature. Physical and occupational therapy is an important part of treatment and eventual recovery.

Assess yourself

STIs: Do You Really Know What You Think You Know?

PEARSON myhealthlab

Fill out this assessment online at www.pearsonhighered.com/myhealthlab or www.pearsonhighered.com/donatelle.

The following quiz will help you evaluate whether your beliefs and attitudes about sexually transmitted infections (STIs) lead you to behaviors that increase your risk of infection. Indicate whether you believe the following items are true or false, then consult the answer key that follows.

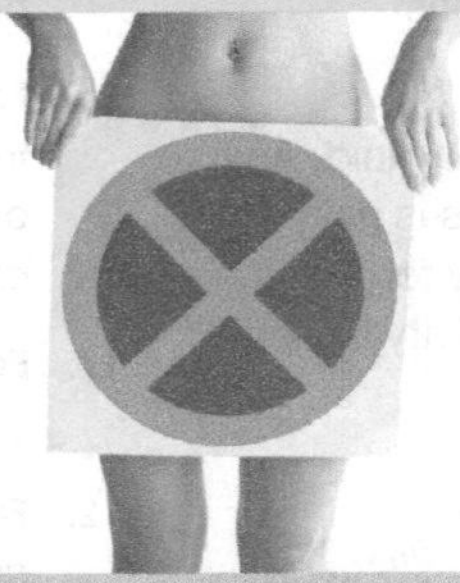
Tomaz Levstek/iStockphoto

	True	False
1. You can always tell when you've got an STI because the symptoms are so obvious.	○	○
2. Some STIs can be passed on by skin-to-skin contact in the genital area.	○	○
3. Herpes can be transmitted only when a person has visible sores on his or her genitals.	○	○
4. Oral sex is safe sex.	○	○
5. Condoms reduce your risk of both pregnancy and STIs.	○	○
6. As long as you don't have anal intercourse, you can't get HIV.	○	○
7. All sexually active females should have a regular Pap smear.	○	○
8. Once genital warts have been removed, there is no risk of passing on the virus.	○	○
9. You can get several STIs at one time.	○	○
10. If the signs of an STI go away, you are cured.	○	○
11. People who get an STI have a lot of sex partners.	○	○
12. All STIs can be cured.	○	○
13. You can get an STI more than once.	○	○

Answer Key

1. **False.** The unfortunate fact is that many STIs show no symptoms. This has serious implications: (1) you can be passing on the infection without knowing it, and (2) the pathogen may be damaging your reproductive organs without you knowing it.
2. **True.** Some viruses are present on the skin around the genital area. Herpes and genital warts are the main culprits.
3. **False.** Herpes is most easily passed on when the sores and blisters are present, because the fluid in the lesions carries the virus. But the virus is also found on the skin around the genital area. Most people contract herpes this way, unaware that the virus is present.

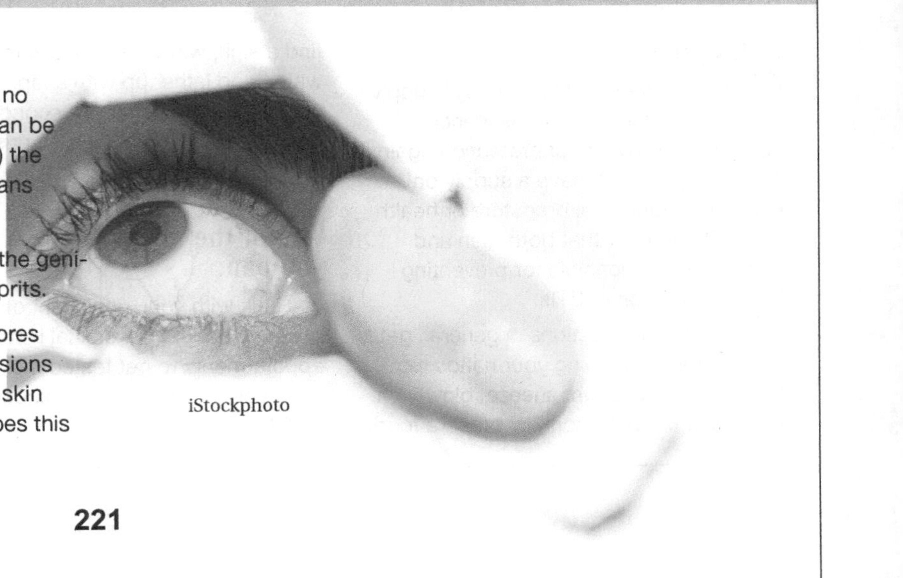
iStockphoto

4. **False.** Oral sex is not safe sex. Herpes, genital warts, and chlamydia can all be passed on through oral sex. Condoms should be used on the penis. Dental dams should be placed over the female genitals during oral sex.

5. **True.** Condoms significantly reduce the risk of pregnancy when used correctly. They also reduce the risk of STIs. It is important to point out that abstinence is the only behavior that provides complete protection against pregnancy and STIs.

6. **False.** HIV is present in blood, semen, and vaginal fluid. Any activity that allows for the transfer of these fluids is risky. Anal intercourse is a high-risk activity, especially for the receptive (passive) partner, but other sexual activity is also a risk. When you don't know your partner's sexual history and you're not in a long-term monogamous relationship, condoms are a must.

7. **True.** A Pap smear is a simple procedure involving the scraping of a small amount of tissue from the surface of the cervix (at the upper end of the vagina). The sample is tested for abnormal cells that may indicate cancer. All sexually active women should have regular Pap smears.

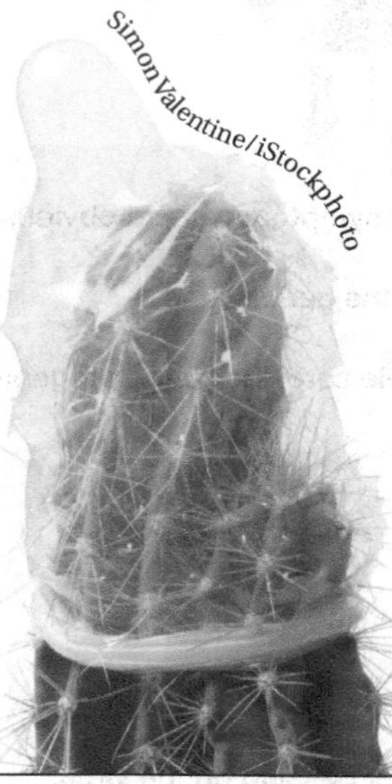

Simon Valentine/iStockphoto

8. **False.** Genital warts, which may be present on the penis, the anus, and inside and outside the vagina, can be removed. However, the virus that caused the warts will always be present in the body and can be passed on to a sexual partner.

9. **True.** It is possible to have many STIs at one time. In fact, having one STI may make it more likely that a person will acquire more STIs. For example, the open sore from herpes creates a place for HIV to be transmitted.

10. **False.** The symptoms may go away, but your body is still infected. For example, syphilis is characterized by various stages. In the first stage, a painless sore called a *chancre* appears for about a week and then goes away.

11. **False.** If you have sex once with an infected partner, you are at risk for an STI.

12. **False.** Some STIs are viruses and therefore cannot be cured. There is no cure at present for herpes, HIV/AIDS, or genital warts. These STIs are treatable (to lessen the pain and irritation of symptoms), but not curable.

13. **True.** Experiencing one infection with an STI does not mean that you can never be infected again. A person can be reinfected many times with the same STI. This is especially true if a person does not get treated for the STI and thus keeps reinfecting his or her partner with the same STI.

Sources: Adapted from Jefferson County Public Health, "STD Quiz," Modified March 2009, www.co.jefferson.co.us/health/health_T111_R69.htm; Family Planning Victoria, "Play Safe," Updated July 2005, www.fpv.org.au/1_2_2.html.

YOUR PLAN FOR CHANGE

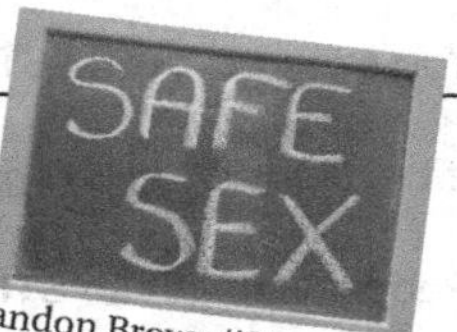

Brandon Brown/iStockphoto

The Assessyourself activity let you consider your beliefs and attitudes about STIs and identify possible risks you may be facing. Now that you have considered these results, you can begin to change behaviors that may be putting you at risk for STIs and for infection in general.

Today, you can:

◯ Put together an "emergency" supply of condoms. Outside of abstinence, condoms are your best protection against an STI. If you don't have a supply on hand, visit your local drugstore or health clinic. Remember that both men and women are responsible for preventing the transmission of STIs.

◯ To prevent infections in general, get in the habit of washing your hands regularly. After you cough, sneeze, blow your nose, use the bathroom, or prepare food, find a sink, wet your hands with warm water, and lather up with soap. Scrub your hands for about 20 seconds (count to 20 or recite the alphabet), rinse well, and dry your hands.

Within the next 2 weeks, you can:

◯ Talk with your significant other honestly about your sexual history. Make appointments to get tested if either of you think you may have been exposed to an STI.

◯ Adjust your sleep schedule so that you're getting an adequate amount of rest every night. Being well rested is one key aspect of maintaining a healthy immune system.

By the end of the semester, you can:

◯ Check your immunization schedule and make sure you're current with all recommended vaccinations. Make an appointment with your health care provider if you need a booster or vaccine.

◯ If you are due for an annual pelvic exam, make an appointment. Ask your partner if he or she has had an annual exam and encourage him or her to make an appointment if not.

Summary

* Your body uses a number of defense systems to keep pathogens from invading. The skin is the body's major protection. The immune system creates antibodies to destroy antigens. Fever and pain play a role in defending the body. Vaccines bolster the body's immune system against specific diseases. Allergies are an overreaction of the body's natural defense system.
* The major pathogens are bacteria, viruses, fungi, protozoans, parasitic worms, and prions. Bacterial infections include staphylococcal infections, streptococcal infections, pneumonia, and tuberculosis. Major viral diseases include the common cold, influenza, and hepatitis. Emerging and resurgent diseases pose significant threats for future generations, as do problems related to antibiotic resistance and superbugs.
* Sexually transmitted infections (STIs) are spread through intercourse, oral sex, anal sex, hand–genital contact, and sometimes mouth-to-mouth contact. Major STIs include chlamydia, gonorrhea, syphilis, herpes, human papillomavirus (HPV) and genital warts, candidiasis, trichomoniasis, and pubic lice.
* Acquired immunodeficiency syndrome (AIDS) is caused by the human immunodeficiency virus (HIV). Globally, HIV/AIDS has become a major threat to the world's population. Anyone can get HIV by engaging in high-risk sexual activities that include exchange of body fluids or by injecting drugs with contaminated needles (or having sex with someone who does).
* Chronic lung diseases include chronic bronchitis, emphysema, and asthma. Lung disease is the third leading cause of death in the United States.
* Headaches may be caused by a variety of factors, the most common of which are tension, dilation and/or rapid contraction of blood vessels in the brain, chemical influences on muscles and vessels that cause inflammation and pain, and underlying physiological and psychological disorders.
* Chronic fatigue syndrome is a complex disorder characterized by profound fatigue. Low back pain is a major cause of disability among Americans, but some risks for it can be addressed by proper posture, supportive shoes, and core-strengthening exercises. Repetitive motion disorders are preventable by proper placement and usage of equipment.

Pop Quiz

1. Which of the following is a *viral* disorder?
   a. the common cold
   b. pneumonia
   c. tuberculosis
   d. streptococcal infections

2. Antibiotic resistance is likely caused by
   a. the overuse of antibiotics in food production.
   b. the improper use of antibiotics by patients for whom they are prescribed.
   c. the overuse of antibacterial soaps and other cleaning products.
   d. all of the above.

3. If you are infected, which one of these STIs will remain in your body for life, regardless of treatment?
   a. chlamydia
   b. gonorrhea
   c. syphilis
   d. herpes

4. The term to best describe infections transmitted through some form of intimate contact is
   a. sexually transmitted diseases.
   b. sexually transmitted infections.
   c. venereal disease.
   d. chronic disease.

5. Jennifer touched her viral herpes sore on her lip and then touched her eye. She ended up with herpesvirus in her eye as well. This is an example of
   a. acquired immunity.
   b. passive immunity.
   c. autoinoculation.
   d. self-vaccination.

6. Which of the following is *not* a true statement about HIV/AIDS?
   a. You can tell whether a potential sex partner has the virus by looking at the person.
   b. The virus can be spread through either semen or vaginal fluids.
   c. You cannot get HIV from a public restroom toilet seat.
   d. Unprotected anal sex increases risk of exposure to the HIV virus.

7. Which of the following is true about HPV?
   a. Genital warts are caused by the low-risk types of HPV.
   b. The HPV vaccine is available for men and women.
   c. There are over 100 different types of HPV that are sexually transmitted.
   d. Antibiotics are used to cure HPV.

8. Which of the following is correct?
   a. There is no increased risk for migraines in children born to parents with migraines.
   b. COPDs include low back pain, asthma, and arthritis.
   c. Fever and inflammation are components of the body's immune response and help fight pathogens.
   d. If you have a low fever, taking aspirin is a good idea.

9. The gradual destruction of the alveoli in a smoker's lungs will usually cause which respiratory condition?
   a. dyspnea
   b. bronchitis
   c. emphysema
   d. asthma
10. Which of the following conditions is the leading cause of employee sick time and lost productivity in the United States?
   a. low back pain
   b. the common cold
   c. asthma
   d. on-the-job injuries

Answers to Chapter Review Questions
1. a; 2. d; 3. d; 4. b; 5. c;
6. a; 7. a; 8. c; 9. c; 10. b

Think about It!

1. What are the major controllable risk factors for contracting infectious diseases? Using this knowledge, how would you change your current lifestyle to prevent such infection?
2. What is a pathogen? What are the similarities and differences between pathogens and antigens?
3. What are the six types of pathogens? What are the various means by which they can be transmitted?
4. How have social conditions among the poor and homeless increased the risks for certain diseases, such as tuberculosis, influenza, and hepatitis? Why are these conditions a challenge to the efforts of public health officials?
5. Identify five STIs and their symptoms. How do they develop? What are their potential long-term effects?
6. Why are women more susceptible to HIV infection than men? What implications does this have for prevention, treatment, and research?
7. List common respiratory diseases affecting Americans. Which of these diseases has a genetic basis? An environmental basis? An individual basis?

Accessing Your Health on the Internet

The following websites explore further topics and issues related to personal health. For links to the websites below, visit the Companion Website for *Health: The Basics,* Green Edition at www.pearsonhighered.com/donatelle.

1. *American Academy of Allergy, Asthma, and Immunology.* Provides an overview of asthma and allergies. Offers interactive quizzes to test your knowledge and an ask-an-expert section. www.aaaai.org
2. *American Social Health Association.* Provides facts, support, resources, and referrals about sexually transmitted infections and diseases. www.ashastd.org
3. *Centers for Disease Control and Prevention (CDC).* Home page for the government agency dedicated to disease intervention and prevention, with links to all the latest data and publications put out by the CDC, including the *Morbidity and Mortality Weekly Report, HIV/AIDS Surveillance Report,* and the *Journal of Emerging Infectious Diseases.* Also provides access to Wonder, the CDC research database. www.cdc.gov
4. *National Center for Preparedness, Detection, and Control of Infectious Diseases (NCPDCID).* Up-to-date perspectives on infectious diseases of significance to the global community. www.cdc.gov/ncpdcid
5. *San Francisco AIDS Foundation.* This community-based AIDS service organization focuses on ending the HIV/AIDS pandemic through education, services for AIDS patients, advocacy and public policy efforts, and global programs. www.sfaf.org
6. *World Health Organization (WHO).* Provides access to the latest information on world health issues, including infectious disease, and direct access to publications and fact sheets, with keywords to help users find topics of interest. www.who.int

References

1. J. R. Pleis and J. W. Lucas, National Center for Health Statistics, "Summary Health Statistics for U.S. Adults: National Health Interview Survey, 2007," *Vital Health and Statistics* 10, no. 240 (2009).
2. Centers for Disease Control and Prevention, National Center for Health Statistics, "FastStats: Allergies and Hay Fever," Updated April 2009, www.cdc.gov/nchs/fastats/allergies.htm.
3. R. Klevens, "Invasive Methicillin-Resistant Staphylococcus Aureus (MRSA) Infections in the United States," *Journal of the American Medical Association* 298, no. 15 (2007): 1763–71.
4. Centers for Disease Control and Prevention, "Group A Streptococcal Disease (GAS)," Accessed August 2009, www.cdc.gov/ncidod/dbmd/diseaseinfo/groupastreptococcal_g.htm.
5. Ibid.
6. J. Tully et al., "Students May Have Higher Risk for Meningococcal Disease Than Other Adolescents," *British Medical Journal* 332, no. 7539 (2006): 1136–42.
7. Centers for Disease Control and Prevention, *Reported Tuberculosis in the United States, 2007* (Atlanta: U.S. Department of Health and Human Services, CDC, 2008).
8. World Health Organization, *WHO Report 2009—Global Tuberculosis Control: Epidemiology, Strategy, Financing* (Geneva, Switzerland: 2009).
9. Centers for Disease Control and Prevention, "Key Facts about Seasonal Influenza (Flu)," Updated October 2009, www.cdc.gov/flu/keyfacts.htm.
10. Centers for Disease Control and Prevention, "Hepatitis A FAQs for Health Professionals," Updated June 2009, www.cdc.gov/hepatitis/HAV/HAVfaq.htm.
11. World Health Organization, "Global Alert and Response: Hepatitis B," 2009, www.who.int/csr/disease/hepatitis/whocdscsrlyo20022/en/index1.html.
12. Centers for Disease Control and Prevention, Division of Viral Hepatitis, National Center for HIV/AIDS, Viral Hepatitis, STD, and TB Prevention, "Viral Hepatitis," 2009, www.cdc.gov/hepatitis/index.htm.
13. Centers for Disease Control and Prevention, National Center for Infectious Diseases, "vCJD (Variant Creutzfeldt-Jakob Disease)," 2007, www.cdc.gov/ncidod/dvrd/vcjd/index.htm.
14. Centers for Disease Control and Prevention, Division of Vector-Borne Infectious Diseases, National Center for Zoonotic, Vector-Borne, and Enteric Diseases, "West Nile Virus: Statistics, Surveillance and Control,"

2009, www.cdc.gov/ncidod/dvbid/westnile/surv&controlCaseCount08_detailed.htm.
15. World Health Organization, "Confirmed Human Cases of Avian Influenza A (H5N1)," Updated September 2009, www.who.int/csr/disease/avian_influenza/country/en.
16. Centers for Disease Control and Prevention, Division of STD Prevention, National Center for HIV/AIDS, Viral Hepatitis, STD, and TB Prevention, "Trends in Reportable Sexually Transmitted Diseases in the United States, 2008," 2009.
17. Centers for Disease Control and Prevention, Division of STD Prevention, National Center for HIV/AIDS, Viral Hepatitis, STD, and TB Prevention, "Trends in Reportable Sexually Transmitted Diseases in the United States, 2008: National Surveillance Data for Chlamydia, Gonorrhea, and Syphilis," 2009, www.cdc.gov/std/stats08/trends.htm; American Social Health Association, "STD/STI Statistics: Fast Facts," Updated October 2006, www.ashastd.org/learn/learn_statistics.cfm.
18. Centers for Disease Control and Prevention, Division of STD Prevention, National Center for HIV/AIDS, Viral Hepatitis, STD, and TB Prevention, "Chlamydia—CDC Fact Sheet," Updated December 2007, www.cdc.gov/std/Chlamydia/STDFact-Chlamydia.htm.
19. National Institute of Allergy and Infectious Diseases, "Chlamydia," Updated April 2009, www3.niaid.nih.gov/topics/chlamydia.
20. Centers for Disease Control and Prevention, Division of STD Prevention, National Center for HIV/AIDS, Viral Hepatitis, STD, and TB Prevention, "Gonorrhea—CDC Fact Sheet," 2008, www.cdc.gov/std/Gonorrhea/STDFact-gonorrhea.htm.
21. U.S. National Library of Medicine, Medline Plus, "Gonorrhea," Updated May 2009, www.nlm.nih.gov/medlineplus/ency/article/007267.htm.
22. National Institute of Allergy and Infectious Diseases, "Gonorrhea," Updated March 2009, www3.niaid.nih.gov/topics/gonorrhea.
23. Centers for Disease Control and Prevention, Division of STD Prevention, National Center for HIV/AIDS, Viral Hepatitis, STD, and TB Prevention, "Syphilis: CDC Fact Sheet," 2008, www.cdc.gov/std/syphilis/STDFact-Syphilis.htm.
24. National Institute of Allergy and Infectious Diseases, "Syphilis," Updated March 2009, www3.niaid.nih.gov/topics/syphilis.
25. Centers for Disease Control and Prevention, Division of STD Prevention, National Center for HIV/AIDS, Viral Hepatitis, STD, and TB Prevention, "Genital Herpes—CDC Fact Sheet," 2008, www.cdc.gov/std/Herpes/STDFact-Herpes.htm.
26. American Society for Microbiology, Fourth Annual Interscience Conference on Antimicrobial Agents and Chemotherapy (San Francisco. September 27–30, 2006); Centers for Disease Control and Prevention, "Genital Herpes—CDC Fact Sheet 2008."
27. National Institute of Allergy and Infectious Diseases, "Human Papillomavirus and Genital Warts" Updated August 2009, www3.niaid.nih.gov/topics/genitalWarts.
28. National Institute of Allergy and Infectious Diseases, "Vaginal Yeast Infection," Updated July 2009, www3.niaid.nih.gov/topics/vaginalYeast.
29. National Institute of Allergy and Infectious Diseases, "Trichomoniasis," Updated March 2009, www3.niaid.nih.gov/topics/trichomoniasis.
30. Joint United Nations Programme on HIV/AIDS (UNAIDS), *2008 Report on the Global AIDS Epidemic* (Geneva, Switzerland: UNAIDS, 2008); AVERT, "Worldwide HIV & AIDS Statistics," Updated November 2009, www.avert.org/worldstats.htm.
31. Centers for Disease Control and Prevention, *HIV/AIDS Surveillance Report, 2007* Vol. 19, (Atlanta: U.S. Department of Health and Human Services, Centers for Disease Control and Prevention, 2009) Available at www.cdc.gov/hiv/topics/surveillance/resources/reports.
32. Centers for Disease Control and Prevention, Divisions of HIV/AIDS Prevention, National Center for HIV/AIDS, Viral Hepatitis, STD, and TB Prevention, "HIV Incidence," Updated September 2008, www.cdc.gov/hiv/topics/surveillance/incidence.htm; H. I. Hall et al., "Estimation of HIV Incidence in the United States," *JAMA:* 300, no. 5 (2008): 520–29.
33. National Institute of Allergy and Infectious Diseases, "HIV/AIDS," Updated August 2009, www3.niaid.nih.gov/topics/HIVAIDS.
34. Centers for Disease Control and Prevention, Divisions of HIV/AIDS Prevention, National Center for HIV/AIDS, Viral Hepatitis, STD, and TB Prevention, "Mother-to-Child (Perinatal) HIV Transmission and Prevention," 2007, www.cdc.gov/hiv/topics/perinatal/resources/factsheets/perinatal.htm; Centers for Disease Control and Prevention, Divisions of HIV/AIDS Prevention, National Center for HIV/AIDS, Viral Hepatitis, STD, and TB Prevention, "HIV/AIDS: Questions and Answers," Updated February 2009, www.cdc.gov/hiv/resources/qa; AVERT, "Preventing Mother to Child Transmission of HIV," Updated August 2009, www.avert.org/motherchild.htm.
35. American Lung Association, "Lung Disease," Accessed November 2009, www.lungusa.org/lung-disease.
36. American Lung Association, "About COPD," Accessed November 2009, www.lungusa.org/lung-disease/copd/about-copd.
37. Ibid.
38. Centers for Disease Control and Prevention, National Center for Health Statistics, FASTSTATS A to Z, "Chronic Obstructive Pulmonary Disease (COPD) Includes: Chronic Bronchitis and Emphysema," Updated May 2009, www.cdc.gov/nchs/fastats/copd.htm.
39. American Lung Association, "About Asthma," Accessed November 2009, www.lungusa.org/lung-disease/asthma/about-asthma.
40. Ibid.
41. Ibid.
42. Ibid.
43. Ibid.
44. National Headache Foundation, "Headache Topic Sheets," 2009, www.headaches.org.
45. National Headache Foundation, "Headache Topic Sheets: Migraine," 2009, www.headaches.org/education/Headache_Topic_Sheets/Migraine.
46. National Headache Foundation, "Headache Topic Sheets: Cluster Headaches," 2009, www.headaches.org/education/Headache_Topic_Sheets/Cluster_Headaches.
47. Centers for Disease Control and Prevention, National Institute of Neurological Disorders and Stroke, "Low Back Pain Fact Sheet," Updated August 2009, www.ninds.nih.gov/disorders/backpain/detail_backpain.htm.
48. Centers for Disease Control and Prevention, National Institute of Neurological Disorders, "NINDS Repetitive Motion Disorders Information Page," Updated February 2007, www.ninds.nih.gov/disorders/repetitive_motion/repetitive_motion.htm?css=print.

Addictions and Addictive Behavior

THREATS TO WELLNESS

Addictions and Addictive Behavior

THREATS TO WELLNESS

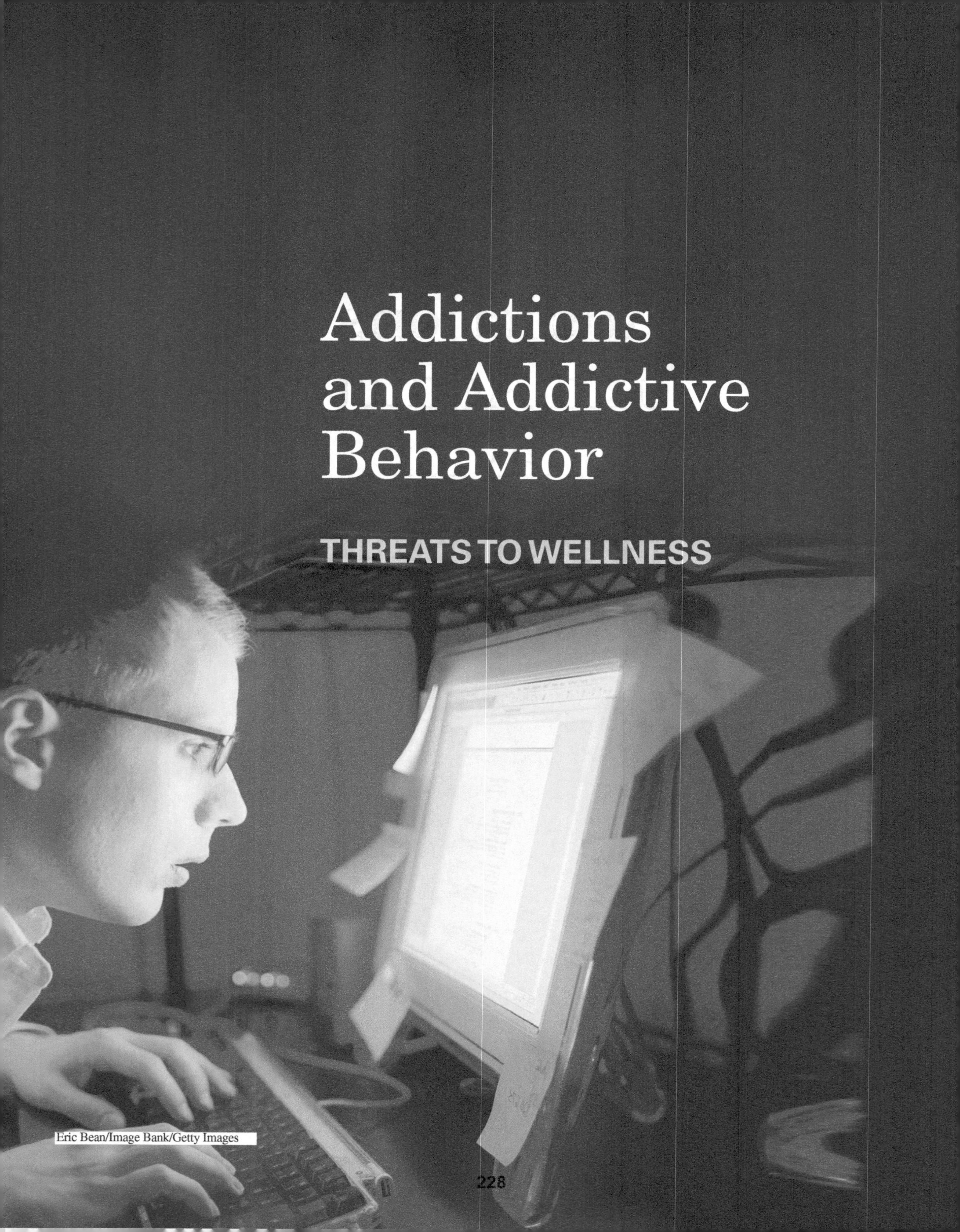

Eric Bean/Image Bank/Getty Images

What makes an **ADDICTION** different from a habit?

How can I **RECOGNIZE** addiction in a loved one or even myself?

Do some people have more addictive **PERSONALITIES** than others?

Is my roommate's **OBSESSIVE** online gaming an addiction?

How can I approach someone who needs help and **TREATMENT?**

Objectives

- Define *addiction.*
- Distinguish addictions from habits, and identify the signs of addiction.
- Discuss the addictive process, the physiology of addiction, and the biopsychosocial model of addiction.
- Describe types of addictions, including gambling, work, exercise, sexual, and Internet addictions, as well as codependence.
- Evaluate treatment and recovery options for addicts, including individual therapy, group therapy, family therapy, and 12-step programs.

These days, it's easy to find high-profile cases of compulsive and destructive behavior. Stories of celebrities and politicians struggling with addictions to alcohol, drugs, and sex are splashed in the headlines and profiled on television news programs. But millions of "everyday" people throughout the world are staging their own battles with addiction as well. People with addictions can sometimes be caught off guard, because many potentially addictive activities may actually enhance the lives of those who engage in them moderately. In addition to alcohol and drugs, the most commonly recognized addictions include food, sex, relationships, shopping, work, exercise, gambling, and using the Internet.

Defining Addiction

Addiction is continued involvement with a substance or activity despite ongoing negative consequences. Addictive behaviors initially provide a sense of pleasure or stability that is beyond the addict's power to achieve in other ways. Eventually, the addicted person needs to be involved in the behavior in order to feel normal.

In this chapter, *addiction* is used interchangeably with *physiological addiction.* However, **physiological dependence,** the adaptive state that occurs with regular addictive behavior and results in withdrawal syndrome, is only one indicator of addiction. Psychological dynamics play an important role, which explains why behaviors not related to the use of chemicals—gambling, for example—may also be addictive. A person with an intense, uncontrollable urge to continue engaging in a particular activity is said to have developed a psychological dependence. In fact, psychological and physiological dependence are so intertwined that it is not really possible to separate the two. For every psychological state, there is a corresponding physiological state. In other words, everything you feel is tied to a chemical process occurring in your body.[1] Thus, addictions once thought to be entirely psychological in nature are now understood to have physiological components.

To be addictive, a behavior must have the potential to produce a positive mood change. Chemicals are responsible for the most profound addictions because they produce dramatic mood changes and cause cellular changes to which the body adapts so well that it eventually requires the chemical in order to function normally. Yet other behaviors, such as gambling, spending money, working, and sex, also create changes at the cellular level along with positive mood changes. Although the mechanism is not well understood, all forms of addiction probably reflect dysfunction of certain biochemical systems in the brain.[2]

Traditionally, diagnosis of an addiction was limited to drug addiction and was based on four criteria as defined by the American Psychological Association:

1. Used for the purpose of relieving **withdrawal** symptoms—a series of temporary physical and psychological symptoms that occurs when the addicted person abruptly stops using the drug.
2. Continued use of the substance despite knowledge of the harm it causes yourself and others (deterioration in work performance, relationships, and social interaction).
3. Unsuccessful efforts to cut down or cease using the drug, including **relapse**—the tendency to return to the addictive behavior after a period of abstinence.
4. **Tolerance,** or an acquired reaction to a drug in which continued intake of the same dose has diminished effects. In response to tolerance, drug users must increase the dose in order to achieve the desired effect.

Until recently, health professionals were unwilling to diagnose an addiction until medical symptoms appeared in the patient. Now we know that although withdrawal, pathological behavior, relapse, and medical symptoms are valid indicators of addiction, they do not characterize all addictive behavior.

addiction Continued involvement with a substance or activity despite ongoing negative consequences

physiological dependence The adaptive state that occurs with regular addictive behavior and results in withdrawal syndrome

withdrawal A series of temporary physical and biopsychosocial symptoms that occur when an addict abruptly abstains from an addictive chemical or behavior

relapse The tendency to return to the addictive behavior after a period of abstinence

tolerance Phenomenon in which progressively larger doses of a drug or more intense involvement in a behavior are needed to produce the desired effects

Habit versus Addiction

How do we distinguish between a harmless habit and an addiction? The stereotypical image of the addict is of someone desperately seeking a fix 24 hours a day. People have the notion that if you aren't doing the behavior every day, you're not addicted. The reality is somewhere between these two extremes.

> What makes an addiction different from a habit?

Addiction certainly involves elements of **habit,** a repeated behavior in which the repetition may be unconscious. A habit can be annoying, but it can be broken without too much discomfort by simply becoming aware of its presence and choosing not to do it. Addiction also involves repetition of a behavior, but the repetition occurs by **compulsion,** and

Addictive substances and the chemical reactions they trigger in our brain mimic the euphoric feeling we have after successfully completing an achievement or when experiencing joy.

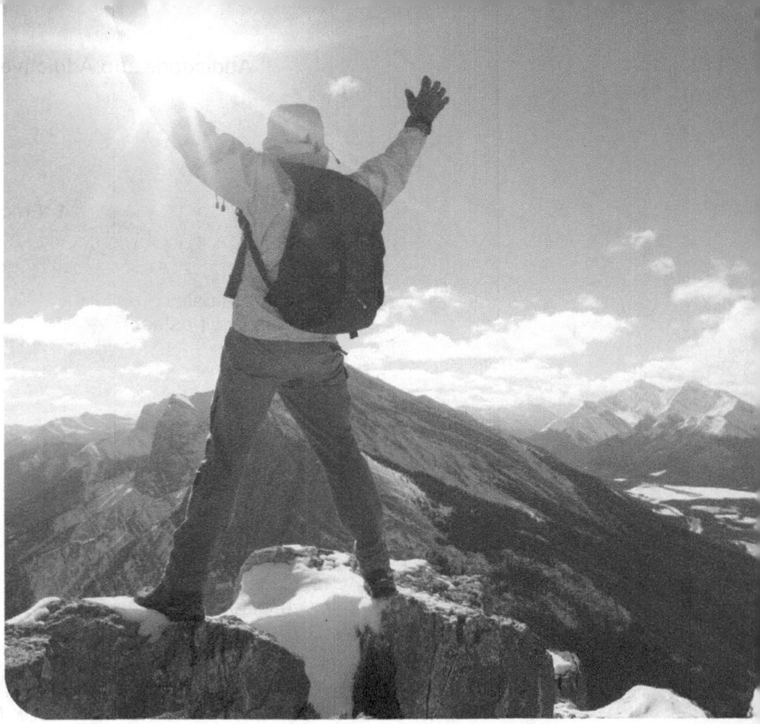

Philip & Karen Smith/Getty Images

considerable discomfort is experienced if the behavior is not performed. An addiction is a habit that has gotten out of control and has negative health effects.

To understand addiction, we must look beyond the amount and frequency of the behavior, because what happens when a person is involved in the behavior is far more meaningful. For example, someone who drinks only rarely and then engages in a night of heavy drinking may experience personality changes, blackouts (drug-induced amnesia), and other negative consequences (i.e., failing a test, missing an important appointment, getting into a fight) that would never have occurred otherwise. On the other hand, someone who has a few martinis every evening may never do anything out of character while under the influence of alcohol but may become irritable, manipulative, and aggressive without those regular drinks. For both of these people, alcohol appears to perform a function (mood control) that they should be able to do without the aid of chemicals, which is a possible sign of addiction. Habits are behaviors that occur through choice and typically do not cause negative health consequences. In contrast, no one decides to become addicted, even though people make choices that contribute to the development of an addiction.

Signs of Addiction

Studies show that most animals share the same basic pleasure and reward circuits in the brain that turn on when they encounter addictive substances or engage in something pleasurable, such as eating or orgasm. We all engage in potentially addictive behaviors to some extent, because some are essential to our survival and are highly reinforcing, such as eating, drinking, and sex. At some point along the continuum, however, some individuals are not able to engage in these or other behaviors moderately—they become addicted.

Addictions are characterized by four common symptoms: (1) compulsion, which is distinguished by **obsession,** or excessive preoccupation with the behavior and an overwhelming need to perform it; (2) **loss of control,** or the inability to reliably predict whether any isolated occurrence of the behavior will be healthy or damaging; (3) **negative consequences,** such as physical damage, legal trouble, financial problems, academic failure, and family dissolution, which do not occur with healthy involvement in any behavior; and (4) **denial,** the inability to perceive that the behavior is self-destructive. These four components are present in all addictions, whether chemical or behavioral.

How can I recognize addiction in a loved one or even myself?

habit A repeated behavior in which the repetition may be unconscious

compulsion Preoccupation with a behavior and an overwhelming need to perform it

obsession Excessive preoccupation with an addictive object or behavior

loss of control Inability to reliably predict whether a particular instance of involvement with the addictive substance or behavior will be healthy or damaging

negative consequences Severe problems associated with addiction, such as physical damage, legal trouble, financial problems, academic failure, or family dissolution

denial Inability to perceive or accurately interpret the self-destructive effects of the addictive behavior

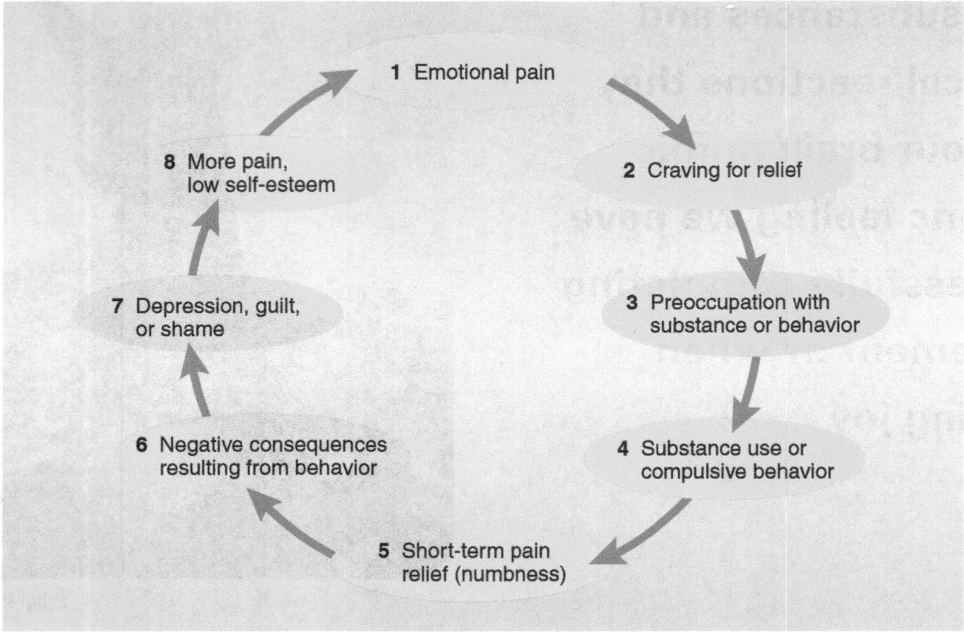

FIGURE 1 Cycle of Psychological Addiction
Source: From Turner, Sizer, Whitney, and Wilks, *Life Choices,* 2nd ed. © 1992 Brooks/Cole, a part of Cengage Learning, Inc. Reproduced by permission. www.cengage.com/permissions

? what do you think?

Have you ever seen signs of addiction in a friend or family member? ● What types of negative consequences have you witnessed? ● Can you think of any habits you have that could potentially become addictive?

The Addictive Process

Addiction is a process that evolves over time. It begins when a person repeatedly seeks the illusion of relief to avoid unpleasant feelings or situations. This pattern is known as *nurturing through avoidance* and is a maladaptive way of taking care of emotional needs. As a person becomes increasingly dependent on the addictive behavior, there is a corresponding deterioration in relationships with family, friends, and coworkers; in performance at work or school; and in personal life. Eventually, addicts do not find the addictive behavior pleasurable but consider it preferable to the unhappy realities they are seeking to escape. Figure 1 illustrates the cycle of psychological addiction.

neurotransmitters Biochemical messengers that bind to specific receptor sites on nerve cells

biopsychosocial model of addiction Theory of the relationship between an addict's biological (genetic) nature and psychological and environmental influences

The Physiology of Addiction

Virtually all intellectual, emotional, and behavioral functions occur as a result of biochemical interactions between nerve cells in the body. Biochemical messengers, called **neurotransmitters,** exert their influence at specific receptor sites on nerve cells. Drug use and chronic stress can alter these receptor sites and cause the production and breakdown of neurotransmitters.

Mood-altering chemicals, for example, fill up the receptor sites for the body's natural "feel-good" neurotransmitters (endorphins) so that nerve cells are fooled into believing they have enough neurotransmitters and shut down production of these substances temporarily. When the drug use stops, those receptor sites empty, resulting in uncomfortable feelings that remain until the body resumes normal neurotransmitter production or the person consumes more of the drug. Some people's bodies naturally produce insufficient quantities of these neurotransmitters, which predisposes them to seeking out chemicals, such as alcohol, as substitutes or to pursuing behaviors such as exercise that increase natural production.

Thus, some may be "wired" to look for substances or experiences that increase pleasure or reduce discomfort, making them more susceptible to addiction.

Mood-altering substances and experiences produce *tolerance,* defined earlier as a phenomenon in which progressively larger doses of a drug or more intense involvement in an experience are needed to obtain the desired effects. All of us develop some degree of tolerance to any mood-altering experience. But because addicts tend to seek intense mood-altering experiences, they eventually increase the amount and intensity to the point of causing negative side effects.

Withdrawal is another phenomenon associated with mood-altering experiences. The drug or activity replaces or causes an effect that the body should normally provide on its own. If the experience is repeated often enough, the body adjusts: It starts requiring the drug or experience to obtain the effect. Stopping the behavior will cause a withdrawal syndrome, because the body cannot naturally create the same effect as the drug.

Withdrawal symptoms of chemical dependencies are generally the opposite of the effects of the drugs. For example, a cocaine addict who feels a high while using the drug, experiences a characteristic "crash" (depression and lethargy) when he stops taking it. Conversely, a heroin addict experiences drowsiness, slowed speech and reactions, and uninhibited behavior while using the drug. When withdrawing from heroin, the addict experiences anxiety, elevated heart rate, trembling, irritability, insomnia, and convulsions. Withdrawal symptoms for addictive behaviors are usually less dramatic. They typically involve psychological discomfort such as anxiety, depression, irritability, guilt, anger, and frustration, with an underlying preoccupation with or craving for the behavior.

Withdrawal syndromes range from mild to severe. The most severe form is delirium tremens (DTs), which occurs in approximately 5 percent of dependent individuals withdrawing from alcohol.

Psychological Factors

A person's psychological makeup also factors into the potential for addiction. People with low self-esteem, a tendency toward risk-taking behavior, or poor coping skills are more likely to develop addictive patterns of behavior.

Do some people have more addictive personalities than others?

Individuals who consistently look outside themselves (who have an external locus of control) for solutions and explanations for life events are more likely to experience addiction.

The complexity of addiction and consistent evidence of multiple contributing factors lead us to conclude that the problem is not the result of a single influence but rather of a variety of influences working together. Biological, psychological, and environmental factors all contribute to its development. Although one factor may play a larger role than another in a specific individual, it is rarely sufficient to explain an addiction. Figure 2 lists risk factors for addiction.

A Model of Addiction

Since ancient times, biological or disease models of addiction have been proposed. However, psychological and environmental factors may also be involved in an addiction's development. The most effective treatment today is being provided by those who rely on the **biopsychosocial model of addiction,** which proposes that addiction is caused by a variety of factors operating together. This model represents a reasonable comprehension of all that we have learned about addiction.

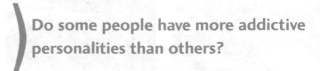

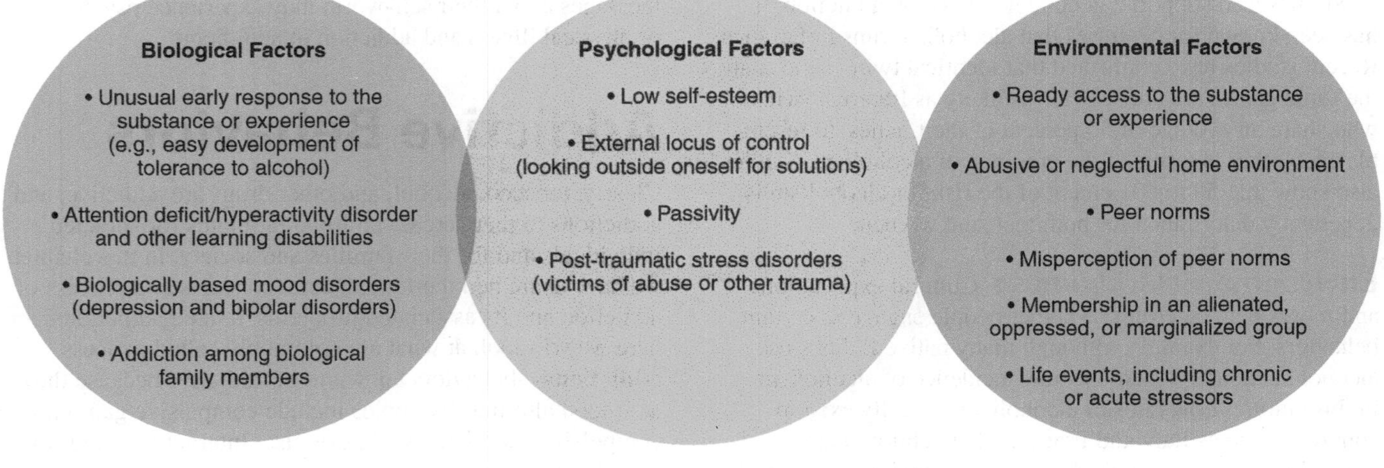

Biological Factors
• Unusual early response to the substance or experience (e.g., easy development of tolerance to alcohol)
• Attention deficit/hyperactivity disorder and other learning disabilities
• Biologically based mood disorders (depression and bipolar disorders)
• Addiction among biological family members
Psychological Factors
• Low self-esteem
• External locus of control (looking outside oneself for solutions)
• Passivity
• Post-traumatic stress disorders (victims of abuse or other trauma)
Environmental Factors
• Ready access to the substance or experience
• Abusive or neglectful home environment
• Peer norms
• Misperception of peer norms
• Membership in an alienated, oppressed, or marginalized group
• Life events, including chronic or acute stressors

FIGURE 2 Risk Factors for Addiction

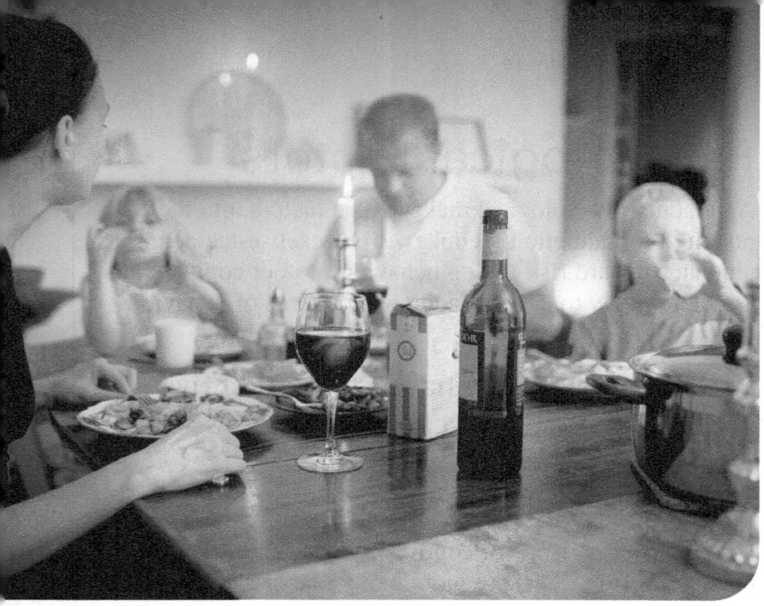

Nordicphotos/Alamy

One predisposing factor for developing an addiction might be environmental influences such as the norms we were taught during childhood.

Biological or Disease Influences For many people, addiction is thought to be based in the brain and involves memory, motivation, and emotional state. The processes that control these aspects of brain function are thus logical subjects for genetic research into a biologically based risk for addiction, particularly to mood-altering substances. Studies show that drug addicts metabolize these substances differently than nonaddicted people. Research suggests that genes affecting the activity of the neurotransmitters serotonin and GABA (gamma-aminobutyric acid) are likely involved in the risk for alcoholism.[3] For example, a study found that college students with a particular variant of the serotonin transporter gene consumed more alcohol per occasion, drank expressly to become inebriated more often, and engaged more frequently in heavy drinking than students with another variant of the gene. The relationships between neurotransmitters and alcoholism are complex, however; not all studies have shown a connection between alcoholism risk and these genes.[4]

Studies also support a genetic influence on addiction. It has been known for centuries that alcoholism runs in families. Recent studies have confirmed that identical twins, who share the same genes, are about twice as likely as fraternal twins, who share an average of 50 percent of their genes, to resemble each other in terms of the presence of alcoholism. Studies also show that 50 to 60 percent of the risk for alcoholism is genetically determined for both men and women.[5]

Environmental Influences Cultural expectations and mores help determine whether people engage in certain behaviors. For example, although many native Italians use alcohol abundantly, there is a low incidence of alcoholism in this culture. Low rates of alcoholism typically exist in countries such as Italy and France, where children are gradually introduced to alcohol in diluted amounts, on special occasions, and within a strong family group. There is deep disapproval of intoxication, which is not viewed as socially acceptable, stylish, or funny.[6] Such cultural traditions and values are less widespread in the United States, where the incidence of alcohol addiction and alcohol-related problems is very high.

Societal attitudes and messages also influence addictive behavior. The media's emphasis on appearance and the ideal body plays a significant role in exercise addiction. Societal glorification of money and material achievement can lead to work addiction, which is often admired. Societal changes, in turn, influence individual norms. People living in cities characterized by rapid social change or social disorganization often feel less connected to social, religious, and civic institutions. The resulting disenfranchisement leads to increased destructive behaviors, including addiction.[7]

Social learning theory proposes that people learn behaviors by watching role models—parents, caregivers, and significant others. The effects of modeling, imitation, and identification with behavior from early childhood on are well documented. Modeling is especially influential when it involves behavior that is mood altering. Many studies show that modeling by parents and by idolized celebrities exerts a profound influence on young people.[8]

On an individual level, major stressful life events, such as marriage, divorce, change in work status, and death of a loved one, may trigger addictive behaviors. Traumatic events in general often instigate addictive behaviors, as traumatized people seek to medicate their pain—pain they may not even be aware of because they've repressed it. One thing that makes addictive behaviors so powerfully attractive is that they reliably alleviate personal pain, at least for a short time. However, over the long-term, addictive behaviors actually cause more pain than they relieve.

Family members whose needs for love, security, and affirmation are not consistently met; who are refused permission to express their feelings, desires, or needs; and who frequently submerge their personalities to "keep the peace" are prone to addiction. Children whose parents are not consistently available to them (physically or emotionally); who are subjected to sexual abuse, physical abuse, neglect, or abandonment; or who receive inconsistent or disparaging messages about their self-worth may experience psychosocial or physical illness and addiction in adulthood.

Addictive Behaviors

Clearly, tobacco, alcohol, and other drugs are addictive, and addictions to them create multiple problems for addicted individuals and for their families and society. In this chapter, we have examined the fundamental concepts and process of addiction and its associated problems, related addictions; here we will look at what are commonly called **process addictions**—behaviors known to be addictive because they are mood altering. Examples include compulsive gambling, compulsive shopping, work, exercise, Internet use, and sexual addictions.

Compulsive or Pathological Gambling

Gambling is a form of recreation and entertainment for millions of Americans. Most people who gamble do so casually and moderately to experience the excitement of anticipating a win.

However, over 2 million Americans are **compulsive (pathological) gamblers,** and 6 million more are considered at risk for developing a gambling addiction.[9] The American Psychiatric Association (APA) recognizes pathological gambling as a mental disorder and lists ten characteristic behaviors, including preoccupation with gambling, unsuccessful efforts to cut back or quit, using gambling to escape problems, and lying to family members to conceal the extent of involvement.

Gamblers and drug addicts describe many similar cravings and highs. A recent study supports what many experts believe to be true: that compulsive gambling is like drug addiction. Compulsive gamblers in this study were found to have decreased blood flow to a key section of the brain's reward system. Much as with people who abuse drugs, it is thought that compulsive gamblers compensate for this deficiency in their brain's reward system by overdoing it and getting hooked.[10] Most compulsive gamblers state that they seek excitement even more than money. They place progressively larger bets to obtain the desired level of exhilaration. See the gambling portion of the Assess Yourself box to evaluate your gambling behavior.

Gambling problems are more prevalent among men than among women. Gambling prevalence is also higher among lower-income individuals, those who are divorced, African Americans, older adults, and people residing within 50 miles of a casino. Residents in Southern states, where opportunities to gamble have increased significantly over the past 20 years, also have higher gambling rates.[11] (See the Green Guide for some of the negative impacts the rise of gambling also has on the environment.)

Among students, gambling is on the rise on college campuses across the nation. Since 2002, the University of Pennsylvania's Annenburg Public Policy Center has been conducting a tracking survey of gambling among young people aged 14 to 22. Their survey reported that in 2005, 15.5 percent of college students reported gambling once a week, up from 8.3 percent in 2002, an 87 percent increase. Men dominated the gambling scene, with 26 percent reportedly doing it each week, whereas 5.5 percent of women reported gambling weekly.[12]

What accounts for this trend? College students have easier access to gambling opportunities than ever before, with the advent of online gambling, a growing number of casinos, scratch tickets, lotteries, and sports-betting networks. In particular, the largest boost has been from the increasing popularity of poker. Access to poker on the Internet and poker tournaments that are frequently televised have revived the game, causing many young people to spend an unhealthy amount of time and money participating in online poker tournaments.

Other characteristics associated with gambling among college students include spending more time watching TV and using computers for nonacademic purposes, spending less time studying, earning lower grades, participating in intercollegiate athletics, engaging in heavy episodic drinking, and using illicit drugs in the past year.[13] See the Health Headlines box for more on college students and gambling.

Whereas casual gamblers can stop anytime they wish and are capable of understanding why they need to stop, compulsive gamblers are unable to control the urge to gamble even in the face of devastating consequences: high debt, legal problems, and the loss of everything meaningful, including homes, families, jobs, health, and even their lives. Gambling can also have a detrimental effect on health: cardiovascular problems affect 38 percent of compulsive gamblers, and their suicide rate is 20 times higher than that of the general population.

Compulsive Shopping and Borrowing

People who "shop till they drop" and run their credit cards to the limit often have a shopping addiction. Since the credit

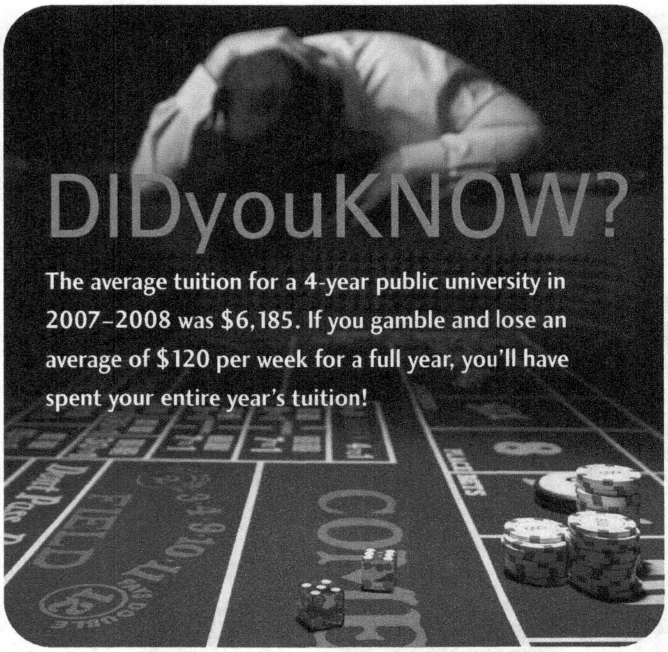

DIDyouKNOW?
The average tuition for a 4-year public university in 2007–2008 was $6,185. If you gamble and lose an average of $120 per week for a full year, you'll have spent your entire year's tuition!

John Howard/Getty Images

Source: Trends in College Pricing, 2007. The College Board, New York.

social learning theory Theory that people learn behaviors by watching role models—parents, caregivers, and significant others

process addictions Behaviors such as money addiction, work addiction, exercise addiction, and sex addiction that are known to be addictive because they are mood altering

compulsive (pathological) gambler A person addicted to gambling

Health Headlines

GAMBLING AND COLLEGE STUDENTS

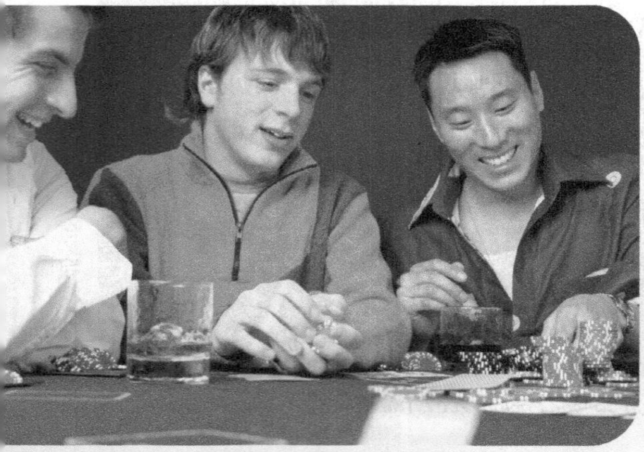

Ike Van de Velde/Digital Vision/Alamy

Although many people gamble occasionally without it ever becoming a problem, many otherwise "model" students can find themselves caught up in the rush of making big bets and winning even bigger money. Consider the story of John,* a Lehigh University sophomore, who is the son of a Baptist minister, a fraternity member, a cellist in the university orchestra, and the sophomore class president—the epitome of a responsible student active in the community and serving as a role model to the student body. When John was arrested for allegedly robbing the Wachovia Bank branch in Allentown, Pennsylvania, making off with $2,781, many wondered why such a good kid would be driven to such an act. According to the Associated Press, his lawyer stated that his client had run up about $5,000 in debt playing online poker. In a desperate move to feed his compulsive gambling addiction, John turned to bank robbery.

Compulsive gambling on college campuses has become a big concern for college administrators as gambling grows ever more popular among students. The National Collegiate Athletic Association (NCAA) estimates that each year during March Madness (the men's college basketball tournament), there are over 1.2 million active gambling pools, with over 2.5 billion dollars gambled. More and more of these dollars come from the pockets of college students. There is growing evidence, in fact, that betting on college campuses is interfering with students' financial and academic futures. In a recent survey, approximately 60 percent of students reported they had gambled, and almost 13 percent reported a significant loss of time and 12 percent a significant loss of money. Consider the following:

- Almost 53 percent of college students have participated in most forms of gambling, including casino gambling, lottery tickets, racing, and sports betting in the past month.
- At least 78 percent of youths have placed a bet by the age of 18.
- An estimated 18 percent of men and 4 percent of women on college campuses could be classified as problem gamblers.
- The three most common reasons college students give for gambling are risk, excitement, and the chance to make money.

Although most college students who gamble are able to do so without developing a problem, warning signs of problem gambling include the following:

- Frequent talk about gambling
- Spending more time or money on gambling than can be afforded
- Borrowing money to gamble
- Encouraging or challenging others to gamble
- Selling sports-betting cards or organizing sports pools
- Possession of gambling paraphernalia such as lottery tickets or poker items
- Missing or being late for school, work, or family activities due to gambling
- Feeling sad, anxious, fearful, or angry about gambling losses

*Not his real name

Sources: W. DeJong et al., "Gambling: The New Addiction Crisis in Higher Education," *Prevention Profile* (March 2006): 11–13; The Annenburg Public Policy Center, "Card-Playing Trend in Young People Continues," Press Release, September 28, 2005, www.annenbergpublicpolicycenter.org; Massachusetts Council on Compulsive Gambling, "Students Know the Limits," www.masscompulsivegambling.org; R. Schachter, "Targeting Student Gambling," *University Business* (January 2008): 35–38.

card's introduction, millions of Americans have found themselves mired in consumer debt. There are 400 million MasterCards and Visas out there, and on average, compulsive spenders are $23,000 in debt, usually in the form of credit card debt or mortgages against their homes.[14] College students may be particularly vulnerable to spending problems, because advertisers and credit card companies aggressively target them.

In our society, people often use shopping as a way to make themselves feel better. However, for compulsive shoppers, it does not make them feel any better but actually worse. Compulsive shopping and spending has many of the same characteristics as alcoholism, gambling, and other addictions. Symptoms that a shopper has crossed the line into addiction include buying more than one of the same item, keeping items in the closet with the tags still attached, repeatedly buying much more than they need or can afford, hiding purchases from relatives and loved ones, and experiencing feelings of euphoria and excitement when shopping.[15]

Green Guide

Gambling can

have enduring and devastating damage on more than just your checkbook. With the growing popularity of casinos, we are becoming increasingly aware of the lasting negative impacts of gambling on the environment—just as it can have lasting impacts on your financial and emotional stability. Here are just some of the ways casinos hurt the environment:

- Building casinos can threaten native plant and animal species by removing or damaging native habitats. By removing soil, trees, foliage, and natural habitat, native species have fewer resources for feeding, living, and reproducing.
- Roads and parking lots essential to casinos also contribute to increased land clearing and diminished water absorption by the earth. Soil particles help filter rainwater on its way to surface and groundwater aquifers. This is a vital step in the natural process of water purification. Nonpermeable surfaces such as roads and parking lots not only restrict water absorption by the earth but also inhibit the natural filtering of soils.
- Chemicals and petroleum products that gather on roads and parking lots are carried into our groundwater and drinking water, leading to contamination. These harmful chemicals can include air-pollution particles, spilled or leaked oil, gasoline, detergents, solvents, de-icing salts during freezing conditions, dead leaves, pesticides, fertilizer, bacteria from pet waste, and others.
- Casinos congregate large numbers of people in areas that are often remote or otherwise unpopulated. All the fossil fuels required to transport people and the supplies they require to a casino add stress to the environment, as do the waste products created by these people.
- Generally casinos operate 24 hours a day—24 hours during which lights, slot machines, air-conditioning systems, TV monitors, and other electricity-requiring systems and appliances are going full force. The combined effect of the glitz and clamor is a heavy drain on energy resources.
- Casinos and the hotels and resorts frequently attached to them also consume large quantities of water. Additionally, many casinos have golf courses that require an exorbitant amount of water to keep green. Water is precious anywhere, but it can be especially difficult to replenish for casinos located in deserts or remote areas where water or other resources are scarce. Las Vegas, for example, barely has enough water to last the next 20 years if consumption rates stay as they are. Currently, Nevada borrows much of its water from neighboring states such as Utah, Colorado, and California. Las Vegas draws 90 percent of its water from the Colorado River at the Hoover Dam (on the border between Nevada and Arizona), which is 104 feet below its 1998 peak and still falling.

In recent years, there have been a few developments toward transitioning to green casinos:

- Online casinos are gaining in popularity—it is estimated that 5 percent of gross gaming yields in 2005 was from online casinos. Because online casinos don't have the physical presence that traditional casinos have, they can have less of a measurable environmental impact. Some online casinos are going an extra step toward minimizing their impact by adopting environmentally sustainable practices in the buildings where they have their offices. However, skeptics have expressed doubts as to the true intentions of such casinos, saying that some casino companies and developers are simply trying to find ways to qualify for lucrative environmentally friendly tax breaks.
- A handful of casinos are jumping on the green building bandwagon. For example, the St. Regis Mohawk Tribe and Empire Resorts have announced that their new casino at Monticello Raceway has taken the first steps toward becoming the first LEED-certified green casino in the Northeast. LEED (Leadership in Energy and Environmental Design) is a registered trademark of the U.S. Green Building Council. To earn a LEED certification, the project must meet benchmarks in five areas of human and environmental health: sustainable site development, water savings, energy efficiency, materials selection, and indoor environmental quality.
- Some companies that produce gaming products are working to create ecofriendly products that reduce waste, use more sustainable materials, and decrease the use of natural resources.
- The EPA has recognized that hotels and casinos represent an excellent but underutilized market for combined heat and power (CHP), also know as *cogeneration*. CHP systems provide efficient and reliable supplies of both electricity and heat from a single fuel source. In September 2006, the EPA's CHP Partnership hosted approximately 40 casino managers, Nevada policymakers, and other stakeholders for a workshop titled "CHP Opportunities for Las Vegas Casinos in Las Vegas." This is just a first step, but it may lead to significant changes in casino energy use in the near future.

Compulsive shopping or spending can be seasonal, such as shopping during the winter months, to alleviate feelings of anxiety and depression. It can also occur when people feel depressed, lonely, or angry. Shopping and spending will not assure more love; increase self-esteem; or heal the hurts, regrets, stresses, and problems of daily living. It generally makes people feel worse because of the increased financial debt the person has obtained from their addiction.

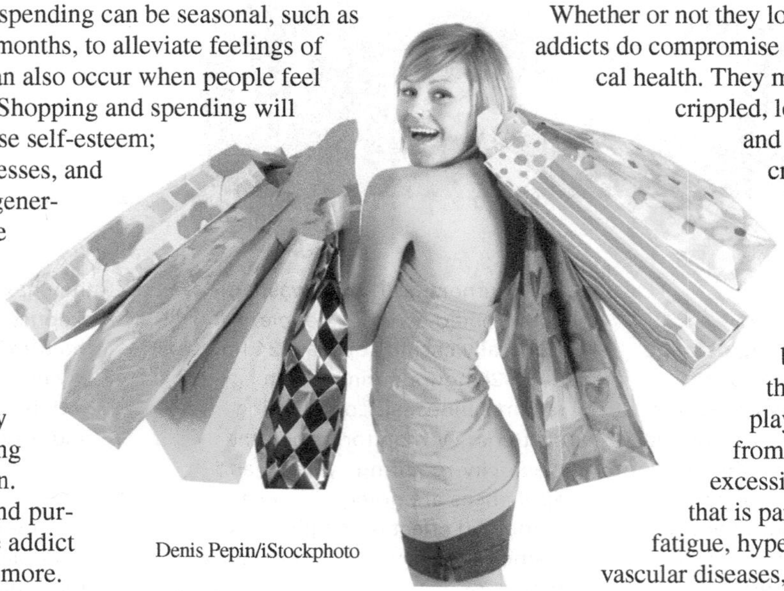

Denis Pepin/iStockphoto

Compulsive gambling and shopping can frequently lead to compulsive borrowing to help support the addiction. Irresponsible investments and purchases lead to debts that the addict tries to repay by borrowing more. Compulsive debtors borrow money repeatedly from family, friends, or institutions in spite of the problems this causes. Although most people who incur overwhelming debt do so through a combination of hardship and ignorance about financial management, compulsive debtors incur debt primarily as a result of buying or gambling behaviors in which they have engaged to relieve painful feelings.

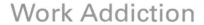

Work Addiction

In order to understand work addiction, we must understand the concept of healthy work. Healthy work provides a sense of identity; helps develop our strengths; and is a means of satisfaction, accomplishment, and mastery of problems. Healthy workers may work passionately for long hours. Although they have occasional projects that keep them away from family, friends, and personal interests for short periods of time, they generally maintain balance in their lives and full control of their schedules. Healthy work does not "consume" the worker.

Conversely, **work addiction** is the compulsive use of work and the work persona to fulfill needs of intimacy, power, and success. It is characterized by obsession, perfectionism, rigidity, fear, anxiety, feelings of inadequacy, low self-esteem, and alienation. Work addiction is more than being unable to relax when not doing something considered "productive." It is the pursuit of the "work persona"—the image that work addicts wish to project onto others. Work addiction is found among all age, racial, and socioeconomic groups, but it typically develops in people in their forties and fifties. Male work addicts outnumber female work addicts, but women are catching up fast as they gain more equality in the workforce.

Although work addicts tend to be admired in our society, the effects on individuals and those around them are far-reaching. Work addiction is a major source of marital discord and family breakup. In fact, most work addicts come from homes that were alcoholic, rigid, violent, or otherwise dysfunctional.

Whether or not they lose their families, work addicts do compromise their emotional and physical health. They may become emotionally crippled, losing the communication and human interaction skills critical to living and working with other people. They are often riddled with guilt and chronic fear—of failure, boredom, laziness, persecution, or being found out. Because they are unable to relax and play, they commonly suffer from chronic fatigue. The excessive pumping of adrenaline that is part of the addiction causes fatigue, hypertension and other cardiovascular diseases, nervousness, trembling, and increased sweating. Work addicts commonly suffer from disorders of the gastrointestinal tract, and they often report a feeling of pressure in the chest, constricted breathing, dizziness, and light-headedness. Figure 3 identifies other typical signs of work addiction.

Exercise Addiction

It may seem odd that a personal health text that advocates exercise would also identify it as a potential addiction. Yet, as

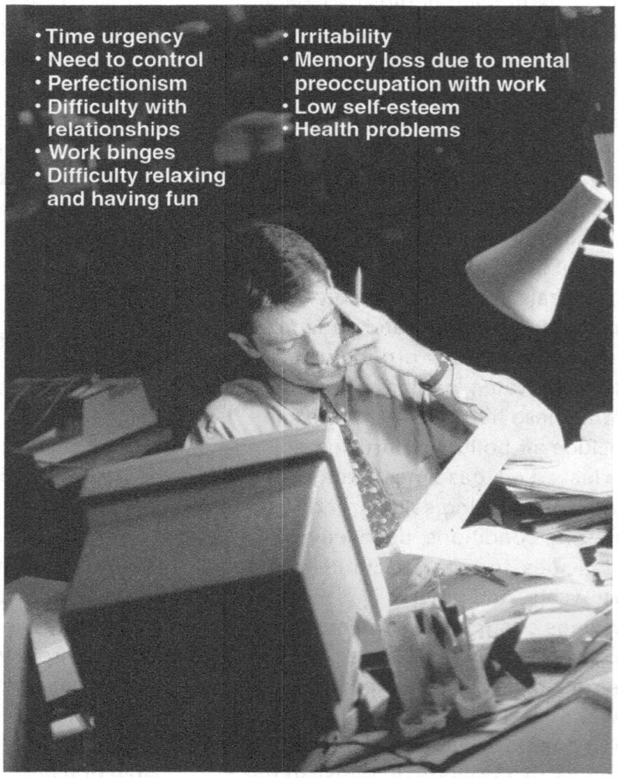

• Time urgency
• Need to control
• Perfectionism
• Difficulty with relationships
• Work binges
• Difficulty relaxing and having fun
• Irritability
• Memory loss due to mental preoccupation with work
• Low self-esteem
• Health problems

Peter Cade/Stone/Getty Images

FIGURE 3 Signs of Work Addiction

a powerful mood enhancer, exercise can be addictive. Statistics on the incidence of this addiction are not available, but one indication of its prevalence is that a large portion of America's 2 million people with the eating disorders anorexia nervosa and bulimia nervosa use exercise to purge instead of, or in addition to, self-induced vomiting.

Addictive exercisers abuse exercise in the same way that alcoholics abuse alcohol or addictive shoppers abuse money. They use it compulsively to try to meet needs—for nurturance, intimacy, self-esteem, and self-competency—that an object or activity cannot truly meet. Consequently, addictive exercise results in negative consequences similar to those found in other addictions: alienation of family and friends, injuries from overdoing it, and a craving for more.

Traditionally, women have been perceived as more at risk for exercise addiction. However, evidence is growing that more men are developing unhealthy exercise patterns. Media images promoting six-pack abs and lean, muscular bodies have influenced society's view of the masculine ideal. However, that body type is as unrealistic for most men as the stick-thin fashion-model figure is for most women. Meanwhile, more men are abusing steroids and overexercising to attain the desired frame. **Muscle dysmorphia,** sometimes referred to as "bigarexia," is a pathological preoccupation with being larger and more muscular.[16] Sufferers view themselves as small and weak even though they may be quite the opposite.[17] Consequences of muscle dysmorphia include excessive weight lifting and exercising as well as steroid or supplement abuse.

Internet Addiction

Have you ever opened your Web browser to quickly check something, and an hour later you were still online? With the practically unlimited access to the Internet we now have with our cell phones, BlackBerries, and laptops, it isn't surprising that surfing the Web can be addictive. An estimated 5 to 10 percent of Internet users will likely experience **Internet addiction,**[18] a blanket term that encompasses five problematic issues: cybersex addiction, cyber relationship addiction, Net compulsions, information overload, and addiction to interactive computer games.[19]

What is normal Internet use? We still don't know. Studies suggest that some college students average 8 hours or so per week, and Web surfers can average 20 hours online without having major problems. What you do online may be as important as how long you spend there. Some online activities seem to be more compelling and potentially "addictive" than others.

Men and women experience Internet addiction differently. Men are interested in information-seeking, games, and cybersex. Women, on the other hand, use the Internet more for support, friendship, and romance.

Internet addicts have multiple signs and symptoms, such as general disregard for one's health, sleep deprivation, neglecting family and friends, lack of physical activity, euphoria when online, lower grades in school, and poor job performance. Approximately 15 percent of college students report that Internet use and computer games have interfered with their academic performance.[20] Internet addicts may feel moody or uncomfortable when they are not online. Online addicts may be using their behavior to compensate for feelings of loneliness, marital or work problems, a poor social life, or financial problems. See the Assess Yourself box to analyze your own Internet use.

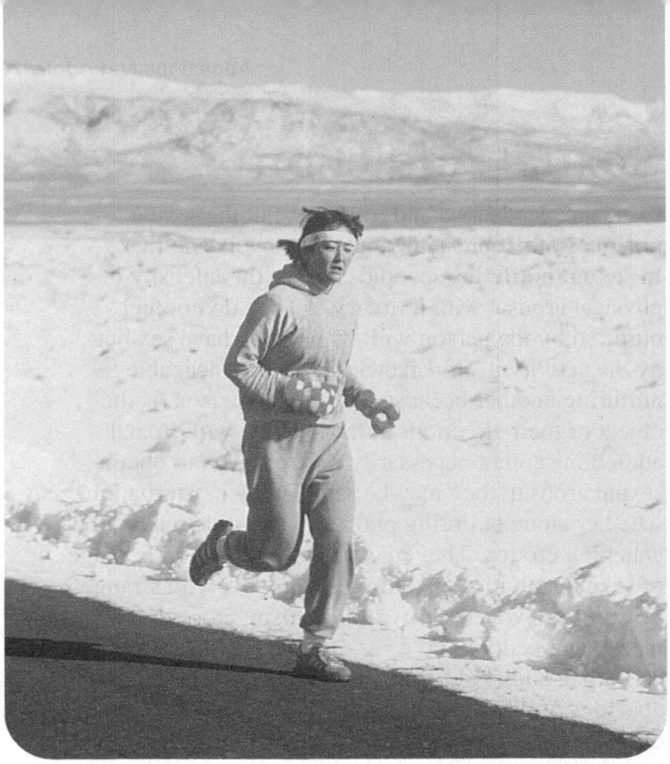

Bonnie Kamin/PhotoEdit

Obsession with a substance or behavior, even a generally positive activity such as exercise, can eventually develop into an addiction.

Is my roommate's obsessive online gaming an addiction?

work addiction The compulsive use of work and the work persona to fulfill needs for intimacy, power, and success

addictive exercisers People who exercise compulsively to try to meet needs of nurturance, intimacy, self-esteem, and self-competency

muscle dysmorphia A pathological preoccupation with being larger and more muscular, which can lead to exercise addiction

Internet addiction Compulsive use of the computer to play online video games, shop online, view websites, and participate in chat rooms

Sexual Addiction

Everyone needs love and intimacy, but the sexual practices of people addicted to sex involve neither. In **sexual addiction,** people confuse the intensity of physical arousal with intimacy.[21] They do not feel nurtured by the person with whom they have sex but by the activity itself. Likewise, they are incapable of nurturing another because sex, not the person, is the object of their affection. In fact, people with sexual addictions do not necessarily seek partners to obtain sexual arousal; they may be satisfied by masturbation, whether alone or during phone sex or while reading or watching erotica. They may participate in a wide range of sexual activities, including affairs, sex with strangers, prostitution, voyeurism, exhibitionism, cross-dressing, rape, incest, and pedophilia.

People addicted to sex frequently experience crushing episodes of depression and anxiety, fueled by the fear of discovery. Suicide is high among this group. The toll that sexual addiction exacts is most clearly seen in loss of intimacy with loved ones, which frequently leads to family disintegration.

No group of people is more or less likely than another to become involved in sexual addictions. They affect men and women of all ages, including married and single people, and people of any sexual preference. Most people with sexual addictions share a similar background: a dysfunctional childhood family, often characterized by chemical dependency or other addictions. Many were physically and emotionally abused. People addicted to sex tend to have a history of sexual abuse.

what do you think?

Do you think any behavior can be addictive? ● For example, can one be a chocolate addict or a study addict? Why or why not? ● What potential dangers lie in using the term *addiction* too loosely?

Multiple Addictions

Health professionals at addiction treatment centers often find that addicts depend on more than one chemical or behavior. Though addicts tend to have a favorite drug or behavior—one that is most effective at meeting their needs—as many as 60 percent of people in treatment have problems with more than one addiction. The figure may be as high as 75 percent for people addicted to chemicals. For example, alcohol addiction and eating disorders are commonly paired in women. Individuals trying to break a chemical dependency frequently resort to compulsive eating to keep themselves abstinent from drugs. Though multiple addictions certainly complicate recovery, they do not make it impossible. As with single addictions, recovery begins with the recognition that there is a problem.

How Addiction Affects Family and Friends

The family and friends of an addicted person also suffer many negative consequences. Often they struggle with **codependence,** a self-defeating relationship pattern in which a person is "addicted to the addict." It is the primary outcome of dysfunctional relationships or families.

Codependence is not accurately defined by isolated incidents, but rather by a pattern of behavior. Codependents find it hard to set healthy boundaries and often live in the chaotic, crisis-oriented mode that naturally occurs around addicts. They place meeting others' needs above their own, to the point that they may even cease being aware of their own needs. They may be unable to perceive their needs because they have repeatedly been taught that their needs are inappropriate or less important than someone else's.

Their behavior goes far beyond performing kind services for another person. Codependents feel less than human if they fail to respond to someone else's needs, even when their help was not requested. Although the term *codependent* is used less frequently today, treatment professionals still recognize the importance of helping addicts see how their behavior affects those around them and of working with family and friends to establish healthier relationships and boundaries.

Family and friends can play an important role in getting an addict to seek treatment. They are most helpful when they refuse to be **enablers**—people who knowingly or unknowingly pro-tect addicts from the natural consequences of their

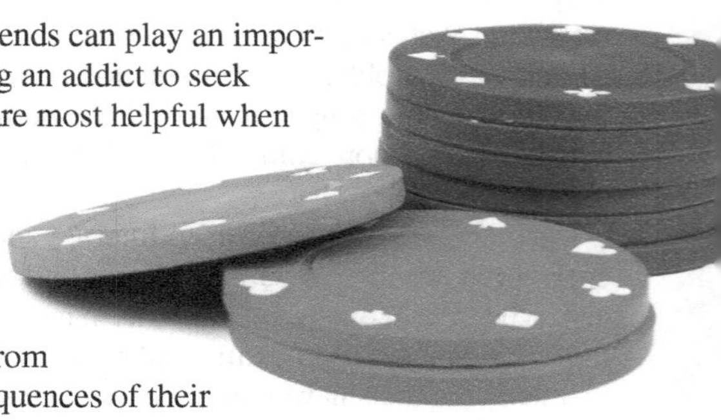

wheatley/Shutterstock

sexual addiction Compulsive involvement in sexual activity

codependence A self-defeating relationship pattern in which a person is "addicted to the addict"

enablers People who knowingly or unknowingly protect addicts from the natural consequences of their behavior

behavior. If they don't have to deal with the consequences, addicts cannot see the self-destructive nature of their behavior and will therefore continue it. Codependents are the primary enablers of their addicted loved ones, although anyone who has contact with an addict can be an enabler and thus contribute (perhaps powerfully) to the behavior's continuation. Enablers are generally unaware that their actions have this effect. In fact, enabling is rarely conscious and certainly not intentional.

what do you think?

Why do we tend to protect others from the natural consequences of their destructive behaviors? • Have you ever confronted someone you were concerned about? If so, was the confrontation successful? • What tips would you give someone who wants to confront a loved one about an addiction?

Treatment and Recovery

A key step in the recovery process is to recognize the addiction. This can be difficult because of the power of denial—the inability to see the truth. Denial is the hallmark of addiction. It can be so powerful that intervention is sometimes necessary to break down the addict's defenses against recognizing the problem.

Intervention

Intervention is a planned process of confrontation by people who are important to the addict, including spouses, parents, children, bosses, and friends. Its purpose is to break down the denial compassionately so that the person can see the addiction's destructive nature. Getting addicts to admit that they have a problem is not enough. They must come to perceive that the behavior is destructive and requires treatment.

How can I approach someone who needs help and treatment?

Individual confrontation is difficult and often futile. However, an addict's defenses generally crumble when significant others collectively share their observations and concerns about the addict's behavior. It is critical that those involved in the intervention clarify how they plan to end their enabling. For example, a wife may state that she will no longer cover bounced checks or make excuses for her compulsive gambling husband's antisocial behavior. She may even close their joint bank account and open a personal account so she will not be legally responsible for his irresponsible acts. All parties involved in the intervention must choose consequences they are ready to actually stick to if the addict refuses treatment. Significant others must also be ready to give support if the addict is willing to begin a recovery program.

Components of effective intervention include (1) emphasizing care and concern for the addicted person; (2) describing the behavior that is the cause for concern; (3) expressing how the behavior affects the addict, each person taking part in the intervention, and others; and (4) outlining specifically what you would like to see happen.

Intervention is a serious step toward assisting someone who probably does not want help. It should therefore be well planned and rehearsed. Most addiction treatment centers have specialists on staff who can help plan an intervention. In addition, books on the subject are available for families and friends who are concerned about an addict. Once the problem has been recognized, recovery can begin.

Treatment

Treatment and recovery for any addiction generally begin with **abstinence**—refraining from the addictive behavior. Whereas complete abstinence is possible for people addicted to chemicals, it obviously is not feasible for people addicted to behaviors like work and sex. For these addicts, abstinence means restoring balance to their lives through noncompulsive engagement in the behaviors, such as avoiding certain activities.

Detoxification refers to the early abstinence period during which an addict adjusts physically and cognitively to being free from the addiction's influence. It occurs in virtually every recovering addict, and, whereas it is uncomfortable for all addicts, it can be dangerous for some. This is primarily true for those addicted to chemicals, especially alcohol, heroin, and painkillers such as OxyContin. For these people, early abstinence may involve profound withdrawal symptoms that require medical supervision. Therefore, most inpatient treatment programs provide a pretreatment component of supervised detoxification to achieve abstinence safely before treatment begins.

Abstinence alone does little to change the psychological, biological, and environmental dynamics that underlie the addictive behavior. Without recovery, an addict is apt to relapse repeatedly or simply to change addictions. Recovery involves learning new ways of looking at oneself, others, and the world. It may require exploring a traumatic past so that

intervention A planned process of confronting an addict; carried out by close family, friends, and significant others

abstinence Refraining from a behavior

detoxification The early abstinence period during which an addict adjusts physically and cognitively to being free from the influences of the addiction

Women's health Men's health

ADDICTION TREATMENT FOR WOMEN: STILL CONFRONTING BARRIERS

The addiction treatment industry has traditionally been based on a male model and has only recently begun to address the unique needs of women. Studies support the need for greater prevention efforts targeted specifically at women at risk and gender-specific treatment for drug and alcohol dependence. Unfortunately, significant barriers remain for women seeking addiction treatment.

Although women entering treatment generally have fewer addiction-related legal problems (arrests for public intoxication or drug dealing, for example) than men, they face more psychological issues and family, financial, and medical problems. Studies consistently indicate that the two primary barriers women face in successfully completing treatment are child care and transportation. One study found that women who were able to bring their children to inpatient treatment were more likely to remain healthy at 6 months after treatment. Additional barriers for women seeking addiction treatment include the following factors:

Individual

- Lack of insurance or inadequate coverage
- Fear of losing child custody
- Low self-esteem
- Low feelings of self-efficacy

Family

- Too many responsibilities
- Lack of family support for treatment
- Abuse in the family environment

Community

- Lack of support from employer
- Lack of gender-sensitive treatment options

A "women-friendly" treatment center should offer the following:

- Educational programs on self-worth, assertiveness, family issues, parenting, and anger management
- Women-only groups, especially for addressing issues of rape, incest, and abuse
- Networking with and support from other women in recovery
- Housing and day care

Clearly, many women have different treatment needs than men. Finding a program that addresses these needs improves the likelihood of long-term success and recovery.

Sources: W. Weschberg, S. Craddock, and R. Hubbard, "How Are Women Who Enter Substance Abuse Treatment Different Than Men? A Gender Comparison from the Drug Abuse Treatment Outcome Study," in *Women and Substance Abuse: Gender Transparency,* eds. S. Stevens and H. Wexler (New York: Haworth, 1998); C. A. Hernandez-Avila, B. J. Rounsaville, and H. R. Kranzler, "Opioid-, Cannabis-, and Alcohol-Dependent Women Show More Rapid Progression to Substance-Abuse Treatment," *Journal of Drug and Alcohol Dependence* 74, no. 3 (2004): 265–72.

psychological wounds can be healed. It also involves learning interdependence with significant others and new ways of taking care of oneself, physically and emotionally—and it involves developing communication skills and new ways of having fun.

Finding Quality Recovery Programs Recovery programs are the fuel that gives addicts the energy to resist relapsing. For a large number of addicts, recovery begins with a period of formal treatment. A good treatment program includes the following characteristics:

- Professional staff familiar with the specific addictive disorder for which help is being sought
- A flexible schedule of both inpatient and outpatient services
- Access to medical personnel who can assess the addict's health and treat all medical concerns as needed
- Medical supervision of addicts who are at high risk for a complicated detoxification

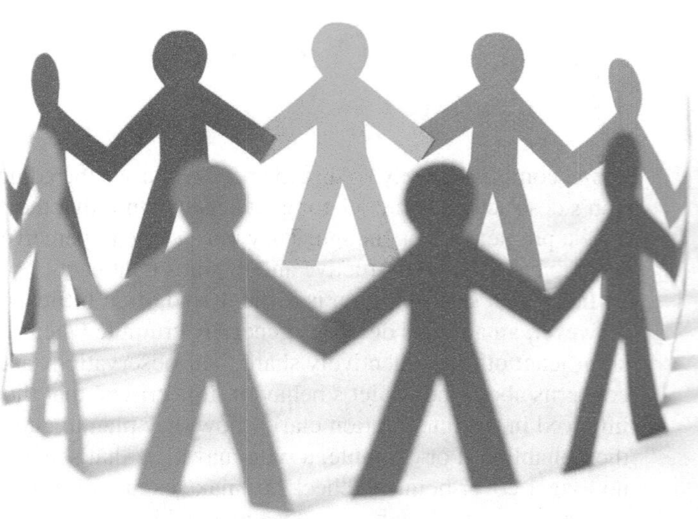

Stefanie Timmermann/iStockphoto

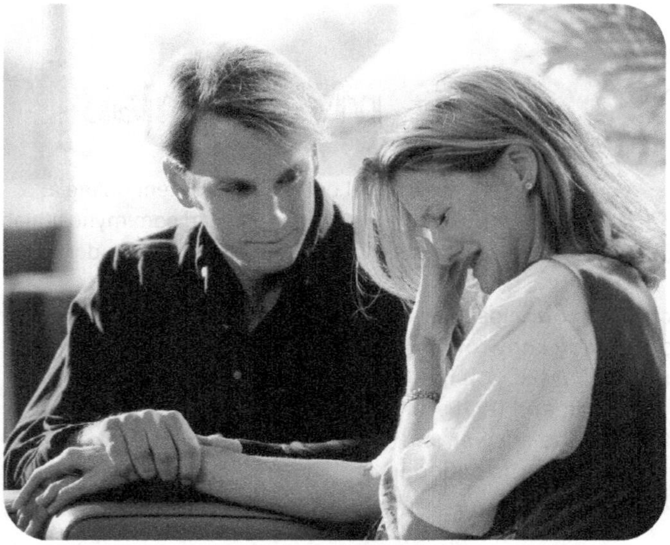

Bostick/Index Stock Imagery

The process of acknowledging and overcoming an addiction is a long and difficult journey for everyone involved.

- Involvement of family members in the treatment process
- A team approach to treating addictive disorders (for example, medical personnel, counselors, psychotherapists, social workers, clergy, educators, dietitians, and fitness counselors)
- Both group and individual therapy options
- Peer-led support groups that encourage the addict to continue involvement after treatment ends
- Structured aftercare and relapse-prevention programs
- Accreditation by the Joint Commission (a national organization that accredits and certifies health care organizations and programs) and a license from the state in which it operates

Most programs apply a combination of family, individual, and group counseling, supplemented with attendance at a 12-step support group. Individuals may also wish to explore alternatives to 12-step groups. Organizations such as Rational Recovery and the Secular Organization for Sobriety provide support without the spiritual emphasis of 12-step groups such as Alcoholics Anonymous.

Choosing a Treatment The National Institute on Alcohol Abuse and Alcoholism (NIAAA) completed Project MATCH (Matching Alcoholism Treatment to Client Heterogeneity), a large-scale study designed to determine if certain types of patients respond better to particular treatments.

The investigators studied three strategies: cognitive-behavior therapy, motivational psychology, and a facilitated 12-step program with sessions run by a therapist. Results showed that patients did equally well in each of the treatment approaches. This outcome was somewhat surprising, given that it has been common practice for treatment professionals to match patients to certain approaches. Researchers concluded that the focus, therefore, should simply be on selecting a competently run treatment program. Large-scale studies on other addictions have yet to occur.[22]

The Women's Health/Men's Health box on the previous page describes factors that are important to address when treating female addicts.

Relapse

Relapse is an isolated occurrence of or full return to addictive behavior. It is one of the defining characteristics of addiction. A person who does not relapse or have powerful urges to do so was probably not addicted in the first place. Relapse is proof that a person is addicted and has abandoned the practice of an ongoing recovery program. Addicts are set up to relapse long before they actually do so because of their tendency to meet change and other forms of stress in their lives with the same kind of denial they once used to justify their addictive behavior (for example, thinking, "I don't have a problem; I can handle this"). This sets off a series of events involving immediate or gradual abandonment of structured recovery plans. For example, the addict may quit attending support group meetings and slip into situations that previously triggered the addictive behavior.

Because treatment programs recognize this strong tendency to relapse, they routinely teach clients and significant others concepts of relapse prevention, including how to recognize the signs of imminent relapse and to develop a plan for responding to these signs. Without such a plan, recovering addicts are likely to relapse more frequently, more completely, and perhaps permanently.

Relapse should not be interpreted as failure to change or lack of desire to stay well. The appropriate response to relapse is to remind addicts that they are addicted and to redirect them to the recovery strategies that have previously worked for them.

In addition to teaching skills, relapse prevention may involve aftercare planning such as connecting the recovering person with support groups, career counselors, or community services.

? what do you think?

Why do you think addicts resist seeking treatment, even when they may admit they have a problem? • What factors need to be considered in helping addicted individuals prevent relapse?

Assess yourself

PEARSON myhealthlab

Fill out this assessment online at www.pearsonhighered.com/myhealthlab or www.pearsonhighered.com/donatelle.

ARE YOU ADDICTED?

We may not always recognize addictive behaviors in ourselves or even our closest friends. This simple exercise will help you in two ways: (1) if you already know or strongly believe you are addicted to one of the behaviors below, this guide will assist you in identifying the areas in your life most impacted by your compulsive behavior, and (2) if you're not sure whether or not you are addicted, this will help you determine the answer and assess the damage. When answering, consider only the time you spend participating in the behavior at the expense of academic, work, and social responsibilities.

PART ONE: Internet Addiction

Circle the answer that most closely describes your behavior.

	Rarely	Occasionally	Frequently	Often	Always
1. How often do you stay online longer than you intended?	1	2	3	4	5
2. How often do you neglect household chores to spend more time online?	1	2	3	4	5
3. How often do you prefer the excitement of the Internet to intimacy with your partner?	1	2	3	4	5
4. How often do you form new relationships with people you meet online?	1	2	3	4	5
5. How often do others in your life complain about the amount of time you spend online?	1	2	3	4	5
6. How often do your grades or schoolwork suffer because of the amount of time you spend online?	1	2	3	4	5
7. How often do you check your e-mail before something else that you need to do?	1	2	3	4	5
8. How often does your job performance or productivity suffer because of the Internet?	1	2	3	4	5
9. How often do you become defensive or secretive when someone asks you what you do online?	1	2	3	4	5
10. How often do you block out disturbing thoughts about your life with soothing thoughts about the Internet?	1	2	3	4	5
11. How often do you find yourself anticipating when you will go online again?	1	2	3	4	5
12. How often do you fear that life without the Internet would be boring, empty, and joyless?	1	2	3	4	5
13. How often do you snap, yell, or act annoyed if someone bothers you while you are online?	1	2	3	4	5
14. How often do you lose sleep to late-night log-ons?	1	2	3	4	5
15. How often do you feel preoccupied with the Internet when offline or fantasize about being online?	1	2	3	4	5
16. How often do you find yourself saying, "Just a few more minutes" when online?	1	2	3	4	5

	Rarely	Occasionally	Frequently	Often	Always
17. How often do you try to cut down the amount of time you spend online and fail?	1	2	3	4	5
18. How often do you try hiding how long you've been online?	1	2	3	4	5
19. How often do you choose to spend more time online rather than go out with others?	1	2	3	4	5
20. How often do you feel depressed, moody, or nervous when you are offline? Do these feelings go away once you are back online?	1	2	3	4	5

Interpreting Your Scores for This Section

After you have answered all the questions, add the numbers you selected for each response to obtain a final score. The higher your score, the greater your level of addiction and the problems your Internet usage causes.

20–49 points: You are an average Internet user. You may surf the Web a bit too long at times, but you have control over your usage.

50–79 points: You are experiencing occasional or frequent problems because of the Internet. You should consider the Internet's full impact on your life.

80–100 points: Your Internet usage is causing significant problems. You should evaluate the Internet's impact on your life and address the problems directly caused by it.

PART TWO: Compulsive Gambling

Answer Yes or No to the following questions:

	Yes	No
1. Do you ever lose time at school or work due to gambling?	❑	❑
2. Do you ever gamble to get money with which to pay debts or otherwise solve financial difficulties?	❑	❑
3. After losing, do you feel you must return to gambling as soon as possible to win back your losses?	❑	❑
4. Do you often gamble until your last dollar is gone?	❑	❑
5. Do you ever borrow to finance your gambling?	❑	❑
6. Have you ever sold anything to finance your gambling?	❑	❑
7. Do you ever gamble longer than you had planned?	❑	❑
8. Have you ever gambled to escape worry or trouble?	❑	❑
9. Has gambling ever made your life unhappy?	❑	❑
10. Has gambling ever made you careless of the welfare of yourself or your family?	❑	❑
11. Has gambling ever affected your reputation?	❑	❑
12. Do arguments, disappointments, or frustrations give you the urge to gamble?	❑	❑
13. Have you ever felt remorse after gambling?	❑	❑
14. After a win, do you have a strong urge to return and win more?	❑	❑
15. Does gambling ever cause you to have difficulty sleeping?	❑	❑
16. Do you ever have an urge to celebrate any good fortune by going gambling?	❑	❑

Continued

	Yes	No
17. Have you ever committed, or considered committing, an illegal act to finance gambling?	❑	❑
18. Have you ever felt self-destructive or suicidal as a result of gambling losses?	❑	❑
19. Has gambling ever caused a decrease in your ambition or efficiency?	❑	❑
20. Have you ever been reluctant to use "gambling money" for normal expenditures?	❑	❑

Interpreting Your Scores for This Section

If you answered Yes to any of these questions, we would encourage you to consider your potential for problem gambling.

3–7: If you answered Yes to three of these questions, you are involved in problem gambling.

8 or more: If you answered Yes to eight or more, you may be a compulsive gambler.

PART THREE: Compulsive Shopping

Answer True or False to each of the following questions:

	True	False
1. I often return items—at least one out of every four purchases.	❑	❑
2. I've lied to my spouse, friends, or colleagues about the cost of things.	❑	❑
3. I've had guilt, insomnia, fatigue, or a sense of hopelessness about my spending.	❑	❑
4. I can correlate my overspending with overeating.	❑	❑
5. My closet has over four or more unworn items with the tags still hanging from them.	❑	❑
6. I'm having trouble making ends meet.	❑	❑
7. I screen my calls so I don't have to talk to creditors.	❑	❑
8. Shopping is my antidote to feeling bored, lonely, angry, or frustrated.	❑	❑
9. When I shop, I can't return home empty-handed.	❑	❑
10. I've made false statements to creditors to get new lines of credit.	❑	❑
11. My shopping habits have interfered with my work.	❑	❑
12. My spending has caused problems in my marriage or my primary relationship.	❑	❑
13. I feel uneasy if I've not shopped for several days.	❑	❑
14. I spend over 30 percent of my income on nonmortgage debt.	❑	❑
15. I have considered illegal or questionable means to raise money to support my shopping habits.	❑	❑
16. I've had issues with eating disorders or sexual, drug, or alcohol addictions.	❑	❑
17. I repeatedly resolve not to spend, only to relapse and binge shop.	❑	❑
18. I have to drive or wear status initials (BMW, DKNY, LV).	❑	❑

Interpreting Your Scores for This Section

Total your True responses and find your corresponding score below.

1–3: You have an indicator or two that trouble could be brewing around the corner, but you know your issues and are in a strong position to keep a check on things. Keep your good habits going!

4–6: You're within shouting distance of having a problem. Make note of any marked changes in your shopping habits. Cognizance of your behavior is your most effective tool for keeping your spending in check.

7–12: You may be close to having a shopping addiction. Take a good look at the motivations driving your behavior. Know what money will buy for you, and get clear about what it won't. Consider seeking advice from a credit counselor or a therapist.

13–18: You likely have a shopping addiction, and it's time to get help. Check out www.debtorsanonymous.org. Relief is only a meeting away.

Sources: Reprinted by permission of Dr. K. S. Young, director of the Center for Online and Internet Addiction, 2004, www.netaddiction.com; Gamblers Anonymous, "Twenty Questions," 2006, www.gamblersanonymous.org; S. Durling, "Am I a Compulsive Shopper?" Copyright © 2002, www.sharondurling.com/Compulsive.htm.

Make it happen!

The Assess Yourself activity above gave you a chance to evaluate signs of Internet, gambling, and spending addictions. Depending on your results, you may need to take steps toward changing certain behaviors that could be detrimental to your health.

Today, you can:

- ❍ Identify any problem areas where you may have an addiction. Be honest with yourself about your behaviors and commit to addressing the issue. The first step in beating an addiction is admitting you have a problem.
- ❍ Write a list of the things that contribute to the behavior you feel may be addictive. Include your reasons for engaging in the behavior and the things about it that are reinforcing. Why do you want to change it? Try to identify barriers that would make it hard to break away from the behavior or bring it under control. What would help you address these barriers?

Within the next 2 weeks, you can:

- ❍ Look into support groups in your area that could possibly help you, such as Gamblers Anonymous or Alcoholics Anonymous. Visit your student health center to find out about programs that may be available on campus.
- ❍ Begin tracking your addictive behavior. Keep a log of dates, time spent engaging in the behavior, the way you are feeling, the amount of money spent (if pertinent), any other people involved, and anything else you think is relevant. Look for patterns in your log, such as particular time of day when you are most vulnerable to the addiction, a specific mood related to it, or certain people or places that trigger your compulsion.

By the end of the semester, you can:

- ❍ Take positive steps to address some of the patterns you noted in your log. Come up with a distraction to turn to when you begin feeling the addictive urge, and try to avoid settings or circumstances that trigger your addictive behavior.
- ❍ Establish new limits for your addictive behavior and strive to enforce them for several days at a time. For example, this could mean setting a time limit on Internet use. Ask a trusted friend to help you enforce these limits—for example, by making plans to play Frisbee after your allotted half hour of Internet surfing.

Taking Charge

Summary

- Addiction is the continued involvement with a substance or activity despite ongoing negative consequences.
- Habits are repeated behaviors, whereas addiction is behavior resulting from compulsion; without the behavior, the addict experiences withdrawal. All addictions share four common symptoms: compulsion, loss of control, negative consequences, and denial.
- Addiction is a process, evolving over time through a pattern known as "nurturing through avoidance." Mood-altering substances and experiences produce biochemical reactions

that make the body feel good; when absent, the person feels a withdrawal effect. The biopsychosocial model of addiction takes into account biological (genetic) factors as well as psychological and environmental influences in understanding the addiction process.

- Addictive behaviors include compulsive gambling, spending, and borrowing; work addiction; Internet addiction; exercise addiction; and sexual addiction. Codependents are typically friends or family members who are "addicted to the addict." Enablers are people who knowingly or unknowingly protect addicts from the consequences of their behavior.
- Treatment begins with abstinence from the addictive behavior or substance, usually instituted through intervention by close family, friends, or other loved ones. Treatment programs may include individual, group, or family therapy, as well as 12-step programs.

Chapter Review

1. Which of the following is not a characteristic of addiction?
   a. Denial
   b. Tolerance
   c. Loss of control
   d. Habit

2. Jason is addicted to the Internet. He is so preoccupied with surfing websites that he skips classes and misses important exams. What symptom of addiction does his preoccupation characterize?
   a. Denial
   b. Compulsion
   c. Loss of control
   d. Negative consequences

3. Which of the following is the definition of *tolerance*?
   a. The human body's rejection of a drug or chemical
   b. The need to consume more of a drug to achieve the same high that was previously achieved with a smaller amount
   c. The need to consume less of the chemical or drug
   d. A person's ability to handle a toxic amount of drugs in their body

4. Chemical dependency *relapse* refers to
   a. a person who is experiencing a blackout.
   b. a gap in one's drinking or drugging patterns.
   c. a full return to addictive behavior.
   d. the failure to change one's behavior.

5. People who excessively and compulsively exercise to meet needs of nurturance, intimacy, and self-esteem have a(n)
   a. money addiction.
   b. work addiction.
   c. shopping addiction.
   d. exercise addiction.

6. When a person repeatedly seeks the illusion of relief to avoid unpleasant feelings, this pattern is known as
   a. neurotransmitter deficiency.
   b. nurturing through avoidance.
   c. a bad habit.
   d. compulsive behavior.

7. The current theory of addiction relies on the biopsychosocial model of addiction. This model proposes that most addictive conditions were influenced by
   a. biological or disease influences.
   b. genetic influences.
   c. environmental influences.
   d. All of the above.

8. Chris was obsessed with his weight-lifting program and constantly checking to see if his 6-pack abs and lean muscles were nicely sculpted. He suffers from
   a. anorexia.
   b. muscle dysmorphia.
   c. exercise addiction.
   d. tolerance.

9. The first step in treating an addiction is to
   a. organize an intervention.
   b. recognize the addiction.
   c. enter a rehabilitation facility.
   d. do nothing.

10. An individual who knowingly tries to protect an addict from natural consequences of his or her destructive behaviors is
    a. enabling.
    b. coddling.
    c. practicing intervention.
    d. controlling.

Questions for Discussion and Reflection

1. What factors distinguish a habit from an addiction? Is it possible for you to tell whether someone else is really addicted?
2. Explain why the biopsychosocial model of addiction is a more effective model for treatment than a single-factor model.
3. Explain the potential genetic, environmental, and psychological risk factors for addiction.
4. Discuss how addiction affects family and friends. What role do family and friends play in helping the addict get help and maintain recovery?
5. What are some key components of an effective treatment program? Do the components vary for men and women? Why or why not?

Accessing Your Health on the Internet

The following websites explore further topics and issues related to personal health. You'll also find links to each organization's website on the Companion Website for *Access to Health,* Green Edition, at www.pearsonhighered.com/donatelle.

1. *Center for Online and Internet Addiction.* Information and assistance for those dealing with Internet addiction. www.netaddiction.com
2. *National Council on Problem Gambling.* Provides information and help for people with gambling problems and their families, including a searchable directory for counselors. www.ncpgambling.org
3. *Keeping the Score (University of Missouri, Columbia).* Provides pertinent information for college students regarding gambling. http://gambling.missouri.edu
4. *Society for the Advancement of Sexual Health.* Provides information, resources, and a self-quiz relating to sexual addiction. www.sash.net

Further Reading

B. Shaw, *Addiction and Recovery for Dummies* (Hoboken: Wiley Publishing Co., 2005).

This compassionate guide helps you identify the problem and work toward a healthy, realistic approach to recovery, explaining the latest clinical and self-help treatments for both adults and teens.

C. Erickson, *The Science of Addiction: From Neurobiology to Treatment* (New York: W.W. Norton & Co., 2007).

This book by a leading addictions specialist discusses the neurobiology and genetics of drug and alcohol addictions. In addition, the book presents research on the ways addicted individuals respond to various therapies.

J. Elster, ed., *Addiction: Entries and Exits* (New York: Russell Sage Foundation, 2000).

Addresses addiction controversies from an international perspective, with authors from the United States and Norway. Topics include whether addicts have a choice in their behavior and current addiction theories.

S. Cheever, *Addiction: Why Can't They Just Stop?* (New York: Rodale, 2007).

A companion to the HBO documentary of the same name, this book blends personal narratives with statistics and expert opinions to shed light on the epidemic of addiction in America. In addition to considering the impact of addiction on addicts, their loved ones, society, and the economy, the book presents recent research on the ways drugs and alcohol alter the chemical composition of the addict's brain.

S. Peele, *Seven Tools to Beat Addiction* (New York: Three Rivers Press, 2004).

A hands-on, practical guide to overcoming any type of addiction.

References

1. H. F. Doweiko, *Concepts of Chemical Dependency.* 6th ed. (Belmont, CA: Wadsworth, 2005), 11.
2. R. Goldberg, *Drugs Across the Spectrum.* 5th ed. (Belmont, CA: Brooks/Cole, 2006).
3. National Institute on Alcohol Abuse and Alcoholism, "Alcohol Alert 60: The Genetics of Alcoholism," July 2003, http://pubs.niaaa.nih.gov/publications/aa60.htm.
4. A. I. Herman et al., "Serotonin Transporter Promoter Polymorphism and Differences in Alcohol Consumption Behavior in a College Student Population," *Alcohol and Alcoholism* 38 (2003): 446–49.
5. National Institute on Alcohol Abuse and Alcoholism, "Alcohol Alert," 2003.
6. J. Kinney, *Loosening the Grip* (Boston: McGraw-Hill, 2005), 106.
7. G. Hansen and P. Venturelli, *Drugs and Society.* 7th ed. (Sudbury, MA: Jones and Bartlett, 2002), 49.
8. Ibid., 4.
9. National Council on Problem Gambling, "FAQs—Problem Gamblers," www.ncpgambling.org/i4a/pages/index.cfm?pageid=3390. Accessed April 2008.
10. C. Holden, "Gambling as Addiction," *Science* 307, no. 5708 (2005): 349, www.sciencemag.org.
11. J. W. Welte et al., "Gambling Participation and Pathology in the United States," *Addictive Behaviors* 29, no. 5 (2004): 983–89.
12. The Annenburg Public Policy Center, "Card-Playing Trend in Young People Continues," Press Release, September 28, 2005, www.annenbergpublicpolicycenter.org.
13. W. DeJong et al., "Gambling: The New Addiction Crisis in Higher Education," *Prevention Profile* (March 2006): 11–13.
14. S. Durling, "Conquer the Compulsive Shopping Blues," Women's Wall Street, June 19, 2004.
15. R. Engs, "How Can I Manage Compulsive Shopping and Spending Addiction?" www.indiana.edu/~engs/hints/shop.html. Updated December 2007.
16. J. Leone et al., "Recognition and Treatment of Muscle Dysmorphia and Related Body Image Disorders," *Journal of Athletic Training* 40, no. 4 (2005): 352–59.
17. M. Maine, *Body Wars: Making Peace with Women's Bodies* (Carlsbad, CA: Gurze, 2000), 282.
18. D. M. Wieland, "Computer Addiction: Implications for Nursing Psychotherapy Practice," *Perspectives in Psychiatric Care* 41, no. 4 (2005): 153–61.
19. Ibid.

20. American College Health Association, *American College Health Association—National College Health Assessment: Reference Group Data Report Fall 2007* (Baltimore: American College Health Association, 2008).
21. C. Nakken, *The Addictive Personality* (Center City, MN: Hazelden, 1996).
22. S. Maisto, P. Clifford, and J. S. Tonigan, "Initial and Long-Term Alcohol Treatment Success: A 10-Year Study of the Project MATCH Albuquerque Sample," *Alcoholism: Clinical and Experimental Research* 26, no. 5 (supplement), 2003.

Answers to Chapter Review Questions

1. d; 2. d; 3. b; 4. c; 5. d; 6. b; 7. d; 8. b; 9. b; 10. a

Savvy Health Care Consumerism

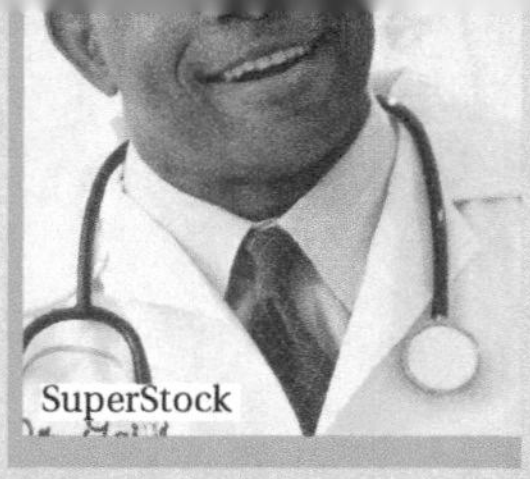
SuperStock

What questions should I ask my health care provider about proposed tests, treatments, or medications?

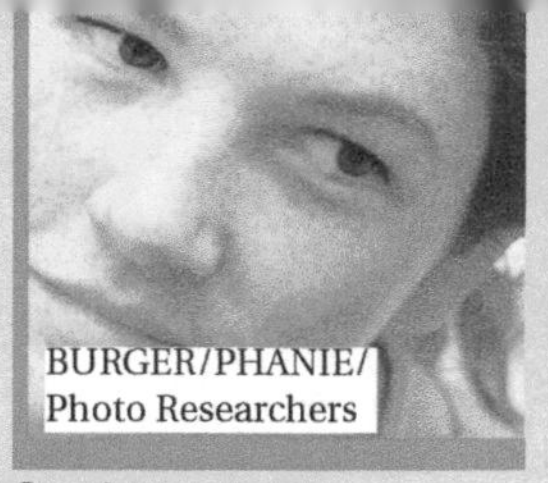
BURGER/PHANIE/ Photo Researchers

Can I count on my school's health care plan to cover my medical needs?

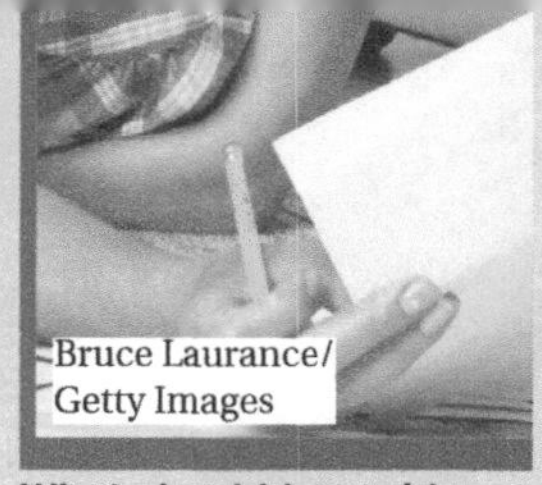
Bruce Laurance/ Getty Images

What should I consider when choosing health insurance?

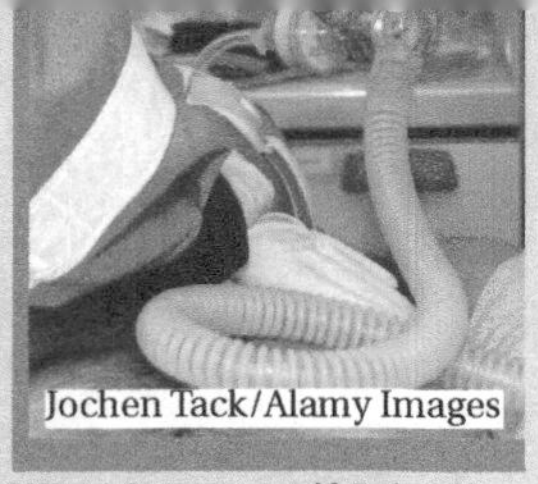
Jochen Tack/Alamy Images

What happens if I don't have insurance and I need medical care?

Savvy Health Care Consumerism

Objectives

* Explain why it is important to be a responsible health care consumer and how to encourage health care consumers to take action.
* Understand what factors to consider when making health care decisions.
* Describe the U.S. health care system in terms of types of insurance; the changing structure of the system; and issues concerning cost, quality, and access to services.
* Understand the role health insurers play in providing health care.

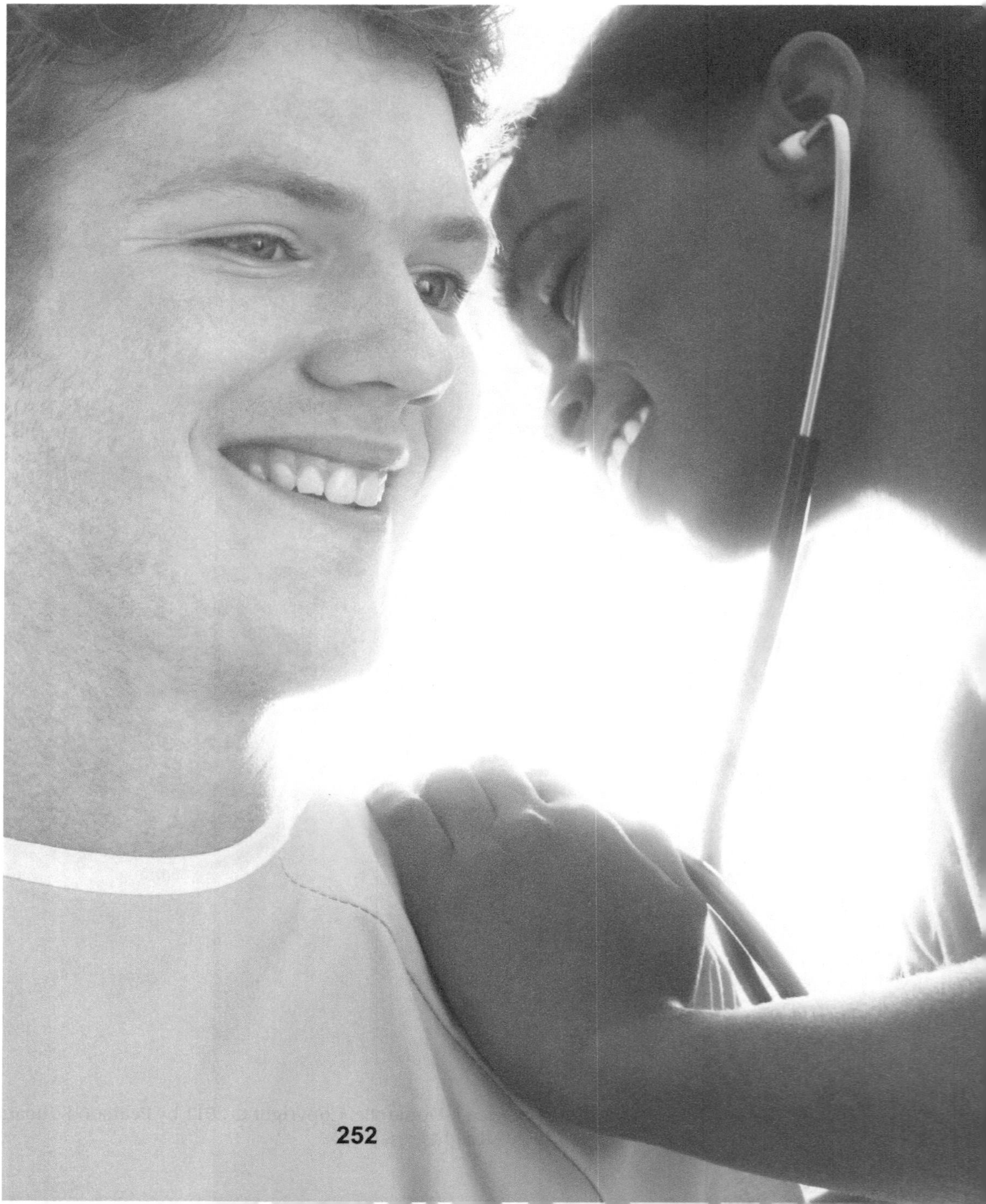
Darren Kemper/Corbis

Have there been times when you wondered whether you were sick enough to go to your campus health clinic? Have you left visits with your health care provider feeling like you had more questions than you did when you arrived? Do you engage in risky behaviors, such as skateboarding without a helmet, and don't know where or how you would be treated if you were injured? Are you one of the 20 percent of college students without health insurance? If any of these is true, you will find the information in this chapter valuable in helping you to become a better health care consumer.

There are many reasons for you to learn to make better decisions about your health and health care. Most important, you have only one body—if you don't treat it with care, you will pay a major price in terms of financial costs and health consequences. Doing everything you can to stay healthy and to recover rapidly when you do get sick will enhance every other part of your life. Throughout this text we emphasize the importance of healthy preventive behaviors. Learning how to navigate the health care system is an important part of taking charge of your health.

Taking Responsibility for Your Health Care

As the health care industry has become more sophisticated in seeking your business, so must you become more sophisticated in purchasing its products and services. Acting responsibly in times of illness can be difficult, but the person best able to act on your behalf is you.

If you are not feeling well, you must first decide whether you really need to seek medical advice. Not seeking treatment, whether because of high costs or limited coverage, or trying to medicate yourself when more rigorous methods of treatment are needed, is potentially dangerous. Being knowledgeable about the benefits and limits of self-care is critical for responsible consumerism.

Self-Help or Self-Care

Individuals can practice behaviors that promote health, prevent disease, and minimize reliance on the formal medical system. We can also treat minor afflictions without seeking professional help. Self-care consists of knowing your body, paying attention to its signals, and taking appropriate action to stop the progression of illness or injury. Common forms of self-care include the following:

- Diagnosing symptoms or conditions that occur frequently but may not require physician visits (e.g., the common cold, minor abrasions)
- Using over-the-counter remedies to treat minor infrequent pains, scrapes, or cold or allergy symptoms.
- Performing monthly breast or testicular self-examinations
- Learning first aid for common, uncomplicated injuries and conditions
- Checking blood pressure, pulse, and temperature
- Using home pregnancy tests and ovulation kits
- Using home HIV test kits
- Doing periodic checks for blood cholesterol
- Learning from reliable self-help books, websites, and DVDs
- Benefiting from meditation and other relaxation techniques and nutrition, rest, and exercise

When to Seek Help

Effective self-care also means understanding when to seek medical attention rather than treating a condition yourself. Deciding which conditions warrant professional advice is not always easy. Generally, you should consult a physician if you experience *any* of the following:

- A serious accident or injury
- Sudden or severe chest pains especially if they cause breathing difficulties
- Trauma to the head or spine accompanied by persistent headache, blurred vision, loss of consciousness, vomiting, convulsions, or paralysis
- Sudden high fever or recurring high temperature (over 102°F for children and 103°F for adults) and/or sweats
- Tingling sensation in the arm accompanied by slurred speech or impaired thought processes
- Adverse reactions to a drug or insect bite (shortness of breath, severe swelling, dizziness)
- Unexplained bleeding or loss of body fluid from any body opening
- Unexplained sudden weight loss
- Persistent or recurrent diarrhea or vomiting
- Blue-colored lips, eyelids, or nail beds
- Any lump, swelling, thickness, or sore that does not subside or that grows for over a month
- Any marked change or pain in bowel or bladder habits
- Yellowing of the skin or the whites of the eyes

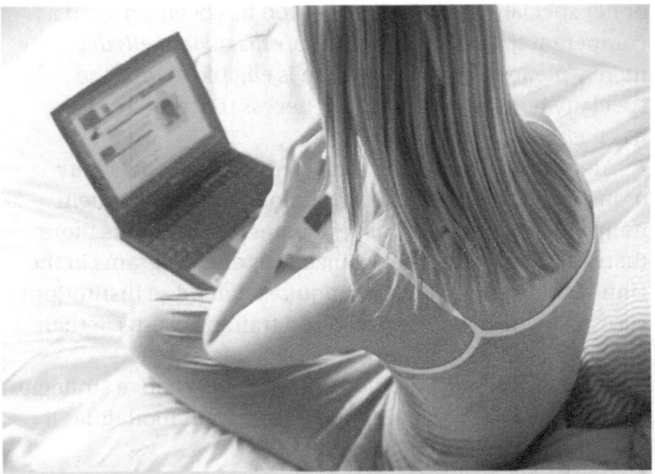

Peter Scholey/Photographer's Choice/Getty Images

Deciding when to contact a physician can be difficult. Most people first try to diagnose and treat a condition themselves.

35 million

Americans are admitted to the hospital each year.

- Any symptom that is unusual and recurs over time
- Pregnancy

With the vast array of home diagnostic devices available, it seems relatively easy for most people to take care of themselves. But some caution is in order here: Although many of these devices are valuable for making an initial diagnosis, home health tests are no substitute for regular, complete examinations by a trained practitioner. See the **Skills for Behavior Change** box at right for information on taking an active role in your own health care.

Assessing Health Professionals

Suppose you decide that you do need medical help. You must then identify what type of help you need and where to obtain it. Selecting a professional may seem simple, yet many people have no idea how to assess the qualifications of a health care provider.

Numerous studies document the importance of good communication skills: The most satisfied patients are those who feel their health care provider explains diagnosis and treatment options thoroughly and involves them in decisions regarding their own care.[1]

When evaluating a health care provider, be sure to consider the following questions:

- What professional educational training have they had? What license or board certification(s) do they hold? Note that there is a difference between "board certified" and "board eligible" physicians. *Board certified* indicates that the physician has passed the national board examination for his or her specialty (e.g., pediatrics) and has been certified as competent in that specialty. In contrast, *board eligible* merely means that the physician is eligible to take the specialty board's exam, but not necessarily that he or she has passed it.
- Are they affiliated with an accredited medical facility or institution? The Joint Commission is an independent nonprofit organization that evaluates and accredits more than 15,000 health care organizations and programs in the United States. Accreditation requires that these institutions verify all education, licensing, and training claims of their affiliated practitioners.
- Are they open to complementary or alternative strategies? Would they refer you for different treatment modalities if appropriate?
- Do they indicate clearly how long a given treatment may last, what side effects you might expect, and what problems you should watch for?

Skills for Behavior Change

Be Proactive in Your Health Care

The more you know about your body and the factors that can affect your health, the better you will be at communicating with health care providers. The following points can help:

- **Know your own and your family's medical history.**
- **Research your condition—causes, physiological effects, possible treatments, and prognosis. Don't rely on the health care provider for this information.**
- **Bring a friend or relative along for medical visits to help you review what the doctor says. If you go alone, take notes.**
- **Ask the practitioner to explain the problem and possible treatments, tests, and drugs in a clear and understandable way. If you don't understand something, ask for clarification.**
- **If the health care provider prescribes any medications, ask whether you can take generic equivalents that cost less.**
- **Ask for a written summary of the results of your visit and any lab tests.**
- **If you have any doubt about the health care provider's recommended treatment, seek a second opinion.**
- **After seeing a health care professional, write down an accurate account of what happened and what was said. Be sure to include the names of the health care provider and all other people involved in your care, the date, and the place.**
- **When filling prescriptions, ask the pharmacist to show you the package inserts that list medical considerations. Request detailed information about potential drug and food interactions.**

- Are their diagnoses, treatments, and general statements consistent with established scientific theory and practice?
- Who will be responsible for your care when your physician is on vacation or off call?
- Do they listen to you, respect you as an individual, and give you time to ask questions? Do they return your calls, and are they available to answer questions?

Asking the right questions at the right time may save you personal suffering and expense. Many patients find that writing their questions down before an appointment helps them get answers to all their questions. You should not accept a defensive or hostile response; asking questions is your right as a patient.

Active participation in your treatment is the only sensible course in a health care environment that encourages

defensive medicine. A recent study examined over 4,000 routine preventive health checkups. In 43 percent of the checkups, doctors ordered a urinalysis, an electrocardiogram, or an X ray, despite the fact that the patient showed no symptoms that would have caused the physician to ask for such tests.[2] Unnecessary drugs and procedures are not likely to improve health outcomes and in some cases may create new health problems.

In addition to asking the suggested questions above, being proactive in your health care also means that you should be aware of your rights as a patient:[3]

1. The right of informed consent means that before receiving any care, you should be fully informed of what is being planned; the risks and potential benefits; and possible alternative forms of treatment, including the option of no treatment. Your consent must be voluntary and without any form of coercion. It is critical that you read any consent forms carefully and amend them as necessary before signing.
2. You are entitled to know whether the treatment you are receiving is standard or experimental. In experimental conditions, you have the legal and ethical right to know if any drug is being used in the research project for a purpose not approved by the Food and Drug Administration (FDA), and if the study is one in which some people receive treatment while others receive a placebo. (See the **Health Today** box for more on placebos and the placebo effect.)

SuperStock

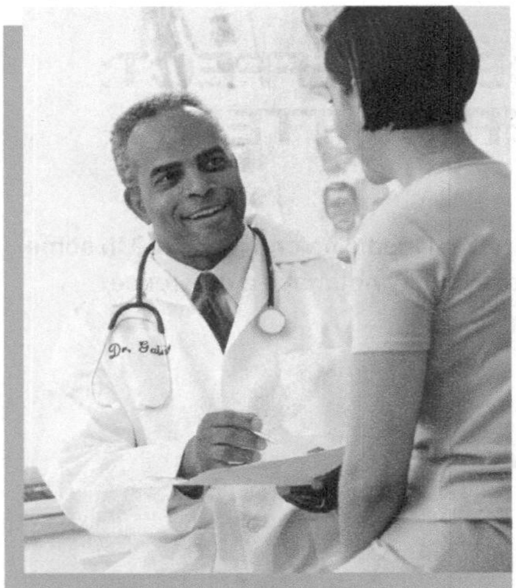

What questions should I ask my health care provider about proposed tests, treatments, or medications?

It's important to understand recommendations that your health care provider makes. Questions to ask include how often the practitioner has performed a procedure, the proportion of successful outcomes for the treatment or procedure, any side effects and whether they can be treated or reduced, whether a hospital stay will be required, and why a test has been ordered.

91% of U.S. physicians admitted that they sometimes order unnecessary medical tests because they are concerned about being sued for malpractice.

3. You have the right to privacy, which includes the source of payment for treatment and care. It also includes protecting your right to make personal decisions concerning all reproductive matters.
4. You have the right to receive care. You also have the legal right to refuse treatment at any time and to cease treatment at any time.
5. You are entitled to have access to all of your medical records and to have those records remain confidential.
6. You have the right to seek the opinions of other health care professionals regarding your condition.

Choosing Health Products

Prescription drugs can be obtained only with a written prescription from a physician, while over-the-counter drugs can be purchased without a prescription. Just as making wise decisions about providers is an important aspect of responsible health care, so is making wise decisions about medications.

Prescription Drugs

In about two-thirds of doctor visits, the physician administers or prescribes at least one medication. In fact, prescription drug use has risen by 25 percent over the past decade. Even though these drugs are administered under medical supervision, the wise consumer still takes precautions. Hazards and complications arising from the use of prescription drugs are common.

Consumers have a variety of resources available to determine the risks of various prescription medicines and can make educated decisions about whether to take a certain drug. One of the best resources is the U.S. FDA Center for Drug Evaluation and Research

defensive medicine Actions taken by a health care provider, such as ordering unnecessary tests, for the sake of avoiding potential malpractice claims rather than for the health of the patient.

Did you Know?

Forty-five percent of Americans report taking at least one prescription drug in the last month, while 18% report taking three or more.

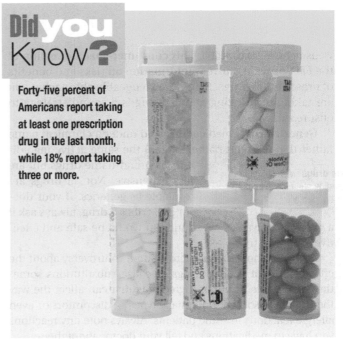

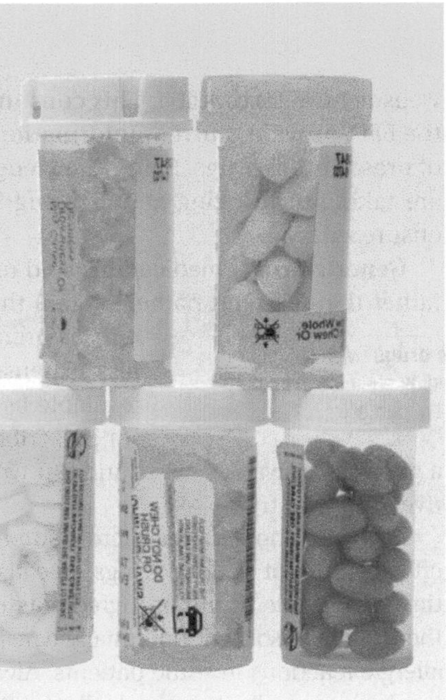

Steve Snowden/Shutterstock

HEALTH Today

THE PLACEBO EFFECT: MIND OVER MATTER?

The *placebo effect* is an apparent cure or improved state of health brought about by a substance, product, or procedure that has no generally recognized therapeutic value. Patients often report improvements in a condition based on what they expect, desire, or were told would happen after receiving a treatment, even though the treatment was, for example, simple sugar pills instead of powerful drugs.

Researchers are investigating how and why placebos work on some people. One theory is that expecting a positive outcome activates the same natural pathways in the brain as some medications do. One recent study involved patients with Parkinson's disease. The patients who thought that they were receiving the real treatment but actually received a placebo had the same changes in their brains on positron-emission tomography (PET) scans as those who received the medication. Similar chemical changes on brain imaging tests were seen with placebos in studies of pain and depression.

In another recent trial, a sample of alcohol-dependent patients received either the drugs naltrexone or acamprosate, or a placebo for a period of 12 weeks. They were also asked whether they thought they were receiving an active medication or a placebo. Those who believed they had been taking medication consumed fewer alcoholic drinks and reported less alcohol dependence and cravings, regardless of whether they really were receiving the drug.

Is it a real medicine or a placebo? In some cases, it may not make a difference.

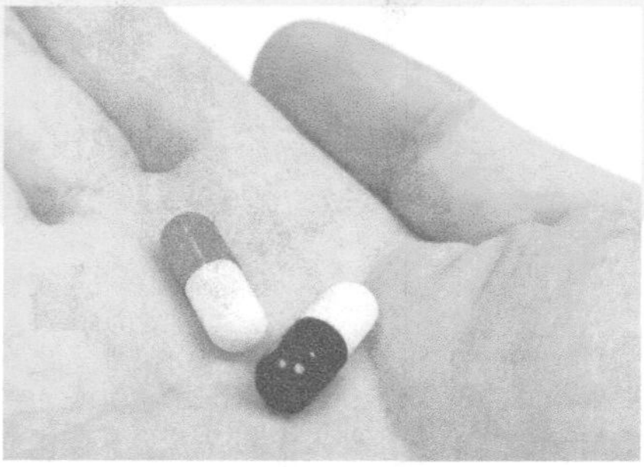

Tatiana Popova/Shutterstock

Placebos are also used in clinical research studies. Patients with a particular condition are given either the treatment that is being tested or a placebo. If the patients receiving the treatment have a more beneficial outcome than the patients receiving the placebo, then the treatment can be considered effective. The patients and the doctors running the study are not told until the study ends who had the real treatment and who had the placebo.

People who mistakenly use placebos when medical treatment is needed increase their risk for health problems. However, what we learn from the ways in which placebos work may someday help us harness the mind's power to treat certain diseases and conditions.

Sources: J. Friedman and R. Dubinsky, "The Placebo Effect," 2008, www.neurology.org/cgi/content/full/71/9/e25#R1-20; R. de la Fuente-Fernandez et al., "Expectation and Dopamine Release: Mechanism of the Placebo Effect in Parkinson's Disease," *Science* 293 (2001): 1164–66; N. Diederich and C. Goetz, "The Placebo Treatments in Neurosciences: New Insights from Clinical and Neuroimaging Studies," *Neurology* 71 (2008): 677–84; *Journal of Psychotherapy and Psychosomatics*, "Learning More about the Placebo Effect," 2009, *ScienceDaily*, www.sciencedaily.com/releases/2009/06/090622064701.htm.

website (www.fda.gov/cder). This consumer-specific section of the FDA provides current information on risks and benefits of prescription drugs. Being knowledgeable about what you are taking or thinking about taking is a sound strategy to ensure safety.

Generic drugs, medications sold under a chemical name rather than a brand name, contain the same active ingredients as brand-name drugs but are less expensive. Not all drugs are available as generics. If your doctor prescribes a drug, always ask if a generic equivalent exists and if it would be safe and effective for you to try.

generic drugs Medications marketed by chemical names rather than brand names.

Be aware, though, that there is some controversy about the effectiveness of generic drugs, because substitutions sometimes are made in minor ingredients that can affect the way the drug is absorbed, potentially causing discomfort or even allergic reactions in some patients. Always note any reactions you have to medications and tell your doctor about them.

Over-the-Counter (OTC) Drugs

Over-the-counter (OTC) drugs are nonprescription substances used in the course of self-diagnosis and self-medication. More than one-third of the time, people treat their routine health problems with OTC medications. In fact, American consumers spend billions of dollars yearly on OTC preparations for relief of everything from runny noses to ingrown toenails.

The FDA has categorized 26 types of OTC preparations. Those most commonly used are analgesics; cold, cough, allergy, and asthma relievers; stimulants; sleeping aids and relaxants; and dieting aids (Table 1).

Despite a common belief that OTC products are safe and effective, indiscriminate use and abuse can occur with these drugs as with all others. For example, people who frequently drop medication into their eyes to "get the red out" or pop

TABLE 1 **Common Over-the-Counter Drugs, Their Uses, and Potential Side Effects**

Type/Name of Drug	Use	Examples	Potential Hazards/Common Side Effects
Acetaminophen	Pain reliever, fever reducer	Tylenol	Bloody urine, painful urination, skin rash, bleeding and bruising, yellowing of the eyes or skin, difficulty in diagnosing overdose because reaction may be delayed up to a week; liver damage from chronic low-level use
Antacids	Relieve "heartburn"	Tums Maalox	Reduced mineral absorption from food; possible concealment of ulcer; reduced effectiveness of anticlotting medications; interference with the function of certain antibiotics (for antacids that contain aluminum); worsened high blood pressure (for antacids that contain sodium); aggravated kidney problems
Anticholinergics	Often added to cold preparations to reduce nasal secretions and tears	atropine scopolamine	None of the preparations tested by the FDA have been found to be Generally Recognized as Effective (GRAE) or Generally Recognized as Safe (GRAS). Some cold compounds contain alcohol in concentrations greater than 40%.
Antihistamines	Central nervous system depressants that dry runny noses, clear postnasal drip and sinus congestion, and reduce tears	Claritin Benadryl Xyzal	Drowsiness, sedation, dizziness, disturbed coordination
Aspirin	Pain reliever; reduces fever and inflammation	Bayer Bufferin	Stomach upset and vomiting; stomach bleeding; worsening of ulcers; enhancement of the action of anticlotting medications; hearing damage from loud noise; severe allergic reaction; association with Reye's syndrome in children and teenagers; prolonged bleeding when combined with alcohol
Decongestants	Reduce nasal stuffiness due to colds	Sudafed DayQuil Allermed	Nervousness, restlessness, excitability, dizziness, drowsiness, headache, nausea, weakness, and sleep problems
Diet pills, caffeine	Aid to weight loss	Dexatrim	Organ damage or death from cerebral hemorrhage; nervousness; irritability; dehydration
Expectorants	Loosen phlegm, which allows the user to cough it up and clear congested respiratory passages.	Mucinex	Safety issues may arise when combined with other medications, particularly in frail or very ill individuals. Effectiveness is sometimes in question.
Ibuprofen	Pain reliever; reduces fever and inflammation	Advil Motrin	Allergic reaction in some people with aspirin allergy; fluid retention or swelling (edema); liver damage similar to that from acetaminophen; enhancement of anticlotting medications; digestive disturbances
Laxatives	Relieve constipation	Ex-lax Citrucel	Reduced absorption of minerals from food; dehydration; dependency
Naproxen sodium	Pain reliever; reduces fever and inflammation	Aleve Naprosyn	Potential bleeding in the digestive tract; possible stomach cramps or ulcers
Sleep aids and relaxants	Help relieve occasional sleeplessness	Nytol Sleep-Eze Sominex	Drowsiness the next day; dizziness; lack of coordination; reduced mental alertness; constipation; dry mouth and throat; dependency

antacids after every meal are likely to become dependent. Many people also experience adverse side effects because they ignore the warnings on the labels or simply do not read them.

The FDA has developed a standard label that appears on most OTC products (see Figure 1 on the next page). It provides directions for use, warnings, and other useful information. Diet supplements, which are regulated as food products, have their own type of label that includes a Supplement Facts panel.

Choices in Medical Care

Most people believe that **allopathic medicine,** or traditional Western medical practice, is based on scientifically validated methods. But be aware that not all allopathic treatments have had the benefit of the extensive clinical trials and long-term studies of outcomes

allopathic medicine Conventional, Western medical practice; in theory, based on scientifically validated methods and procedures.

ACTIVE INGREDIENT
Therapeutic substance in product; amount of active ingredient per unit

USES
Symptoms or diseases the product will treat or prevent

WARNINGS
When not to use the product; conditions that may require advice from a doctor before taking the product; possible interactions or side effects; when to stop taking the product and when to contact a doctor; if you are pregnant or breast-feeding, seek guidance from a health care professional; keep product out of children's reach

PURPOSE
Product action or category (such as an antihistamine, antacid, or cough suppressant)

DIRECTIONS
Specific age categories, how much to take, how to take, and how often and how long to take

OTHER INFORMATION
How to store the product properly and required information about certain ingredients (such as the amount of calcium, potassium, or sodium the product contains)

INACTIVE INGREDIENTS
Substances such as color or flavors

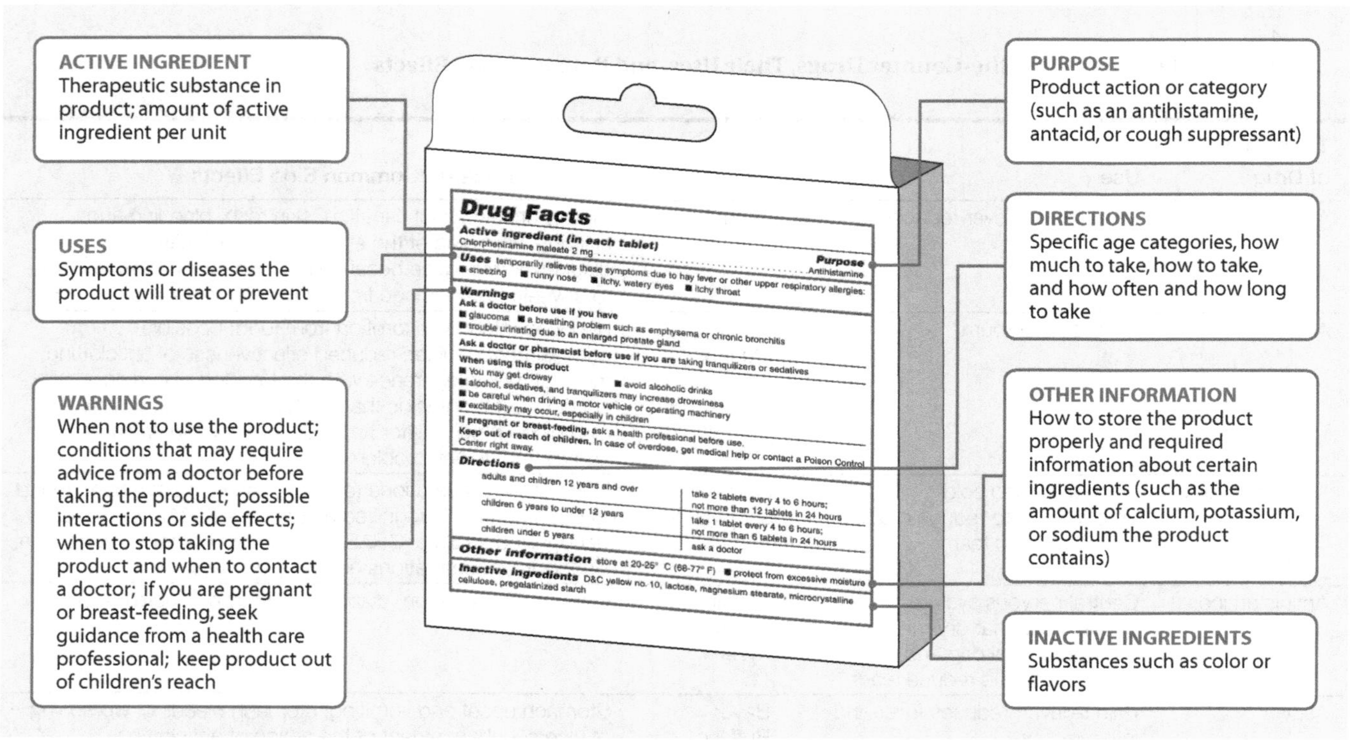

FIGURE 1 **The Over-the-Counter Medicine Label**

Source: Adapted from Consumer Healthcare Products Association, "Check the OTC Label," 2009, www.otcsafety.org/publications.

that would be necessary to conclusively prove effectiveness in different populations. Even when studies appear to support the health benefits of a particular treatment or product, other studies with equal or better scientific validity often refute these claims. Also, today's recommended treatment may change dramatically in the future as new technologies and medical advances replace older practices. Like other professionals, medical doctors are only as good as their training, continued acquisition of knowledge, and resources allow them to be.

Selecting a **primary care practitioner (PCP)**—a medical practitioner whom you can visit for routine ailments, preventive care, general medical advice, and appropriate referrals—is not an easy task. The PCP for most people is a family practitioner, an internist, a pediatrician, or an obstetrician/gynecologist (OB/Gyn). Many people routinely see nurse practitioners or physician assistants who work for an individual doctor or a medical group, and others use nontraditional providers as their primary source of care. As a college student, you may opt to visit a PCP at your campus health center. The reputation of health care providers on college campuses is

excellent. In national surveys, students have indicated that the health center medical staff is their most trusted source of health information.[4]

Doctors undergo rigorous training before they can begin practicing. After 4 years of undergraduate work, students typically spend 4 years studying for their medical degree (MD). After this general training, some students choose a specialty, such as pediatrics, cardiology, cancer, radiology, or surgery, and spend 1 year in an internship and several years doing a residency. Some specialties also require a fellowship; in all, the time spent in additional training after receiving an MD can be up to 8 years.

Other specialists include **osteopaths,** general practitioners who receive training similar to that of a medical doctor but who place special emphasis on the skeletal and muscular systems. Their treatments may involve manipulation of the muscles and joints. Osteopaths receive the degree of doctor of osteopathy (DO) rather than MD.

Eye care specialists can be either ophthalmologists or optometrists. An **ophthalmologist** holds a medical degree and can perform surgery and prescribe medications. An **optometrist** typically evaluates visual problems and fits glasses but is not a trained physician. If you have an eye infection, glaucoma, or other eye condition needing diagnosis and treatment, you need to see an ophthalmologist.

Dentists are specialists who diagnose and treat diseases of the teeth, gums, and oral cavity. They attend dental school for 4 years and receive the title of doctor of dental surgery (DDS) or doctor of medical dentistry (DMD). They must also pass

primary care practitioner (PCP) A medical practitioner who treats routine ailments, advises on preventive care, gives general medical advice, and makes appropriate referrals when necessary.

osteopath General practitioner who receives training similar to a medical doctor's but with an emphasis on the skeletal and muscular systems; often uses spinal manipulation as part of treatment.

ophthalmologist Physician who specializes in the medical and surgical care of the eyes, including prescriptions for glasses.

optometrist Eye specialist whose practice is limited to prescribing and fitting lenses.

dentist Specialist who diagnoses and treats diseases of the teeth, gums, and oral cavity.

both state and national board examinations before receiving their licenses to practice. The field of dentistry includes many specialties. For example, *orthodontists* specialize in the alignment of teeth. *Oral surgeons* perform surgical procedures to correct problems of the mouth, face, and jaw.

Nurses are highly trained and strictly regulated health professionals who provide a wide range of services for patients and their families, including patient education, counseling, community health and disease prevention information, and administration of medications. They may choose from several training options. There are over 2.4 million licensed registered nurses (RNs) in the United States who have completed either a 4-year program leading to a bachelor of science in nursing (BSN) degree or a 2-year associate degree program. More than half a million lower-level licensed practical or vocational nurses (LPN or LVN) have completed a 1- to 2-year training program, which may be based in either a community college or a hospital.

Nurse practitioners (NPs) are nurses with advanced training obtained through either a master's degree program or a specialized nurse practitioner program. Nurse practitioners have the training and authority to conduct diagnostic tests and prescribe medications (in some states). They work in a variety of settings, particularly in HMOs (health maintenance organizations), clinics, and student health centers. Nurses and nurse practitioners may also earn the clinical doctor of nursing degree (ND), doctor of nursing science (DNS and DNSc degrees), or a research-based PhD in nursing.

More than 68,000 **physician assistants (PAs)** currently practice in the United States. Physician assistants are licensed to examine and diagnose patients, offer treatment, and write prescriptions under a physician's supervision. An important difference between a PA and an NP is that the PA must practice under a physician's supervision. Like other health care providers, PAs are licensed by state boards of medicine.

Health Insurance

Whether you're visiting your regular doctor, consulting a specialist, or preparing for a hospital stay, chances are that you'll be using some form of health insurance to pay for your care. Insurance typically allows you, the consumer, to pay into a pool of funds and then bill the insurance carrier for health care charges you incur. The fundamental principle of insurance underwriting is that the cost of health care can be predicted for large populations. This is how health care premiums (payments) are determined. Policyholders pay premiums into a pool, which is held in reserve until needed. When you are sick or injured, the insurance company pays out of the pool, regardless of your total amount of contribution. Depending on circumstances, you may never pay for what your medical care costs, or you may pay much more for insurance than your medical bills ever total. The idea is that you pay affordable premiums so that you never have to face catastrophic bills. In today's profit-oriented system, insurers prefer to have healthy people in their plans who pour money into risk pools without taking money out.

Unfortunately, not everyone has health insurance. Over 46 million Americans are uninsured—that is, they have no private health insurance and are not eligible for Medicare, Medicaid, or other government health programs.[5] Lack of health insurance has been associated with delayed health care and increased mortality. *Underinsurance* (i.e., the inability to pay out-of-pocket expenses despite having insurance) also may result in adverse health consequences. Another 25 million Americans between the ages of 19 and 64 are estimated to be underinsured (at risk for spending more than 10% of their income on medical care because their insurance is inadequate).[6]

nurse Health professional who provides many services for patients and who may work in a variety of settings.

nurse practitioner (NP) Professional nurse with advanced training obtained through either a master's degree program or a specialized nurse practitioner program.

physician assistant (PA) A midlevel practitioner trained to handle most standard cases of care under the supervision of a physician.

Contrary to the common belief that the uninsured are unemployed, 75 percent of them are either workers or the dependents of workers. One-quarter of all the uninsured are children under age 16. Among young adults 18 to 24 years of age, 30 percent reported being uninsured at some point in time. This age group is more than twice as likely to be uninsured as are people 45 to 64 years of age. However, for young adults who are college students, the statistics are different. According to a recent survey, approximately 8 percent of college students report not having health insurance, and another 5 percent are unsure whether they have health insurance.[7]

For the uninsured and many of the underinsured, health care from any source may be too expensive to be obtainable. People without health care coverage are less likely than other

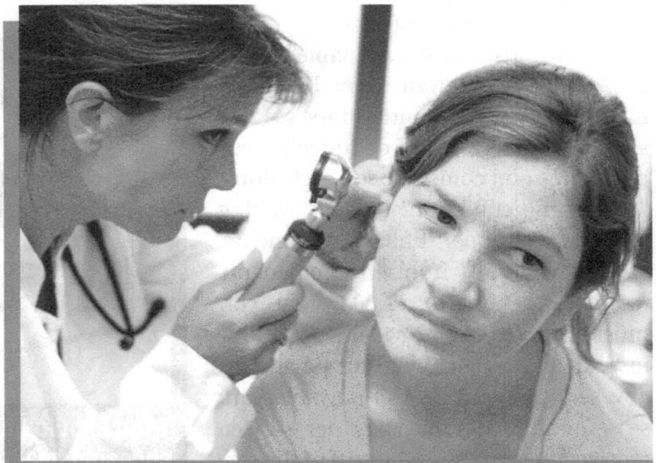

BURGER/PHANIE/Photo Researchers

Can I count on my school's health care plan to cover my medical needs?

If you are enrolled in your parents' health insurance plan, coverage will end at age 23 or if you are not enrolled in school full time. Most university insurance plans are short term and noncatastrophic and have low upper limits of benefits, all of which are problematic in the event of an emergency illness or accident. If you are covered only under your school's health care plan, you should consider buying a higher level catastrophic plan in case of costly illness or accident.

Americans to have their children immunized, seek early prenatal care, obtain annual blood pressure checks, and seek attention for serious symptoms. Experts believe that this ultimately leads to higher system costs, because their conditions deteriorate to a more debilitating and costly stage before they are forced to seek help.

Private Health Insurance

Originally, health insurance consisted solely of coverage for hospital costs (it was called *major medical*), but gradually it was extended to cover routine physicians' treatment and other areas, such as dental services and pharmaceuticals. These payment mechanisms laid the groundwork for today's steadily rising health care costs. Hospitals were reimbursed for the costs of providing care plus an amount for profit. This system provided no incentive to contain costs, limit the number of procedures, or curtail capital investment in redundant equipment and facilities. Physicians were reimbursed on a fee-for-service (indemnity) basis determined by "usual, customary, and reasonable" fees. This system encouraged physicians to charge high fees, raise them often, and perform as many procedures as possible. At the same time, because most insurance did not cover routine or preventive services, consumers were encouraged to use hospitals whenever possible (the coverage was better) and to wait until illness developed to seek care instead of seeking preventive care. Consumers were also free to choose any provider or service they wished, including even inappropriate—and often very expensive—levels of care.

managed care Cost-control procedures used by health insurers to coordinate treatment.
capitation Prepayment of a fixed monthly amount for each patient without regard to the type or number of services provided.

Private insurance companies have increasingly employed several mechanisms to limit potential losses: cost sharing (in the form of deductibles, co-payments, and coinsurance), exclusions, "preexisting condition" clauses, waiting periods, and upper limits on payments. *Deductibles* are front-end payments (commonly $250 to $1,000) that you must make to your provider before your insurance company will start paying for any services you use. *Co-payments* are set amounts that you pay per service received, regardless of the cost of the service (e.g., $20 per doctor visit or per prescription). *Coinsurance* is the percentage of the bill that you must pay throughout the course of treatment (e.g., 20% of the total bill). *Preexisting condition clauses* limit the insurance company's liability for medical conditions that a consumer had before obtaining coverage (i.e., if a woman takes out coverage while she is pregnant, the insurance company may cover pregnancy complications and infant care but may not cover charges related to "normal pregnancy"). Because many insurance companies use a combination of these mechanisms, keeping track of the costs you are responsible for can become very difficult.

Group plans of large employers (e.g., government agencies, school districts, and corporations) generally do not have preexisting condition clauses in their plans, but smaller group plans (a group may be as small as two people) often do. Some plans never cover preexisting conditions, whereas others specify a *waiting period* (e.g., 6 months) before they will provide coverage. All insurers set some limits on the types of services they cover (e.g., most exclude cosmetic surgery, private rooms, and experimental procedures). Some insurance plans may also include an *upper* or *lifetime limit,* after which coverage will end. Although $250,000 may seem like an enormous sum, medical bills for a sick child or chronic disease can easily run this high within a few years.

what do you think?

Why is it important that private insurance cover preventive or lower-level care as well as hospitalization and high-technology interventions?
● What kinds of incentives would cause you to seek care early rather than delay care?

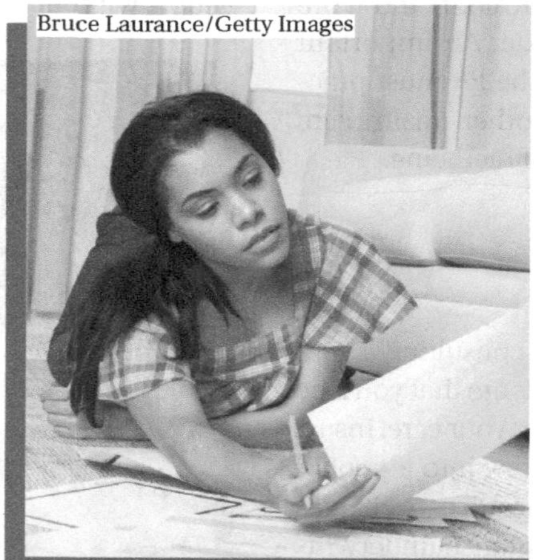

Bruce Laurance/Getty Images

What should I consider when choosing health insurance?

Choosing a health insurance plan can be confusing. Some things to think about include how comprehensive your coverage needs to be, how convenient your care must be, how much you are willing to spend on premiums and co-payments, what the overall cost will be, and whether the services of the plan meet your needs.

Managed Care

Managed care describes a health care delivery system consisting of the following elements:

1. A network of physicians, hospitals, and other providers and facilities linked contractually to deliver comprehensive health benefits within a predetermined budget, sharing economic risk for any budget deficit or surplus
2. A budget based on an estimate of the annual cost of delivering health care for a given population
3. An established set of administrative rules requiring patients to follow the advice of participating health care providers in order to have their health care paid for under the terms of the health plan

Types of managed care plans include health maintenance organizations (HMOs), preferred provider organizations (PPOs), and point of service (POS). Approximately 64 million Americans are enrolled in HMOs, the most common type.[8]

Many managed care plans pay their contracted health care providers through **capitation,** that is, prepayment of a fixed monthly amount for each patient without regard for the type or number of health services provided. Some plans pay health care providers a salary, and some are still fee-for-service plans. As with other insurance plans, enrollees are members of a risk pool, and it is expected that some persons will use no services, some will use a modest amount, and others will have high-cost usage over a given year. Doctors have the incentive to keep their patient pool healthy and avoid catastrophic ailments that are preventable; usually such incentives come back in terms of increased salaries, bonuses, and other benefits. As such, prevention and health education to reduce risk and intervene early to avoid major problems are often capstone components of such plans.

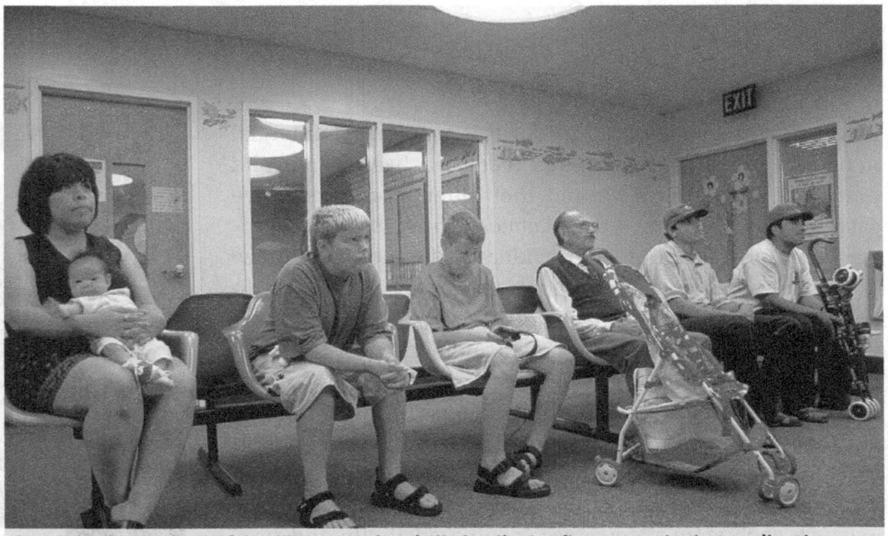

One downside to the HMO health care system is that patients often encounter long waits when they need to see their health care provider.

Spencer Grant/PhotoEdit

Managed care plans have grown steadily over the past decade with a proportionate decline of enrollment in traditional indemnity insurance plans. The reason for this shift is that indemnity insurance, which pays providers and hospitals on a fee-for-service basis with no built-in incentives to control costs, has become unaffordable or unavailable for most Americans.

Health Maintenance Organization Health maintenance organizations (HMOs) provide a wide range of covered health benefits (e.g., checkups, surgery, doctor visits, lab tests) for a fixed amount prepaid by the patient, the employer, Medicaid, or Medicare (discussed later). Usually, HMO premiums are the least expensive form of managed care (saving between 10 and 40 percent more than other plans) but also are the most restrictive (offering little or no choice in doctors and certain services). These premiums are 8 to 10 percent lower than for traditional plans, there are low or no deductibles or coinsurance payments, and co-payments are approximately $20 per office visit.

The downside of HMOs is that patients are typically required to use the plan's doctors and hospitals and to get approval from a "gatekeeper" or PCP for treatment and referrals. As more and more people enroll in HMOs, criticisms about them are mounting. Concerns about HMOs include questions about care allocation, profit-motivated medical decision making, and the degree of focus on prevention and intervention.

Preferred Provider Organization Preferred provider organizations (PPOs) are networks of independent doctors and hospitals that contract to provide care at discounted rates. Although they offer greater choices in doctors than HMOs do, they are less likely to coordinate a patient's care. Members do have a choice of seeing doctors who are not on the preferred list, but this choice may come at considerable cost (e.g., having to pay 30% of the charges out of pocket, rather than 10 to 20% for PPO doctors and services).

Point of Service Point of service (POS)—a hybrid of the HMO and PPO types—provides a more acceptable form of managed care for people used to the traditional indemnity plan of insurance, which probably explains why it is among the fastest growing of the managed care plans. Under POS plans, patients can go to providers outside their HMO for care but must pay for the extra cost.

Medicare and Medicaid

Medicare is a federal insurance program that covers a broad range of services except long-term care. Medicare covers 99 percent of individuals over age 65, all totally and permanently disabled people (after a waiting period), and all people with end-stage kidney failure—currently over 45 million people, or one in seven Americans, in all.[9] By 2030, it is estimated that one in five—or 77 million—Americans will be insured by Medicare. As the costs of medical care have continued to increase, Medicare has placed limits on the amount of reimbursement to providers. As a result, some physicians and managed care programs have stopped accepting Medicare patients.

To control hospital costs, in 1983 the federal government set up a prospective payment system based on **diagnosis-related groups (DRGs)** for Medicare. Using a complicated formula, nearly 500 groupings of diagnoses were created to establish how much a hospital would be reimbursed for a particular patient. If a hospital can treat the patient for less than that amount, it can keep the difference. However, if a patient's care costs more than the set amount, the hospital must absorb the difference (with a few exceptions that must be reviewed by a panel). This system gives hospitals the incentive to discharge patients quickly after doing as little as possible for them, to provide more ambulatory care, and to admit only patients with favorable (profitable) DRGs. Many private health insurance companies have followed the federal government in adopting this type of reimbursement. In 1998, the federal Health Care Financing Administration (HCFA) expanded the prospective payment system to include payments for outpatient surgery and skilled nursing care.

diagnosis-related groups (DRGs) Diagnostic categories established by the federal government to determine in advance how much hospitals will be reimbursed for the care of a particular Medicare patient.

In its continuing effort to control rising costs, the HCFA has encouraged the growth of prepaid HMO senior plans for

Medicare-eligible persons. Under this system, commercial managed care insurance plans receive a fixed per capita premium from the HCFA and then offer more preventive services with lower out-of-pocket co-payments. These managed care plans encourage providers and patients to utilize health care resources under administrative rules similar to commercial HMO plans.

In contrast to Medicare, Medicaid, covering approximately 46 million people, is a federal–state matching funds welfare program for people who are defined as poor, including many who are blind, disabled, elderly, or receiving Aid to Families with Dependent Children. Medicaid relies on matching funds provided by federal and state sources.[10] Because each state determines income eligibility and payments to providers, there are vast differences in the way Medicaid operates from state to state.

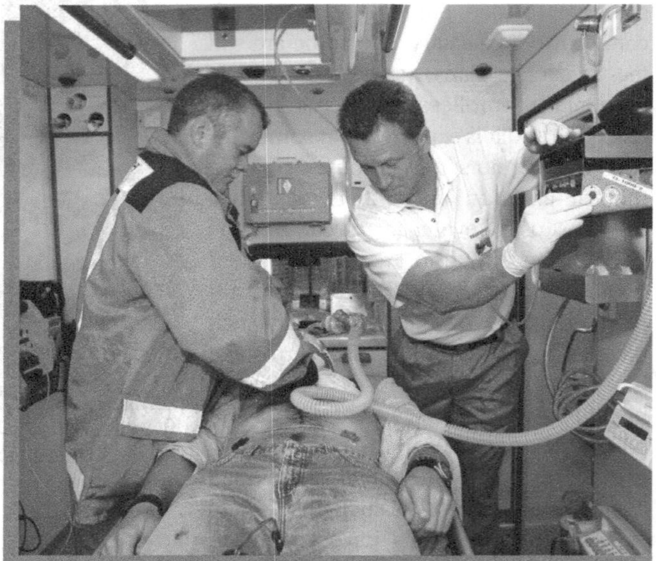

Jochen Tack/Alamy Images

What happens if I don't have insurance and I need medical care?

People without insurance can't gain access to preventive care, so they seek care only in an emergency or crisis. Because emergency care is extraordinarily expensive, they often are unable to pay, and the cost is absorbed by those who can pay—the insured or taxpayers. Using the emergency room for anything other than a real crisis contributes to higher health care costs and diminished access to emergency care for everyone. If you need nonemergency health care, there are often community-based resources, such as free or low-cost clinics, that can provide preventive care.

Issues Facing Today's Health Care System

Many Americans believe that our health care system needs fundamental reform. In recent years, the number of individuals who are underinsured has risen dramatically, and, without reform, the rise will likely continue. Individuals with preexisting conditions, and those who are self-employed are just two groups who often find themselves unable to find or afford health care. The significant costs of a major procedure, course of treatment, or hospital stay mean many families are one catastrophic illness or accident away from financial ruin. In addition to cost and access, malpractice, restricted choices in providers and treatments, unnecessary procedures, complicated and cumbersome insurance rules, and dramatic ranges in quality are also issues of concern. See the **Green Guide** on the next page for a discussion of another concern about the health care system: the amount of waste it produces and its impact on the environment.

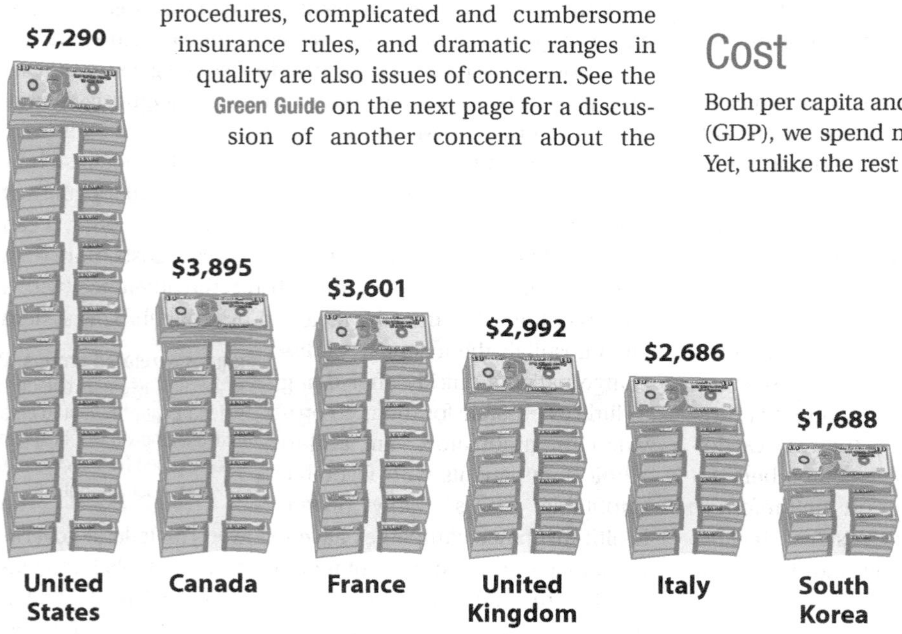

FIGURE 2 **Health Care Spending per Person, 2007 (in thousands of U.S. dollars)**

Source: Data are from Organisation for Economic Co-operation and Development, *OECD Health Data 2009*, 2009, www.oecd.org/health.

Cost

Both per capita and as a percentage of gross domestic product (GDP), we spend more on health care than any other nation. Yet, unlike the rest of the industrialized world, we do not provide access for our entire population. Already, we spend over $2 trillion annually on health care, over $7,200 for every man, woman, and child (Figure 2). This translates into 16.3 percent of our GDP. Does this sound like a lot? Consider that health care expenditures are projected to grow by 6.2 percent each year, reaching over $4 trillion annually by 2018—nearly 20 percent of our projected GDP.[11]

Why do health care costs continue to skyrocket? Many factors are involved: excess administrative costs; duplication of services; an aging population; growing rates of obesity, inactivity, and related health problems; demand for new diagnostic and treatment technologies; an emphasis on crisis-oriented care instead

GREEN GUIDE

The Perils of Medical Waste

The health care system in the United States is massive, and it affects many aspects of our daily lives, including our environment. Medical and pharmaceutical waste have been shown to have negative environmental impacts on air and water resources, as well as on human and animal health.

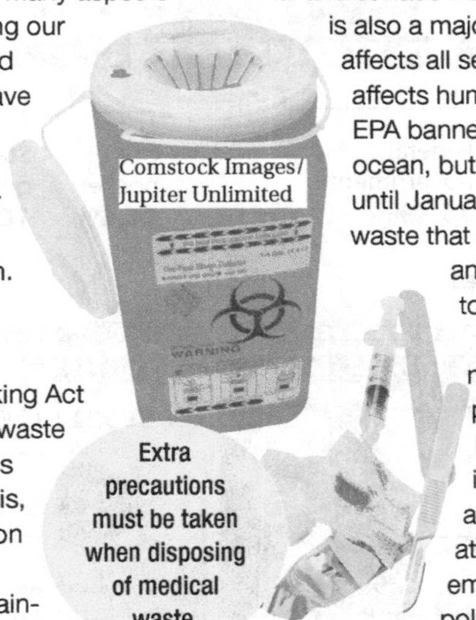

Comstock Images/ Jupiter Unlimited

Extra precautions must be taken when disposing of medical waste.

MEDICAL WASTE

The Medical Waste Tracking Act of 1988 defines medical waste as "any solid waste that is generated in the diagnosis, treatment, or immunization of human beings or animals, in research pertaining thereto, or in the production or testing of biologicals." This definition includes, but is not limited to, blood-soaked bandages; culture dishes and other glassware; discarded surgical gloves; discarded surgical instruments; discarded needles used to give shots or draw blood (e.g., medical sharps); cultures, stocks, or swabs used to inoculate cultures; removed body organs (e.g., tonsils, appendices, limbs); and discarded lancets.

Due to concern about the spread of infectious diseases, especially in hospital and clinic settings, there is a vital need for sterility. This leads to excessive one-time-use items such as latex gloves, needles, bandages, and much more. All these items contribute substantially to the amount of medical waste.

Some estimate that the volume of hospital-generated medical waste is as much as 2 million tons each year. Approximately 10 percent of potentially infectious medical waste is combined with medical waste that is not deemed infectious and then disposed of in landfills. As water percolates through solid-waste disposal sites such as landfills, it collects contaminants and forms a substance called *leachate*. This can contaminate groundwater and surface water. Pollution in the ocean is also a major problem, as it directly affects all sea life and indirectly affects human health. In 1988, the EPA banned dumping waste into the ocean, but the ban wasn't enforced until January 1992. Most of the waste that was dumped in the 1980s and early 1990s is still there today.

Currently, the vast majority—over 90 percent—of potentially infectious medical waste in the United States and around the world is incinerated, resulting in carbon emissions and other pollution such as particulate matter. Alternatives to incineration of medical waste include thermal treatment, such as microwave technologies; steam sterilization, such as autoclaving; and chemical mechanical systems that break down organic and inorganic wastes without polluting.

PHARMACEUTICAL WASTE

In addition to medical waste, hospitals generate a substantial amount of pharmaceutical waste—both hazardous and nonhazardous—that requires proper disposal. Generally, this waste comprises drugs that have been dispensed but not completely used. There is also a large amount of individual-generated pharmaceutical waste. Studies have shown that nearly 54 percent of consumers put unwanted medications in the trash, and 35 percent flush them down the toilet.

Prescription drug waste can contaminate our water supply through a number of avenues. First, medicines disposed of down the toilet or drain can easily be incorporated into groundwater, lakes, rivers, and streams. This may harm fish and wildlife that live in lakes, rivers, and the ocean. In addition, these drugs can end up back in our drinking water supply. This leads to elevated levels of chemicals that many water treatment facilities are not equipped to filter. Pharmaceutical drugs have been detected in the drinking water supplies of major metropolitan areas all across the United States. To date, the federal government has not set limits on the amount of pharmaceutical drugs in drinking water and doesn't require any testing for their presence.

Prescription drugs that are thrown away rather than flushed add to our growing landfills and can contribute to the toxicity of leachate. However, many sources still encourage throwing away unused prescription drugs, as it is a better method of disposal than flushing or dumping down the drain. Alternatively, here are some more green ways to manage unused medications:

* Send your medicine to those in need. Some organizations collect unused, unexpired medicine to send to other countries where prescription drugs are harder to access. Recently, nine states (Florida, Nebraska, Nevada, New Jersey, Oklahoma, Texas, Wisconsin, Indiana, and South Dakota) have passed legislation for recycling unused medications in nursing homes with nine more considering similar practices. Nonprofits, like the Iowa Prescription Drug Corporation (www.iowapdc.org), have developed and administered statewide drug-donation programs.
* Take your drugs back to the pharmacy. Many community pharmacies are starting take-back programs for unused or unneeded prescriptions. The pharmacy then disposes of these drugs safely. In some cases, pharmacies return unused pharmaceuticals to manufacturers for processing; in other cases, unused prescription medications are destroyed safely. It is still recommended to throw away (instead of flush) nonprescription drugs such as aspirin or ibuprofen.

of prevention; and inappropriate use of services by consumers.

Our system has more than 2,000 health insurance companies, each with different coverage structures and administrative requirements. This lack of uniformity prevents our system from achieving the *economies of scale* (bulk purchasing at a reduced cost) and administrative efficiency realized in countries where there is a single-payer delivery system. According to the Health Insurance Association of America, commercial insurance companies commonly experience administrative costs greater than 10 percent of the total health care insurance premium, whereas the administrative cost of the government's Medicare program is less than 4 percent. These administrative expenses contribute to the high cost of health care and force companies to require employees to share more of the costs, cut back on benefits, and drop some benefits altogether. These costs are largely passed on to consumers in the form of higher prices for goods and services. See Figure 3 for a breakdown of how health care dollars are spent.

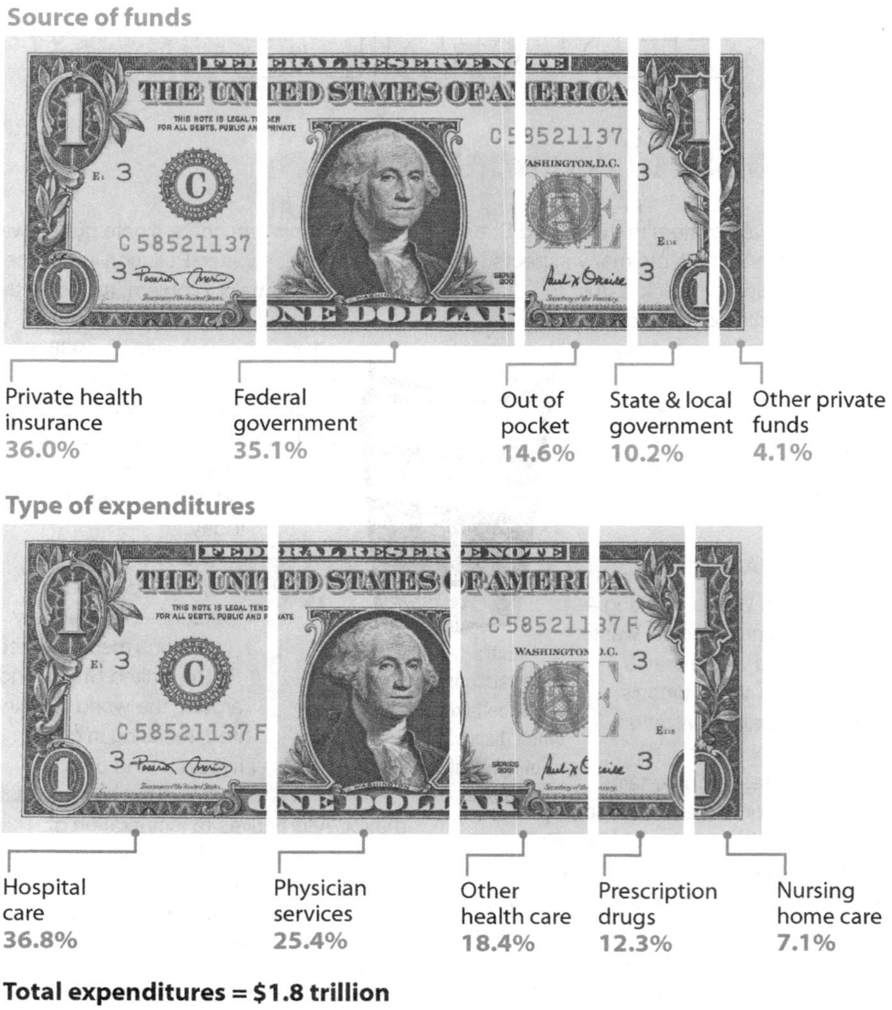

FIGURE 3 **Where Do We Spend Our Health Care Dollars?**

Source: Data are from National Center for Health Statistics, *Health, United States, 2008, with Chartbook on Trends in the Health of Americans* (Hyattsville, MD: National Center for Health Statistics, 2009).

Access

Over 90 million people in the United States suffer from chronic health conditions that should be at least monitored by medical practitioners.[12] Their access to care is largely determined by whether they have health insurance. Catastrophic or chronic illness among only 10 percent of the population accounts for 75 percent of all health expenditures.[13] Since we cannot perfectly predict who will fall into that 10 percent, every American is potentially vulnerable to the high cost and devastating effects of such illnesses.

Access to health care is determined by numerous factors, including the supply of providers and facilities, proximity to care, ability to maneuver in the system, health status, and insurance coverage. Although there are approximately 700,000 physicians in the United States, many Americans lack adequate access to health services because of insurance barriers or maldistribution of providers. There is an oversupply of higher-paid specialists and a shortage of lower-paid primary care physicians (family practitioners, pediatricians, internists, OB/Gyns, geriatricians). Inner cities and some rural areas face constant shortages of physicians.

Until recently, many employees lost their insurance benefits when they changed jobs; this led the federal government to pass legislation mandating the "portability" of health insurance benefits from one job to the next, thereby guaranteeing coverage during the transition. Today, individuals who leave their jobs can continue their group health insurance benefits under the Consolidated Omnibus Budget Reconciliation Act (COBRA). COBRA allows former employees, retirees, spouses, and dependents to continue their insurance at group rates. COBRA beneficiaries pay a higher amount than when they were employed, as they're covering both the personal premium and the amount previously covered by the employer. As a result, COBRA benefits are more expensive than benefits through an employer, but less expensive than purchasing individual insurance. COBRA coverage is only temporary, and usually lasts for up to 18 months.

Managed care health plans determine access on the basis of participating providers, health plan benefits, and administrative rules. Often this means that consumers do not have the freedom to choose specialists, facilities, or treatment options beyond those contracted with the health plan and recommended by their PCP. In the United States, consumer demand has led to an expansion of benefits to include nonallopathic therapies such as chiropractic and acupuncture.

However, many nonallopathic treatments remain unavailable, even to a limited degree, through current health plans.

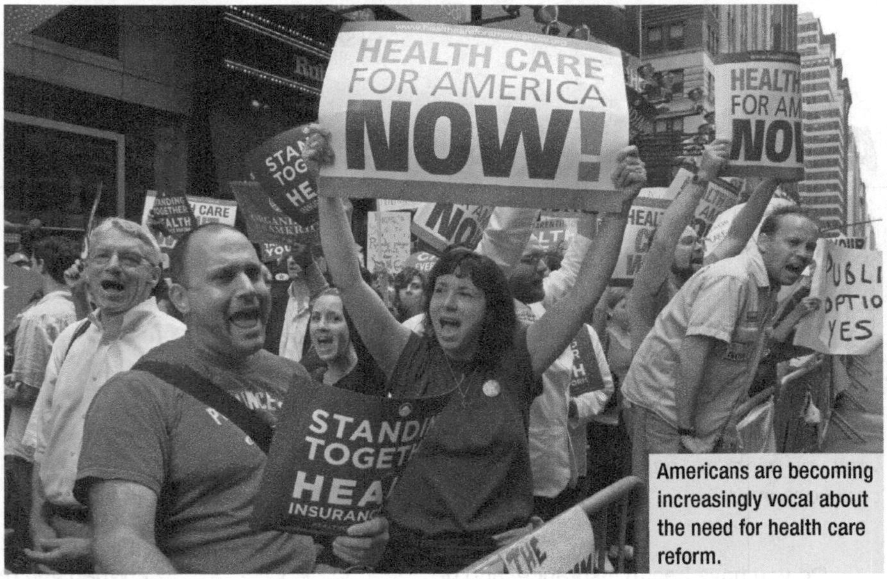

Americans are becoming increasingly vocal about the need for health care reform.

Viviane Moos/Corbis

Quality and Malpractice

The U.S. health care system has several mechanisms for ensuring quality services: education, licensure, certification/registration, accreditation, peer review, and the legal system of malpractice litigation. Some of these mechanisms are mandatory before a professional or organization may provide care, whereas others are purely voluntary. (Be aware that licensure, although mandated by the state for some practitioners and facilities, is only a minimum guarantee of quality.) Insurance companies and government payers may also require a higher level of quality by linking payment to whether a practitioner is board certified or a facility is accredited by the appropriate agency. In addition, most insurance plans now require prior authorization and/or second opinions, not only to reduce costs but also to improve quality of care.

Consumer, provider, and advocacy groups focus on the great variation in quality as a major problem. A new form of quality measurement uses "outcome" as the primary indicator for measuring health care quality at the individual level. With outcome measurements, we don't look just at what is done to the patient, but at what subsequently happens to the patient's health status. Thus, mortality rates and complication rates (e.g., infections) become important in assessing individual practitioners and facilities.

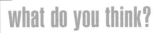

what do you think?

Do you believe prospective patients should have access to information about practitioners' and facilities' malpractice records? ● How about their success and failure rates or outcomes of various procedures?

Medical errors and mistakes do happen. An Institute of Medicine report indicates that as many as 44,000 to 98,000 people die in U.S. hospitals each year as the result of medical errors.[14] Clearly, we must be proactive in our health care.

The Debate over National Health Insurance

The United States has seen four major political movements supporting national health insurance during the past century, but none has succeeded. Most recently, the Obama administration put health care reform at the top of its domestic agenda. Whether universal coverage will—or should—be achieved and through what mechanism remain hotly debated topics.

Proponents of reform argue that health care should be available and affordable for everyone, and often state the view that health care is a right, not a privilege. They point to other Western countries, such as Canada and France, that currently have successful universal coverage. Opponents of health care reform feel that the high cost of changing the system is more than the United States can afford, and often state that the government should not interfere in what has been a largely free-market industry. Both sides of the debate have articulated valid arguments and concerns.

However, analysts believe that health care reform has failed in the past due to a combination of less valid factors that have little to do with the quality of the nation's health. Lobbying efforts by the insurance industry and the medical community, proposed plans that were too complicated, and interest groups that contended that the plans either went "too far" or "not far enough" have all played a role in thwarting reform in the past. Some people also believe that our current system serves people well.

One critical point must be made, though: We are paying for the most expensive system in the world without obtaining full coverage. We pay for people who don't have insurance through increased premiums and taxes, and we spend more than necessary, because prevention and early treatment are not emphasized. We also pay for much duplication of services and technologies, for practitioners who practice defensive medicine, and for the vast bureaucracy made inevitable by the vast number of private health insurance companies.

The Institute of Medicine, a nonpartisan organization that advises the federal government on health issues, recommends a single-payer, tax-financed scheme that severs insurance ties from employment.[15] Similar to the Canadian model, it would cover everyone—regardless of income or other factors such as health status. It would offer many different ways to tailor a plan to the needs of U.S. citizens. A single federal plan or a privately administered plan paid for by general tax funds or earmarked taxes could be created. Thus, all (or most) private insurers would be eliminated or would see their role limited to that of fiscal administrators. While a single-payer system might be the most equitable and efficient health care model, it is not realistically on the table for the United States, due to the size and influence of the current health care industry. The closest viable alternative is the "public option," which would implement a government-run insurer, similar to Medicare, that consumers could choose instead of a traditional provider.

Assess yourself

Are You a Smart Health Care Consumer?

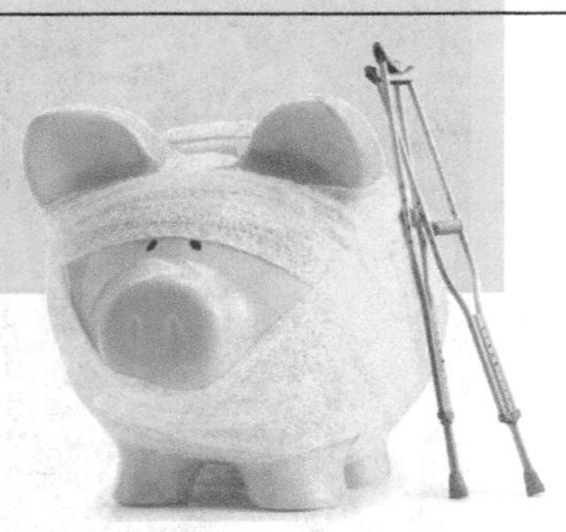
iStockphoto

PEARSON myhealthlab

Fill out this assessment online at www.pearsonhighered.com/myhealthlab or www.pearsonhighered.com/donatelle.

Answer the following questions to determine what you might do to become a better health care consumer.

	Yes	No
1. Do you have health insurance, and do you understand the coverage available to you under your plan?	◯	◯
2. Do you know which health care services are available for free or at a reduced cost at your student health center or local clinic? If so, what are they?	◯	◯
3. When you receive a prescription, do you ask the doctor or pharmacist if a generic brand could be substituted?	◯	◯
4. When you receive a prescription, do you ask the doctor or pharmacist about potential side effects, including possible food and drug interactions?	◯	◯
5. Do you report any unusual drug side effects to your health care provider?	◯	◯
6. Do you take medication as directed?	◯	◯
7. When you receive a diagnosis, do you seek more information about the diagnosis and treatment?	◯	◯
8. If your health care provider recommends surgery or an invasive type of treatment, do you seek a second opinion?	◯	◯
9. Do you seek health information only from reliable and credible sources? Can you name three examples of such sources?	◯	◯
10. Do you read labels carefully before buying over-the-counter (OTC) medications?	◯	◯
11. Do you have a health care provider?	◯	◯

12. How much of a role do you think advertising plays in your decision to purchase a new product?

None ◯ Some ◯ A lot ◯

YOUR PLAN FOR CHANGE

Once you have considered your responses to the Assess yourself questions, you may want to change or improve certain behaviors in order to get the best treatment from your health care provider and the heath care system.

Today, you can:

◯ Research the insurance plan under which you're covered. Find out which health care providers and hospitals you can visit, the amounts of any co-payments and premiums you will be responsible for, and the drug coverage of your plan.

◯ Clean out your medicine cabinet. Get rid of any expired prescriptions or OTC medications (for information on safe drug disposal) and take stock of what you have. Keep on hand a supply of basic items, such as pain relievers, antiseptic cream, bandages, cough suppressants, and throat lozenges, and replenish the supply if you're running low.

Within the next 2 weeks, you can:

◯ Find a regular health care provider if you do not have one and make an appointment for a general checkup and interview.

◯ Think about health conditions you would benefit from knowing more about—such as those that run in your family or that you've experienced in the past—and do some research on them. Write down any unanswered questions so you can discuss them with your health care provider.

By the end of the semester, you can:

◯ Ask if a generic version is available when filling your next prescription.

◯ Become an advocate for health insurance for all. Write to your congressperson or state legislature to express your interest in health care reform.

Summary

- Self-care and individual responsibility are key factors in reducing rising health care costs and improving health status. Advance planning can help you navigate health care treatment in unfamiliar situations or emergencies. Assess health professionals by considering their qualifications, their record of treating problems like yours, and their ability to work with you.
- In theory, allopathic (conventional Western) medicine is based on scientifically validated methods and procedures. Medical doctors, specialists of various kinds, nurses, physician assistants, and other health care professionals practice allopathic medicine.
- Prescription drugs are administered under medical supervision. Generic drugs often can be substituted for more expensive brand name products. Over-the-counter (OTC) drugs include analgesics; cold, cough, allergy, and asthma relievers; stimulants; sleeping aids and relaxants; and dieting aids. Consumers should be aware of the potential side effects and interactions of both prescription and OTC drugs.
- Health insurance is based on the concept of spreading risk. Insurance is provided by private insurance companies (which charge premiums) and the government Medicare and Medicaid programs (which are funded by taxes). Managed care (in the form of HMOs, POS plans, and PPOs) attempts to control costs by streamlining administrative procedures and stressing preventive care, among other initiatives.
- Concerns about the U.S. health care system include cost, access, choice of treatment modality, quality and malpractice, and fraud and abuse.

Pop Quiz

1. Which of the following is not a condition that would indicate a visit to a physician is needed?
   a. recurring high temperature (over 103°F in adults)
   b. persistent or recurrent diarrhea
   c. the common cold
   d. yellowing of the skin or the whites of the eyes

2. Which is a common type of over-the-counter drug?
   a. antibiotics
   b. hormonal contraceptives
   c. antidepressants
   d. antacids

3. What medical practice is based on procedures whose objective is to heal by countering the patient's symptoms?
   a. allopathic medicine
   b. nonallopathic medicine
   c. osteopathic medicine
   d. chiropractic medicine

4. Jack evaluates visual problems and fits glasses but is not a trained physician. Jack is a(n)
   a. osteopath.
   b. ophthalmologist.
   c. optometrist.
   d. physician assistant.

5. What mechanism used by private insurance companies requires that the subscriber pay a certain amount directly to the provider before the insurance company will begin paying for services?
   a. coinsurance
   b. cost sharing
   c. co-payments
   d. deductibles

6. Deborah, 28, is a single parent on welfare. Her medical bills are paid by a federal health insurance program for the poor. This agency is
   a. an HMO.
   b. Social Security.
   c. Medicaid.
   d. Medicare

7. The federal insurance program that covers 99 percent of adults over 65 years of age is
   a. Medicare.
   b. Medicaid.
   c. COBRA.
   d. HMO.

8. The most restrictive type of managed care is
   a. fee-for-service.
   b. health maintenance organizations.
   c. point of service.
   d. preferred provider organizations.

9. Lauren has diabetes, and because of a job change she had to choose a new health insurance provider. The new insurance company refused to cover her diabetic care expenses under a clause in the contract which stated that Lauren has
   a. a coinsurance limit.
   b. a preexisting health condition.
   c. already exceeded the lifetime upper limit.
   d. no major medical coverage on her policy.

10. A specialist who diagnoses and treats diseases of the teeth, gums, and oral cavity is a(n)
    a. dentist.
    b. orthodontist.
    c. oral surgeon.
    d. osteopath.

Answers to Chapter Review Questions
1. c; 2. d; 3. a; 4. c; 5. d;
6. c; 7. a; 8. b; 9. b; 10. a

Think about It!

1. List several conditions (resulting from illness or accident) for which you wouldn't need to seek medical help. When would you consider each condition to be bad enough to require medical attention? How would you decide to whom and where to go for treatment?
2. Describe your rights as a patient. Have you ever received treatment that violated these rights? If so, what action, if any, did you take?
3. What are the inherent benefits and risks of managed care organizations?
4. Explain the differences between traditional indemnity insurance and managed health care. Which would you feel more comfortable with? Should insurance companies dictate rates for various medical tests and procedures in an attempt to keep prices down?
5. Discuss how medical and pharmaceutical waste has a negative impact on the environment. What are two ways in which you personally can reduce such waste?

Accessing Your Health on the Internet

The following websites explore further topics and issues related to personal health. For links to the websites below, visit the Companion Website for *Health: The Basics,* Green Edition at www.pearsonhighered.com/donatelle.

1. *Agency for HealthCare Research and Quality (AHRQ).* A gateway to consumer health information. Provides links to sites that can address health care concerns and provide information on what questions to ask, what to look for, and what you should know when making critical decisions about personal care. www.ahrq.gov
2. *Food and Drug Administration (FDA).* News on the latest government-approved home health tests and other health-related products. www.fda.gov
3. *HealthGrades.* This company provides quality reports on physicians as well as hospitals, nursing homes, and other health care facilities. www.healthgrades.com
4. *The Leapfrog Group.* A nationwide coalition of more than 150 public and private organizations, the Leapfrog Group focuses on identifying problems in the U.S. hospital system that can lead to medical errors and on devising solutions. www.leapfroggroup.org
5. *National Committee for Quality Assurance (NCQA).* The NCQA assesses and reports on the quality of managed care plans, including HMOs. www.ncqa.org
6. *National Library of Medicine.* Supports Medline/Pubmed information retrieval systems in addition to providing public health information for consumers. www.nlm.nih.gov
7. *HealthReform.Gov.* Provides up-to-date information regarding health care reform in America. www.healthreform.gov

References

1. American Academy of Orthopaedic Surgeons, "Information Statement: The Importance of Good Communication in the Physician-Patient Relationship," September 2005, www.aaos.org/about/papers/advistmt/1017.asp.
2. D. Merenstein et al., "Use and Costs of Nonrecommended Tests during Routine Preventive Health Exams," *American Journal of Preventive Medicine,* 30 (2006): 521–27.
3. Consumer Health, "Patient Rights: Informed Consent," 2008, www.emedicinehealth.com/informed_consent/article_em.htm.
4. American College Health Association, *American College Health Association-National College Health Assessment (ACHA-NCHA) Reference Group Data Report Fall 2008* (Baltimore: American College Health Association, 2009).
5. C. DeNavas-Walt, B. Proctor, and J. Smith, *Income, Poverty, and Health Insurance Coverage in the United States: 2008,* U.S. Census Bureau, Current Population Reports, P60-236 (Washington, DC: U.S. Government Printing Office, 2009).
6. C. Schoen et al. "How Many Are Underinsured? Trends among U.S. Adults, 2003 and 2007," *Health Affairs* Web Exclusive (June 10, 2008): w298–w309.
7. National Center for Health Statistics, *Health, United States, 2007, with Chartbook on Trends in the Health of Americans* (Hyattsville, MD: National Center for Health Statistics, 2008).
8. Kaiser Family Foundation, "Total HMO Enrollment, June 2008," Statehealthfacts.org, 2009, www.statehealthfacts.org/comparemaptable.jsp?ind=348&cat=7.
9. Centers for Medicare and Medicaid Services, "Medicare Enrollment: National Trends 1966–2008," 2009, www.cms.hhs.gov/MedicareEnRpts/Downloads/HISMI08.pdf.
10. Centers for Medicare and Medicaid Services, "Medicaid Data Sources," 2008, www.cms.hhs.gov/MedicaidDataSourcesGenInfo.
11. National Center for Health Statistics, *Health, United States, 2008 with Chartbook on Trends in the Health of Americans,* 2009; Centers for Medicare and Medicaid Services, "National Health Care Expenditures Projections: 2008–2018," 2008, www.cms.hhs.gov/NationalHealthExpendData/Downloads/proj2008.pdf.
12. Centers for Disease Control and Prevention, "Indicators for Chronic Disease Surveillance," *Morbidity and Mortality Weekly Report, Recommendations and Reports* 53, no. RR11 (2004): 1–6, www.cdc.gov/mmwr/preview/mmwrhtml/rr5311a1.htm.
13. National Center for Chronic Disease Prevention and Health Promotion, "Chronic Disease Overview," 2008, www.cdc.gov/nccdphp/overview.htm.
14. Institute of Medicine, "The Chasm in Quality: Select Indicators from Recent Reports," May 2006, www.iom.edu.
15. Institute of Medicine, "Insuring America's Health: Principles and Recommendations," January 2004, www.iom.edu/CMS/3809/4660/17632.aspx.

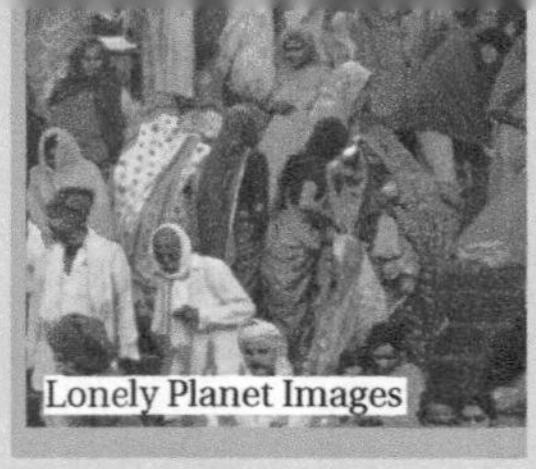

Why is population growth an environmental issue?

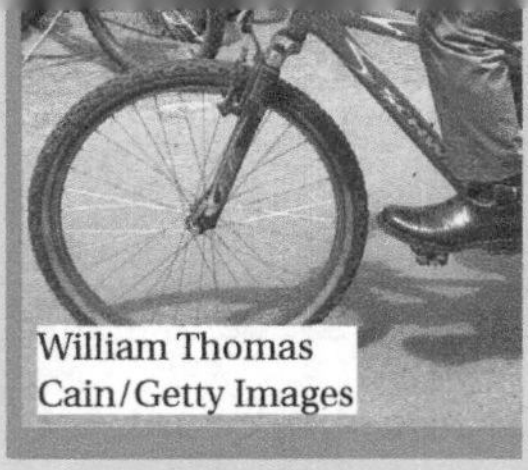

How can I reduce my carbon footprint?

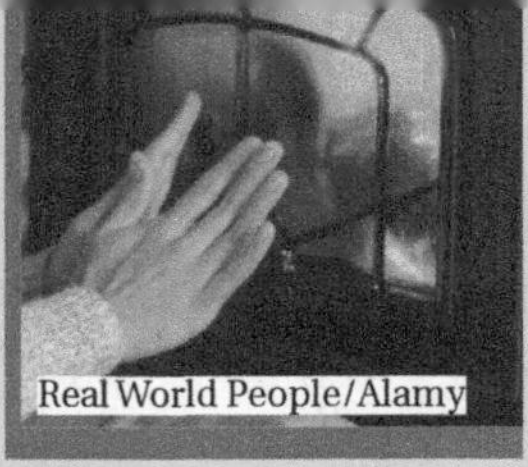

How can air pollution be a problem indoors?

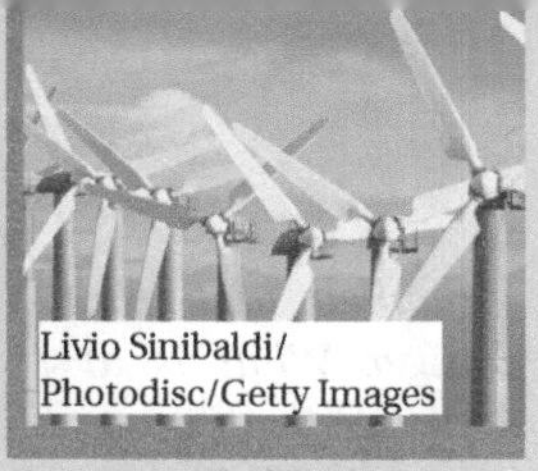

How can I help prevent global warming?

Environmental Health

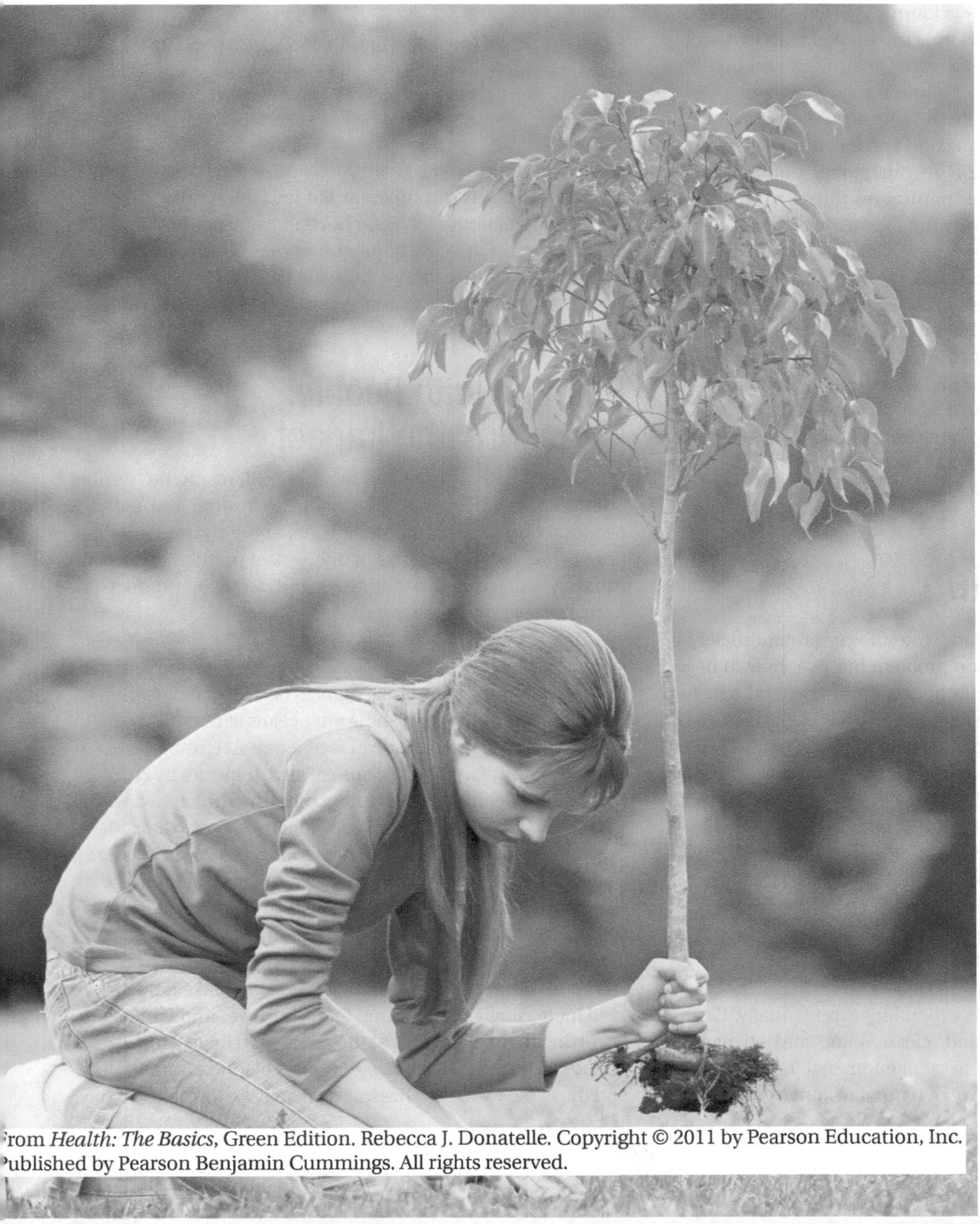

Alix Minde/Getty Images

Objectives

* Explain the environmental impact associated with the current global population and its projected growth.
* Discuss major causes of air pollution and the global consequences of the accumulation of greenhouse gases and ozone depletion.
* Identify sources of water pollution and chemical contaminants often found in water.
* Distinguish municipal solid waste from hazardous waste, and list strategies for reducing land pollution.
* Discuss the health concerns associated with ionizing and nonionizing radiation.
* Describe the physiological consequences of noise pollution.

"We have arrived at a moment of decision. Our home—Earth—is in grave danger. What is at risk of being destroyed is not the planet itself, of course, but the conditions that have made it hospitable for human beings."

—Al Gore, opening statement before the Senate Foreign Relations Committee, January 28, 2009

We live in an especially dangerous time—dangerous for us, dangerous for future generations, and dangerous to our very existence. Our global population has grown more in the past 50 years than at any other time in human history. Population growth poses a potentially devastating threat to the water we drink, the air we breathe, the food we eat, and our capacity to survive. Our polar ice caps and glaciers are melting at rates that defy even the most dire predictions of just a decade ago, and threats of rising sea levels loom large. One in four existing mammals in the world is now threatened with extinction as humans destroy habitat, exacerbate drought and flooding due to climate change, and pollute the environment. Clean water is becoming scarce, fossil fuels are being depleted at unprecedented rates, and our solid and hazardous wastes are growing in direct proportion to our global population. In short, we are plundering our natural resources, and greedily consuming and throwing away the future life of all species.

Individuals, communities, and political powers must take action now to make positive change. We must reduce consumption, waste less, be less selfish when it comes to personal comfort and perceived needs, and force governments to enact and enforce environmentally responsible legislation. This chapter provides an overview of the factors contributing to our global environmental crisis. It also provides a blueprint for action—by individuals, communities, policymakers, and governments. Staying informed and becoming involved in the process are key things you can do to help.

Overpopulation

Anthropologist Margaret Mead wrote, "Every human society is faced with not one population problem but two: how to beget and rear enough children and how not to beget and rear too many."[1] As noted health scientist Robert H. Friis has described it, "Every day we share Earth and its resources with 250,000 more people than the day before. Every year, there are another 90 million mouths to feed. This is the equivalent to adding a city the size of Philadelphia to the world population every week, a Los Angeles every 2 weeks, a Mexico every year, and a United States and Canada every 3 years."[2] The United Nations projects that the world population will grow from 7 billion in 2011 to 9.4 billion by 2050 and to 11.5 billion by 2150 (Figure 1).[3]

ecosystem The collection of physical (nonliving) and biological (living) components of an environment and the relationships between them.

Though our population is expanding exponentially, Earth's resources are not. Fertile land, clean water, and all natural resources are disappearing at a phenomenal rate. There is heavy pressure on the capacity of natural resources to support human life and world health. According to a recent United Nations Global Environmental Outlook report (GEO-4), the human population is living far beyond its means and is inflicting damage on the environment that may already be irreparable.[4] Population experts believe that the most critical environmental challenge today is to slow the world's population growth.

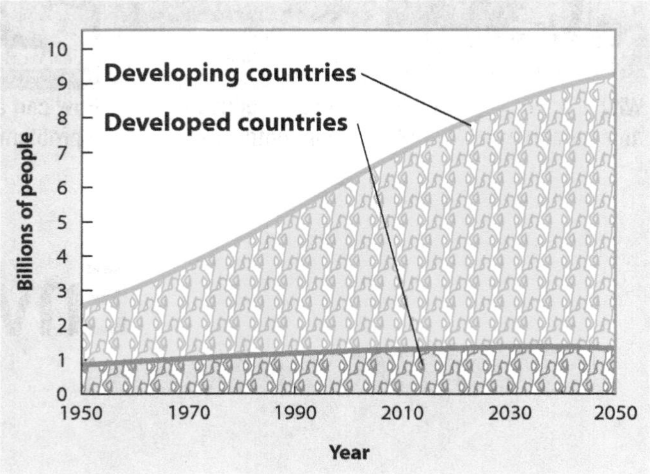

FIGURE 1 **World Population Growth, 1950–2050 (Projected)**

Source: Data are from Population Division of the Department of Economic and Social Affairs of the United Nations Secretariat, *World Population Prospects: The 2008 Revision*, 2009, http://esa.un.org/unpp.

Bursting with People: Measuring the Impact

While many people question *when* we will reach the "tipping point" at which we will be unable to restore the balance between humans and nature, others argue that it is too late now. Evidence of the effects of unchecked population growth, runaway consumption patterns, and toxic by-products of human use and waste is everywhere:

- **Impact on other species.** Based on current reporting, changes in the **ecosystem** are resulting in mass destruction of many species. We are currently fishing our oceans at rates that are 250 percent more than they can regenerate. At current rates, scientists project a global collapse of all fish species by 2050.

  At the same time, 12 percent of birds are threatened with extinction, and 23 percent of mammals and more than 30 percent of amphibians are already gone or nearly gone. Many that survive are sick, have chemically induced ailments, or have genetic disfigurement that will hasten their demise.
- **Impact on our food supply.** In addition to overfishing, aquatic ecosystems continue to be heavily exploited by chemical and human waste. Drought and erosion make growing food increasingly difficult, and food shortages and famine are occurring in many regions of the world with increasing frequency. Faced with decreasing supplies of food products, fish, and the capacity to feed livestock, we may be forced to change

the way we think about food. Many experts have long advocated for humans to "eat lower on the food chain" by eating fewer high-resource animal products.

- **Land degradation and contamination of drinking water.** The per capita availability of freshwater is declining rapidly, and contaminated water remains the greatest single environmental cause of human sickness and health. Unsustainable land use and climate change are increasing land degradation, including erosion, nutrient depletion, deforestation, and other problems that will inevitably affect human life.
- **Excessive energy consumption.** "Use it *and* lose it" is an apt saying for our vast greed in using nonrenewable energy sources in the form of **fossil fuels** (oil, coal, natural gas). Although we are seeing a shift toward renewable energy sources, such as hydropower, solar and wind power, and biomass power, the predominant energy sources are still fossil fuels. In many developing regions of the world, demand for limited fossil fuels is growing at unprecedented rates.
- **Impact on our lives.** Imagine waking up in the morning and finding that you have no water for a shower, that your lights can be used only a few hours each day or not at all, that you have to choose between using electricity for your flat-screen TV or your refrigerator. Imagine having very little gas for your car, and going to the grocery store to find half-empty shelves of items you can't afford. Imagine the news filled with stories about long lines at gas stations; natural disasters; and wars over water rights, food, and fuel. Such scenarios are not the imaginings of science fiction. Major difficulties loom unless we take action to change our current rate of population growth and our consumption of natural resources, and unless the global community acts together to enforce policies and programs to check rampant population growth.

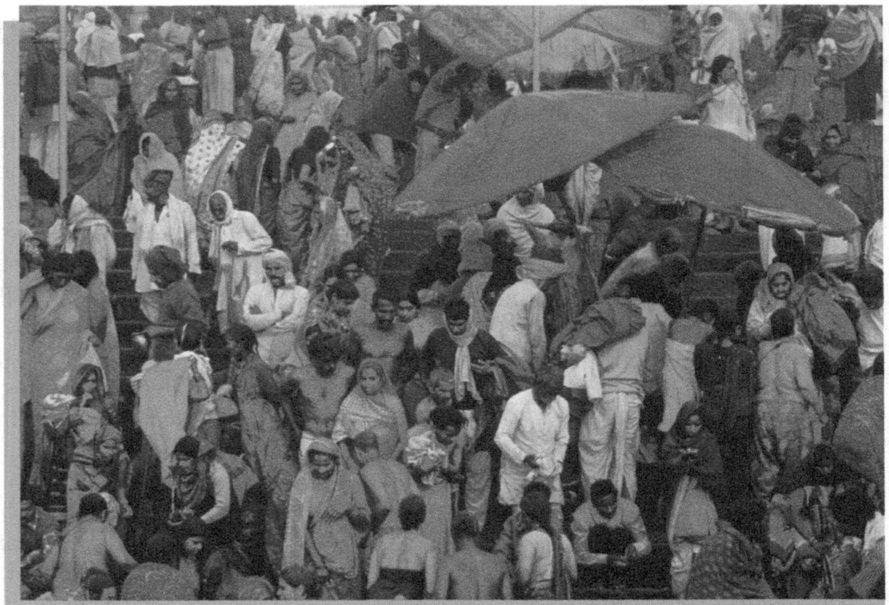

Lonely Planet Images

Why is population growth an environmental issue?

Every year the global population grows by 90 million, but Earth's resources are not expanding. Population increases are believed to be responsible for most of the current environmental stress.

Factors That Affect Population Growth

Before we consider how to slow the growing tide of people, we must first understand the factors that have led to the world population's increase. Key among them are changes in fertility and mortality rates.

Fertility rate refers to how many births a woman has by the end of her reproductive life. In the United States today, the fertility rate is just over 2 births per woman, as compared to nearly 3.5 births per woman during the baby boom years after World War II. In other regions of the world, particularly in India and in many Asian, Latin American, and African countries, birth rates are about four per woman; this leads to rapid increases in overall population in these poorer countries. In countries where women have little say over reproductive choices, where birth control is either not available or frowned upon, pregnancy rates continue to rise.

Mortality rates from both chronic and infectious diseases have declined in both developed and developing regions of the world as a result of improved public health infrastructure, increased availability of drugs and vaccines, better disaster preparedness, and other factors. Consequently, people are living longer and consuming more over the course of their lifetimes. This, too, contributes to pressure on the environment.

97% of global growth in the next four decades will happen in Asia, Africa, Latin America, and the Caribbean.

Different Nations, Different Growth Rates

By 2050, India is projected to be the most populous nation at 1.7 billion, overtaking current leader China, which will grow to 1.4 billion.[5] The continued preference for large families in many developing nations is related to several factors: high infant mortality rates; the traditional view of children as "social security" (working from a young age to assist families in daily survival and supporting parents when they grow too old to work); the low educational and economic status of women, which often leaves women with few reproductive

fossil fuels Carbon-based material used for energy; includes oil, coal, and natural gas.

fertility rate The average number of births a female in a certain population has during her reproductive years.

choices; and the traditional desire for sons, which keeps parents of daughters reproducing until they have male offspring.

In contrast to developing nations, the population sizes in wealthier nations are static or declining, with one notable exception—the United States. With a population of 305 million, and an expected 439 million people by 2050, the United States is the only industrialized country in the world currently experiencing significant population growth.[6] Last year, the U.S. growth rate was nearly 1 percent, far greater than that of Canada, England, or other industrialized nations. Each year, the United States adds 3 million more people, or 8,000 per day.[7] This is particularly noteworthy because the United States also has the largest "ecological footprint"—that is, the United States exerts greater impact on many of the planet's resources and ecosystems than any other nation on Earth. Overall, we are the world's largest single emitter of greenhouse gases, the world's largest forest-product consumers, and the generators of the most municipal solid waste per person in the world.[8]

Although the United States makes up only 5 percent of the world's population, it is responsible for nearly 25 percent of total global resource consumption. We consume 2.3 billion metric tons of oil equivalents for energy per year; the rest of the world consumes 10 billion tons per year. Per capita, Americans consume nearly 8,000 kg of oil equivalents for energy, compared to 3,600 kg consumed by Europeans and 900 kg by Asians (see Figure 2).[9]

Zero Population Growth

Recognizing that population control will be essential in the decades ahead, many countries have already enacted strict population control measures or have encouraged their citizens to limit the size of their families. Proponents of *zero population growth (ZPG)* believe that each couple should produce only two offspring. When the parents die, these two children are their replacements, allowing the population to stabilize. By 2000, Italy, Spain, Portugal, Greece, and Sweden were among the first to achieve zero population growth.[10] Germany, Russia, Ukraine, Hungary, and Bulgaria had actually achieved negative population growth, causing some people in these countries to worry that they may have gone too far in their population control campaigns.

Education may be the single biggest contributor to ZPG. As education levels of women increase and women achieve equality in pay, job status, and social status with men, fertility rates decline. Access to information about family planning and contraception can also make a big difference.

what do you think?

Should individuals get tax breaks for having fewer children? ● How would such policies compare to our current policies? ● Can you think of other policies that might be effective in encouraging population control and resource conservation in the United States?

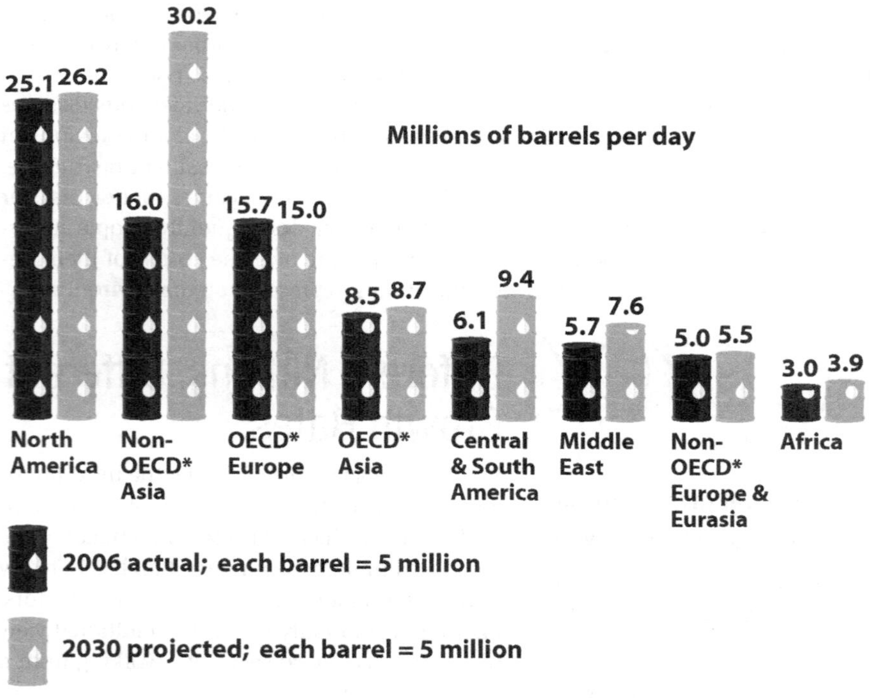

FIGURE 2 **World Liquid Fuels Consumption by Region and Country Group, 2006 and 2030 (Projected)**

*OECD is the Organization for Economic Cooperation and Development.

Source: Data are from Energy Information Administration (EIA), *International Energy Annual 2006* (June-December 2008), www.eia.doe.gov/iea; and EIA World Energy Projections Plus (2009).

Air Pollution

The term *air pollution* refers to the presence, in varying degrees, of those substances (suspended particles and vapors) not found in perfectly clean air. From the beginning of time, natural events, living creatures, and toxic by-products have been polluting the environment. As such, air pollution is not a new phenomenon. What is new is the vast array of **pollutants** that exist today and the potential interactive effects of many of these substances.

Generally, air pollutants are either *naturally occurring* or *anthropogenic* (human caused). Naturally occurring air pollutants include particulate matter, such as the dust spread from windstorms, smoke and ash from major forest fires, salt spray from the oceans, ash from volcanic eruptions, and others. Anthropogenic sources include those caused by stationary sources (e.g., electric-generating plants, factories, manufacturing complexes, chemical plants, oil and natural gas refineries, coal plants, chemical plants, and incinerators) and mobile sources (e.g., cars, trucks, buses, ATVs, airplanes, ships, and trains). According to Environmental Protection Agency (EPA) estimates, mobile sources produce over half of two major sources of smog—hydrocarbons and nitrogen oxides (NO)—almost 90 percent of carbon monoxide and more than half of hazardous air pollution.[11]

Components of Air Pollution

Concern about air quality prompted Congress to pass the Clean Air Act in 1970 and to amend it in 1977 and again in 1990. The goal was to develop standards for six of the most widespread air pollutants that seriously affect health: sulfur dioxide, particulates, carbon monoxide, nitrogen dioxide, ground-level ozone, and lead. Other common air pollutants include carbon dioxide and hydrocarbons. Today, ozone and particle air pollution are the most widespread and most dangerous of the air pollutants.[12] Table 1 ranks the ten best and the ten worst cities in the United States in terms of these two air pollutants.

Sulfur Dioxide **Sulfur dioxide (SO_2)** is a yellowish brown gas that forms when fuel containing sulfur, particularly coal and oil, is burned; when gasoline is extracted from oil; or when metals are extracted from ore.

Sulfur dioxide is also derived from fertilizers and livestock wastes. More than 65 percent (or more than 13 million tons) of SO_2 released into the air each year comes from electric and coal-fired power plants. Other sources of SO_2 are industrial facilities, locomotives, large ships, and previous-generation diesel engines.

Sulfur dioxide dissolves in water vapor to form acid rain and interacts with other gases and particles in the air to form sulfates and other products. In humans, sulfur dioxide aggravates symptoms of heart and lung disease; obstructs breathing passages; and increases the incidence of respiratory diseases such as colds, asthma, bronchitis, and emphysema. Sulfur dioxide is toxic to plants, destroys some paint pigments, corrodes metals, impairs visibility, and is a precursor to acid deposition (discussed later).

In 2007, a new generation of engines that burn an ultralow sulfur diesel fuel became available in the United States.[13] This new cleaner-burning diesel has been readily available in European countries and has the potential to drastically reduce sulfur-dioxide pollution in the United States, particularly as newer diesel engine technology is developed that will prevent virtually all SO_2 emissions.

Particle Pollution *Particle pollution* refers to a mix of very tiny solid or liquid particles in the air we breathe. **Particulates** vary in size, from coarse to fine to ultrafine; coarse particulates may make you sneeze or cough; fine particles can make your eyes water, or your lungs feel congested. Some of these particles are so small that they can pass through the lungs into the bloodstream. Whether found in solid or liquid form, particle pollution poses one of the greatest health risks to humans today. Depending on the part of the country you live in, the season, or a variety of other factors, you may be exposed to a variety of particle health threats daily. Most particle pollution comes from either mechanical or chemical processes. Dust storms (particularly in drought-ridden areas), construction and demolition, mining, and agriculture are among the most common sources; however, engine exhausts and many industrial and chemical processing releases are also key sources.

How risky is it to breathe particulate pollution? It depends on the size and nature of the particle, the length of and time of exposure, and the concentration in the air. For those prone to asthma, particulate inhalation can be deadly. When combined with SO_2, they can make all respiratory diseases worse.

pollutant A substance that contaminates some aspect of the environment and causes potential harm to living organisms.
sulfur dioxide (SO_2) A yellowish brown gaseous by-product of the burning of fossil fuels.
particulates Nongaseous air pollutants.

TABLE 1
The Cleanest and Dirtiest U.S. Cities in Terms of Air Pollution

Top 10 Highest Ozone Pollution	Top 10 Highest Year-Round Particle Pollution	Lowest Ozone Pollution (Not Ranked)	Top 10 Lowest Year-Round Particle Pollution
1. Los Angeles, CA	1. Bakersfield, CA	Billings, MT	1. Cheyenne, WY
2. Bakersfield, CA	2. Pittsburgh, PA	Carson City, NV	2. Santa Fe, NM
3. Visalia, CA	3. Los Angeles, CA	Coeur D'Alene, ID	3. Honolulu, HI
4. Fresno, CA	4. Visalia, CA	Fargo, ND	4. Great Falls, MT
5. Houston, TX	5. Birmingham, AL	Honolulu, HI	5. Farmington, NM
6. Sacramento, CA	6. Hanford, CA	Laredo, TX	6. Anchorage, AK
7. Dallas–Fort Worth, TX	7. Fresno, CA	Lincoln, NE	7. Tucson, AZ
8. Charlotte, NC	8. Cincinnati, OH	Port St. Lucie, FL	8. Bismark, ND
9. Phoenix, AZ	9. Detroit, MI	Sioux Falls, SD	9. Flagstaff, AZ (tie)
10. El Centro, TX	10. Cleveland, OH		10. Salinas, CA (tie)

Source: American Lung Association, "State of the Air," 2009, www.stateoftheair.org/2009/city-rankings.

Symptoms may be similar to those of a long-term smoker. Although risks to the lungs and cardiovascular system are significant, these particles can also corrode metals, damage homes and plant life, and decrease visibility. Short-term spikes in particulate levels can be deadly, particularly for the very young and for older adults who are suffering from chronic illnesses.

carbon monoxide (CO) An odorless, colorless gas that originates primarily from motor vehicle emissions.
nitrogen dioxide An amber-colored gas found in smog; can cause eye and respiratory irritations.
ozone A gas composed of 3 atoms of oxygen; occurs at ground level and in the upper atmosphere.
carbon dioxide (CO_2) Gas created by the combustion of fossil fuels, exhaled by animals, and used by plants for photosynthesis; the primary greenhouse gas in Earth's atmosphere.
greenhouse gases Gases that accumulate in the atmosphere, where they contribute to global warming by trapping heat near Earth's surface.
carbon footprint The amount of greenhouse gases produced, usually expressed in equivalent tons of carbon dioxide emissions.
hydrocarbons Chemical compounds that contain carbon and hydrogen.

Carbon Monoxide **Carbon monoxide (CO)** in our atmosphere originates primarily from motor vehicle emissions. Carbon monoxide is an odorless, colorless gas that interferes with the blood's ability to absorb and carry oxygen. It can impair thinking, slow reflexes, and cause drowsiness, unconsciousness, and death. Carbon monoxide poisoning is the third leading cause of death due to unintentional poisoning in the United States, killing nearly 1,400 and injuring 15,000 to 40,000 Americans each year.[14] Carbon monoxide is a major component of both indoor and outdoor air pollution.

Nitrogen Dioxide Coal-powered electrical utility boilers and motor vehicles emit **nitrogen dioxide,** an amber-colored gas. High concentrations of nitrogen dioxide can be fatal to humans. Lower concentrations increase susceptibility to colds and flu, bronchitis, and pneumonia. Nitrogen dioxide is also toxic to plant life and causes a brown discoloration of the atmosphere.

Ground-Level Ozone Ground-level **ozone** is a gas and one of the molecular forms of oxygen. When it occurs in nature, ozone has a sharp smell akin to sparks from electrical equipment. Ground-level ozone is produced when nitrogen dioxide reacts with sunlight and oxygen molecules, and it is a main component of smog. (Note, however, that ozone in the upper atmosphere is essential to protecting Earth from the sun's heat and ultraviolet light, as we discuss later.) Ground-level ozone irritates the respiratory system's mucous membranes, causing coughing and choking. It can impair lung function; reduce resistance to colds and pneumonia; and aggravate heart disease, asthma, bronchitis, and pneumonia. Ozone corrodes rubber and paint and can kill vegetation.

Carbon Dioxide **Carbon dioxide (CO_2)** is one of the most plentiful gases in Earth's atmosphere, and, as the primary fuel for plant respiration, it is essential to all life. However, CO_2 is also a principal component of emissions from internal combustion engines. Much of the rise in air pollution is directly related to excess CO_2 released from burning carbon-containing fossil fuels. CO_2 is also the most prominent **greenhouse gas** and thus the major culprit in global warming (discussed later).

As one of the largest CO_2 emitters in the world, the United States has the largest **carbon footprint**—the measure of impact that human activities have on the environment in terms of greenhouse gases produced, measured in units of CO_2.[15] When you drive your car or heat your house with oil, gas, or coal, the burning of these fossil fuels emits CO_2 into the atmosphere. Each time you turn up your thermostat or leave lights on in your house, the fuel burned adds to your individual carbon footprint. For each gallon of gasoline burned in your car, you emit 8.7 kg of CO_2 into the atmosphere. Multiply that by millions of people driving cars that burn lots of fuel and you can see how the problem escalates. Reducing our individual carbon footprint is a key goal in the struggle to combat air pollution, global warming, and climate change, and has been the purpose of several Green Guide tips throughout this book.

Hydrocarbons **Hydrocarbons** are chemical compounds containing different combinations of carbon and hydrogen. They encompass a wide variety of pollutants in the air and play a major part in forming smog. Most automobile engines emit hundreds of different hydrocarbon compounds. By themselves, hydrocarbons seem to cause few problems, but when they combine with sunlight and other pollutants, they form such poisons as formaldehyde, ketones, and peroxyacetyl nitrate, all of which are respiratory irritants. Hydrocarbon combinations such as benzene and benzo[*a*]pyrene are

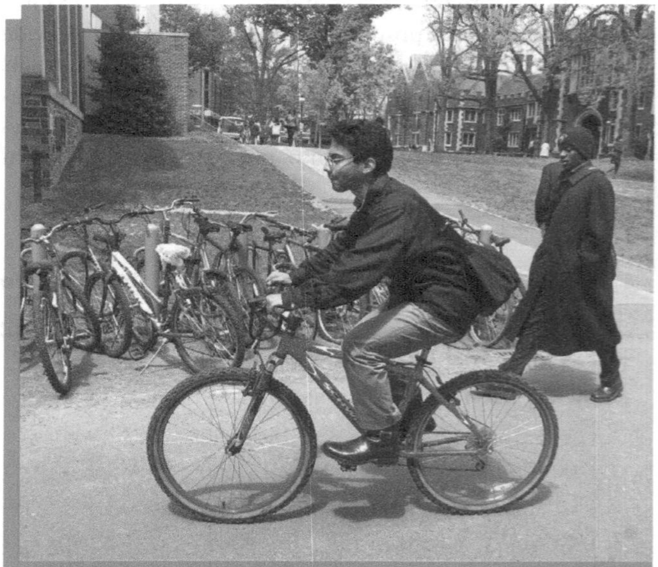

William Thomas Cain/Getty Images

How can I reduce my carbon footprint?

Reducing our individual carbon footprints is a key goal in the struggle to combat air pollution, global warming, and climate change. Making small changes such as driving less, riding your bike more, taking public transportation or carpooling, turning off lights when you leave a room, and recycling and composting can all help reduce your carbon footprint.

When the AQI is in this range:	... air quality conditions are	... as symbolized by this color:
0 to 50	Good	Green
51 to 100	Moderate	Yellow
101 to 150	Unhealthy for sensitive groups	Orange
151 to 200	Unhealthy	Red
201 to 300	Very unhealthy	Purple
301 to 500	Hazardous	Maroon

FIGURE 3 **Air Quality Index (AQI)**

The Environmental Protection Agency (EPA) provides individual AQIs for ground-level ozone, particle pollution, carbon monoxide, sulfur dioxide, and nitrogen dioxide. All of the AQIs are presented using the general values, categories, and colors of this figure.

Source: U.S. Environmental Protection Agency, "Air Quality Index: A Guide to Air Quality and Your Health," Updated April 2009, www.airnow.gov/index.cfm?action=aqibasics.aqi.

carcinogenic. All of these pollutants are also commonly known as *volatile organic compounds (VOCs).*

Air Quality Index

A measure of daily air quality, the Air Quality Index (AQI) tells you how clean or polluted your air is and what associated health concerns you should be aware of. The AQI focuses on health effects that can happen within a few hours or days after breathing polluted air.

The AQI runs from 0 to 500: The higher the AQI value, the greater the level of air pollution and associated health risks. An AQI value of 100 generally corresponds to the national air quality standard for the pollutant, which is the level the EPA has set to protect public health. Air Quality Index values below 100 are generally considered satisfactory. When AQI values rise above 100, air quality is considered unhealthy—at first for certain groups of people, then for everyone.

As shown in Figure 3, the EPA has divided the AQI scale into six categories and color codes. This is the best way for the public to assess the daily quality of the air we breathe.

Indoor Air Pollution

In the past several years, a growing body of scientific evidence has indicated that the air within homes and other buildings can be 10 to 40 times more hazardous than outdoor air, even in the most industrialized cities. Potentially dangerous chemical compounds can increase risks of cancer, contribute to respiratory problems, reduce the immune system's ability to fight disease, and increase problems with allergies and allergic reactions: The higher the dose of these pollutants and the more airtight the house, the greater the risk for individuals.

Skills for Behavior Change

Shopping to Save the Planet

* Look for products with less packaging or with refillable, reusable, or recyclable containers.
* Bring your own reusable cloth grocery bags to the store.
* Buy foods that are produced with minimal or sustainable energy.
* Purchase organic foods or foods produced with fewer chemicals and pesticides.
* Do not buy plastic bottles of water or other beverages. Purchase a hard plastic or steel, wide-mouth water bottle and fill it from a filtered source.
* Do not use caustic cleansers. Simple vinegar is usually just as effective and less harsh on your home and the environment.
* Buy laundry products that are free of dyes, fragrances, and sulfates.
* Use soap and water to clean surfaces, not disposable cleaning cloths and spray-on shower cleaners.
* Purchase appliances with the Energy Star logo.
* Buy CFLs (compact fluorescent lights) instead of less energy-efficient incandescent bulbs.
* Use reusable mugs, plates, and silverware rather than disposable products.
* Buy recycled paper products.
* Purchase bed linens and bath towels that are made from bamboo, hemp, or organic cotton.

20–100

potentially dangerous chemical compounds can be found in the air of the average American home.

Indoor air pollution comes primarily from these sources: woodstoves, furnaces, passive cigarette smoke exposure, asbestos, formaldehyde, radon, and lead. An emerging source of indoor air pollution is mold. In addition, that "new car" smell we like is often related to potentially harmful chemicals found in interior fabrics, upholstery, and glues. Today, more and more manufacturers are offering green building products and furnishings, such as natural fiber fabrics, untreated wood for furniture and floors, low-VOC paints, and many other products in an attempt to reduce potential pollutants. The **Skills for Behavior Change** box above offers ideas for being an environmentally conscious consumer of products for yourself and your home.

Several factors, including age, preexisting medical conditions, individual sensitivity, room temperature and humidity, and functioning of the liver and immune and respiratory systems contribute to one's risk for being affected by indoor air pollution. Those with allergies may be particularly vulnerable. Health effects may develop over years of exposure or may occur in response to toxic levels of pollutants.

Preventing indoor air pollution should focus on three main areas: *source control* (eliminating or reducing individual contaminants), *ventilation improvements* (increasing the amount of outdoor air coming indoors), and *air cleaners* (removing particulates from the air).[16]

Environmental Tobacco Smoke Perhaps the greatest source of indoor air pollution is *environmental tobacco smoke (ETS)*, which contains carbon monoxide and cancer-causing particulates. The level of carbon monoxide in cigarette smoke contained in enclosed places has been found to be 4,000 times higher than that allowed in the clean air standard established by the EPA. Moreover, the Surgeon General has reported that there are more than 50 carcinogens in environmental tobacco smoke. Ten to 15 percent of nonsmokers are extremely sensitive to tobacco smoke. These people experience itchy eyes, difficulty in breathing, painful headaches, nausea, and dizziness in response to minute amounts of smoke. The only truly effective way to eliminate ETS in public places is to enact strict no-smoking policies; ventilation and separate smoking areas are not sufficient. Today, many major U.S. cities have banned smoking in public places, in worksites, and in automobiles where children are present.

asbestos A mineral compound that separates into stringy fibers and lodges in the lungs, where it can cause various diseases.
formaldehyde A colorless, strong-smelling gas released through outgassing; causes respiratory and other health problems.
radon A naturally occurring radioactive gas resulting from the decay of certain radioactive elements.
lead A highly toxic metal found in emissions from lead smelters and processing plants; also sometimes found in pipes or paint in older houses.

Home Heating Woodstoves emit significant levels of particulates and carbon monoxide in addition to other pollutants, such as sulfur dioxide. If you rely on wood for heating, make sure that your stove is properly installed, vented, and maintained. Burning properly seasoned wood reduces particulates. People who rely on oil- or gas-fired furnaces also need to make sure that these appliances are properly installed, ventilated, and maintained.

Asbestos **Asbestos** is a mineral compound that was once commonly used in insulating materials, but it also found its way into vinyl flooring, shingles/roofing materials, heating pipe coverings, and many other products in buildings constructed before 1970. When bonded to other materials, asbestos is relatively harmless, but if its tiny fibers become loosened and airborne, they can embed themselves in the lungs. Their presence leads to cancer of the lungs, stomach, and chest lining, and other life-threatening lung diseases called *mesothelioma* and *asbestosis*. If asbestos is detected in the home, it must be removed or sealed off by a professional.

Formaldehyde **Formaldehyde** is a colorless, strong-smelling gas present in some carpets, draperies, furniture, particleboard, plywood, wood paneling, countertops, and many adhesives. It is released into the air in a process called *outgassing*. Outgassing is highest in new products, but the process can continue for many years. Exposure to formaldehyde can cause respiratory problems, dizziness, fatigue, nausea, and rashes. Long-term exposure can lead to central nervous system disorders and cancer.

How can you limit the amount of formaldehyde in your home? Ask about the formaldehyde content of products you purchase, and avoid those that contain it. Some houseplants, such as philodendrons and spider plants, help clean formaldehyde from the air.

Radon **Radon,** an odorless, colorless gas, penetrates homes through cracks, pipes, sump pits, and other openings in the basement or foundation. The EPA, National Cancer Institute (NCI), and the American Lung Association estimate that radon causes 7,000 to 30,000 preventable deaths per year.[17] The number of lung cancer deaths per year attributed to radon make it second only to smoking as a cause of lung cancer.[18]

The EPA estimates that as many as 7.7 million homes throughout the country have elevated levels of radon.[19] Short-term testing, taking from 2 to 90 days to complete, is the quickest way to determine whether a potential problem exists. Low-cost radon test kits are available by mail order, in hardware stores, and through other retail outlets. Since 1988, the EPA and the Office of the Surgeon General have recommended that homes below the third floor be tested for radon and that Americans test their homes every 2 years or when they move into a new home.

Lead **Lead** is a metal pollutant sometimes found in paint, batteries, drinking water, pipes, dishes with lead-based

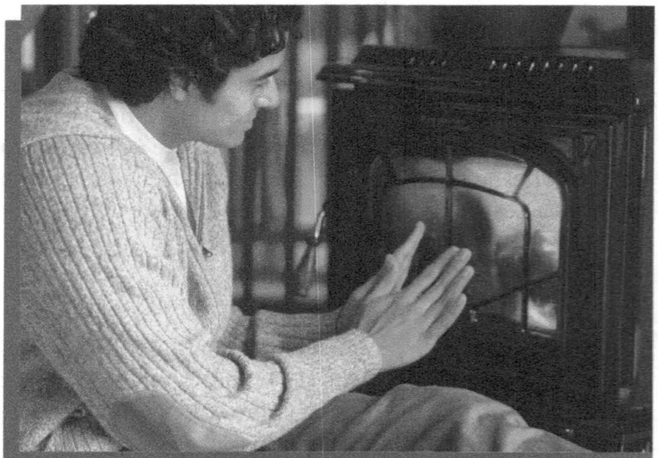

Real World People/Alamy

How can air pollution be a problem indoors?

The air within homes can be 10 to 40 times more hazardous than outside air. Indoor air pollution comes from woodstoves, furnaces, cigarette smoke, asbestos, formaldehyde, radon, lead, mold, and household chemicals.

glazes, dirt, soldered cans, and some candies made in Mexico. Recently, toys produced in China and other regions of the world have been recalled due to unsafe levels of lead in their paint.

Lead affects the circulatory, reproductive, urinary, and nervous systems and can accumulate in bone and other tissues. It is particularly detrimental to children and fetuses, and can cause birth defects, learning problems, behavioral abnormalities, and other health problems. By some estimates, as many as 25 percent of U.S. homes still have lead-based paint hazards, and an estimated 250,000 American children aged 1 to 5 have unsafe blood lead levels.[20]

Mold Molds are fungi that live both indoors and outdoors in most regions of the country. Molds produce tiny reproductive spores, which waft through the indoor and outdoor air continually. When they land on a damp spot indoors, they may begin growing and digesting whatever they are on, including wood, paper, carpet, and food. In general, molds are harmless; however, some people are sensitive or allergic to them. In such people, exposure to molds may lead to nasal stuffiness, running nose and eyes, and itchy skin. For those who are really sensitive, molds may cause fever, headache, shortness of breath, nausea, light-headedness, or severe respiratory problems.[21] For ways to reduce your exposure to mold, see the **Skills for Behavior Change** box at right.

Ozone Layer Depletion

As mentioned earlier, the ozone layer forms a protective stratum in Earth's stratosphere—the highest level of our atmosphere, located 12 to 30 miles above Earth's surface. The ozone layer in the stratosphere protects our planet and its inhabitants from ultraviolet B (UVB) radiation, a primary cause of skin cancer. Such radiation damages DNA and weakens immune systems in both humans and animals (radiation in general is discussed later in the chapter).

In the 1970s, scientists began to warn of a breakdown in the ozone layer. Instruments developed to test atmospheric contents indicated that chemicals used on Earth, especially **chlorofluorocarbons (CFCs),** were contributing to the ozone layer's rapid depletion. Chlorofluorocarbons were used as refrigerants, aerosol propellants, and cleaning solvents, and were also used in medical sterilizers, rigid foam insulation, and Styrofoam. When released into the air through spraying or outgassing, CFCs migrate into the ozone layer, where they decompose and release chlorine atoms. These atoms cause ozone molecules to break apart and levels to be depleted.

The U.S. government banned the use of aerosol sprays containing CFCs in the 1970s. The discovery of an ozone "hole" over Antarctica led to the 1987 Montreal Protocol treaty, whereby the United States and other nations agreed to further reduce the use of CFCs and other ozone-depleting chemicals. The treaty was amended in 1995 to ban CFC production in developed countries. Today, over 160 countries have signed the treaty as the international community strives to preserve the ozone layer.[22] Although the ban on CFCs is believed to be responsible for slowing the depletion of the ozone layer, some CFC replacements may also be damaging because they contribute to the enhanced greenhouse effect.

Skills for Behavior Change

Be Mold Free

* Keep the humidity level in your home between 40 and 60 percent.
* Use an air conditioner or a dehumidifier during humid months.
* Be sure your home has adequate ventilation, including exhaust fans in the kitchen and bathrooms. If there are no fans, open windows.
* Add mold inhibitors to paints before application.
* Use mold-killing products to clean bathrooms.
* Do not carpet bathrooms and basements.
* Wash rugs used in entryways and other areas where moisture can accumulate.
* Get rid of mattresses and other furniture that may have been exposed to moisture during moving or through bed-wetting or other situations where slow drying may occur.
* Dry clothing thoroughly before folding and putting in drawers or hanging in dark closets.

Global Warming

More than 100 years ago, scientists theorized that carbon dioxide emissions from the burning of fossil fuels would create a buildup of greenhouse gases in Earth's atmosphere that could have a warming effect on Earth's surface.[23] In recent years, these predictions have been supported by reports of leading international scientists in the field and accounts in the popular media, such as the documentary *An Inconvenient Truth,* all detailing startling indicators of a planet in trouble.

The *greenhouse effect* is a natural phenomenon in which greenhouse gases form a gaseous layer in the atmosphere, encircling Earth, allowing solar heat to pass through, and then trapping some of the heat close to Earth's surface, where it warms the planet. Human activities such as burning fossil fuels and land clearing have increased greenhouse gases in the atmosphere, resulting in the **enhanced greenhouse effect,** in which excess solar heat is trapped, raising the planet's temperature (see Figure 4 on the next page). According to data from the National Oceanic and Atmospheric Administration (NOAA) and the National Aeronautics and Space Administration (NASA), Earth's surface temperature has risen about 1.2 to 1.4 degrees

chlorofluorocarbons (CFCs) Chemicals that contribute to the depletion of the atmospheric ozone layer.

enhanced greenhouse effect The warming of Earth's surface as a direct result of human activities that release greenhouse gases into the atmosphere, trapping more of the sun's radiation than is normal.

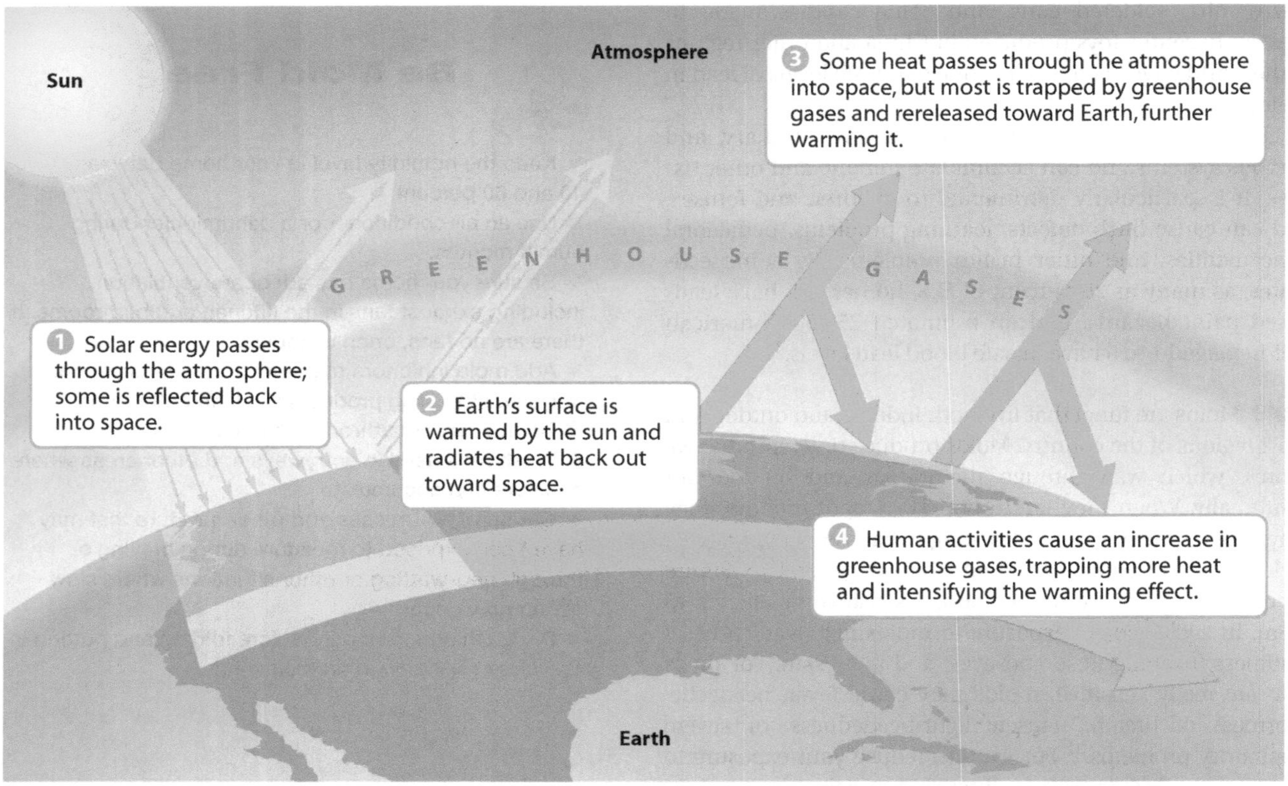

Sun
Atmosphere
Some heat passes through the atmosphere into space, but most is trapped by greenhouse gases and rereleased toward Earth, further warming it.
GREENHOUSE GASES
Solar energy passes through the atmosphere; some is reflected back into space.
Earth's surface is warmed by the sun and radiates heat back out toward space.
Human activities cause an increase in greenhouse gases, trapping more heat and intensifying the warming effect.
Earth

FIGURE 4 **The Enhanced Greenhouse Effect**
The natural greenhouse effect is responsible for making Earth habitable; it keeps the planet 33 degrees Celsius (60 degrees Fahrenheit) warmer than it would otherwise be. An increase in greenhouse gases resulting from human activities is creating the enhanced greenhouse effect, trapping more heat and causing dangerous global climate change.

Fahrenheit since 1900, with accelerated warming in the past two decades.[24] Furthermore, the consensus is that temperatures will continue to rise, perhaps by as much as 5 to 10 degrees in the next 100 years, unless immediate steps are taken to reverse the trend. Results of such a temperature increase—which might include rising sea levels (potentially flooding entire countries), glacier retreat, arctic shrinkage at the poles, altered patterns of agriculture (including changes in growing seasons and alterations of climatic zones), deforestation, drought, extreme weather events, increases in tropical diseases, changes in disease trends and patterns, loss of biological species, and economic devastation—would be catastrophic.

The greenhouse gases include carbon dioxide, nitrous oxide, methane, CFCs, and hydrocarbons. The most predominant is carbon dioxide, which accounts for 49 percent of all greenhouse gases. The United States is the greatest producer of greenhouse gases, responsible for over 22 percent of all output, and this output is expected to increase by 43 percent by 2025.[25] Rapid deforestation of the tropical rain forests of Central and South America, Africa, and southeast Asia also contributes to the rapid rise in greenhouse gases. Trees take in carbon dioxide, transform it, store the carbon for food, and release oxygen into the air. As we lose forests, at the rate of hundreds of acres per hour, we lose the capacity to dissipate carbon dioxide.

A United Nations treaty signed in Kyoto in 1997 outlined an international plan to reduce the manmade emissions responsible for climate change. The Kyoto Protocol, which came into effect in 2005, requires participating countries to reduce their emissions between 2008 and 2012 by at least 5 percent below 1990 levels.[26] More than 160 countries signed on to the Kyoto Protocol, including more than 30 industrialized countries.[27] The treaty would require the United States to reduce emissions by 33 percent, but the United States has so far refused to ratify it, stating concerns that major developing nations, including India and China, are not required to reduce emissions under the treaty.

Reducing Air Pollution and the Threat of Global Warming

Air pollution and climate change problems are rooted in our energy, transportation, and industrial practices. Clearly, we must develop comprehensive national strategies that encourage the use of renewable resources such as solar, wind, and water power. Because industrial production is a key contributor to fossil fuel emission, clean energy, green factories, improved technology, and governmental regulation are necessary for preventing climate change.

Most experts agree that reducing consumption of fossil fuels in cars and shifting to alternative fuels, improving gas mileage, and using mass transportation are crucial to air pollution reduction. Many cities have taken steps in this direction by setting high parking fees and road-usage tolls in congested areas and by imposing bans on city driving. Local governments should be encouraged to provide convenient and inexpensive public transportation and to motivate people to use it regularly.

Although stricter laws on vehicular carbon emissions and the development of new cars that operate on electricity, hydrogen, biodiesel, ethanol, or other alternative energy sources are promising, we have a long way to go to reduce fossil-fuel consumption.

Meanwhile, many U.S. communities are creating bicycle lanes and holding "bike to work" days. Scooters and other-low-energy modes of transportation are becoming increasingly popular. Some college campuses have enacted new policies allowing increased skateboard and Rollerblade use on campus. Other campuses provide scooter and bike garages to protect students from theft and vandalism and to encourage students to bring energy-efficient vehicles to campus. See the **Green Guide** on the following page for more ideas about reducing energy use on campus.

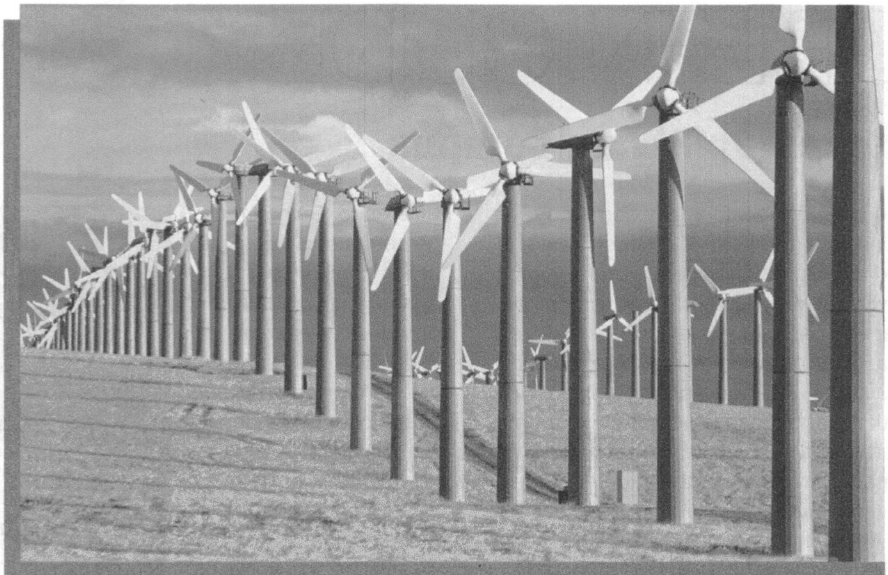

Livio Sinibaldi/Photodisc/Getty Images

How can I help prevent global warming?

Global warming is a global problem. We need to work with other nations to ensure that everyone does their part. By reducing your use of fossil fuels; using high-efficiency vehicles; and supporting increased use of renewable resources such as solar, wind, and water power, you can help combat global warming.

Water Pollution and Shortages

Seventy-five percent of Earth is covered with water in the form of oceans, seas, lakes, rivers, streams, and wetlands. Beneath the landmass are reservoirs of groundwater. We draw our drinking water from this underground source and from surface freshwater; however, just 1 percent of the world's entire water supply is available for human use. The rest is too salty, too polluted, or locked away in polar ice caps.

99% of the world's water is unavailable for human use.

We cannot take the safety of our water supply for granted. Over half the global population faces a shortage of clean water. More than 2.6 billion people, about 40 percent of the planet's population, have no access to basic sanitation or adequate toilet facilities. More than 1 billion have no access to clean water, and over 4,000 children die every day from illnesses caused by lack of safe water and sanitation.[28]

Ironically, two regions of the world that have the most severe water shortages also have some of the highest population growth rates—Africa and the Near East, which comprise 20 countries. Estimates suggest that by the year 2025, approximately 2.8 billion people will live in countries with severe water shortages. By 2050, these numbers will increase to 4 billion people in 54 countries.[29]

Considering how little water is available to meet the world's agricultural, manufacturing, community, personal, and sanitation needs, it is no wonder that clean water is a precious commodity that must not be wasted. Each U.S. resident uses an average of 1,500 gallons of water daily for all purposes—domestic consumption, recreation, energy (primarily from cooling at power plants), food production, and industry—about three times the world average.[30] The **Skills for Behavior Change** box presents simple conservation measures you can adopt to save water in your home.

Water Contamination

Any substance that gets into the soil can potentially enter the water supply. Industrial pollutants and pesticides eventually work their way into the soil, then into groundwater. Underground storage tanks for gasoline may leak. A recent survey by a group of U.S. Geological Survey researchers discovered the presence of low levels of many chemical compounds in a network of 139 targeted streams across the United States. Steroids, prescription and nonprescription drugs, hormones, insect repellent, and wastewater compounds were all detected.[31]

Tap water in the United States is among the safest in the world. The Safe Drinking Water Act (SDWA) is the main federal

GREEN GUIDE

Sustainability on Campus

You are moving into a new dorm room, along with hundreds of other students, and are excited to decorate, meet your new roommate, and make your room the place to be. As a student, this is also your chance to make a positive difference and minimize your ecological footprint. Your actions, and those of your friends, roommates, and school can have a lasting impact on your life and the future of the environment.

More and more universities and colleges are recognizing that students want to attend schools that reflect their values and beliefs around sustainable movements. Several organizations publish annual rankings of the "greenest" schools, including the College Sustainability Report Card and the Sierra Club's "Cool Schools" list (see table below).

The green sustainability movement is picking up steam and turning ideas into realities. You do not need to be an environmental science major or a self-proclaimed "hippie" to make a difference. Going green on campus can be part of the goal for your apartment, your sorority or fraternity, or your residence hall.

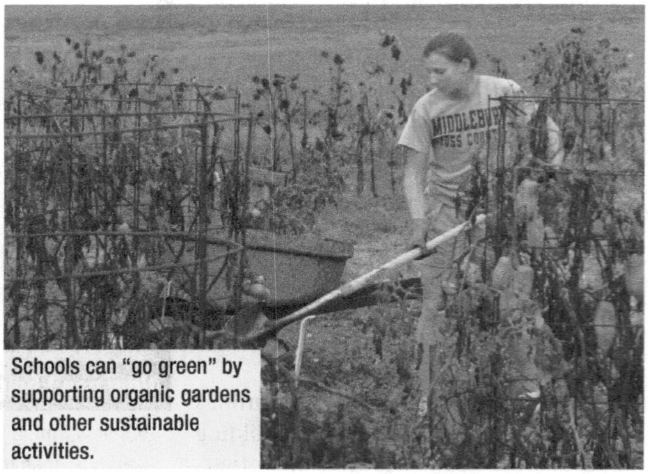

Schools can "go green" by supporting organic gardens and other sustainable activities.

Ari Joseph/Middlebury College

Start making a positive impact by turning off lights when you leave a room or bathroom. See if your residence has a way of minimizing the amount of lights used on a floor. Sometimes lights might be connected through several outlets, and turning off a strand might still provide enough light but minimize the amount of energy consumed. Find out whether your administration supports the use of CFLs—compact fluorescent lights—which are typically longer-lasting energy-conserving bulbs that give off the same amount of light as an incandescent bulb at a fraction of the energy used. Next time you go to the store, buy a couple for your new lighting fixtures and start making a positive impact.

When buying a new appliance, look for the Energy Star logo, indicating that the appliance meets energy-efficiency standards set by the EPA and U.S. Department of Energy. Adjust the controls on your new appliances so they do not run at full power all the time. This will help curb unnecessary energy usage and lower the cost of your monthly energy bills. Better yet, consider unplugging items such as iPods, TVs, laptops, desktop computers, hair dryers, and cell phones, all of which still consume energy when not in use.

So what about your computer? While in school, you will probably use it for everything from checking your e-mail to writing your papers. Fortunately, you have many options to help you make better energy-conserving choices when it comes to your computer use. When buying your computer, always look for the Energy Star logo. (Go to www.energystar.gov/index.cfm?c=news.nr_dormroom&Layout=print for more information about creating an Energy Star dorm room.)

Consider buying a laptop rather than a desktop computer, as laptops use less energy. You can also set your computer to sleep or hibernate mode when not in use. When you look for a printer, choose one that prints double-sided, which will help reduce the amount of paper you use. Do not print unnecessary documents, and make sure you recycle used paper—don't just throw it away.

The Ten Most Eco-Enlightened U.S. Colleges and Universities*

1.	University of Colorado at Boulder
2.	University of Washington at Seattle
3.	Middlebury College (VT)
4.	University of Vermont
5.	College of the Atlantic (ME)
6.	Evergreen State College (WA)
7.	University of California at Santa Cruz
8.	University of California at Berkeley
9.	University of California at Los Angeles
10.	Oberlin College (OH)

*As ranked by the Sierra Club in their third annual Cool Schools list.

Source: Sierra Club, "Cool Schools: Third Annual List," *Sierra Magazine* September 2009, www.sierraclub.org/sierra/200909/coolschools.

Skills for Behavior Change

Waste Less Water!

IN THE KITCHEN

* Turn off the tap while washing dishes.
* Check faucets and pipes for leaks. Leaky faucets can waste more than 3,000 gallons of water each year.
* Equip faucets with aerators to reduce water use by 4 percent.
* Run dishwashers only when they are full, and use the energy-saving mode.

IN THE LAUNDRY ROOM

* Wash only full laundry loads.
* Upgrade to a high-efficiency washing machine to use 30 percent less water per load.

IN THE BATHROOM

* Detect and fix leaks. A leaky toilet can waste about 200 gallons of water every day.
* Take showers instead of baths and limit showers to the time it takes to lather up and rinse off.
* Replace old showerheads with new efficient models that use 60 percent less water per minute.
* Turn off the tap while brushing your teeth to save up to 8 gallons of water per day.
* Replace your old toilet with a high-efficiency model that uses 60 percent less water per flush.

law that ensures the quality of Americans' drinking water. Under SDWA, the EPA sets standards for drinking water quality and oversees the states, localities, and water suppliers who implement those standards. Cities and municipalities have strict policies and procedures governing water treatment, filtration, and disinfection to screen out pathogens and microorganisms.

Congress has coined two terms, *point source* and *nonpoint source,* to describe the general sources of water pollution. **Point source pollutants** enter a waterway at a specific location through a pipe, ditch, culvert, or other conduit. The two major sources of point source pollution are sewage treatment plants and industrial facilities. **Nonpoint source pollutants**—commonly known as *runoff* and *sedimentation*—drain or seep into waterways from broad areas of land rather than through a discrete conduit. Nonpoint source pollution results from a variety of human land use practices. It includes soil erosion and sedimentation, construction wastes, pesticide and fertilizer runoff, urban street runoff, acid mine drainage, wastes from engineering projects, leakage from septic tanks, and sewage sludge. Among the pollutants causing the most concern and the greatest potential harm are the following:

- **Gasoline and petroleum products.** There are more than 2 million underground storage tanks for gasoline and petroleum products in the United States, most of which are located at gasoline filling stations. One-quarter of them are thought to be leaking after years of corrosion.
- **Chemical contaminants.** *Organic solvents* are chemicals designed to dissolve grease and oil. These extremely toxic substances are used to clean clothing, painting equipment, plastics, and metal parts. Many household products (e.g., stain and spot removers, degreasers, drain cleaners, septic system cleaners, and paint removers) also contain these toxic chemicals. Organic solvents work their way into the water supply in different ways. Consumers often dump leftover products into the toilet or into street drains. Industries pour leftovers into large barrels, which are then buried. After a while, the chemicals eat through the barrels and leach into groundwater.
- **Polychlorinated biphenyls.** Fire resistant and stable at high temperatures, **polychlorinated biphenyls (PCBs)** were used for many years as insulating materials in high-voltage electrical equipment, such as transformers and older fluorescent lights. The human body does not excrete ingested PCBs but rather stores them in fatty tissues and the liver (i.e., they *bioaccumulate*). Exposure to PCBs is associated with birth defects, cancer, and various skin problems. The manufacture of PCBs was discontinued in the United States in 1977, but approximately 500 million pounds of them have been dumped into landfills and waterways, where they continue to pose an environmental threat.[32]
- **Dioxins. Dioxins** are chlorinated hydrocarbons found in herbicides (chemicals that are used to kill vegetation) and are produced during certain industrial processes. Dioxins have the ability to bioaccumulate and are much more toxic than PCBs. Long-term effects include possible damage to the immune system and increased risk of infections and cancer. Exposure to high concentrations of PCBs or dioxins for a short period of time can also have severe consequences, including nausea, vomiting, diarrhea, painful rashes and sores, and chloracne, an ailment in which the skin develops hard, black, painful pimples that may never go away.
- **Pesticides. Pesticides** are chemicals that are designed to kill insects, rodents, plants, and fungi. There are over 1,055 active ingredients sold as pesticides, marketed as thousands of products sold in stores throughout the world.[33] Americans use more than 1.2 billion pounds of pesticides each year, but only 10 percent actually reach the targeted organisms. The other 90 percent settle on the land and in our air and water. Pesticides evaporate readily, often being dispersed by winds over a large area or carried to the sea. This is particularly true in tropical regions, where many farmers use pesticides heavily and the climate promotes their rapid release into the

point source pollutants Pollutants that enter waterways at a specific point.

nonpoint source pollutants Pollutants that run off or seep into waterways from broad areas of land.

polychlorinated biphenyls (PCBs) Toxic chemicals that were once used as insulating materials in high-voltage electrical equipment.

dioxins Highly toxic chlorinated hydrocarbons contained in herbicides and produced during certain industrial processes.

pesticides Chemicals that kill pests, such as insects or rodents.

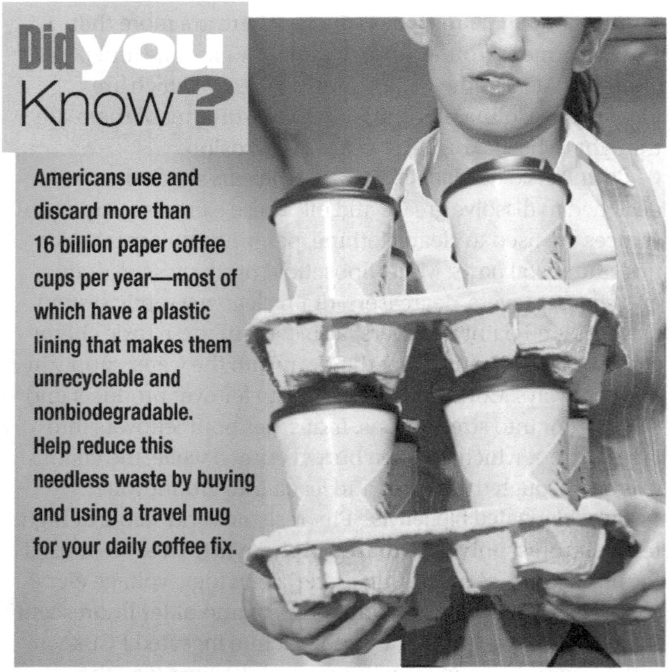

Did you Know?

Americans use and discard more than 16 billion paper coffee cups per year—most of which have a plastic lining that makes them unrecyclable and nonbiodegradable. Help reduce this needless waste by buying and using a travel mug for your daily coffee fix.

Image Source/Corbis

atmosphere. Pesticide residues cling to fresh fruits and vegetables and can accumulate in the body when people eat these items. Potential hazards associated with exposure to pesticides include birth defects, liver and kidney damage, and nervous system disorders.

- **Lead.** Lead can sometimes leach into tapwater from lead pipes or water lines, usually in older homes. The EPA has issued new standards to dramatically reduce the levels of lead in drinking water. The new rules stipulate that tap water lead values must not exceed 15 parts per billion (ppb). (The previous standard allowed an average lead level of 50 ppb.) If lead is present in your home's water, you can reduce your risk by running tap water for several minutes before taking a drink or cooking with it. This flushes out water that has been standing overnight in lead-contaminated lines.

municipal solid waste (MSW) Solid waste such as durable goods; nondurable goods; containers and packaging; food waste; yard waste; and miscellaneous waste from residential, commercial, institutional, and industrial sources.

Land Pollution

Much of the waste that ends up polluting the water starts out polluting the land. The more people there are on the planet, the more waste they create, and the more pressure is put on the land to accommodate increasing amounts of refuse, much of which is nonbiodegradable, and some of which is directly harmful to living organisms.

Solid Waste

Each day, every person in the United States generates more than 4.62 pounds of **municipal solid waste (MSW)** more commonly known as trash or garbage—containers and packaging; discarded food; yard debris; and refuse from residential, commercial, institutional, and industrial sources (Figure 5).[34] The total comes to over 254 million tons of MSW each year.[35] Although experts believe that up to 90 percent of our trash is recyclable, we still fall far short of this goal with respect to most types of trash (Figure 6). Currently in the United States, 32 percent of all MSW is recovered and recycled or composted, 14 percent is burned at combustion facilities, and the remaining 54 percent is disposed of in landfills.[36]

68% of all MSW in the United States is burned or buried in landfills.

The number of landfills in the United States has actually decreased in the past decade, but their sheer mass has increased. Many people worry that we are rapidly losing our ability to dispose of all of the waste we create. As communities run out of landfill space, it is becoming more common to haul garbage out to sea to dump, where it contaminates ocean ecosystems, or to ship it to landfills in developing countries, where it becomes someone else's problem. In today's throwaway society, we need to become aware of the amount of waste we generate every day and to look for ways to recycle, reuse, and—most desirable of all—reduce what we consume.

Communities, businesses, and individuals can adopt several strategies to control the growing MSW:

- **Source reduction** (*waste prevention*) involves altering the design, manufacture, or use of products and materials to reduce the amount and toxicity of what gets thrown away.

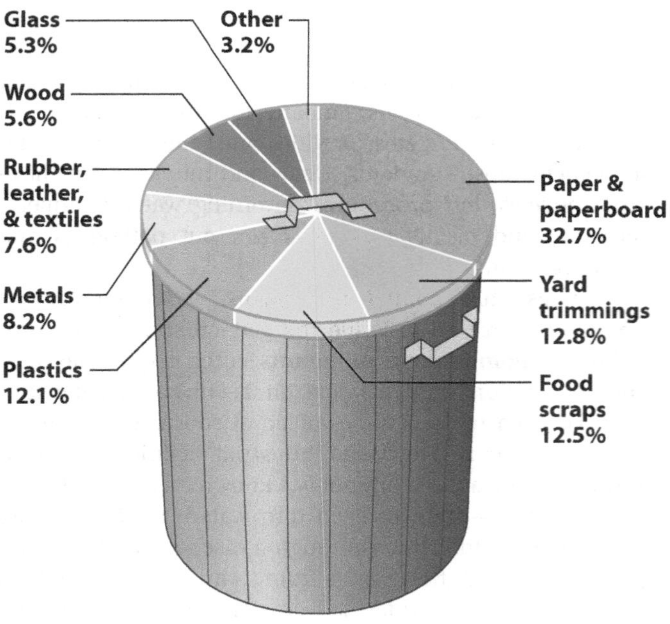

FIGURE 5 **What's in Our Trash?**

Source: Data are from U.S. Environmental Protection Agency, *Municipal Solid Waste Generation, Recycling, and Disposal in the United States: Facts and Figures for 2007,* EPA-503-F-08-018 (Washington, DC: EPA, 2008), www.epa.gov/epawaste/nonhaz/municipal/msw99.htm.

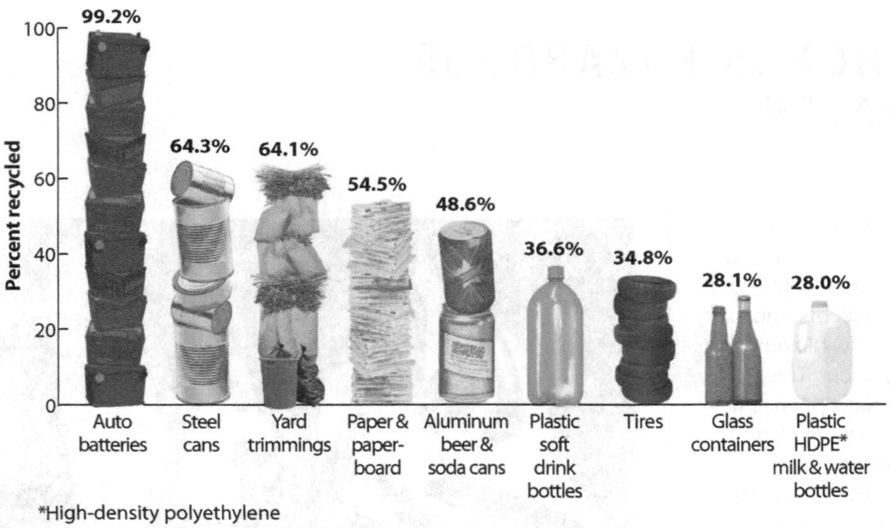

*High-density polyethylene

FIGURE 6 **How Much Do We Recycle?**

Source: Data are from U.S. Environmental Protection Agency, *Municipal Solid Waste Generation, Recycling, and Disposal in the United States: Facts and Figures for 2007,* EPA-530-F-08-018 (Washington, DC: EPA, 2008), www.epa.gov/epawaste/nonhaz/municipal/msw99.htm.

The most effective MSW-reducing strategy is to prevent waste from ever being generated in the first place.

- **Recycling** involves sorting, collecting, and processing materials to be reused in manufacturing new products. This process diverts items such as paper, glass, plastic, and metals from the waste stream.
- **Composting** involves collecting organic waste, such as food scraps and yard trimmings, and allowing it to decompose with the help of microorganisms (mainly bacteria and fungi). This process produces a humus-like substance that is suitable for use in gardens and for soil enhancement.
- **Combustion with energy recovery** typically involves the use of boilers and industrial furnaces to generate energy and material recovery or incinerators, which primarily destroy waste but can also recover waste for material use.

what do you think?

Do you know anyone who throws items away rather than recycles them? ● What do you think motivates their behavior? ● What might encourage them to recycle more than they do now?

Hazardous Waste

Hazardous waste is defined as waste with properties that make it capable of harming human health or the environment. In 1980, the *Comprehensive Environmental Response and Liability Act,* known as the **Superfund,** was enacted to provide funds for cleaning up hazardous waste dump sites that endanger public health and land. This fund is financed through taxes on the chemical and petroleum industries (87%) and through general federal tax revenues (13%). To date, 32,500 potentially hazardous waste sites have been identified across the nation, and 90 percent of these have been cleared or "recovered." Currently there are 50 priority sites being actively cleared, with thousands more sites, costing billions of dollars, possible for future clean up.[37] Newer technologies for cleanup are being investigated, including nanotechnologies that could reduce these costs by as much as 75 percent.

The large number of hazardous waste dump sites in the United States indicates the severity of our toxic chemical problem. American manufacturers generate more than 1 ton of chemical waste per person per year (approximately 275 million tons). Many wastes are now banned from land disposal or are being treated to reduce their toxicity before they become part of land disposal sites. The EPA has developed protective requirements for land disposal facilities, such as double liners, detection systems for substances that may leach into groundwater, and groundwater monitoring systems.

Radiation

Radiation is energy that travels in waves or particles. There are many different types of radiation, ranging from radio waves to gamma rays, all making up the electromagnetic spectrum. Exposure to radiation is an inescapable part of life on this planet, and only some of it poses a threat to human health.

Nonionizing Radiation

Nonionizing radiation is radiation at the lower end of the electromagnetic spectrum. This radiation moves in relatively long wavelengths and has enough energy to move atoms around, or cause them to vibrate, but not enough to remove electrons or alter molecular structure. Examples of nonionizing radiation are radio waves, TV signals, microwaves, infrared waves, and visible light.

Concerns have been raised about the safety of the radio frequency waves generated by cell phones, discussed in the **Consumer Health** box on the next page. The potential for exploiting fearful consumers is probably greater than the real hazard to health from this nonionizing form of exposure.

Ionizing Radiation

Ionizing radiation is caused by the release of particles and electromagnetic rays from atomic

hazardous waste Waste that, because of its toxic properties, poses a hazard to humans or to the environment.

Superfund Fund established under the Comprehensive Environmental Response Compensation and Liability Act to be used for cleaning up toxic waste dumps.

nonionizing radiation Electromagnetic waves having relatively long wavelengths and enough energy to move atoms around, or cause them to vibrate.

ionizing radiation Electromagnetic waves and particles having short wavelengths and energy high enough to ionize atoms.

CONSUMER HEALTH

ARE CELL PHONES HAZARDOUS TO YOUR HEALTH?

Although everyone today seems to have a cell phone, most users are unaware that their phone may pose a health risk. Depending on how close the cell phone antenna is to the head, as much as 60 percent of the microwave radiation emitted by the phone may actually penetrate the area around the head, some of it reaching an inch to an inch-and-a-half into the brain.

At high power levels, radio-frequency energy (the energy used in cell phones) can rapidly heat biological tissue and cause damage. However, cell phones operate at power levels well below the level at which such heating occurs. Many countries, including the United States and most European nations, use standards set by the Federal Communications Commission (FCC) for radio-frequency energy based on research by several scientific groups. These groups identified a whole-body *specific absorption rate (SAR)* value for exposure to radio-frequency energy. Four watts per kilogram was identified as a threshold level of exposure at which harmful biological effects may occur. The FCC requires wireless phones to comply with a safety limit of 1.6 watts per kg.

The U.S. Food and Drug Administration, the World Health Organization, and other major health agencies agree that the research to date has not shown radio-frequency energy emitted from cell phones to be harmful. However, they also point to the need for more research, because cell phones have only been in widespread use for less than two decades, and no long-term studies have been done to determine that cell phones are risk free. Three large studies have compared cell phone use among brain cancer patients and individuals free of brain cancer, finding no correlation between cell phone use and brain tumors. However, preliminary results from smaller, well-designed studies have continued to raise questions.

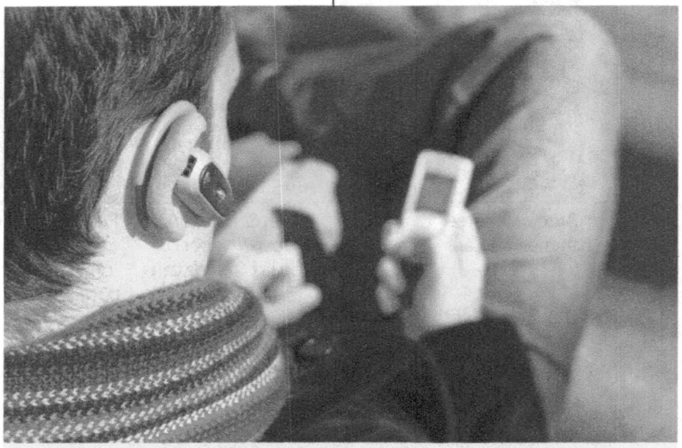

Lawrence Lawry/Getty Images

A hands-free device lets you keep your phone—and any radio-frequency energy it may emit—away from your head.

To lower any potential risk of problems related to cell phone use, limit your cell phone usage, and purchase a hands-free device that keeps the phone farther from your head. Use landlines whenever possible, or send a text message or e-mail rather than talking on the phone. In addition, check the SAR level of your phone (for instructions, see www.fcc.gov/cgb/sar). Purchase one with a lower level if yours is near the FCC limit.

Sources: Committee on Identification of Research Needs Relating to Potential Biological or Adverse Health Effects of Wireless Communications Devices, National Research Council (Washington, DC: National Academies Press, 2008); American Cancer Society, "Cellular Phones," 2008, www.cancer.org/docroot/PED/content/PED_1_3X_Cellular_Phones.asp.

nuclei during the normal process of disintegration. This type of radiation has enough energy to remove electrons from the atoms it passes through. Some naturally occurring elements, such as uranium, emit ionizing radiation. The sun is another source of ionizing radiation, in the form of high-frequency ultraviolet rays—those against which the ozone layer protects us.

radiation absorbed doses (rads) Units that measure exposure to radioactivity.

Reactions to radiation differ from person to person. Exposure is measured in **radiation absorbed doses,** or **rads** (also called *roentgens*). Radiation can cause damage at dosages as low as 100 to 200 rads. At this level, signs of radiation sickness include nausea, diarrhea, fatigue, anemia, sore throat, and hair loss. At 350 to 500 rads, these symptoms become more severe, and death may result because the radiation hinders bone marrow production of the white blood cells we need to protect us from disease. Dosages above 600 to 700 rads are invariably fatal.

Recommended maximum "safe" dosages range from 0.5 to 5 rads per year. Approximately 50 percent of the radiation to which we are exposed comes from natural sources, such as building materials. Another 45 percent comes from medical and dental X rays. The remaining 5 percent is nonionizing radiation that comes from such sources as computer monitors, microwave ovens, television sets, and radar screens. Most of us are exposed to far less radiation than the safe maximum dosage per year. The effects of long-term exposure to relatively low levels of radiation are unknown. Some scientists believe that such exposure can cause lung cancer, leukemia, skin cancer, bone cancer, and skeletal deformities.

Nuclear Power Plants

Although nuclear power plants account for less than 1 percent of the total radiation to which we are exposed, the number of plants may increase in the next decade. Proponents of nuclear energy believe that it is a safe and efficient way to generate electricity. Initial costs of building nuclear power plants are high, but actual power generation is relatively inexpensive. A 1,000-megawatt reactor produces enough energy for 650,000 homes and saves 420 million gallons of fossil fuels each year. In some areas where nuclear power plants were decommissioned, electricity bills tripled when power companies turned to hydroelectric or fossil fuel sources to generate electricity. Nuclear reactors discharge fewer carbon oxides into the air than fossil fuel–powered generators. Advocates believe that converting to nuclear power could help slow global warming.

The advantages of nuclear energy must be weighed against the disadvantages. Currently, disposal of nuclear waste is extremely problematic. In addition, a reactor core meltdown could pose serious threats to a plant's immediate environment and to the world in general. A **nuclear meltdown** occurs when the temperature in the core of a nuclear reactor increases enough to melt both the nuclear fuel and the containment vessel that holds it. Most modern facilities seal their reactors and containment vessels in concrete buildings with pools of cold water on the bottom. If a meltdown occurs, the building and the pool are supposed to prevent the escape of radioactivity.

One serious nuclear accident in particular contributed to a steep decline in public support for nuclear energy: the 1986 reactor core fire and explosion at the Chernobyl nuclear power plant in Russia, which killed 48 people, hospitalized another 200, and led officials to evacuate towns near the plant. Some medical workers estimate that the eventual death toll from radiation-induced cancers related to the Chernobyl incident topped 100,000.

Noise Pollution

Our bodies have definite physiological responses to noise, and it can become a source of physical and mental distress. Sounds are measured in decibels. A sound with a decibel level of 110 is 10 times louder than one at 100 decibels (dB). A jet takeoff from 200 feet has a noise level of approximately 140 dB, whereas the human voice in normal conversation has a level of about 60 dB (Figure 7). Short-term exposure to loud noise reduces productivity and concentration and may affect mental and emotional health. Symptoms of noise-related distress include disturbed sleep patterns, headaches, and tension. Prolonged exposure to loud noise can lead to hearing loss; the risks depend on both the decibel level and the length of exposure.

Unfortunately, despite increasing awareness that noise pollution is more than just a nuisance, noise control programs have received low budgetary priority in the United States. According to the National Institute for Occupational Safety and Health, 30 million Americans are exposed to hazardous noise at work, and 10 million suffer from permanent hearing loss.[38] Clearly, to protect your hearing, you must take it upon yourself to avoid voluntary and involuntary exposure to excessive noise. Playing stereos in your car and home at reasonable levels, keeping the volume down on your iPod, wearing earplugs when you use power equipment, and establishing barriers such as closed windows between you and noise will help keep your hearing intact.

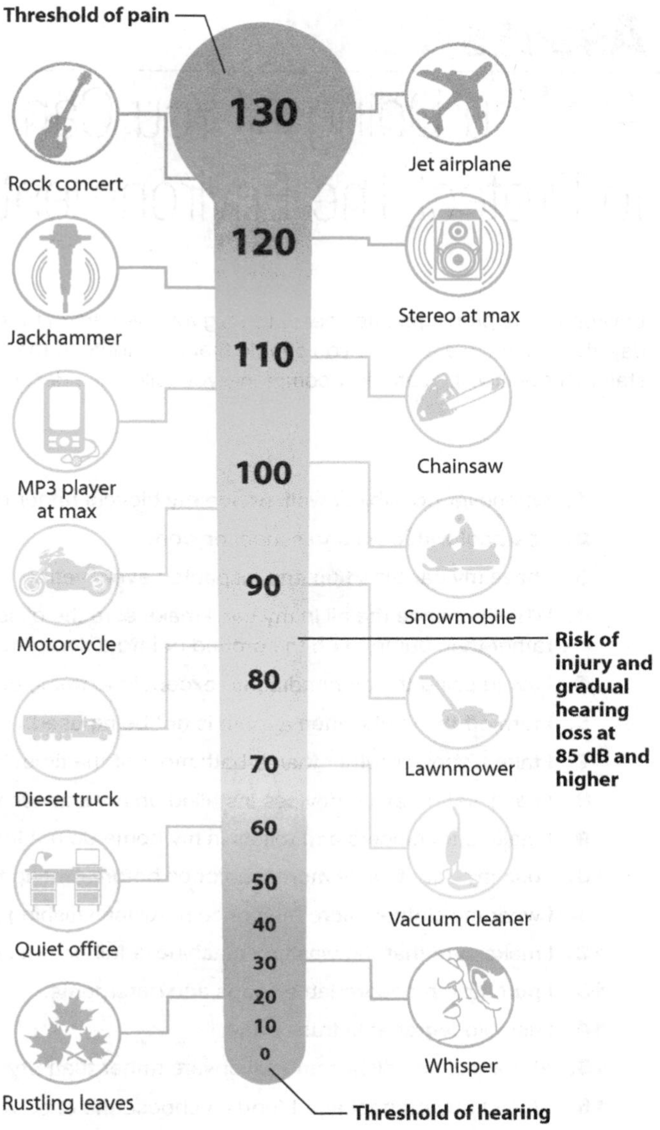

FIGURE 7 **Noise Levels of Various Sounds (dB)**

Decibels increase logarithmically, so each increase of 10 db represents a tenfold increase in loudness.

Source: Adapted from National Institute on Deafness and Other Communication Disorders, "How Loud Is Too Loud? Bookmark," 2006, www.nidcd.nih.gov/health/hearing/ruler.asp.

nuclear meltdown An accident that results when the temperature in the core of a nuclear reactor increases enough to melt the nuclear fuel and the containment vessel housing it.

Assess yourself

Are You Doing All You Can to Protect The Environment?

PEARSON myhealthlab

Fill out this assessment online at www.pearsonhighered.com/myhealthlab or www.pearsonhighered.com/donatelle.

Environmental problems often seem too big for one person to make a difference. Each day, though, there are things you can do that contribute to the planet's health. For each statement below, indicate how commonly you follow the described behavior.

	Always	Usually	Sometimes	Never
1. Whenever possible, I walk or ride my bicycle rather than drive a car.	1	2	3	4
2. I carpool with others to school or work.	1	2	3	4
3. I have my car tuned up and inspected every year.	1	2	3	4
4. When I change the oil in my car, I make sure the oil is properly recycled, rather than dumped on the ground or into a floor drain.	1	2	3	4
5. I avoid using the air conditioner except in extreme conditions.	1	2	3	4
6. I turn off the lights when a room is not being used.	1	2	3	4
7. I take a shower rather than a bath most of the time.	1	2	3	4
8. I have water-saving devices installed on my shower, toilet, and sinks.	1	2	3	4
9. I make sure faucets and toilets in my home do not leak.	1	2	3	4
10. I use my bath towels more than once before putting them in the wash.	1	2	3	4
11. I wear my clothes more than once between washings when possible.	1	2	3	4
12. I make sure that the washing machine is full before I wash a load of clothes.	1	2	3	4
13. I purchase biodegradable soaps and detergents.	1	2	3	4
14. I use biodegradable trash bags.	1	2	3	4
15. At home, I use dishes and silverware rather than Styrofoam or plastic.	1	2	3	4
16. When I buy prepackaged foods, I choose the ones with the least packaging.	1	2	3	4
17. I do not subscribe to newspapers and magazines that I can view online.	1	2	3	4
18. I do not use a hair dryer.	1	2	3	4
19. I recycle plastic bags that I get when I bring something home from the store.	1	2	3	4
20. I don't run water continuously when washing the dishes, shaving, or brushing my teeth.	1	2	3	4
21. I use unbleached or recycled paper.	1	2	3	4
22. I use both sides of printer paper and other paper when possible.	1	2	3	4
23. If I have items I do not want to use anymore, I donate them to charity so someone else can use them.	1	2	3	4
24. I carry a reusable mug for my coffee or tea and have it filled rather than using a new paper cup each time I buy a hot beverage	1	2	3	4
25. I carry and use a refillable water bottle rather than frequently buying bottled water.	1	2	3	4
26. I clean up after myself while enjoying the outdoors (picnicking, camping, etc.).	1	2	3	4
27. I volunteer for cleanup days in the community in which I live.	1	2	3	4
28. I consider candidates' positions on environmental issues before casting my vote.	1	2	3	4

christopher conrad/iStockphoto

For Further Thought

Review your scores. Are your responses mostly 1s and 2s? If not, what actions can you take to become more environmentally responsible? Are there ways to help the environment on this list that you had not thought of before? Are there behaviors not on the list that you are already doing?

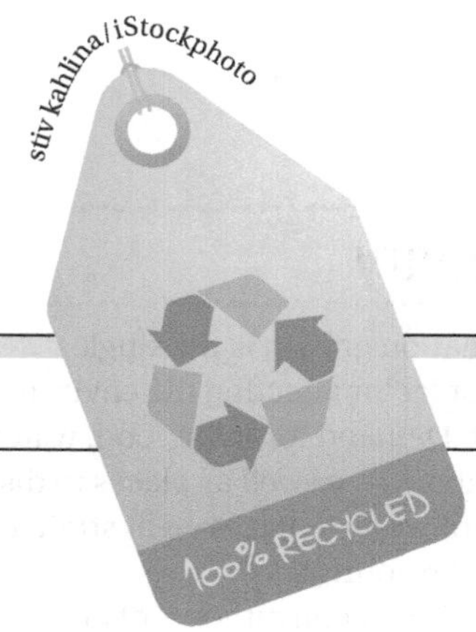

stiv kahlina/iStockphoto

YOUR PLAN FOR CHANGE

The Assess yourself activity gave you the chance to look at your behavior and consider ways to conserve energy, save water, reduce waste, and otherwise help protect the planet. Now that you have considered these results, you can take steps to become more environmentally responsible.

Today, you can:

◯ Find out how much energy you are using. Visit www.carbonfund.org, www.carbonoffsets.org, or www.greatestplanet.org to find out what your carbon footprint is and to learn about projects you can support to offset your own emissions and energy usage. New carbon offset programs and organizations are popping up all the time, so watch for other opportunities to counter your carbon usage.

◯ Reduce the amount of paper waste in your mailbox. You can stop junk mail, such as credit card offers and unwanted catalogs, by visiting the Direct Marketing Association's Mail Preference Service site at www.dmachoice.org. You can also call 1-888-5 OPT OUT to put an end to unwanted mail. In addition, the website www.catalogchoice.org is a free service that lets you decline paper catalogs you no longer want to receive.

Within the next 2 weeks, you can:

◯ Look into joining an on-campus environmental group, attending an environmental campus event, or taking an environmental science course.

◯ Take part in a local cleanup day or recycling drives. These can be fun opportunities to meet like-minded people while benefiting the planet.

By the end of the semester, you can:

◯ Start a compost pile for all your organic waste. You don't need a yard to do this; the EPA provides information on setting up an indoor compost bin at www.epa.gov/epawaste/conserve/rrr/composting/by_compost.htm.

◯ Make a habit of recycling everything you can rather than adding things to the trash. Find out what items can be recycled in your neighborhood and designate a box or trash can in your apartment or dorm to hold recyclable materials—cans, bottles, newspapers, junk mail, and so on—until you can carry them out to the curbside bins or a drop-off center.

◯ Work to influence the environment on a larger scale. Take part in an environmental activism group on campus or in your community. Listen carefully to what political candidates say about the environment. Let your legislators know how you feel about environmental issues and that you will vote according to their record on the issues.

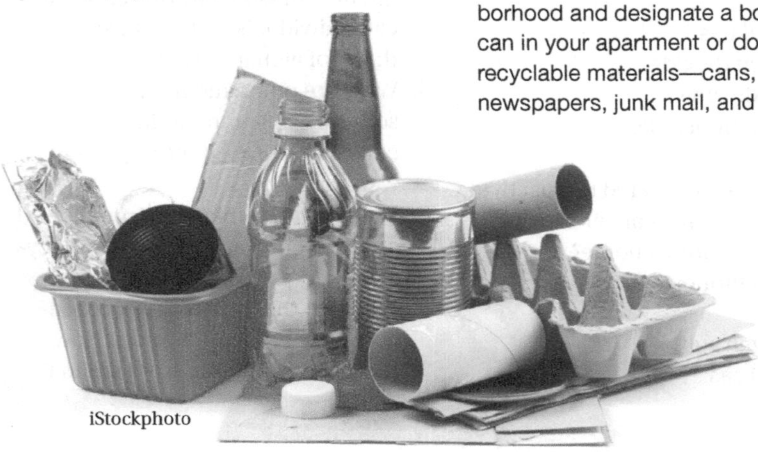

iStockphoto

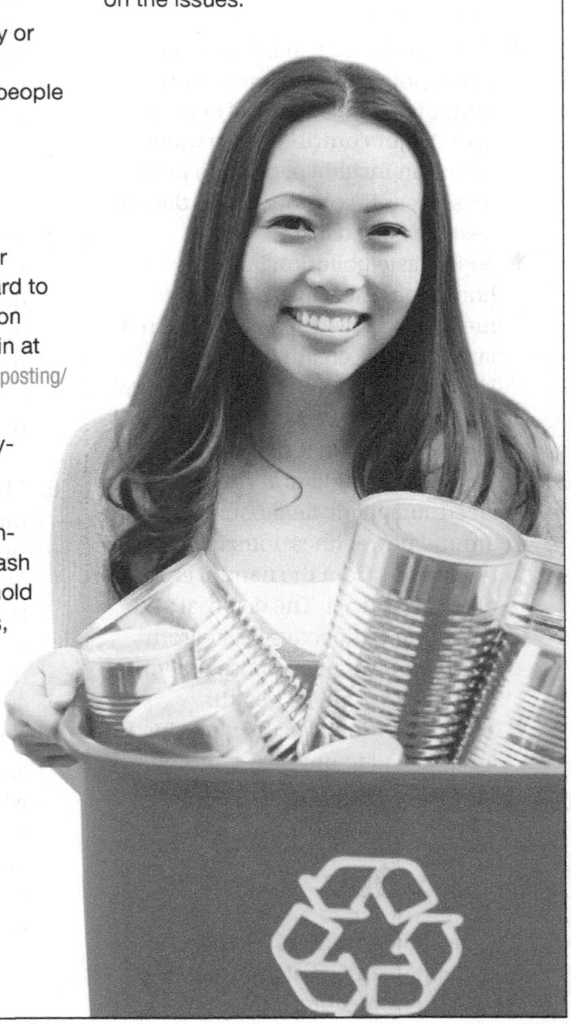

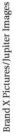

Brand X Pictures/Jupiter Images

Summary

- Population growth is the single largest factor affecting the environment. Demand for more food, water, and energy—as well as places to dispose of waste—places great strain on Earth's resources.
- The primary constituents of air pollution are sulfur dioxide, particulate matter, carbon monoxide, nitrogen dioxide, ozone, carbon dioxide, and hydrocarbons. Indoor air pollution is caused primarily by tobacco smoke, woodstove smoke, furnace emissions, asbestos, formaldehyde, radon, lead, and mold. Pollution is depleting Earth's protective ozone layer and contributing to global warming by enhancing the greenhouse effect.
- Water pollution can be caused by either point sources (direct entry) or nonpoint sources (runoff or seepage). Major contributors to water pollution include petroleum products, organic solvents, PCBs, dioxins, pesticides, and lead.
- Solid waste pollution includes household trash, plastics, glass, metal products, and paper. Limited landfill space creates problems. Hazardous waste is toxic; improper disposal creates health hazards for people in surrounding communities.
- Nonionizing radiation comes from electromagnetic fields, such as those around power lines. Ionizing radiation results from the natural erosion of atomic nuclei. The disposal and storage of radioactive waste from nuclear power plants pose potential problems for public health.
- Noise pollution can affect productivity, and lead to physical symptoms including hearing loss.

Pop Quiz

1. The United States is responsible for what percentage of total global resource consumption?
   a. 10 percent
   b. 25 percent
   c. 50 percent
   d. 70 percent

2. The single biggest influence on zero population growth is
   a. income.
   b. gender.
   c. education.
   d. ethnicity.

3. One possible source of indoor air pollution is a gas present in some carpets called
   a. lead.
   b. asbestos.
   c. radon.
   d. formaldehyde.

4. What substance separates into stringy fibers, embeds itself in lungs, and causes mesothelioma?
   a. asbestos
   b. particulate matter
   c. radon
   d. formaldehyde

5. The terms *point source* and *nonpoint source* are used to describe the two general sources of
   a. water pollution.
   b. air pollution.
   c. noise pollution.
   d. ozone depletion.

6. The air pollutant that originates primarily from motor vehicle emissions is
   a. particulates.
   b. nitrogen dioxide.
   c. sulfur dioxide.
   d. carbon monoxide.

7. Which gas is considered radioactive and could become cancer causing when it seeps into a home?
   a. carbon monoxide
   b. radon
   c. hydrogen sulfide
   d. natural gas

8. The phenomenon that creates a barrier to protect us from the sun's harmful ultraviolet radiation rays is
   a. photochemical smog.
   b. ozone layer.
   c. gray air smog.
   d. greenhouse effect.

9. Intensity (exposure) to sound is measured in
   a. foot candles.
   b. noise volume.
   c. hertz.
   d. decibels.

10. Some herbicides contain toxic substances called
    a. THMs.
    b. PCPs.
    c. dioxins.
    d. PCBs.

Answers to Chapter Review Questions

1. b; 2. c; 3. d; 4. a; 5. a;
6. d; 7. b; 8. b; 9. d; 10. c

Think about It!

1. How are the rapid increases in global population and consumption of resources related? Is population control the best solution? Why or why not?
2. What are the primary sources of air pollution? What can be done to reduce air pollution?
3. What are the causes and consequences of global warming? What can individuals do to reduce the threat of global warming?
4. What are point and nonpoint sources of water pollution? What can be done to reduce or prevent water pollution?
5. How do you think communities and governments could encourage recycling efforts in the United States?
6. What are the physiological consequences of noise pollution? How can you lessen your exposure to it?

Accessing Your Health on the Internet

The following websites explore further topics and issues related to personal health. For links to the websites below, visit the Companion Website for *Health: The Basics*, Green Edition at www.pearsonhighered.com/donatelle.

1. *Environmental Literacy Council.* This website is an excellent source of information about environmental issues in general. Topics range from how the ozone layer works to why the rain forests are important ecosystems. www.enviroliteracy.org
2. *Environmental Protection Agency (EPA).* The EPA is the government agency responsible for overseeing environmental regulation and protection issues in the United States. www.epa.gov
3. *National Center for Environmental Health (NCEH).* This site provides information on a wide variety of environmental health issues, including a series of helpful fact sheets. www.cdc.gov/nceh
4. *National Environmental Health Association (NEHA).* This organization provides educational resources and opportunities for environmental health professionals. www.neha.org

References

1. R. Caplan, *Our Earth, Ourselves* (New York: Bantam, 1990), 247.
2. R. H. Friis, *Essentials of Environmental Health* (Boston: Jones and Bartlett, 2007), 7.
3. Population Reference Bureau, "2009 World Population Data Sheet," www.prb.org/Publications/Datasheets/2009/2009wpds.aspx.
4. United Nations, *Global Environment Outlook: Environment for Development (GEO-4)* (United Nations Environment Programme, 2007), www.unep.org/geo/geo4/media.
5. U.S. Census Bureau, "U.S. and World Population Clocks," 2008, www.census.gov/main/www/popclock.html.
6. Ibid.
7. V. Markham, "U.S. Population, Energy and Climate Change," 2009, Center for Environment and Population, www.cepnet.org/documents/USPopulationEnergyandClimateChangeReportCEP.pdf.
8. Ibid.
9. Ibid.
10. Ibid.
11. U.S. Environmental Protection Agency, "Mobile Source Emissions—Past, Present and Future," 2008, www.epa.gov/otaq/invntory/overview/pollutants/index.htm.
12. American Lung Association, "State of the Air. 2009 Health Risks Overview," www.stateoftheair.org/2009/health-risks/overview.html.
13. U.S. Environmental Protection Agency, "SO_2—How Sulfur Dioxide Affects the Way We Live and Breathe," 2008, www.epa.gov/air/sulfurdioxide.
14. E. Lavonas, "Focus On: Carbon Monoxide Poisoning," American College of Emergency Physicians, 2007, www3.acep.org/publications.aspx?id=26590.
15. V. Markham, "U.S. Population, Energy and Climate Change," 2009.
16. U.S. Environmental Protection Agency, "The Inside Story: A Guide to Indoor Air Quality," 2009, www.epa.gov/iaq/pubs/insidest.html.
17. Ibid.
18. National Cancer Institute, "Lung Cancer Prevention (PDQ)," 2007, www.cancer.gov/cancertopics/pdq/prevention/lung/healthprofessional.
19. Environmental Protection Agency, "U.S. Homes above EPA's Radon Action Level," 2009, http://cfpub.epa.gov/eroe/index.cfm?fuseaction=detail.viewInd&lv=list.listByAlpha&r=201747.
20. Centers for Disease Control Lead Prevention Program, 2009, www.cdc.gov/nceh/lead.
21. National Center for Environmental Health, "Environmental Hazards and Health Effects: Mold," 2009, www.cdc.gov/mold.
22. U.S. Environmental Protection Agency, *Questions and Answers on Ozone Depletion* (Washington, DC: Stratospheric Protection Division, 2008).
23. S. Arrhenius, "On the Influence of Carbonic Acid in the Air upon the Temperature of the Ground," *Philosophical Magazine and Journal of Science* (fifth series) 41 (1896): 237–75.
24. U.S. Environmental Protection Agency, "Climate Change: Basic Information," 2007, http://epa.gov/climatechange/basicinfo.html.
25. U.S. General Accounting Office, *Climate Change: Trends in Greenhouse Gas Emissions and Emissions Intensity in the United States and Other High-Emitting Nations,* GAQ04.146R, 2003.
26. United Nations Framework Convention on Climate Change, "Kyoto Protocol," 2007, http://unfccc.int/kyoto_protocol/items/2830.php.
27. D. Malakoff and E. M. Williams, "Q & A: An Examination of the Kyoto Protocol," NPR.org (June 6, 2007), www.npr.org/templates/story/story.php?storyId=5042766.
28. World Health Organization, "World in Danger of Missing Sanitation Target; Drinking-Water Target Also at Risk, New Report Shows," 2006, www.who.int/mediacentre/news/releases/2006/pr47/en.
29. R. H. Friis, *Essentials of Environmental Health,* 2007, 204.
30. V. Markham, "U.S. National Report on Population and the Environment," 2006, Center for Environment and Population, www.cepnet.org/documents/USNatlReptFinal_000.pdf.
31. U.S. Geological Survey, "National Reconnaissance of Pharmaceuticals, Hormones, and Other Organic Wastewater Contaminants in Streams of the U.S., 1999–2000," 2006, http://toxics.usgs.gov/regional/emc_surfacewater.html.
32. Agency for Toxic Substances and Disease Registry (ATSDR), "Polychlorinated Biphenyls (PCBs)," 2009, www.atsdr.cdc.gov/substances/toxsubstance.asp?toxid=26.
33. U.S. Environmental Protection Agency, "Assessing Health Risks of Pesticides," 2007, www.epa.gov/pesticides/factsheets/riskassess.htm.
34. U.S. Environmental Protection Agency, "Municipal Solid Waste: Basic Facts," 2007, www.epa.gov/msw/facts.htm.
35. U.S. Environmental Protection Agency, "Municipal Solid Waste in the United States—Facts and Figures," 2007, www.epa.gov/osw/nonhaz/municipal/pubs/msw07-rpt.pdf.
36. Ibid.
37. U.S. Environmental Protection Agency, "Superfund National Accomplishments Summary, 2008," 2009. www.epa.gov/superfund/accomp/numbers08.htm.
38. National Institute for Occupational Safety and Health, "Noise and Hearing Loss Prevention: At-Work Solutions for Noise," 2009, www.cdc.gov/niosh/topics/noise/solutions/atworkSolutions.html.

Index

Page references followed by "f" indicate illustrated figures or photographs; followed by "t" indicates a table.

2

2005 Dietary Guidelines for Americans, 100

A

ABCD rule for melanomas, 178fig
abdominal fat, 122
Academic performance, impediments to, 3fig
Access, to health care, 264-265
Acomplia (rimonabant), 124
ACTH, 31, 32f
Action, 17
Activities of daily living (ADLs), 5
Activity reinforcers, 18
adaptation(s), 141f, 142
  defined, 141
  dose-response relationship and, 142
  general adaptation syndrome, 33f
  individuality and variation in, 143
Adequate Intake, 98
adrenalin (epinephrine), 31
Adrenocorticotropic hormone (ACTH), 31, 32f
Adult attention deficit/hyperactivity disorder (ADHD), 60
Adult-onset diabetes (type 2), 88
advertising, overeating and, 120
African Americans
  asthma, 218
  overweight in, 121
age
  designing fitness program for, 149
  overweight and obesity and, 120
agility, 140
Aging
  cardiovascular disease and, 167
  infectious diseases and, 192
Agreeableness, 56
Air pollution
  air quality index (AQI), 275
  carbon dioxide, 274
  carbon monoxide, 274
  cleanest and dirtiest U.S. cities, 273t
  defined, 272
  ground-level ozone, 274
  hydrocarbons, 274-275
  nitrogen dioxide, 274
  ozone layer depletion, 277
  particulates, 273-274
  reducing, 278-279
  sulfur dioxide, 272-273
Air quality index (AQI), 275
alarm stage of GAS, 33
Alcohol
  gender differences and, 4
alcohol use and abuse
  stress management and avoiding, 39
Allergens, 196, 219
Allergies, 196-197
Allergy shots, 197
Allopathic medicine (traditional Western medical practice), 257
Allostasis, 33-34
Allostatic load, 34
alternatives, considering, 44
Alveoli, 217
American College Health Association's National College Health Assessment (ACHA-NCHA), 3fig, 59fig, 62
American College of Obstetrics and Gynecology, guidelines for exercise during pregnancy, 151
American College of Sports Medicine (ACSM), 86
  recommended levels of activity, 144, 146t
American Dietetic Association, 106p
American Heart Association
American Medical Association (AMA), 90
American Psychiatric Association (APA), 59, 67, 72t
American Self-Harm Information Clearinghouse, 63
Amino acids, 86
Aneurysm, 162
anger, managing, 44
Angina pectoris, 160-161
Angiography, 168
Angioplasty, 169
Animalborne pathogens, 193
Anorexia nervosa, 131
Antecedents, 20
Antianxiety drugs, 65t, 256
Antibiotic resistance, 198, 200-201
Antibiotics, 2, 198, 200-201
Antidepressants, 64, 65t, 66, 256
Antigens, 194, 196
Antimicrobial agents, 107
Antioxidants, 92, 107
Antipsychotics, 65t
Anxiety disorders, 66-68
  defined, 66
  generalized anxiety disorder (GAD), 66
  obsessive-compulsive disorder (OCD), 67
  panic disorders, 66p
  phobic disorders, 67p
  post-traumatic stress disorder (PTSD), 67
  sources of, 67-68
Anxiolytics (antianxiety drugs), 65t, 256
appetite suppressants, 124
appraisal, of stress, 38
Armstrong, Lance, 181p
Arrhythmias, 161
Arteries, 157-158
Arterioles, 157-158
Arteriosclerosis, 159
Asian Americans
  overweight among, 121
Aspirin
  for heart disease, 169
Assess Yourself
  cardiovascular disease and cancer, 184-186
  consumer of health care, 266
  eating habits, 109-110
  environmental health, 286-287
  health questionnaire, 22-24
  psychosocial health status, 73-74
  sexually transmitted infections, 221-222
assessment
  of current weight, 125
  of how you spend time, 43
  of stress, 45
  of stressor, 39-40
Asthma, 217, 218p
Atherectomy, 169
Atria, 158
Attention deficit/hyperactivity disorder (ADHD), 60
attitudes
  weight management and, 132
Attitudes, defined, 14
Autoimmune diseases, 195
Autoinoculation, 193
Avian (bird) flu, 204

B

B lymphocytes (B cells), 195
Back pain, 220
Bacteria, 199fig
  antibiotic resistance to, 198, 200-201
  chlamydia, 206
  defined, 197-198
  gonorrhea, 206-208
  meningitis, 199
  pneumonia, 199
  staphylococcal infections, 198-199
  streptococcus infections, 199
  syphilis, 208-209
  tickborne diseases, 202
  tuberculosis, 199-202
balance, 140
Balloon angioplasty, 169
Barriers, to behavior change, 14fig
barriers to change
  weight management and, 132-133
Basal cell carcinoma, 178fig
Behavior change
  barriers to, 14fig
  Behavior Change Contract, 21fig
  beliefs and attitudes and, 13-14
  controlling the situation, 18
  enabling factors and, 13
  external vs. internal locus of control, 15
  modeling and, 18
  motivation and readiness to change, 16p, 17
  planning for, 20-21
  positive reinforcement and, 18
  predisposing factors and, 13
  reinforcing factors and, 13
  self-efficacy and, 15
  self-talk and, 18-20
  shaping and, 17
  significant others/family and, 15p, 16
  Transtheoretical Model of Health Behavior Change (Stages of Change model), 16-17
  visualization and, 17
Behavior Change Contract, 21fig
behavior change contract
  for stress management, 45
  for weight management, 132-134
Behavioral Risk Factor Surveillance System (BRFSS), 12
behavior(s)
  behavioral responses to stress, changing, 39-41
  inconsistent goals and, 37
beliefs
  weight management and, 132
Beliefs, defined, 14
Benign tumors, 170
Binge eating disorder (BED), 131
Biofeedback, 42
biofeedback
  for stress management, 42-43
Biological factors
  anxiety and, 67-68
biological factors
  in overweight and obesity, 120
Bipolar disorder, 61
Blocking/thought stopping, 19-20
Blood clots, 159
blood pressure
  hypertension, 34
Blood transfusions, HIV/AIDS and, 214
Blueberries, 92p
BMR, 124
Body art, infections and, 216
Body dysmorphic disorder (BDD), 131
body fat
  abdominal, 122
  accumulation around waist, metabolic syndrome and, 123
  percent, 118
body image
  eating disorders and, 130f, 131
body mass index (BMI)
  by height and weight, 117f
Body mass index (BMI)
  cancer and, 171-172
body mass index (BMI)
  cancer and high, 123
  ideal range for health, 122
  stable throughout adulthood, 122
Body piercing, infection and, 216

Body's defenses against pathogens, 193fig
Bone mass, gender differences in, 4
Borderline personality disorder, 68
Bradycardia, 161
Brain
gender differences in, 4
Braxton, Toni, 158p
BRCA1 and BRCA2 genes for breast cancer, 176
Breast self-exams, 177, 183t
breathing
relaxation, 41-42
Bulimia nervosa, 131
Burger King hamburger, increasing portion size of, 119, 120p
Burnout, 37
Bypass surgery, 169

C
Calcium, 96t, 98
calorie-counting programs, 126
Calories, 82, 83t
calories
in pound of fat, 118f, 125-126
isocaloric balance, 134
Calories (kilocalories)
basal metabolic rate (BMR) and use of, 124
burned through activity, 126, 127t
Cancer
assessing yourself, 184-186
cervical and endometrial (uterine), 174, 181
chemicals in food, 174
classifications of, 174
colon and rectal, 176-177
common sites of and deaths from each type, 174fig
detecting, 181, 182t, 183p
five-year survival rates, 169
genetic and physiological risks, 172
go green against, 173
cancer
high body mass index and, 123
Cancer
infectious diseases and, 174
leading sites of new cancer causes and deaths (2009 estimates), 175fig
liver, 174
metastasis, 170fig
occupational and environmental risks, 172-174
poor nutrition, physical inactivity, and obesity and, 171-172
probability of developing invasive cancers by age and sex (2003–2005), 172t
radiation and, 173-174
screening guidelines for early detection, 182t
skin, 177, 178p, 179
stress and psychosocial risks, 172
testicular, 181p
tobacco use and, 171p
treatments for, 183
websites for, 188
Cancer pathway, 183
Cancer-fighting vaccines, 183
Candida albicans, 199fig, 211
Candidiasis (moniliasis), 211
Capillaries, 157-158
Capitalization, 58
Capitation, 260-261
Carbohydrates
complex, 87p
defined, 87
glycemic index and glycemic load, 87
simple, 87
Carbon dioxide, 274
Carbon footprint, 274p
Carbon monoxide, 274
Carcinogens
in foods, 174
Carcinomas, 174
Cardiac catheterization, 168
Cardiometabolic risks, 163
cardiorespiratory fitness/endurance, 139-140
Cardiovascular disease (CVD)
age and, 167
angina pectoris, 160-161
arrhythmias, 161
aspirin and, 169
atherosclerosis, 159
body weight and, 165-166
bypass surgery and angioplasty, 169
congestive heart failure (CHF), 161-162
coronary heart disease (CHD), 159-160
diagnosis techniques, 168-169
epidemiological overview of, 157
exercise and, 166
gender and, 167
heredity and, 167
hypertension (high blood pressure) and, 166
inflammation and C-reactive protein and, 168
overweight/obesity and, 171-172
race/ethnicity and, 167
saturated fat and cholesterol and, 164t, 165
stress and, 34, 166-167
stroke, 162-163
tobacco use and, 163-164
websites for, 188
Cardiovascular system, 157-158
gender differences in, 4
parts of, 157
the heart, 158
CD4 cells, 213-214
Cell phones, health and, 174, 284
Cell-mediated immunity, 195
Center for Environment and Population, 12
Centers for Disease Control and Prevention, 3fig, 7t, 19, 196, 203, 206, 212-213
Cerebrovascular accident (stroke), 162-163
Certified Health Education Specialist (CHES), 11
Cervical cancer, 181, 183t
HPV and, 174, 210-211
Chancre, 208
change
as natural part of living, perceiving, 44
as psychosocial stressor, 36
Chemicals, in foods, 174
Chemotherapy, 183
Chernobyl nuclear plant (Russia), 285
Children
depression in, 64
children
overweight or obese, 119
Children and Adults with Attention-Deficit Hyperactivity Disorder (CHADD), 60
Chlamydia, 206
Chlorofluorocarbons (CFCs), 277
Chocolate, 165, 166p
Cholesterol
high-density lipoproteins (HDLs), 89, 164t, 165
low-density lipoproteins (LDLs), 88-89, 164t, 165
Chronic disease, defined, 157
chronic diseases
body weight and risk for, 123
Chronic fatigue syndrome (CFS), 219-220
Chronic lung diseases, 216-218
asthma, 217, 218p
bronchitis, 217
emphysema, 217
Chronic mood disorder, 61
Chronic obstructive pulmonary disease (COPD), 216-217
bronchitis, 217
emphysema, 217
Cities, dirtiest and cleanest in U.S. (air pollution), 273t
Clean Air Act, 273
Climate change, 12
clothing for exercise, 149
Cluster headaches, 219
Cognitive behavioral therapy, 64
cognitive coping strategies, 40-41
college students
hours of sleep per night, 40
overweight or obese, 116-117
stress felt by, 30, 36-37
traditional vs. nontraditional, 37
College students/campuses
depression in, 62
eating, 104, 105p
mental health and, 59
suicide, 69
sustainability on campus, 280
ten most eco-enlightened U.S. colleges and universities, 280
Colon cancer, 176-177
Colonization, 198
Combustion, 283
commitment
weight management and, 133
Complete (high-quality) protein, 86
Composting, 283
Comprehensive Environmental Response and Liability Act (Superfund), 283
Computed tomography (CT scan), 169, 183
Condoms
reduction of STIs and, 207, 217
conflict, as stressor, 37
Congenital syphilis, 209
Congestive heart failure (CHF), 161-162
Conscientiousness, 56
Consequences, 20
Consolidated Omnibus Budget Reconciliation Act (COBRA), 264
Consumable reinforcers, 18
Consumer Health
artificial tanning, 179
body piercing and tattooing, 216
cell phones, 284
nutrition hype, 100
online sources, 19
Contemplation, 16
Cool-down, 148
coordination, 140
coping strategies, cognitive, 40-41
Coronary artery bypass graft (CABG), 169
Coronary artery disease, 159
Coronary heart disease (CHD), 159-160
Cortisol, 31
Costs
of health care, 262, 264
Cryosurgery, 178
cultural isolation, stress and, 38
Cutting, 63
cytokines, 35
Cytomegalovirus, 168

D
Daily Reference Values, 99
Daily Values, 99
Death
due to flu, 202
from cancer, 169
leading causes of by age, 10t
leading causes of in developing nations, 12
leading causes of preventable, 11fig
death rate, body weight and, 122
Decibels (dB), 285
Defensive medicine, 255
Deforestation, 12
Dentists, 258-259
Deoxyribonucleic acid (DNA), 202
depression
stress and, 35
Depressive disorders, 61, 62p, 63-64
causes of, 62
gender differences and, 4
in children, 64
in college students, 62
in men, 63-64
in older adults, 64
in women, 62-63
pharmacological treatment for, 64, 65t, 66
professional treatment for, 70-71, 72t
psychotherapeutic treatment for, 64
symptoms of, 61
types of, 61
Desertification, 12
Developed countries, population growth, 270fig
Developing countries, population growth, 270fig
Diabetes mellitus
diet and, 87
type 2, 88
Diagnosis related groups (DRGs), 261
Diagnostic and Statistical Manual of Mental Disorders (DSM-IVTR), 59, 67-68
Diaphragmatic breathing, 42
Diet aids, 257t
diet drugs, 124, 128
Dietary Reference Intakes (DRIS), 98
diethylpropion (Tenuate), 124
diets, dieting
flexible, 129, 134
ineffective diet products and plans, 129
reasons for failure of, 128-129
rigid, 128-129, 134
weight cycling and, 128-129
yo-yo, 129
Digestive process, 84fig
Digitalis, 162
diminished returns, 142
Dioxins, 281

Disabilities, health disparities and, 9
disabilities, persons with
designing fitness program for, 150
Diseases/disorders
cancer, 169-183
cardiovascular disease (CVD), 157-169
chronic fatigue syndrome, 219-220
chronic lung diseases, 216-218
emerging and resurgent diseases, 204-205
headaches, 218-219
HIV/AIDS, 212-216
infectious diseases, 192-205
low back pain, 219-220
mental illnesses, 59-72
noninfectious diseases, 216-220
repetitive motion disorders, 220
sexually transmitted infections (STIs), 205-212
disordered eating
continuum of thought associated with healthy eating to, 130f
Disparities, in health, 8-9
Distress, 31
distress
exercise and ability to tolerate, 39
Doctor of dental surgery (DDS), 258
Doctor of medical dentistry (DMD), 258
dose-response relationship, 142
downshift, 41
drills
for skill-related fitness, 141
drinking during exercise, guidelines for, 149
Drug abuse
gender differences and, 4
drug use and abuse
diet drugs, 124, 128
Drugs
antianxiety, 65t, 256
antidepressants, 64, 65t, 66, 256
antipsychotics, 65t
for cardiovascular disease, 162
for treating mental illness, 64, 65t, 66
for tuberculosis, 199
injecting and HIV/AIDS, 213
mood stabilizers, 65t
stimulants, 65t
du Toit, Natalie, 6p
Dubos, René, 3-4
Dysfunctional families, 55
Dyspnea, 217
Dysthymic disorder, 61

E

eating disorders
recognizing, 130-131
symptoms, 131
treatment, 131-132
eating for exercise, guidelines for, 149
eating habits/patterns
disordered, 129-132
flexible diets and better long-term, 129
stress management through good, 39
Ecological footprint, 271
Ecosystem, 270
Ectopic pregnancy, 208
Edamame, 95p
eDiets.com, 129
education, as factor in both weight and exercise, 121
Electrocardiogram (ECG), 168
Electrodessication, 178
ELISA (enzyme-linked immunosorbent assay), 214
Emerging and resurgent diseases, 204-205
Emotional health, defined, 5, 53
Emotional stability, 56
Emotions, defined, 53
emotions, managing negative, 44
Enabling factors, behavior and, 13
Endangered species, 12
Endemic viruses, 202
Endometrial cancer, 181, 183t
energy
natural tendencies to conserve or use, 120
energy balance, 118
calculating, 126
rigid diets and, 128
Energy consumption, 271
energy equation, balancing, 125-126
energy imbalance, 119f, 120-121
Enhanced greenhouse effect, 277-278
Environment
anxiety and, 68
cancer and, 172-174
challenges to, 12
infectious diseases and, 192
Environmental health, 5
air pollution, 272-273, 274p, 275, 276p, 277-279
assessing yourself, 286-287
global warming, 277-278, 279p
land pollution, 282-283
noise pollution, 285
overpopulation, 270-272, 273p
radiation, 283, 284p, 285
water pollution and shortages, 279, 280p, 281-282
websites for, 289
environmental stressors, 36f, 38
Environmental tobacco smoke (ETS), 163, 276
ephedra (phenylpropanolamine, ma huang), 124, 129
Epidemics, 192
Esteem needs, 52
Eustress, 31
eustress
of exercise, 39
Exercise, 57, 102-103
infectious disease prevention and, 194
exercise training, principles of, 141-144
exercise(s)
as stress management tool, 39
clothing and footwear for, 149
defined, 138
designing fitness program, 149-152
during pregnancy, 151
energy imbalance and too little, 120
FITT formula for, 145-146
general recommendations for, 144, 146, 147t
guidelines for enough, 144-147
Physical Activity Pyramid, 144, 145f
reducing injuries, 147-149
weight management and regular program of, 126
exercise-to-rest transition, 148
exhaustion stage of GAS, 33
expectations, moderating, 44
Extensively drug resistant tuberculosis, 202
External locus of control, 15
Extroversion, 56

F

Fallopian tubes, 206-208
Families
behavior change and, 15p, 16
dysfunctional, 55
psychosocial health and, 55
Fat soluble vitamins, 92, 94t
fat tissue
chemicals triggering inflammation, 123
percent body fat, 118
Fats
avoiding trans fatty acids, 8, 89-90
cholesterol, 89
high-density lipoproteins (HDLs), 89
low-density lipoproteins (LDLs), 89
seafood, 91
triglycerides, 89
types of, 89
Federal Communications Commission (FCC), 284
fen-phen, 124
Fertility
rates, 271
Fever, infection and, 195-196
Fiber, 87, 88p, 89, 165
Fibrillation, 161
Fight-or-flight response, 31, 32f, 33
fight-or-flight response
prolonged, immune system and, 35
fitness
body weight and, 122-123
mortality risk and, 122f
FITT formula, 145-146
Five-year survival rates (cancer), 169
flexible dieting, 129, 134
Food
chemicals in, 174
functional, 92
infectious disease prevention and, 194
organic, 108
population growth and, 270-271
Food additives, 106-107
Food Allergen Labeling and Consumer Protection Act, 107
Food and Drug Administration (FDA), 64, 85, 90, 94-95, 99, 106, 210, 212, 255-256, 257t, 284
on diet drugs, 124
on diet products, 129
Food intolerances, 107
Food irradiation, 106p
Food labels, 99fig
Food preferences, 81
Food safety
allergies and food intolerance, 107p
avoiding risks in the home, 106
food additives, 106-107
food irradiation, 106p
foodborne illnesses, 105-106
organics, 108p
Foodborne illnesses, 105-106
food(s)
easy access to, 119-120
nutrient-dense, 39, 134
relatively low price of, 120
Footwear, 149
Formaldehyde, 173, 276
Fossil fuels, 12, 271
frequency
in FITT formula, 145
Fruit sugar, 87
Fungi, 199fig, 204
candidiasis (moniliasis), 211

G

GAS, 33f
gender
weight and, 121
Gender and Health
breast self-exams, 177
complications from STIs, 208
health/physical, 4
HIV/AIDS, 215
nutrition needs, 103
testicular self-exams, 182
Gender, defined, 8
Gender differences
alcohol and, 4
bone mass, 4
brain, 4
cardiovascular disease and, 167
depression, 4
drug effects, 4
health disparities and, 9
health/physical, 4
heart attacks, 4
HIV/AIDS, 4
nutrition needs, 103
sexually transmitted infections (STIs), 4
smoking, 4
General adaptation syndrome (GAS), 33f
general cool-down, 148
general warm-up, 147-148
Generalized anxiety disorder (GAD), 66
genes/genetic factors
diminished returns approaching limits of, 142
individual differences in training adaptations and, 143
overweight and obesity and, 120
"thrifty genes", 121
Genetic factors
cancer and, 172
Genital herpes, 209-210
Genital warts, 210
Geographic location/transportation, health disparities and, 9
Global health issues, 11p, 12
leading causes of death in developing nations, 12
Global warming, 277-278, 279p
globesity, 119
glucose
stress response and production of, 31
goals
behaviors inconsistent with, 37
Goals
setting realistic, 20-21
Gonorrhea, 206-208
Gore, Al, 270
An Inconvenient Truth, 277
Gratitude, 58
Green Guide
bottled water, 85
cancer and, 173
eco-clean and allergen free, 219
environmental challenges, 12

medical waste, 263
seafood, 91
sustainability on campus, 280
Greenhouse effect, 277-278
Greenhouse gas, 274
Ground-level ozone, 274
Group A streptococci, 199
Group plans (health insurance), 260

H
H1N1 flu virus (swine flu), 202-203
Hand-washing, 194, 200-201, 203, 207
Happiness
health and, 57-58
laughter and, 58p
positive psychology and, 58-59
hardiness, psychological, 38
Hassles, 36
Hay fever, 197
Hazardous waste, 283
Headaches, 218-219, 220p
Health, 2p
defined, 2-4
health
designing fitness program for special health concerns, 150-152
Health
dimensions of, 5fig
gender differences, 4
global issues, 11p, 12
health disparities, 8, 9p
Healthy People initiatives, 6p, 7t, 8
Internet information on, 19, 26
public health achievements, 2, 3fig
questionnaire for, 22-24
types of, 5
U.S. Surgeon General's definition of mental health, 5
Health Belief Model (HBM), 14
Health care
assessing yourself, 266
being proactive in, 254
debate over national insurance, 265
health professionals, 254-255, 257-259
seeking help, 113
self-help/self-care, 253p
websites for, 268
Health Care Financing Administration (HCFA), 261-262
Health care reform, 265p
Health care system
access to, 264-265
cost of, 262, 264
quality and malpractice, 265
Health disparities, 8-9
Health Headlines
adult attention deficit/hyperactivity disorder (ADHD), 60
heart-healthy superfoods, 165
human papillomavirus vaccine, 212
soy intake, 95
vaccines, 198
Health in a Diverse World
challenge of health disparities, 9
global nutrition, 82
Health insurance
managed care, 260-261
Medicaid, 262
Medicare, 261-262
national health insurance, 265
private, 260
underinsured, 259
uninsured, 8-9
Health maintenance organizations (HMOs), 261
Health professionals
assessing, 254-255
types of, 258-259
when to seek help, 253-254
Health promotion, defined, 8
Health Today
antibiotic resistance, 200
placebo effect, 256
self-harm, 63
health-related components of physical fitness, 139-140
Healthy life expectancy, 6
Healthy People 2020, 8
Heart, 158
Heart attacks, 159-160
gender differences and, 4
Heart-healthy superfoods, 165
height, recommended range of weight by, 117f
Helicobacter pylori, 168
Hepatitis A (HAV), 203
Hepatitis B (HBV), 203
liver cancer and, 174
Hepatitis C (HCV), 203
Heredity
cardiovascular disease and, 167p
infectious diseases and, 192
Herpes simplex virus, 168, 209-210
Hierarchy of needs (Maslow), 52
High-density lipoprotein (HDL), 89, 163, 164t, 165-166
High-fructose corn syrup, 87
High-level wellness, 4fig
hippocampus damage, stress and, 35
Hispanics
percentages of overweight among, 121
HIV/AIDS
definition and statistics, 212-213
epidemic, 213p
gender differences and, 4
new hope and treatments, 215
preventing infection, 215-216
symptoms of, 214
testing for HIV antibodies, 214-215
transmission of, 213-214
women and, 215
Holistic approach, 5
Home heating pollution, 276
Homeostasis, 33
Homocysteine, cardiovascular disease and, 168
hormones
stress, 31, 32f, 34, 44
hs-CRP tests, 168
Human immunodeficiency virus (HIV), 212
Human papillomavirus (HPV)
cancer and, 174
vaccine against, 174, 198, 212
Humoral immunity, 194
Hunger, 81
Hydrocarbons, 274-275
Hygiene, 2
Hyperlipidemia, 159
Hypersensitivity reaction, 196
hypertension
stress-induced, 34
Hypertension (high blood pressure), 158
classifications, 167t
heart disease and, 166
metabolic syndrome and, 163
Hypnosis, 43
hypnosis
for stress management, 43

I
Imagined rehearsal, 17
Immune system
autoimmune disorders, 195
gender differences in, 4
happiness and, 58
response to infectious diseases, 194-196
stress and, 35
Immunocompromised system, 192
Immunotherapy, 183, 197
Incidence, defined, 11
inconsistent goals and behaviors, as stressors, 37
Inconvenient Truth, An (Gore), 277
Incubation period, 202, 206
individuality, 143
factors in designing fitness program, 149-152
Indoor air pollution
asbestos, 276
chemical compounds (number of in average home), 275
environmental tobacco smoke, 276
formaldehyde, 276
home heating, 276
lead, 276-277
mold, 277
radon, 276
Infectious diseases, 2
antibiotic resistance and, 200-201
assessing yourself, 221-222
bacteria and, 197-202
body's defenses against, 192
cancer and, 174
emerging and resurgent diseases, 204-205
immune system responses, 194-196
pathogens, 199fig, 204
risk factors for, 192-193
transmission routes, 193, 194t
vaccines, 196p
viruses and, 202-203
websites for, 224
Inflammation
heart disease and, 168
immune response, 195
inflammation
risk of chronic diseases with weight gain due to, 123
stress response and, 35
initial values principle, 142
injuries
exercise-related, reducing, 147-149
Inner well-being, 54
Institute of Medicine, on recommended levels of activity, 147t
Intellectual health, 5
intensity
in FITT formula, 145
Internal locus of control, 15
Internet
surfing for latest in health, 19
Interpersonal therapy, 64
interruptions, avoiding, 43
Interspecies transmission, 193
Ionizing radiation, 283-284
Irradiation, 106p
Ischemia, 160
isocaloric balance, 118f
weight management and attaining, 125-126
Isolated systolic hypertension (ISH), 166

J
Jenny Craig, 129
Journal of the American Medical Association, 19, 100
journaling
charting stress management progress in, 45-46

K
Kaposi's sarcoma, 213-214
kegels, 151
Killer T cells, 35, 195
Kobasa, Susanne, 38
Kyoto Protocol, 278

L
Lacto-ovo-vegetarians, 103
Lacto-vegetarians, 103
Land pollution
hazardous waste, 283
recycling rates, 283fig
solid waste, 282-283
Laser angioplasty, 169
Laughter, 58p
Lead, 276-277, 282
Learned helplessness, 55-56
Learned optimism, 56
learning, sleep loss and, 40
Leukemias, 174
Levine, James, 120
life expectancy
body weight and, 122
Life expectancy
definition of a healthy, 6
statistics, 6
Life span, 56
Lifestyle behaviors
health disparities and, 9
lifestyle/lifestyle choices
downshift in lifestyle, 41
overweight or obesity and, 121
lifestyle/light physical activities, 138, 139f
Liver cancer, 174, 203
Liver failure, 203
Liver transplants, 203
Locavore, 108
Locus of control, 15
Low back pain, 220
low self-esteem, 38
Low-density lipoprotein (LDL), 88-89, 164t, 165
Lung cancer, 172t, 175
Lung diseases, 216-218
Lyme disease, 202
Lymphocytes, 195
Lymphomas, 174

M

Ma huang (ephedra), 124, 129
Macro environment, 55
Macrominerals, 94, 96t
Madden, John, 66
Magnetic resonance imaging (MRI), 168-169, 181
Maintenance, 17
Major depressive disorder, 61
Malpractice, 265
Managed care, 260-261
  health maintenance organizations (HMOs), 261
  point of service (POS), 261
  preferred provider organizations (PPOs), 261
Manic depression, 61
Manipulative reinforcers, 18
Maslow, Abraham, hierarchy of needs, 52
Mead, Margaret, 270
Medicaid, 262
Medical degree (MD), 258
Medical waste, 263
Medicare, 261-262
Medications
  allergy shots, 197
  antibiotic resistance, 200-201
  antibiotics, 198
  for mental illness, 64, 65t, 66
  placebo effect, 256p
medications, designing fitness program and, 152
Meditation, 42
Melanomas, 177-178
  ABCD rule for, 178
memory, sleep loss and, 40
Memory T and B cells, 195
Men
  depression in, 63-64
  health gender differences, 4
  nutrition needs, 103
Meningitis, 199
Meningococcal meningitis, 199
mental disorders, stress and, 35
Mental health
  defined, 5, 53
Mental health professionals, 70-71, 72t
  evaluations, 70-71
  what to expect in therapy, 71-72
Mental illnesses
  adult attention deficit/hyperactivity disorder (ADHD), 60
  anxiety disorders, 66p, 67-68
  college students and, 59
  defined, 59
  depressive disorders, 61, 62p, 63-64
  mood disorders, 61-66
  nonsuicidal self-injury (NSSI), 63
  obsessive-compulsive disorder (OCD), 67
  panic disorders, 66p
  personality disorders, 68
  pharmacological treatment for, 64, 65t, 66
  phobic disorders, 67p
  post-traumatic stress disorder (PTSD), 67
  psychotherapeutic treatment for, 64
  schizophrenia, 68p, 69
  seeking professional help, 70-71, 72t
  statistics, 59
  suicide, 69p, 70
mental skills, stress management and development of, 43-44
Mental status examination, 71
Meridia (sibutramine), 124
MET (metabolic equivalent), 138
metabolic rate
  basal (BMR), 124
  resting (RMR), 124-125
  role in weight management, 124-125
metabolism
  ethnicity and, 121
  exercise boosting, 126
  set point and, 125
Metastasis, 170
Microvascular angina, 158
Migraine headaches, 218-219
Millimeters of mercury, 166
mind, stress and the, 35
Mind–body connection, 57p, 58-59
mindfulness meditation, 42
Minerals, 94-95, 96t, 97t, 98p
mode, defined, 146
Modeling, 18
moderate physical activities, 138, 139f
Mold, 277
Monosaccarides, 87
Monounsaturated fat, 89
Montreal Protocol, 277
Mood disorders
  pharmacological treatment for, 64, 65t, 66
  psychotherapeutic treatment for, 64
Mood stabilizers, 65t
Morbidity, defined, 3
Mortality
  defined, 3
mortality risk, fitness and, 122f
Motivation, 16-17
motivation(s)
  for weight change, 127
  weight management and, 132
Multidrug resistant tuberculosis, 202
multitasking, 43
Municipal solid waste, 282
muscle wasting, underweight and, 123
muscle(s)
  progressive muscle relaxation (PMR), 42
Muscular endurance, 140
Muscular strength, 140
Mutant cells, 170
Myers-Briggs Type Indicator personality test, 56
Myocardial infarction (MI, heart attack), 162
MyPyramid Food Guide, 100
MyPyramid Plan, 100-103
MyPyramid.gov website, 126

N

Narcissistic personality disorder, 68
National Aeronautics and Space Administration (NASA), 277
National Center for Complementary and Alternative Medicine (NCCAM), 57
National College Health Association, 117
National health insurance, 265
National Heart, Lung, and Blood Institute (NHLBI), 167t
National Institutes of Health (NIH)
  website for, 19
National Oceanic and Atmospheric Administration, 277
Natural resources, exploitation of, 12
natural rhythms, accommodating your, 43
Necrotizing faciitis, 199
Needs, hierarchy of (Maslow), 52
negative caloric balance, 118f
Negative stress, 31
Neisseria gonorrhoeae, 207-208
Neoplasm, 170
Nitrogen dioxide, 274
Nitrosamines, 174
Noise pollution, 285
non-exercise activity, 120
Noninfectious conditions
  asthma, 217, 218p
  bronchitis, 217
  chronic fatigue syndrome (CFS), 219-220
  chronic lung diseases, 216-218
  chronic obstructive pulmonary disease (COPD), 217
  emphysema, 217
  headaches, 218-219, 220p
  low back pain, 220
  repetitive motion disorders, 220
  websites for, 224
Nonionizing radiation, 283
Nonpoint source pollutants, 281
Nonsuicidal self-injury (NSSI), 63
Norepinephrine, 31
Nuclear meltdown, 285
Nuclear power plants, 284-285
Nuclear stress test, 168
Nurse practitioners (NPs), 259
Nurses, 259
nutrient-dense foods, 134
  reducing stress by eating, 39
Nutrients
  calories, 82, 83t
  daily needs, 102fig
  fats, 88-92
Nutrition
  allergies and food intolerance, 107p, 108
  assessing yourself, 109-110
  avoiding risks in the home, 106
  budget tips, 105
  cancer and, 171-172
  college students and, 104, 105p
  food additives, 106-107
  food irradiation, 106p
  food labels (Nutrition Facts), 99
  foodborne illnesses, 105-106
  MyPyramid Food Guide, 100-103
  organic foods, 108p
  Recommended Dietary Allowances (RDAs), 98
  supplements, 99, 100p
  vegetarianism, 103, 104p
  websites for, 112
Nutrition Facts (food label), 99fig
Nuts, and reducing heart disease, 165

O

obese, defined, 116
obesity, 118-121
  energy imbalance and, 119-121
  in college students, 116-117
  increasing trends of, 117
  worldwide trend in, 119
Obsessive-compulsive disorder (OCD), 67
Occupational risks, cancer and, 172-174
Office of the Surgeon General
  recommended levels of activity, 147t
Older adults
  depression in, 64
Omega-3 fatty acids, 165
Oncogenes, 172
Ophthalmologist, 258
Optifast, 129
Optometrist, 258
Oral herpes, 210fig
Organic food, 108p
Organic solvents, 281
orlistat (Xenical), 124
Orthodontist, 259
Osteopath, 258
overcommitment, avoiding, 43
overconsumption, 119-120
overload, 141f, 142
  as stressor, 37
  defined, 141
  progression and optimal level of, 142
  rest and recovery after, 143-144
Over-the-counter (OTC) drugs, 256-257
  medicine label, 258fig
  types and potential side effects, 257t
overtraining, 144
overweight
  designing fitness program for, 149-150
  downward fitness spiral caused by, 122-123
  in children, 119
  in college students, 116-117
  increasing trends of, 117
  race/ethnicity and, 121
Overweight/obesity, 3
  cancer and, 171-172
  cardiovascular disease and, 171-172
  fiber and, 88
Ovo-vegetarians, 103
Ozone
  ground-level, 273t, 274
  layer depletion, 277

P

Pain
  infection and, 195
  low back, 220
Palliative care
  flu and, 202
Pandemic flu, 11, 192, 202p, 203
Pandemics, 192
Panic disorders, 66p
Pap test, 181, 183t
Paranoid personality disorder, 68
Parasitic worms, 199fig, 204
Particulates, 273-274
Pathogens
  bacteria, 197-202, 204-205
  body's defenses against, 193fig
  defined, 192
  fungi, 199fig, 204
  parasitic worms, 199fig, 204
  prions, 204
  protozoans, 199fig, 204
  viruses, 199fig, 202-205

eanut allergy, 107p
elvic inflammatory disease (PID), 208
ercent body fat
reducing, 118
erformance demands, as stressor, 37
erformance, sleep loss and, 40
ericarditis, 158
erinatal transmission of HIV/AIDS, 214
eriods of communicability, 206
eripheral artery disease, 159
ersonality
psychosocial health and, 56
ersonality
Type A, 38
Type B, 38
ersonality disorders, 68
esco-vegetarians, 103
etroleum products, as leakage pollutant, 281
harmaceutical waste, 263
hentride (phentermine), 124
henylpropanolamine (ephedra), 124, 129
hobic disorders, 67p
hysical activity
goal for increasing, 7
hysical activity(ies)
as stress management tool, 39
defined, 138
easy ways to get more active, 144
FITT formula for, 145-146
general recommendations for, 144, 146, 147t
lifestyle, 138, 139f
MET levels of, 138, 139f
hysical checkup, 70-71
hysical fitness
guidelines to reduce risk of exercise injury, 147-149
health-related components of, 139-140
individual factors in designing fitness program, 149-152
levels of activity for, 144-147
preparing to exercise, 152
principles of fitness, 141-144
skill-related components of, 140-141
hysical health, 5
hysician assistants (PAs), 259
hysiological factors
cancer and, 172
lant stanols/sterols, 165
laque, 89, 159
MR, 42
neumococcal meningitis, 199
neumocystis carinii pneumonia, 214
neumonia, 199
oint of service (POS), 261
oint source pollutants, 281
ollen allergy, 197
ollution
population growth and, 271
olychlorinated biphenyls, 281
olysaccarides, 87
olyunsaturated fat, 89
opulation
differing rates among nations, 271
factors that affect growth of, 271
impact of overpopulation, 270-271
oil consumption and, 271
world growth, 270fig
zero population growth, 271-272
ortion sizes
increase in, 119
ortions, 101
ositive affirmations, 56
ositive caloric balance, 118f
ositive psychology, 58-59
ositive reinforcement, 18
ositive stress, 31
ositron emission tomography (PET), 168
ossessional reinforcers, 18
ost-traumatic stress disorder (PTSD), 35, 67
ower, 141
recontemplation, 16
redisposing factors, behavior and, 13
referred provider organizations (PPOs), 261
regnancy
designing fitness program for, 151
reparation, 16-17
rescription drugs, 255p, 256
resident's Council on Physical Fitness, 144
revalence, defined, 11
revention
breast cancer, 176
colon and rectal cancers, 176-177
HIV/AIDS, 215-216
lung cancer, 175
prostate cancer, 180
skin cancer, 178-179
Primary care practitioner (PCP), 258
principles of fitness, 141-144
priorities, time management and setting, 43
Private health insurance, 260
progression, 142
recording and tracking, 45-46
progressive muscle relaxation (PMR), 42
Prostate cancer, 172t, 179-180, 183t
Prostate gland, 179
Prostate-specific antigen (PSA) test, 180, 183t
Proteins
amino acids, 86
complementary, 86fig
defined, 86
soy, 95
Protozoans, 199fig, 204
trichomoniasis, 211
Psychiatric history, 71
Psychiatric medications, 64, 65t, 66
Psychological hardiness, 38
Psychoneuroimmunology (PNI), 35, 57
Psychosocial health
adult attention deficit/hyperactivity disorder (ADHD) and, 60
anxiety disorders, 66-68
assessing, 73-74
cancer and, 172
characteristics of, 51-52
defined, 51-53
depressive disorders, 61, 62p, 63-64
emotional health, 53
factors influencing, 54-56
happiness and, 57-58
hierarchy of needs (Maslow), 52
mental health, 53
mental health threats to college students, 59
mind–body connection, 57p, 58-59
mood disorders, 61-66
personality disorders, 68
positive psychology and, 58-59
schizophrenia, 68p, 69
seeking professional help for, 70, 71p, 72t
sleep and, 57
social health, 53, 54p
spiritual health, 54
strategies to enhance, 56p, 57-59
suicide, 69p, 70
websites for, 76
Psychosocial stressors, 36f, 37
Psychotherapeutic treatment, 64
PTSD, 35
Pubic lice, 211-212
Public health, achievements in, 3fig
Purpose, in life, 54

Q

Quality of life, 3
goals for improving, 6, 7t, 8-10

R

race/ethnicity
stress and, 38
weight and, 121
Race/ethnicity differences
cardiovascular disease and, 167
Radiation
cancer and, 173-174
cell phones and, 284
ionizing radiation, 283-284
nonionizing radiation, 283
nuclear power plants, 284-285
Radiation absorbed doses (rads), 284
Radiotherapy, 183
Radon, 276
Rads (radiation absorbed doses), 284
Range of motion, 148
Rational-emotive therapy, 19
reaction time, 141
readiness
for weight change, 127-128
Recommended Dietary Allowances (RDAs), 98
Rectal cancer, 176-177
Recuperation, principle of, 143-144
Recycling, 283
Red wine, 165
Reference Daily Intakes, 99
Reinforcement, 18
Reinforcing factors, behavior and, 13
relaxation breathing, 41-42
Relaxation techniques, 41-43
Remote Area Medical (RAM) clinics, 9
Repetitive motion disorders (RMDs), 220
Resiliency, 56
Resistance, infectious diseases and, 192
resistance stage of GAS, 33
resistance training
rest and recovery after, 144
Resolutions, 12
responder vs. nonresponder, 143
rest and recovery, 143-144
Resting metabolic rate (RMR), 124-125
rest-to-exercise transition, 147-148
reversibility, 143
rewards
time management and, 43
Rickettsia, 202
rigid diets, 128-129, 134
rimonabant (Acomplia), 124
Risk behaviors, 8
cancer and, 171-172
HIV/AIDS, 213
Risk factors
for cancer, 172-181
for infectious diseases, 192-193
for sexually transmitted infections, 205-206
Risk reduction
for cardiovascular disease, 163-168
for infectious diseases, 194
RMR, 124-125
Rocky Mountain spotted fever, 202
Runoff, 281
Russert, Tim, 159

S

S.A.F.E. Alternatives, 63
Safe Drinking Water Act (SDWA), 279, 281
Safer sex, 205-207
communicating about, 217
Sarcomas, 174
satiety
misreading of "fullness signals", 119
Schizophrenia, 68p, 69
Seafood, 91
Seasonal affective disorder (SAD), 61-62
Security needs, 52
Sedimentation, 281
Selective serotonin reuptake inhibitors (SSRIs), 64t
Self-actualization, 52
Self-assessment
analyzing personal behavior, 20
antecedents and consequences, 20
Self-care, 253
Self-efficacy, 15, 38, 55
Self-esteem
building, 55
defined, 55
self-esteem
low, 38
Self-harm, 63
Self-help, 253
Self-Injury Support, 63
Self-talk, 18-20, 56
Self-transcendence, 52
Seligman, Martin, 55-56
Selye, Hans, 33
Semivegetarians, 103
Serving sizes, 101-102
set point, 125
Sex, of an individual, 8
Sexual behavior
safer sex, 207, 217
Sexual orientation
health disparities and, 9
Sexually transmitted infections (STIs)
candidiasis (moniliasis), 211
chlamydia, 206-207
complications in women, 208
defined, 205
gender differences and, 4
gonorrhea, 206-208
herpes, 209-210

human papillomavirus and genital warts, 210
pubic lice (crabs), 211-212
risk factors for, 205-206
syphilis, 208-209
trichomoniasis, 211
Shaping, 17
sibutramine (Meridia), 124
Signature strength, 58-59
Significant others
as change agents, 15p, 16
Simple carbohydrates, 87
Simple sugars, 87
single-tasking, 43
Sinoatrial node, 158
Situational inducement, 18
skills
required for activity, learning, 148-149
skill-related components of fitness, 140-141
Skills for behavior change
being proactive in your health care, 254
budget nutrition tips, 105
building self-esteem, 55
depression, 71
fiber, 89
foodborne illness, 107
health practices, 13
heart attacks, 160
mold-free homes, 277
reducing fat intake, 90
reducing risk of flu, 203
reducing risk of infectious disease, 194
safe sunning, 180
safer sex, 207, 217
shopping to save the planet, 275
stroke warning signs, 162
wasting less water, 281
Skin cancer, 172t, 177, 178p, 179
Sleep
infectious disease prevention and, 194
sleep
poor, 40
Sleep
psychosocial health and, 57
stress management and, 39-40
sleep
weight loss and, 134
Smoking
gender differences and, 4
smoking
stress management by avoiding, 39
Smoking
years of life lost to, 10
Social bonds, 15p, 16, 54
Social health, 5
defined, 53, 54p
Social needs, 52
Social reinforcers, 18
Social support, 54
social support
stress management through, 41
support groups, 41, 129, 134
weight management and, 133
Social/cultural roles, anxiety and, 68
Society for Women's Health Research, 4
Sodium nitrate, 174
Solid waste, 282-283
Soy protein, 95
specific cool-down, 148
specific warm-up, 148
specificity, 142
speed, 141
Spiritual health
defined, 5, 54
psychosocial health and, 51fig, 54
spiritual wellness
stress management and spiritual practice, 44
sports and recreational activities
skill-related components of fitness, 140-141
Squamous cell carcinoma, 178fig
Staphylococcal infections, 192, 198-199
Statistics
air pollution, 273t, 275-278
behavior change, 17
breast cancer, 175-176
calories, 83
cancer, 169, 172t, 175-181
cardiovascular disease, 157, 160-163, 167
chronic lung disease, 216-218
disabilities, 9
extroversion, 56
flu deaths, 202p, 203
food allergies, 105
foodborne illness, 105
global nutrition, 82
hay fever, 197
hazardous waste, 283
headaches, 218-219
health care spending, 262
health insurance, 259, 261
heart attacks, 160
HIV/AIDS, 212-213
hospital admittances, 254
infectious disease, 198-203
leading causes of death, 10t
life expectancies, 3, 6
low back pain, 220
lung cancer, 175
mental disorders, 59, 61, 66-68
nutrient consumption, 83fig
panic disorders, 66
population growth, 270-272
prescription drugs, 255p
recycling, 283fig
self–harm, 63
sexually transmitted infections, 205-211
solid waste, 282
suicide and mental illness, 69
trans fats, 89
uninsured Americans, 8
unnecessary medical tests, 255
U.S. energy consumption, 12
vegetarianism, 103
vitamins, 100
water use and pollution, 279, 281
years lost to cigarette smoking, 10
steady state, 33
Stem cell research, 183
Stent, 169
Stimulants
for mental illness, 65t
Streptococcal infections, 199
Stress, 30
stress
among college students, 30, 36-37
Stress
assessment of, 45
stress
body's response to, 31, 32f
Stress
cancer and, 172
cardiovascular disease (CVD) and, 166-167
defined, 30
stress
harm from, 32-36
Stress
infectious diseases and, 194
stress
major sources of, 36-39
negative, 31
positive, 31
stress hormones, 31, 32f, 34
anger and, 44
stress management
avoiding alcohol use and, 39
basic wellness measures for, 39
creating plan for, 45-46
preparation before stressful events, 41
tools for, 39-44, 45f
Stress response, 31, 32f
stress response
allostatic load and, 34
defined, 30
inflammation promoted by cytokines in, 35
Stressor(s), 30
stressor(s)
assessing, 39-40
environmental, 36f, 38
general adaptation syndrome (GAS) to, 33f
psychosocial, 36f, 37
stretching
during cool-down process, 148
during warm-up, 148p
Subjective well-being, 57
suburban living, decreased activity and, 120
Suicide
college students and, 69
gender differences and, 4
preventing, 70
statistics, 69
warning signs of, 69-70
Sun protection factor (SPF), 178-179
Superfund (Comprehensive Environmental Response and Liability Act), 283
Supplements, 99-100
supplements, dietary
claims as weight-loss aids, 124
support
weight management and, 133
Support groups, 56p, 57
support groups
dieting, 129, 134
stress, 41
Suppressor T cells, 195
Survival needs, 52
Sustainable seafood, 91
Swine flu (H1N1 virus), 202-203
Syphilis, 208-209

T

T cells, killer, 35
T lymphocytes (T cells), 195
Tanning, artificial, 179
target cells, 31
Tattoos, infection and, 216
Td/Tdap vaccine, 197fig, 198
Tension headaches, 218, 220p
Tenuate (diethylpropion), 124
Termination, 17
Testicular cancer, 181p
self-exam for, 182
thinking, managing your, 43-44
threat, stress response to, 31
threshold, increasing physical activity to, 142f
Tickborne bacterial diseases, 202
time
in FITT formula, 145
Time management, 43
Tobacco
cancer and, 171p
cardiovascular disease and, 163-164
tobacco use
stress management and avoiding, 39
Tolerable Upper Intake Level, 98
Toxins, 194
Trace minerals, 94, 97t
training effects, 141-142
Transient ischemic attacks (TIAs), 162
Transmission, routes of infectious diseases, 193, 194t, 206, 213-214
Transtheoretical Model of Health Behavior Change (Stages of Change model), 16-17
trauma
post-traumatic stress disorder (PTSD) and, 35
Treatments
for cancer, 175-181, 183
for cardiovascular disease, 169
for HIV/AIDS, 215
for sexually transmitted infections, 206-212, 215
immunotherapy, 197
Trichomonas vaginalis, 199fig, 211
Trichomoniasis, 211
Tuberculosis (TB), 199-202
resistant, 11
Tumor, defined, 170
Type 2 diabetes, 88
Type A personality, 38
Type B personalities, 38
type, in FITT formula, 145-146
Typhus, 202

U

Ultrafast computed tomography (CT scan), 169, 183
Underweight, 116
underweight
death rate and, 122
designing fitness program for, 150
health risks of, 122
muscle wasting and reduced fitness with, 123
Uninsured/underinsured, 8-9, 259
University of New Hampshire, weight problems among students at, 116
URAC Accredited Health website, 19
Urinary tract infection (UTI), 208
U.S. Department of Agriculture (USDA)
recommended levels of activity, 146t
U.S. Department of Health and Human Services

terine cancer, 172t, 181

accines, 2, 196p
against human papillomavirus, 174, 210, 212
cancer-fighting, 183
safety and necessity of, 198
asodilators, 162
egans, 103
egetarianism, 86fig, 103-104, 105p
eins, 157-158
entricles, 158
enules, 157-158
gorous physical activities, 138, 139f
rulence, 192
iruses
avian (bird) flu, 204
common cold, 202
defined, 202
H1N1 (swine flu), 202-203
hepatitis, 203
herpes, 209-210
human immunodeficiency virus (HIV), 212, 213p, 214-216
human papillomavirus and genital warts, 210
influenza, 202p, 203
West Nile virus, 204
isualization, 17
sualization
weight management and, 133
itamins, 92, 93t, 94t

V

/aiting period, for health insurance, 260
arm-up
phases, 147-148
/ater
as nutrient, 84, 85p, 86
bottled, 85
tap, 85, 279, 281
/ater pollution and shortages, 279, 280p, 281-282
deaths in developing nations and, 12
tips for wasting less water, 281
/ater soluble vitamins, 92, 93t
/ebsites
Accessing Your Health on the Internet, 26, 76, 112, 188, 224, 268, 289
cancer, 188
cardiovascular disease, 188
Centers for Disease Control and Prevention, 19
Children and Adults with Attention-Deficit Hyperactivity Disorder (CHADD), 60
Energy Star logo, 280
environmental health, 289
FDA Center for Drug Evaluation and Research, 256
government- and education-based sites, 19
health care, 268
health information, 19, 26
infectious and noninfectious conditions, 224
National Institute of Mental Health, 19
nutrition, 112
professional journals, 19
psychosocial health, 76
self-harm, 63
URAC, 19
World Health Organization, 19
/eight
choosing realistic goal, 125, 127-128
designing fitness program for, 149-150
recommended range of, by height, 117f
set point, 125
/eight cycling, 128-129
/eight loss
anorexia nervosa and, 131
diet drugs and, 124
health benefits, 123
ineffective diet products and plans, 129
modifying behavior for long-term weight change, 126-128
rate of, 128, 134
reasons for dieting failure, 128-129
resetting one's set point for, 125
tips for, 134
/eight management, 115-135
achieving weight maintenance, 133
behavior change plan for, creating, 132-134
defined, 118
disordered eating and, 129-132
effective tools for, 123-128
Weight management
heart disease and, 165-166
weight management
strategies, 117-118
successful weight maintainers, characteristics of, 125
wellness and, 122-123
Well-being, 2
Wellness, 2p
wellness
basic wellness measures for stress management, 39
body weight and, 122-123
Wellness
continuum of, 4fig
defined, 2
evolution toward, 3-5
West Nile virus (WNV), 204
Western blot, 214
Western medical practice (allopathic medicine), 257
White Americans
asthma, 218
whole foods
nutrient-dense foods, 39, 134
Women
complications of sexually transmitted infections, 208
depression in, 62-63
health gender differences, 4
HIV/AIDS and, 215
nutrition needs, 103
Women's Health Initiative (WHI), 4
World Health Organization, 6, 19, 200
World Health Organization (WHO), 119
recommended levels of activity, 146t
worry, constructive, 43

X

Xenical (orlistat), 124

Y

Yeast infections, 211
yo-yo dieting, 129

Z

Zero population growth (ZPG), 271-272